Pharmacology

Pharmacology

Edited by **Brendon Krauss**

FOSTER ACADEMICS
New Jersey

Published by Foster Academics,
61 Van Reypen Street,
Jersey City, NJ 07306, USA
www.fosteracademics.com

Pharmacology
Edited by Brendon Krauss

International Standard Book Number: 978-1-63242-320-7 (Hardback)

Printed in China.

Contents

Preface IX

Chapter 1 **Evaluation of Adverse Effects of Mutein Forms of Recombinant Human Interferon Alpha-2b in Female Swiss Webster Mice** 1
H. Rachmawati, A. Merika, R. A. Ningrum, K. Anggadiredja, and D. S. Retnoningrum

Chapter 2 **Alantolactone Induces Apoptosis in HepG2 Cells through GSH Depletion, Inhibition of STAT3 Activation, and Mitochondrial Dysfunction** 12
Muhammad Khan, Ting Li, Muhammad Khalil Ahmad Khan, Azhar Rasul, Faisal Nawaz, Meiyan Sun, Yongchen Zheng, and Tonghui Ma

Chapter 3 **The Protective Effect of Fasudil on the Structure and Function of Cardiac Mitochondria from Rats with Type 2 Diabetes Induced by Streptozotocin with a High-Fat Diet Is Mediated by the Attenuation of Oxidative Stress** 23
Rong Guo, Baoxin Liu, Shunping Zhou, Buchun Zhang, and Yawei Xu

Chapter 4 **Therapeutic Effect of Exendin-4, a Long-Acting Analogue of Glucagon-Like Peptide-1 Receptor Agonist, on Nerve Regeneration after the Crush Nerve Injury** 32
Koji Yamamoto, Masatoshi Amako, Yoritsuna Yamamoto, Toyokazu Tsuchihara, Hitoshi Nukada, Yasuo Yoshihara, Hiroshi Arino, Masanori Fujita, Maki Uenoyama, Shoichi Tachibana, and Koichi Nemoto

Chapter 5 **Protective Effect of Egyptian Propolis against Rabbit Pasteurellosis** 39
Somia A. Nassar, Amira H. Mohamed, Hamdy Soufy, and Soad M. Nasr

Chapter 6 **Antiproliferative Activity of Xanthones Isolated from *Artocarpus obtusus*** 48
Najihah Mohd Hashim, Mawardi Rahmani, Gwendoline Cheng Lian Ee, Mohd Aspollah Sukari, Maizatulakmal Yahayu, Winda Oktima, Abd Manaf Ali, and Rusea Go

Chapter 7 **Antilipogenic and Anti-Inflammatory Activities of *Codonopsis lanceolata* in Mice Hepatic Tissues after Chronic Ethanol Feeding** 57
Areum Cha, Youngshim Choi, Yoojeong Jin, Mi-Kyung Sung, Yun-Chang Koo, Kwang-Won Lee, and Taesun Park

Chapter 8 **Trace Level Determination of Polyether Ionophores in Feed** 70
Mervi Rokka, Marika Jestoi, and Kimmo Peltonen

Chapter 9 **Management of Cosmetic Embarrassment Caused by *Malassezia* spp. with Fruticose Lichen *Cladia* Using Phylogenetic Approach** 82
Anand Pandey, Rohit K. Mishra, Amit K. Tiwari, Awadhesh Kumar, A. K. Bajaj, and Anupam Dikshit

Chapter 10 **Tramadol Pretreatment Enhances Ketamine-Induced Antidepressant Effects and Increases Mammalian Target of Rapamycin in Rat Hippocampus and Prefrontal Cortex** 90
Chun Yang, Wen-Yuan Li, Hai-Yin Yu, Zhi-Qin Gao, Xiang-Liu Liu, Zhi-Qiang Zhou, and Jian-Jun Yang

Chapter 11 **Amikacin Population Pharmacokinetics in Critically Ill Kuwaiti Patients** 96
Kamal M. Matar, Yousef Al-lanqawi, Kefaya Abdul-Malek, and Roger Jelliffe

Chapter 12 **Plasma and Ocular Prednisolone Disposition after Oral Treatment in Cats** 104
María J. Del Sole, Paula Schaiquevich, Marcelo A. Aba, Carlos E. Lanusse, and Laura Moreno

Chapter 13 **Involvement of Nrf2-Mediated Upregulation of Heme Oxygenase-1 in Mollugin-Induced Growth Inhibition and Apoptosis in Human Oral Cancer Cells** 110
Young-Man Lee, Q-Schick Auh, Deok-Won Lee, Jun-Yeol Kim, Ha-Jin Jung, Seung-Ho Lee, and Eun-Cheol Kim

Chapter 14 **Antitumor Activity of Artemisinin and Its Derivatives: From a Well-Known Antimalarial Agent to a Potential Anticancer Drug** 124
Maria P. Crespo-Ortiz and Ming Q. Wei

Chapter 15 **Therapeutic Approach in the Improvement of Endothelial Dysfunction: The Current State of the Art** 142
Miroslav Radenković, Marko Stojanović, Tatjana Potpara, and Milica Prostran

Chapter 16 **The Indolic Diet-Derivative, 3,3′-Diindolylmethane, Induced Apoptosis in Human Colon Cancer Cells through Upregulation of NDRG1** 154
A. Lerner, M. Grafi-Cohen, T. Napso, N. Azzam, and F. Fares

Chapter 17 **Comparative Study of the Effect of Baicalin and Its Natural Analogs on Neurons with Oxygen and Glucose Deprivation Involving Innate Immune Reaction of TLR2/TNFα** 159
Hui-Ying Li, Jun Hu, Shuang Zhao, Zhi-Yi Yuan, Hong-Jiao Wan, Fan Lei, Yi Ding, Dong-Ming Xing, and Li-Jun Du

Chapter 18 **Screening of α-Glucosidase Inhibitory Activity from Some Plants of Apocynaceae, Clusiaceae, Euphorbiaceae, and Rubiaceae** 168
Berna Elya, Katrin Basah, Abdul Mun'im, Wulan Yuliastuti, Anastasia Bangun, and Eva Kurnia Septiana

Chapter 19 **Pharmacokinetic Models for FcRn-Mediated IgG Disposition** **174**
Jim J. Xiao

Chapter 20 ***In Vivo* Clearance of Alpha-1 Acid Glycoprotein Is Influenced by the Extent of Its N-Linked Glycosylation and by Its Interaction with the Vessel Wall** **187**
Teresa R. McCurdy, Varsha Bhakta, Louise J. Eltringham-Smith, Sharon Gataiance, Alison E. Fox-Robichaud, and William P. Sheffield

Chapter 21 **Fructation *In Vivo*: Detrimental and Protective Effects of Fructose** **198**
H. M. Semchyshyn

Permissions

List of Contributors

Preface

Pharmacology is derived from the ancient Greek word 'pharmakon' or 'poison'. It is the branch of biology and medicine that concerns itself with the study of drug action. A drug can be broadly explained to be any chemical substance that exerts a biochemical or physiological effect on an organism. To be more specific, it is a field which studies the interactions that occur between a living organism and chemicals that affect their biochemical function. This arena also aims to understand the properties of drugs and their actions. These include the interactions between drug molecules and receptors and how it coaxes an effect. Pharmacology provides the scientific foundation and principles for various applications, like the study of drug actions in the health sciences, as tools in scientific research, as the use of drugs as therapeutic agents in medicine and the development and regulation of pharmaceuticals. It is a multi-disciplinary scientific field with many sub divisions that include clinical pharmacology, behavioural pharmacology, pharmacogenetics, neuropsychopharmacology, pharmacoeconomics and cardiovascular pharmacology. There are still many challenges that remain in this field even though there has been rapid progress. There are always new drugs to be discovered and researched on that affect our way of living.

This book attempts to compile and collate the research and data available in the field of pharmacology. I am grateful to those who put in effort and hard work in this field. I am also thankful to those who supported me in this endeavour. I especially wish to thank my publisher who considered me worthy of this great opportunity and gave me the liberty to edit the text as per my interpretation of the researches. Lastly, I wish to acknowledge the support of my friends and family.

Editor

1

Evaluation of Adverse Effects of Mutein Forms of Recombinant Human Interferon Alpha-2b in Female Swiss Webster Mice

H. Rachmawati,[1] A. Merika,[1] R. A. Ningrum,[1] K. Anggadiredja,[2] and D. S. Retnoningrum[1]

[1] *Research group of Pharmaceutics, School of Pharmacy, Bandung Institute of Technology, Ganesha 10, Bandung 40132, Indonesia*
[2] *Research group of Pharmacology and Clinical Pharmacy, School of Pharmacy, Bandung Institute of Technology, Bandung 40132, Indonesia*

Correspondence should be addressed to H. Rachmawati; hrachma@yahoo.com

Academic Editor: Ayman El-Kadi

Purpose. We successfully developed recombinant human interferon alpha-2b (rhIFN-α2b) and mutein forms through the site-directed mutagenesis technique. The mutein forms were developed by substituting cysteins at positions 2 and 99 with aspartic acids. The potential adverse effects of these rhIFN-α2bs were assessed by acute and subchronic studies. *Methods.* In the acute study, rhIFN-α2bs were subcutaneously administered to mice at a single dose of 97.5 μg/kg, 975 μg/kg, and 9.75 mg/kg BW and were observed for 14 days. In the subchronic study, single dose of 1.95 μg/kg and 19.5 μg/kg, respectively, was given subcutaneously every 3 days for 45 days. *Results.* No death as well as abnormality in body weight, behavior, presentation of main organs, and value of plasma SGPT and SGOT was observed. Wild type and mutein rhIFN-α2bs did not show significant adverse effects at dose up to 9.75 mg/kg BW. Administration of these rhIFN-α2bs given repeatedly did not induce any adverse effect. *Conclusion.* These results suggest that our rhIFN-α2bs are safe. However, further study is still needed to clarify the safety issue before use in clinical trial.

1. Introduction

Hepatitis B and C viruses are highly infectious, and the infections are transmitted almost 100 times more effective than HIV/AIDS. It attacks the liver and is a major cause of liver cancer. Of the estimated 50 million new cases of hepatitis B viral infection diagnosed annually, 5–10% of adults and up to 90% of infants will become chronically infected; 75% of these occur in Asia where hepatitis B is the leading cause of chronic hepatitis, cirrhosis, and hepatocellular carcinoma [1, 2]. Hepatitis C virus, referred to as parentally transmitted non-A non-B hepatitis, has been reported to be the most common transfusion-associated hepatitis in many countries worldwide. Hepatitis C virus infection has been characterized by longer incubation time and chronic, persistent infections and has sevenfolds increased risk of hepatocellular carcinoma [2–4]. Until recently, WHO recommends interferon alpha 2 as a standard therapy for hepatitis B/C virus, either as monotherapy or in combination with nucleotide/nucleoside analogs [5, 6].

Human alpha interferons (hIFN-α) comprise a family of closely related proteins that block viral infection, inhibit cell proliferation, and modulate cell differentiation. Recombinant hIFN-α2 has proven useful for the treatment of a variety of human viral diseases and cancers. However, the clinical use of this cytokine has been restricted due to its short circulating half-life, which makes frequent dosing over an extended period necessary. One main problem of using interferon as a therapy is that interferon exhibits short plasma half-life so that it is not effective to deliver sufficient amount to the target tissue. This short plasma half-life is commonly due to fast renal clearance which is related to the hydrophilic properties of this agent as well as its small size or to enzymatic degradation caused by enzymes present in blood, liver, and kidney. To improve its properties, several approaches have been performed such as chemical modification through pegylation and protein engineering [7]. Our report described a novel strategy on this protein by replacing nonpotential aminoacids influencing the biological activity of the protein with more negative aminoacid, hence increasing the net negative charge of the protein.

Protein charge is a crucial factor for kidney elimination, hence; any effort of modifying this charge will alter its

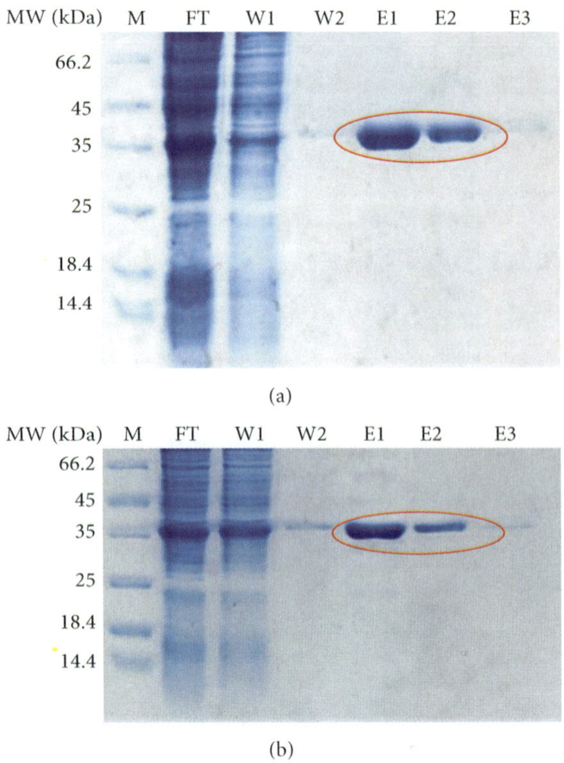

FIGURE 1: SDS-PAGE analysis of wild type rIFN-α2b and rIFN-α2bC$_2$DC$_{99}$D. (a) Wild type rIFN-α2b; (b) rhIFN-α2bC$_2$DC$_{99}$D; M: protein marker; FT: flow through; W1: washing 1; W2: washing 2; E1: elution 1; E2: elution 2; E3: elution 3.

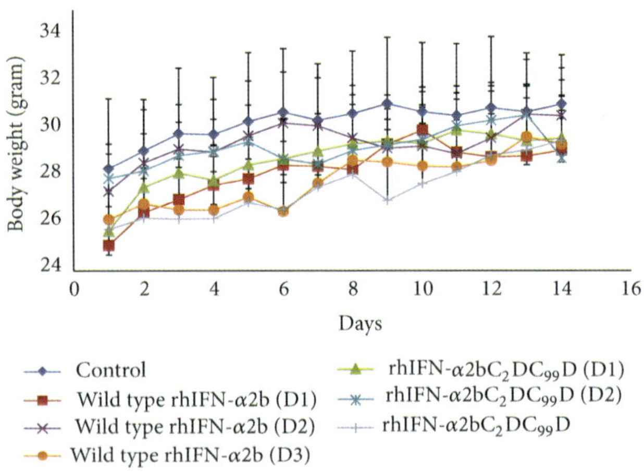

FIGURE 2: Body weight of the mice after a single dose administration of wild type rIFN-α2b and mutein rIFN-α2bC$_2$DC$_{99}$D.

half-life. Negatively charged proteins will be repulsed by glomerular cells that are positively charged. Therefore, the negatively charged proteins will be recirculated into the blood. Diminished kidney elimination and increased blood circulation will prolong protein half-life. This in turn will decrease protein dosing and consequently will lower its toxicity [8].

There are 12 aminoacids (Leu30, Lys31, Arg33, His34, Phe36, Arg120, Lys121, Gln124, Tyr122, Tyr129, Lys131, and Glu132) in hIFN-α2b that are involved in its biological activity [9]. Among 4 cysteine residues, cysteines at positions 1 and 98 which form a disulfide bridge are not required for biological activity of IFN-α2b [10]. Even the disruption of this disulfide bridge by serine substitutions resulted in higher antiviral activity [11]. We have previously cloned the gene encoding wild type human IFN-α2b using synthetic gene approach and have successfully overproduced the protein in *Escherichia coli* [12, 13]. The recombinant protein has been purified and confirmed by nano-LC mass spectrometry to be the right IFN-α2b. We further engineered the protein to generate rhIFN-α2bs that are more negatively charged than the wild type counterpart. The technique developed was site-directed mutagenesis of gene encoding IFN-α2b. The site-directed mutagenesis was focused on two cystein codons (at positions 2 and 99) to be replaced by aspartic acids using mutagenic primers. Our previous results demonstrated that all engineered rhIFN-α2bs (C$_2$D, C$_{99}$D, C$_2$DC$_{99}$D) exhibited longer elimination half-life than their wild type counterpart [14]. The aim of this study was to evaluate the safety of our novel IFN-α2bs. As an earlier step on this matter, we studied whether any potential adverse effects developed on these mutein forms when administered in higher dose for longer period of time.

2. Materials and Methods

2.1. Bacterial Strains and Culture Media. E. coli strain BL21(DE3) containing IFN-α2b wild type and muteins open reading frame previously constructed was used for gene expression [12]. Luria-Bertani (LB) broth and agar containing 100 μg/mL of ampicillin was applied for bacterial growth, and 0.5 mM of isopropyl d-1-thiogalactopyranoside (IPTG) was for protein overproduction.

2.2. Interferon Preparation. The wild type and a mutein IFN-α2b (C$_2$DC$_{99}$D) were each overproduced using optimized condition previously described [12, 13]. The crude and purified proteins (as soluble protein) were analyzed using 15% sodium dodecyl sulphate polyacrylamide gel electrophoresis (SDS-PAGE) under denaturing condition. All IFN-α2bs were affinity purified using Nickel column, and imidazole was removed from purified protein using nanosep centrifugal concentration with 10 kDa cutoff (Pall Life Science) [12]. Protein concentration was determined using Bradford method based on coomassie blue staining.

2.3. Animals. Female Swiss Webster mice, 2-3 months of age, were obtained from the Animal Laboratory, School of Pharmacy, Bandung Institute of Technology, Indonesia. The mice were housed under the barrier-sustained condition in a well-ventilated animal room according to standard laboratory condition with free access to standard diet. Animals used in the experiments received care in compliance with the "Principles of Laboratory Animal Care" and "Guide for the Care and Use of Laboratory Animals." They were acclimatized for about 1 week prior to administration of the test substances. Standard mouse pellet and tap sterilized water were given ad libitum.

2.4. Experimental Design. Studies were conducted under Good Laboratory Practice conditions at Animal Laboratory School of Pharmacy, Bandung Institute of Technology, Bandung, Indonesia. Animals were sacrificed under anaesthesia with 40% $O_2 : 60\%$ N_2O combined with 0.5% Isoflurane (Abbot Laboratoriesb Ltd. Queensborough, Kent, UK).

2.5. Evaluation of Acute Adverse Effect. Acute and subchronic adverse effects study was performed according to OECD Guide Lines for the Testing of Chemicals, Test no. 425 (2008). Thirty-five female mice were divided into 3 groups: control and 2 test groups each receiving either rhIFN-α2b wild type or mutein. The mice in test groups were further divided into 3 groups, each was given 97.5 μg/kg, 975 μg/kg, or 9.75 mg/kg BW rhIFN-α2b in a single subcutaneous injection. The control group only received similar treatment with water for injection. Observations of pharmacotoxic signs were carried out at 0.5, 1, 2, 4, and 24 h after dosing during the first day and daily thereafter for 14 days. The time of onset, intensity, and duration of these symptoms, if any, was recorded. All animals were observed twice daily for mortality during the 14-day period of study. The weight of each mouse was recorded daily throughout the course of the study. The group's mean body weights were calculated. At the termination of the study (14 days), all animals were sacrificed, and a complete organ analysis with both macroscopic and microscopic observations was performed. Histological analysis was carried out using haematoxylin/eosin staining on the vital organs including liver, kidney, and heart.

2.6. Evaluation of Subchronic Adverse Effect. Fifty-four female mice were divided into five groups: control; two test groups, each receiving either rhIFN-α2b wild type or mutein, and two satellite groups. Mice in test groups were further divided into two groups receiving either 1.95 μg/kg or 19.5 μg/kg BW of interferons. The interferons were given subcutaneously every 3 days as a single dose during a 45-day period. The control group only received water for injection through the same route.

At the end of the 45-day period, the animals were fasted overnight. In the following morning, blood sample was collected from the retro-orbital sinus. All animals except the satellite groups were then sacrificed. Vital organs including liver, kidney, lymph, ovary, uterus, and heart were isolated and analyzed. Both macroscopic and microscopic observations were performed in a similar way to those performed in acute study. In addition, the activities of serum glutamic pyruvic transaminase (SGPT) and serum glutamic oxaloacetic transaminase (SGOT) were assayed. Animals in satellite groups were allowed to survive to check the reversibility of the adverse effects.

2.7. Statistical Analysis. The data which were expressed as mean ± standard deviation were analyzed using analysis of variance (ANOVA). Significant difference was considered if $P < 0.05$.

3. Results

3.1. SDS-PAGE Analysis of Wild Type and Mutein Forms of Interferon Alpha-2bs. Figure 1 shows a single band of wild type and mutein forms of rhIFN-α2b; all exhibited correct size as calculated. SDS-PAGE analysis was performed to check the quality of proteins prior to the study.

3.2. Acute Adverse Effect Evaluation. The aim of this evaluation was to observe the potential adverse effect on the wild type as well as the mutein form of interferon alpha-2b during short period of administration.

3.2.1. Mortalities. There was no death observed in all groups (Table 1). Therefore, the LD_{50} value in mice was higher than 9.75 mg/kg BW which is equivalent to 2500 times therapeutic dose of interferon through subcutaneous administration.

3.2.2. Behavioral Findings. The parameters observed during the study included performances in general behavior, respiratory, autonomic, and central nervous systems, digestive system (defecation and urination), and the motor activity. No unusual changes were observed in behavior or locomotor activity. Furthermore, no ataxia and signs of intoxication were found in all groups during the 14-day observation period.

3.2.3. Body Weight. Decrease in body weight can be an early sign of toxic effect of the test drugs. In this study, no significant difference was observed in the body weights between treated and the control groups (Figure 2).

3.2.4. Organ Indices. Organ indices refer to the weight of the organ(s) relative to the body weight. This observation was performed at the end of the study to check whether any alteration occurred on vital organs after the animal received the rhIFN-α2bs. As shown in Table 2, in particular for liver and kidney, there was an increase in organ index when the mice were given the highest dose of both forms of interferon. However, this difference was not significant statistically ($P > 0.05$).

3.2.5. Microscopic Observation. As shown in Figures 3, 4, and 5, there were no significant differences in the microscopic evaluation of the heart, liver, and kidney between control and treated groups.

3.3. Subchronic Adverse Effect Evaluation

3.3.1. Behavioral Findings. The parameters observed during the study included performances in general behavior and body weight. As previously recorded in acute study, no unusual changes in behavior or locomotor activity were found, and no signs of intoxication were seen in all groups during the 45-days observation period.

TABLE 1: Mortalities and LD_{50} values of female Swiss Webster mice after a single subcutaneous administration of wild type rIFN-α2b or mutein rIFN-$\alpha 2bC_2DC_{99}D$.

Group	Substances	N	Σ mortality	Response (%)	LD_{50}
Control	Water for injection	6	0	0	
I	Wild type rIFN-α2b D1	6	0	0	
II	Wild type rIFN-α2b D2	6	0	0	
III	Wild type rIFN-α2b D3	6	0	0	>9.75 mg/kg BW
IV	rIFN-$\alpha 2bC_2DC_{99}D$ D1	6	0	0	
V	rIFN-$\alpha 2bC_2DC_{99}D$ D2	6	0	0	
VI	rIFN-$\alpha 2bC_2DC_{99}D$ D3	6	0	0	

D1 = 97.5 μg/kg BW, D2 = 975 μg/kg BW, and D3 = 9.75 mg/g BW.

TABLE 2: Organ indices of female mice after a single dose of wild type rIFN-α2b or rIFN-$\alpha 2bC_2DC_{99}D$.

Organ	Groups						
	Control	Wild type rIFN-α2b (D1)	rIFN-$\alpha 2bC_2DC_{99}D$ (D1)	Wild type rIFN-α2b (D2)	rIFN-$\alpha 2bC_2DC_{99}D$ (D2)	Wild type rIFN-α2b (D3)	rIFN-$\alpha 2bC_2DC_{99}D$ (D3)
Heart	0.43 ± 0.04	0.45 ± 0.03	0.42 ± 0.02	0.43 ± 0.04	0.44 ± 0.04	0.43 ± 0.04	0.42 ± 0.04
Liver	4.91 ± 0.97	4.18 ± 1.81	4.57 ± 0.27	4.94 ± 0.50	5.53 ± 0.30	5.27 ± 0.50	5.05 ± 0.91
Kidney	1.07 ± 0.14	1.39 ± 0.09	1.17 ± 0.04	1.15 ± 0.11	1.12 ± 0.09	1.25 ± 0.15	1.16 ± 0.08
Limp	0.37 ± 0.14	0.36 ± 0.05	0.33 ± 0.06	0.34 ± 0.04	0.42 ± 0.13	0.63 ± 0.14	0.65 ± 0.28
Ovary-uterus	0.62 ± 0.21	0.73 ± 0.17	0.65 ± 0.11	0.63 ± 0.21	0.62 ± 0.15	0.62 ± 0.08	0.80 ± 0.26
Lung	0.54 ± 0.06	0.62 ± 0.09	0.54 ± 0.04	0.57 ± 0.12	0.58 ± 0.12	0.62 ± 0.06	0.59 ± 0.07

TABLE 3: Organ indices of female mice after subcutaneous administration of wild type rIFN-α2b or rIFN-$\alpha 2bC_2DC_{99}D$ once every 3 days during a 45-day period.

Organ	Groups				
	Control	Wild type rIFN-α2b (D4)	rIFN-$\alpha 2bC_2DC_{99}D$ (D4)	Wild type rIFN-α2b (D5)	rIFN-$\alpha 2bC_2DC_{99}D$ (D5)
Heart	0.43 ± 0.03	0.41 ± 0.013	0.41 ± 0.04	0.43 ± 0.03	0.41 ± 0.03
Liver	5.81 ± 0.39	5.95 ± 0.33	6.14 ± 1.06	5.97 ± 0.55	5.39 ± 0.26
Kidney	1.37 ± 0.16	1.39 ± 0.16	1.48 ± 0.07	1.34 ± 0.05	1.30 ± 0.12
Limp	0.66 ± 0.15	0.59 ± 0.14	0.72 ± 0.18	0.58 ± 0.14	0.48 ± 0.09
Ovary-uterus	0.69 ± 0.16	0.64 ± 0.12	0.78 ± 0.14	0.72 ± 0.19	0.69 ± 0.19
Lung	0.59 ± 0.07	0.58 ± 0.02	0.60 ± 0.09	0.61 ± 0.05	0.59 ± 0.07

D4 = 1.95 μg/kg BW, D5 = 19.5 μg/kg BW.

TABLE 4: Enzyme activities in plasma of the mice after injection of the interferons once every 3 days during a 45-day period.

	Control	Wild type rIFN-α2b (D4)	rIFN-$\alpha 2bC_2DC_{99}D$ (D4)	Wild type rIFN-α2b (D5)	rIFN-$\alpha 2bC_2DC_{99}D$ (D5)
SGPT	54 ± 2	50.67 ± 14.04	54 ± 1	50.33 ± 16.01	53.33 ± 22.36
SGOT	215.67 ± 24.58	231 ± 19.52	219.67 ± 44.76	215.67 ± 41.88	205 ± 44.03

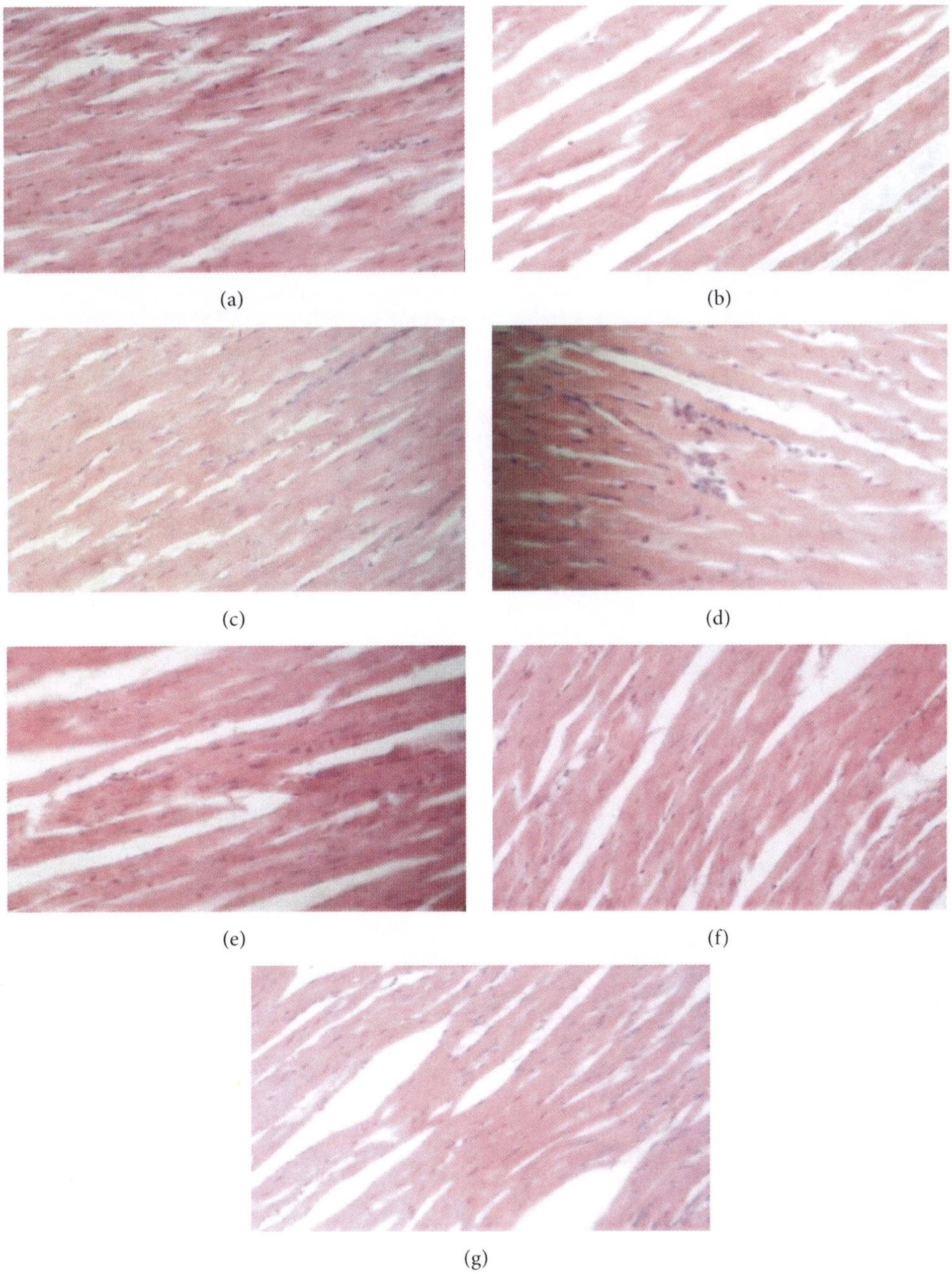

FIGURE 3: Histological presentation after H/E staining of heart tissue of the mice treated with a single dose of subcutaneous wild type rIFN-α2b or rhIFN-$\alpha 2bC_2DC_{99}D$ (magnification 400x). (a) Control; (b) wild type rhIFN-α2b (D1); (c) rhIFN-$\alpha 2bC_2DC_{99}D$ (D1); (d) wild type rhIFN-α2b (D2); (e) rhIFN-$\alpha 2bC_2DC_{99}D$ (D2); (f) wild type rhIFN-α2b (D3); (g) rhIFN-$\alpha 2bC_2DC_{99}D$ (D3).

3.3.2. Body Weights and Organ Indices. As observed in the acute adverse effect evaluation, no differences were found in body weight as well as organ indices between mice in the control group and those treated with various doses of wild type or mutein forms of rhIFN-α2bs (Figure 6 and Table 3).

3.3.3. Microscopic Observation. H/E staining analysis as seen in Figures 7, 8, and 9 clearly shows no difference in the histology of heart, liver, and the kidney tissues between control and treated groups. This was in line with the observations of gross pathology performed in all mice immediately after dissection, demonstrating the uniformity in health, and the lack of any apparent pathological abnormalities. These results indicated that administration of these rhIFN-α2bs at the tested doses did not result in any adverse toxicological effects on these organs.

Table 4 shows the activities of two major hepatic enzymes analyzed in plasma. No significant differences were observed in the enzyme activities between the control and rhIFN-α2bs-treated groups. SGPT and SGOT are the intracellular

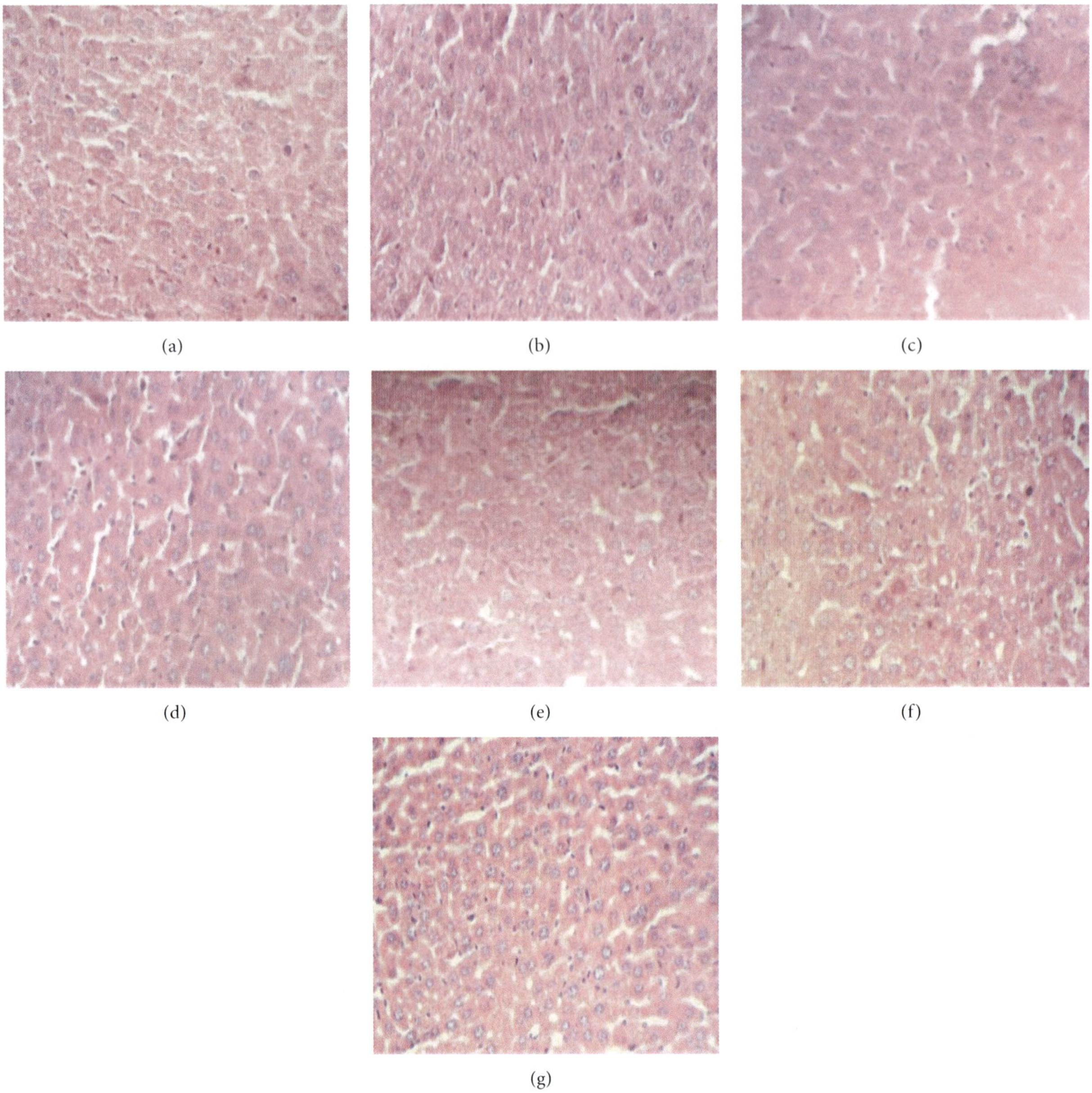

Figure 4: Histological presentation after H/E staining of liver of the mice treated with a single dose of subcutaneous wild type rhIFN-α2b or rhIFN-$\alpha 2bC_2DC_{99}D$ (magnification 400x). (a) Control; (b) wild type rhIFN-α2b (D1); (c) rhIFN-$\alpha 2bC_2DC_{99}D$ (D1); (d) wild type rhIFN-α2b (D2); (e) rhIFN-$\alpha 2bC_2DC_{99}D$ (D2); (f) wild type rhIFN-α2b (D3); (g) rhIFN-$\alpha 2bC_2DC_{99}D$ (D3).

enzymes expressed constitutively with biochemical catalytic functions in the cells. Induction of these enzymes may indicate the imbalance in the liver function due to pathological stress.

4. Discussion

The purpose of this study was to assess the safety of our rhIFN-α2bs either as wild type or mutein form when they were given acutely or repeatedly. The rhIFN-α2bs expressed from synthetic gene and in particular the novel mutein form (rhIFN-$\alpha 2bC_2DC_{99}D$) used in this study is of chemically unique. Unlike other engineered rhIFN-α2bs, $C_2DC_{99}D$ has only one disulphide bridge due to aspartic acid substitutions on cysteines 2 and 99 and therefore has more negative charge. A distinguishing feature of this mutein form of rhIFN-α2b is the lack of charged-mediated renal clearance, which is expected to prolong its presence in the systemic circulation. This charge-modified type is expected to have improved pharmacokinetic profile compared to the wild type form of the interferon [14].

The acute adverse effect evaluation revealed that the value of LD_{50} was higher than 9.75 mg/kg BW for the tested rhIFN-α2b which is equivalent to 2500 times as much therapeutic

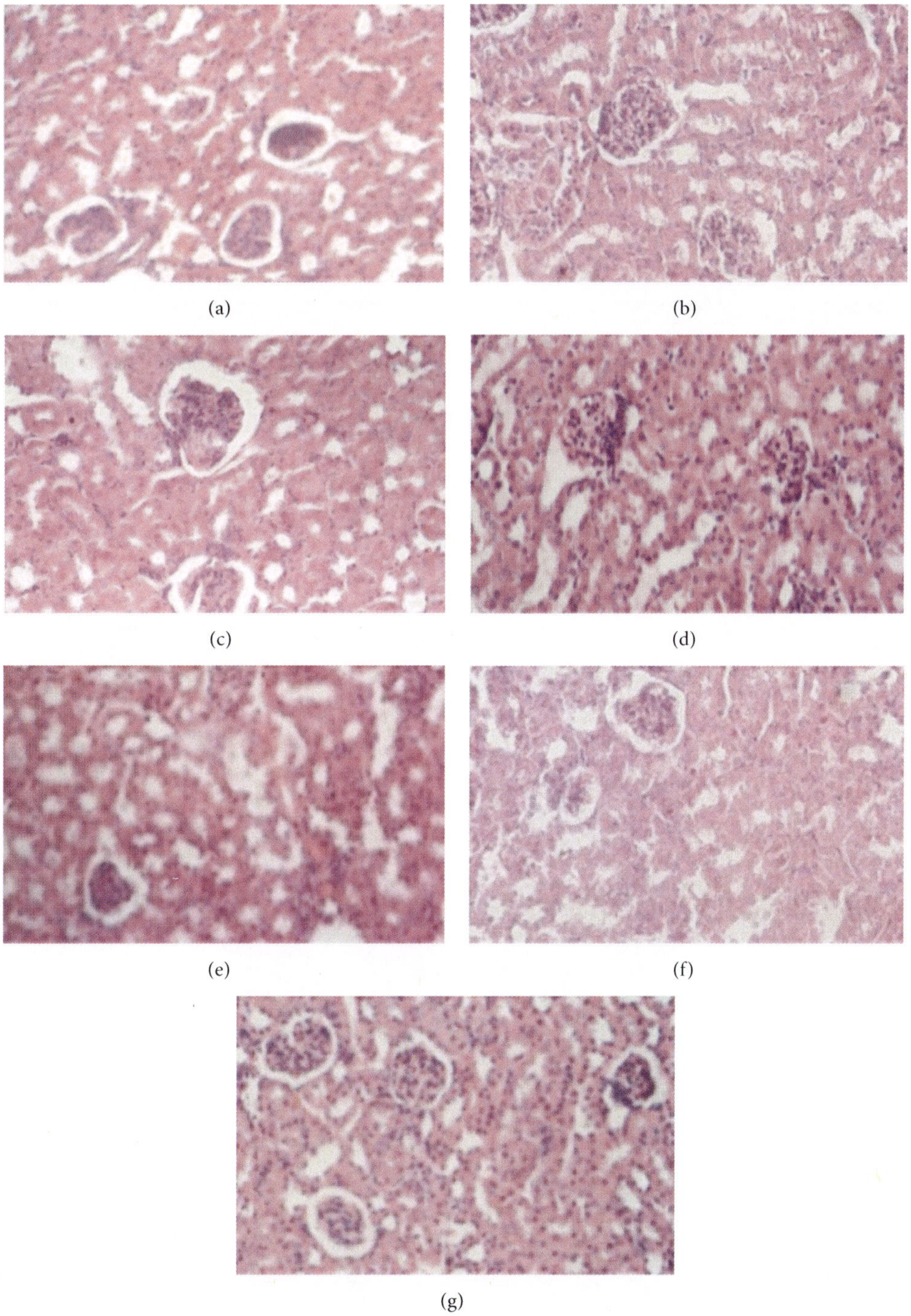

Figure 5: Histological presentation after H/E staining of kidney of the mice treated with a single dose of subcutaneous wild type rhIFN-α2b or rhIFN-α2bC$_2$DC$_{99}$D (magnification 400x). (a) Control; (b) wild type rhIFN-α2b (D1); (c) rhIFN-α2bC$_2$DC$_{99}$D (D1); (d) wild type rhIFN-α2b (D2); (e) rhIFN-α2bC$_2$DC$_{99}$D (D2); (f) wild type rhIFN-α2b (D3); (g) rhIFN-α2bC$_2$DC$_{99}$D (D3).

human dose of interferon given subcutaneously. This result further corroborates a previous study (personal communication) showing no acute toxicological reaction or death when interferon was administered i.v. or intraabdominally to mice at doses up to 10^4 to 10^5 times of human dosage. Furthermore, recent work showed no effect on general signs, body weight, food consumption, and blood chemistry when interferon was given acutely to rat and monkey [11].

Our present results further showed that repeated administration of the rhIFN-α2bs did not induce significant changes in behavioral findings, blood chemistry, and histological presentation of the main organs. Again, these results further supported previous works demonstrating the good tolerability of interferon. Thus, Meng et al. [15] showed that after repeated dose of IFNalpha-2a-NGR (Asn-Gly-Arg), all the clinical chemistry changes were of minor severity there

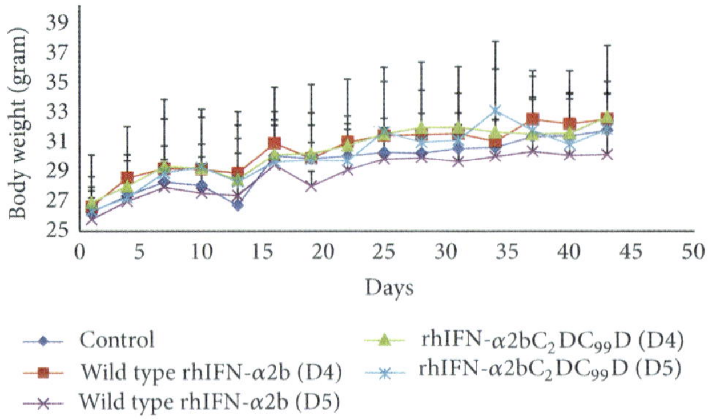

Figure 6: Body weight of the mice after subcutaneous administration of wild type rhIFN-α2b and rhIFN-$\alpha 2bC_2DC_{99}D$ once every 3 days in the subchronic study period that lasted for 45 days.

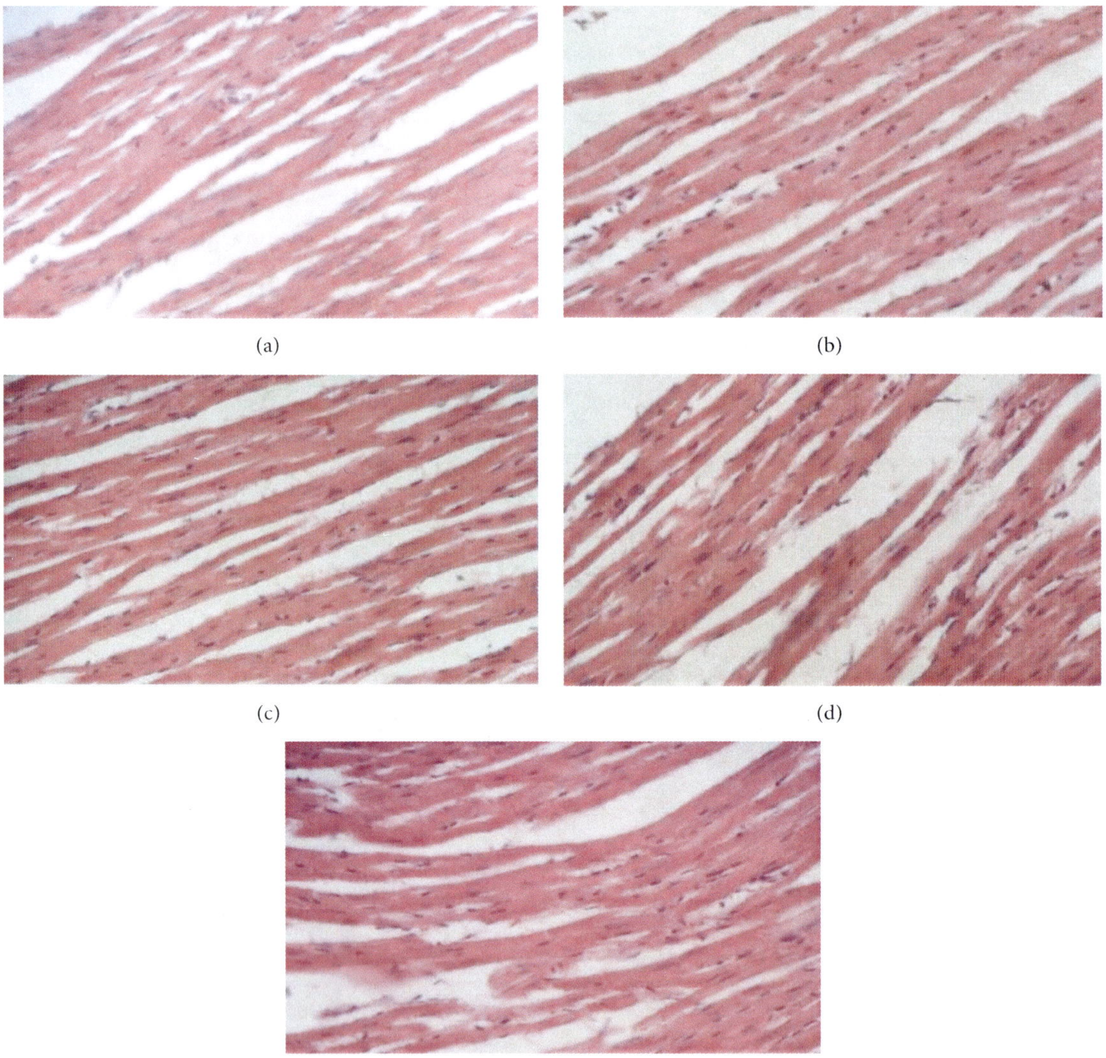

(a) (b) (c) (d) (e)

Figure 7: Histological presentation of H/E staining of heart tissue of the mice after subcutaneous administration of wild type rhIFN-α2b or rhIFN-$\alpha 2bC_2DC_{99}D$ once every 3 days during a 45-day period (magnification 400x). (a) Control; (b) wild type rhIFN-α2b (D4); (c) rhIFN-$\alpha 2bC_2DC_{99}D$ (D4); (d) wild type rhIFN-α2b (D5); (e) rhIFN-$\alpha 2bC_2DC_{99}D$ (D5).

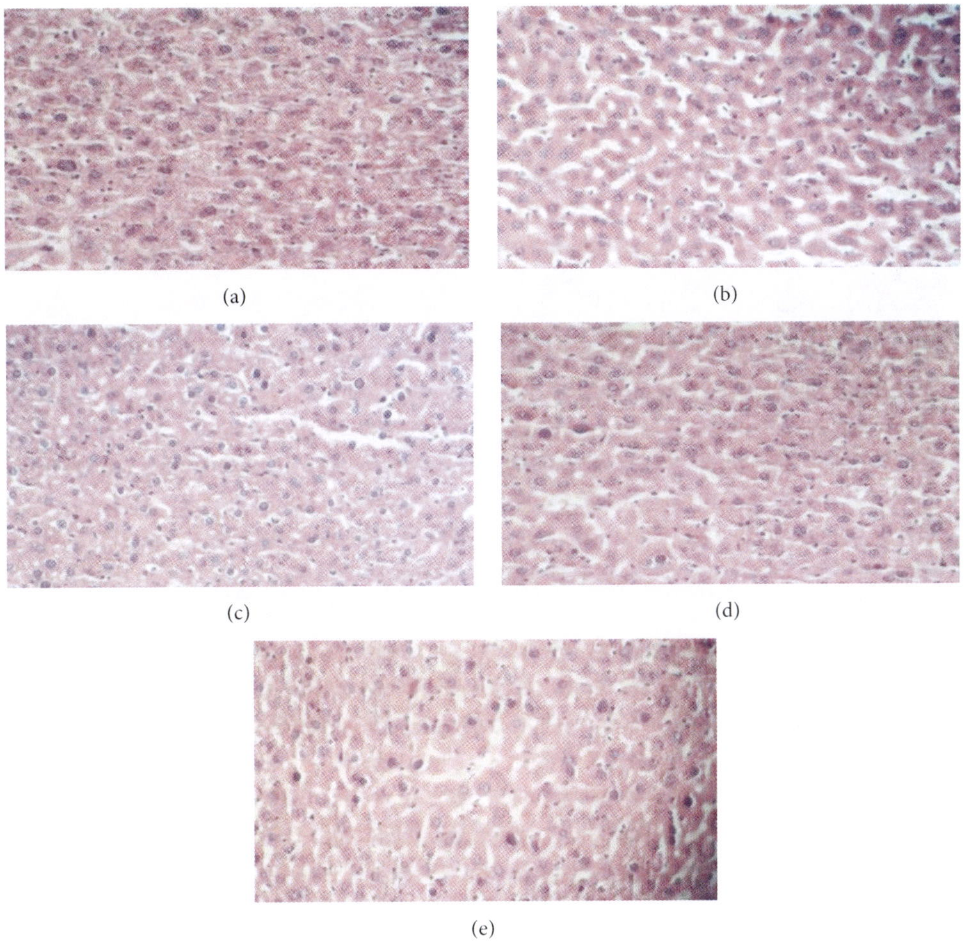

FIGURE 8: Histological presentation of H/E staining of liver tissue of the mice after subcutaneous administration of wild type rhIFN-α2b or rhIFN-α2bC$_2$DC$_{99}$D once every 3 days during a 45-day period (magnification 400x). (a) Control; (b) wild type rhIFN-α2b (D4); (c) rhIFN-α2bC$_2$DC$_{99}$D (D4); (d) wild type rhIFN-α2b (D5); (e) rhIFN-α2bC$_2$DC$_{99}$D (D5).

were no pertinent abnormal parameters or results observed [15]. Furthermore, these authors found that the increase in spleen and thymus organ-to-body weight ratios and decrease in menses were mild, reversible, and likely related to the pharmacology of the interferon. In addition, a recent study showed that administration of up to 100 μg/kg (11 MIU/kg) PEG (Polyethylene Glycol)-IFN β-1a given subcutaneously or intramuscularly once weekly for 5 weeks in monkeys resulted in no drug-related adverse effects.

As indicated previously, the good safety feature of our modified interferons might be closely related to the improved pharmacokinetic properties, affecting mainly the distribution and elimination of the substance. Indeed, Hu and colleagues [16] have reported that polyethylene glycol- (PEG-) IFN β-1a showed greater exposure, longer half-life, lower clearance, and reduced volume of distribution than unmodified IFN β-1a, and this was accompanied with the elevation of neopterin (pharmacodynamic marker of interferon) concentration [16]. In line with this finding, it has been demonstrated that anchoring IFN-α to ApoA-I prolongs the half-life of IFN-α and promotes targeting to the liver, which might be responsible for the increased immunostimulatory properties and lower hematological toxicity [17].

In conclusion, results of our present work demonstrated that the wild type interferon as well as the novel mutein that we developed does not result in adverse effects and is well tolerated when administered during a 45-day study period, which suggests the potential for their safe use. Further work toward evaluating their efficacy is in progress and shall be reported elsewhere.

Conflict of Interests

The author(s) declared no conflict of interests with respect to the authorship and/or publication of this paper.

Authors' Contribution

All authors contributed to the work described in this paper and take responsibility for it. Moreover, none of the works described in this paper has been published elsewhere.

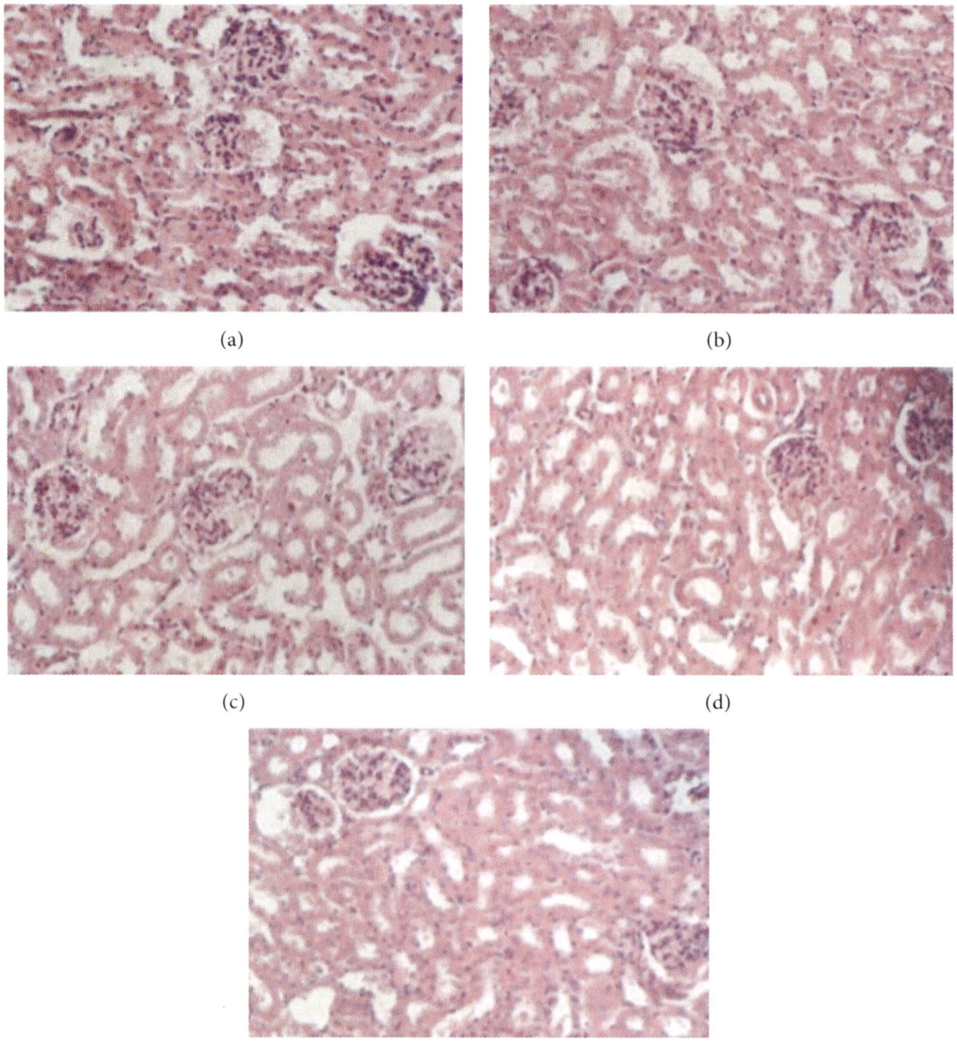

(a) (b) (c) (d) (e)

Figure 9: Histological presentation of H/E staining of kidney tissue of the mice after subcutaneous administration of wild type rhIFN-α2b or rhIFN-$\alpha 2bC_2DC_{99}D$ once every 3 days during a 45-day period (magnification 400x). (a) Control; (b) wild type rhIFN-α2b (D4); (c) rhIFN-$\alpha 2bC_2DC_{99}D$ (D4); (d) wild type rhIFN-α2b (D5); (e) rhIFN-$\alpha 2bC_2DC_{99}D$ (D5).

Acknowledgments

Funding for this work was partly supported by research grant of Incentive Program from the Ministry of Research and Technology of the Republic of Indonesia 2009 and competency research grant DIKTI-Indonesia.

References

[1] C. W. Shepard, L. Finelli, and M. J. Alter, "Global epidemiology of hepatitis C virus infection," *Lancet Infectious Diseases*, vol. 5, no. 9, pp. 558–567, 2005.

[2] T. Utsumi, Y. Yano, M. I. Lusida et al., "Serologic and molecular characteristics of hepatitis B virus among school children in East Java, Indonesia," *American Journal of Tropical Medicine and Hygiene*, vol. 83, no. 1, pp. 189–193, 2010.

[3] H. B. El-Serag, "Epidemiology of hepatocellular carcinoma," *Clinics in Liver Disease*, vol. 5, no. 1, pp. 87–107, 2001.

[4] V. Fensterl and G. C. Sen, "Interferons and viral infections," *BioFactors*, vol. 35, no. 1, pp. 14–20, 2009.

[5] B. Gao, F. Hong, and S. Radaeva, "Host factors and failure of interferon-α treatment in Hepatitis C virus," *Hepatology*, vol. 39, no. 4, pp. 880–890, 2004.

[6] P. J. Gow and D. Mutimer, "Treatment of chronic hepatitis," *British Medical Journal*, vol. 323, pp. 1164–1167, 2001.

[7] E. Jonasch and F. G. Haluska, "Interferon in oncological practice: review of interferon biology, clinical applications, and toxicities," *Oncologist*, vol. 6, no. 1, pp. 34–55, 2001.

[8] N. Ceaglio, M. Etcheverrigaray, R. Kratje, and M. Oggero, "Novel long-lasting interferon alpha derivatives designed by glycoengineering," *Biochimie*, vol. 90, no. 3, pp. 437–449, 2008.

[9] R. Radhakrishnan, L. J. Walter, A. Hruza et al., "Zinc mediated dimer of human interferon-α(2b) revealed by X-ray crystallography," *Structure*, vol. 4, no. 12, pp. 1453–1463, 1996.

[10] C. Weissmann and H. Weber, "The interferon genes," *Progress in Nucleic Acid Research & Molecular Biology*, vol. 33, pp. 251–300, 1986.

[11] F. O. Neves, P. L. Ho, I. Raw, C. A. Pereira, C. Moreira, and A. L. T. O. Nascimento, "Overexpression of a synthetic gene encoding human alpha interferon in *Escherichia coli*," *Protein Expression and Purification*, vol. 35, no. 2, pp. 353–359, 2004.

[12] D. S. Retnoningrum, R. A. Ningrum, Y. N. Kurniawan, A. Indrayati, and H. Rachmawati, "Construction of synthetic open reading frame encoding human interferon alpha 2b for high expression in *Escherichia coli* and characterization of its gene product," *Journal of Biotechnology*, vol. 145, no. 2, pp. 193–198, 2010.

[13] R. A. Ningrum, D. S. Retnoningrum, Y. Cahyati, and H. Rachmawati, "Optimization of human interferon α2b soluble protein overproduction and primary recovery of its inclusion bodies," *Microbiology Indonesia*, vol. 5, no. 1, pp. 27–32, 2011.

[14] R. A. Ningrum, D. E. Rahmatika, D. S. Retnoningrum, A. H. Wangsaatmadja, Y. C. Sumitrapura, and H. Rachmawati, "Development of novel interferon alpha 2b muteins and study the pharmacokinetic and biodistribution profiles in animal model," *Journal of Biomedical Science and Engineering*, vol. 5, pp. 104–112, 2012.

[15] J. Meng, Z. Yan, Y. Wu et al., "Preclinical safety evaluation of IFNα2a-NGR," *Regulatory Toxicology and Pharmacology*, vol. 50, no. 3, pp. 294–302, 2008.

[16] X. Hu, K. Olivier, E. Polack et al., "In vivo pharmacology and toxicology evaluation of polyethylene glycol-conjugated interferon beta-1a," *Journal of Pharmacology and Experimental Therapeutics*, vol. 338, no. 3, pp. 984–996, 2011.

[17] J. Fioravanti, I. González, J. Medina-Echeverz et al., "Anchoring interferon alpha to apolipoprotein A-I reduces hematological toxicity while enhancing immunostimulatory properties," *Hepatology*, vol. 53, no. 6, pp. 1864–1873, 2011.

2

Alantolactone Induces Apoptosis in HepG2 Cells through GSH Depletion, Inhibition of STAT3 Activation, and Mitochondrial Dysfunction

Muhammad Khan,[1,2] Ting Li,[1] Muhammad Khalil Ahmad Khan,[2] Azhar Rasul,[1] Faisal Nawaz,[3] Meiyan Sun,[1] Yongchen Zheng,[1] and Tonghui Ma[1]

[1] *Central Research Laboratory, Jilin University Bethune Second Hospital, Changchun 130041, China*
[2] *Department of Zoology, University of the Punjab, Quaid-e-Azam Campus, Lahore 54590, Pakistan*
[3] *Key Laboratory of Inorganic Synthesis and Preparative Chemistry, Jilin University, Qianjin Street, Changchun 130012, China*

Correspondence should be addressed to Yongchen Zheng; jlzyc@yahoo.com.cn

Academic Editor: D. M. Clarke

Signal transducer and activator of transcription 3 (STAT3) constitutively expresses in human liver cancer cells and has been implicated in apoptosis resistance and tumorigenesis. Alantolactone, a sesquiterpene lactone, has been shown to possess anticancer activities in various cancer cell lines. In our previous report, we showed that alantolactone induced apoptosis in U87 glioblastoma cells via GSH depletion and ROS generation. However, the molecular mechanism of GSH depletion remained unexplored. The present study was conducted to envisage the molecular mechanism of alantolactone-induced apoptosis in HepG2 cells by focusing on the molecular mechanism of GSH depletion and its effect on STAT3 activation. We found that alantolactone induced apoptosis in HepG2 cells in a dose-dependent manner. This alantolactone-induced apoptosis was found to be associated with GSH depletion, inhibition of STAT3 activation, ROS generation, mitochondrial transmembrane potential dissipation, and increased Bax/Bcl-2 ratio and caspase-3 activation. This alantolactone-induced apoptosis and GSH depletion were effectively inhibited or abrogated by a thiol antioxidant, N-acetyl-L-cysteine (NAC). The data demonstrate clearly that intracellular GSH plays a central role in alantolactone-induced apoptosis in HepG2 cells. Thus, alantolactone may become a lead chemotherapeutic candidate for the treatment of liver cancer.

1. Introduction

Hepatocellular carcinoma is currently the fifth most common cancer and third leading cause of cancer-related deaths in the world. Over 600000 patients die because of liver cancer in the world every year. Despite significant advances in surgery and chemotherapy, the majority of patients with hepatocellular carcinoma die within one year of diagnosis [1–4]. At present, the hepatocellular carcinoma is mainly treated with surgery and chemotherapy [5, 6]. Currently, doxorubicin is the most widely used drug against liver cancer either as single agent or in combination with other chemotherapeutics like cisplatin. However, the outcomes of the existing conventional chemotherapeutic drugs remain considerably low due to their severe toxicity on normal hepatocytes [7, 8]. Therefore, searching for highly efficient anticancer drugs with low hepatotoxicity remains a hot research area.

A causal link between chronic inflammation and development of cancer is well established. Many transcription factors such as NF-κB and STAT3 are key to innate inflammation. The constitutive activation of signal transducers and activators of transcription 3 (STAT3) has been frequently detected in many types of human cancers such as glioblastoma, myeloma, colorectal, and hepatocellular carcinoma where it plays an important role in cell proliferation, tumor invasion, metastasis, and drug resistance [9, 10]. Therefore, blockage of STAT3 may have a therapeutic potential in preventing and treating these cancers.

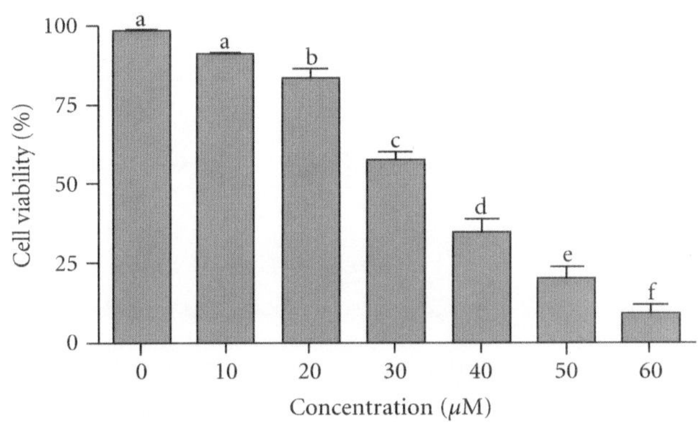

FIGURE 1: Growth inhibition of HepG2 cells after the treatment with alantolactone. Cells were cultured for 24 h before drug treatment in 96 well plates. Cells were treated with alantolactone (0, 10, 20, 30, 40, 50, and 60 μM) for 12 h and cell viability was measured by MTT assay. Data are expressed as mean ± SD ($n = 3$). Columns not sharing the same superscript letter differ significantly ($P < 0.05$).

Sesquiterpene lactones are plant-derived bioactive constituents often used in traditional medicines against inflammation and cancer [11, 12]. Alantolactone, a sesquiterpene lactone component of *Inula helenium* and *Inula racemosa,* has been shown to exhibit multiple pharmacological activities including anticancer effect [13, 14]. In our previous report, we have shown that alantolactone induces apoptosis in U87 glioblastoma cells via GSH depletion and mitochondrial dysfunction. However, the molecular mechanism of GSH depletion by alantolactone remained largely unknown. Furthermore, we showed that alantolactone did not induce hepatotoxicity and nephrotoxicity in mice [15]. Additionally, Butturini et al. showed that GSH depletion is involved in the inhibition of STAT3 activation [16].

Keeping in mind the antiinflammatory effect and GSH depleting activity of sesquiterpene lactones, we hypothesized that alantolactone can inhibit STAT3 activation and induce apoptosis in HepG2 cells. To evaluate this, we investigated the effect of alantolactone on GSH depletion and STAT3 and its downstream target gene Bcl-2 expressions. The data demonstrated that alantolactone-induced apoptosis in HepG2 cells via GSH depletion, STAT3 inhibition, modulation of Bcl-2 family proteins, and caspase-3 activation.

2. Materials and Methods

Alantolactone was obtained from Tauto Biotech Co., Ltd., (Shanghai, China) and purity (>99%) was determined by HPLC (see Supplementary material available online at doi:10.1155/2013/719858, Figure 1). Propidium iodide (PI) calcein acetoxymethyl ester (Calcein AM), Rhodamine 123, Dimethyl Sulfoxide (DMSO), MTT, Dulbecco's Modified Eagle's Medium (DMEM), fatal bovine serum (FBS), penicillin, and streptomycin were purchased from Sigma (Beijing, China). Apoptosis assay kit was purchased from KeyGen (Shanghai, China) while reactive oxygen species kit, and GSH/GSSG assay kit were purchased from Beyotime Institute of Biotechnology (Haimen, Jiangsu, China). Antibodies specific to Bax, Bcl-2, caspase-3, and β-actin were obtained from Beyotime while pTyr^{705} STAT3 was obtained from Wuhan Boster Biological Technolgy, Ltd., (Wuhan, China). Antibody specific to glutathione reductase was obtained from BIOSS Beijing Biosynthesis Biotechnology, Co., ltd. Horseradish peroxidase-conjugated secondary antibodies (goat-antirabbit, goat-antimouse) were purchased from Sigma Aldrich.

2.1. Cell Culture and Treatment. The human HepG2 cells were obtained from Shanghai Cell Bank, China, and were cultured in Dulbecco's Modified Eagle's Medium (DMEM) supplemented with 10% fatal bovine serum (FBS), 100 units/mL penicillin and 100 μg/mL streptomycin and maintained at 37°C with 5% CO_2 in humidified atmosphere. Cells were treated with alantolactone dissolved in DMSO with a final DMSO concentration of 1%. DMSO treated cells were used as control in all the experiments.

2.2. Determination of Cell Viability. Cell viability was determined by MTT assay as described by us previously [17]. Briefly HepG2 cells were treated with different concentrations of alantolactone for 12 h. Following treatment, the MTT reagent was added (500 μg/mL) and cells were further incubated at 37°C for 4 h. Subsequently 150 μL DMSO was added to dissolve farmazan crystals and absorbance was measured at 570 nm in a microplate reader (Thermo Scientific). The percentage of cell viability was calculated as follows:

$$\text{Cell viability (\%)} = \frac{\left(A570_{\text{sample}} - A570_{\text{blank}}\right)}{\left(A570_{\text{control}} - A570_{\text{blank}}\right)} \times 100. \quad (1)$$

The IC_{50} values were calculated using GraphPad Prism 5.

2.3. Observation of Morphological Changes. HepG2 cells were treated with 40 μM alantolactone in the presence or absence of NAC for 0, 3, 6, and 12 h. Cell morphological changes were observed by phase contrast microscopy (Olympus 1x71).

2.4. Live/Dead Assay. HepG2 cells were treated with 40 μM alantolactone in the presence or absence of NAC for 0, 3, 6, and 12 h. Live and dead cells were quantified using fluorescent probe calcein AM and PI and fluorescence microscope as described by us previously [18]. Calcein AM is cell membrane permeable and stains only viable cells whereas PI is cell membrane impermeable and stains only dead cells. Treated and untreated cells were collected, washed with phosphate buffered saline (PBS), and incubated with PBS solution containing 2 μM calcein AM and 4 μM PI in the dark for 20 min at room temperature. Finally, 100 cells were counted microscopically for the percentage of live and dead cells.

2.5. Apoptosis Assay by Annexin V-FITC and Propidium Iodide (PI) Staining. HepG2 cells were treated with 40 μM alantolactone for 0, 3, 6, and 12 h. After treatment, cells were harvested, washed with PBS, and resuspended in 500 μL of binding buffer containing 5 μL Annexin V and 5 μL PI and

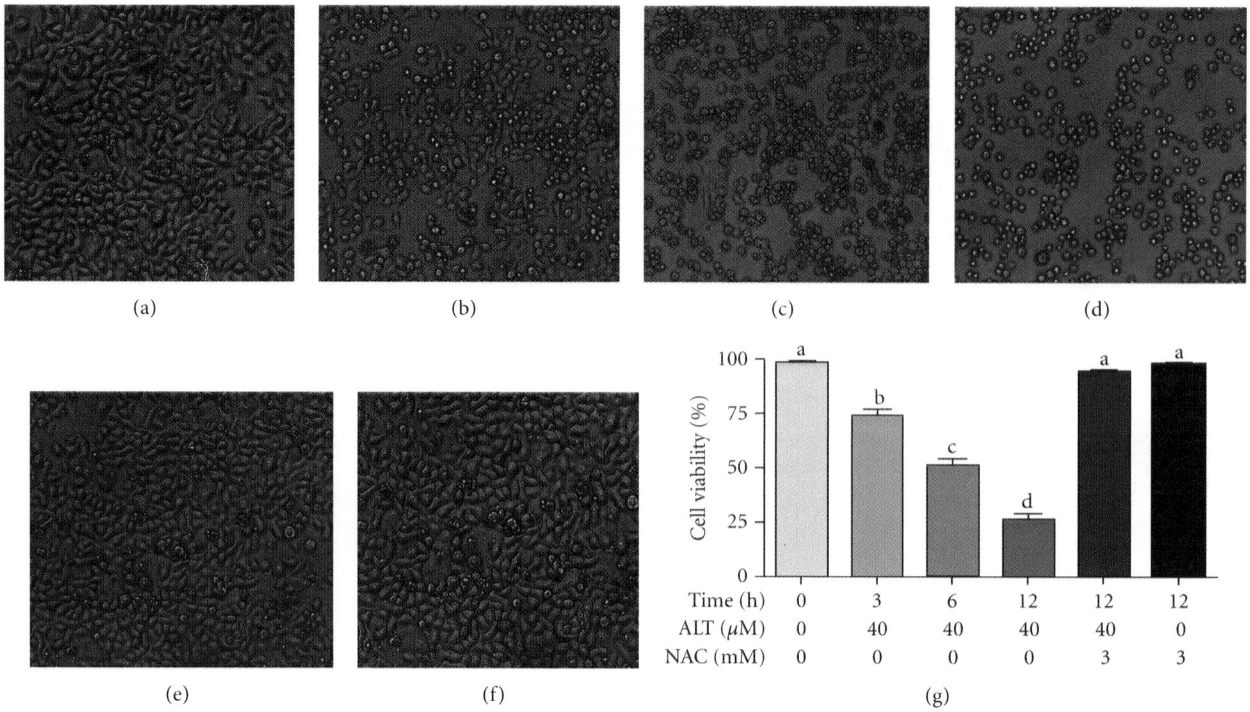

FIGURE 2: Changes in HepG2 cell morphology during alantolactone-induced cell death. HepG2 cells were treated with 40 μM alantolactone in the presence or absence of 3 mM NAC for various time intervals and morphological changes were observed by phase contrast microscopy. (a) control, ((b), (c) and (d)) cells were treated with 40 μM alantolactone for 3, 6, and 12 h, (e) cells were treated with 40 μM alantolactone in the presence of 3 mM NAC for 12 h, and (f) cells were treated with NAC alone for 12 h, respectively. (g) Cells were treated with 40 μM alantolactone as described above and live and dead cells were quantified using fluorescent probe calcein AM and PI as described in Section 2. Data are expressed as mean ± SD ($n = 3$). Columns not sharing the same superscript letter differ significantly ($P < 0.05$).

put in the dark for 15 min according to the kit instructions (KeyGen, Shanghai, China). After incubation, samples were immediately analyzed by flow cytometry (Beckman Coulter, Epics XL).

2.6. Measurement of Reactive Oxygen Species (ROS). The intracellular changes in ROS generation were measured by staining the cells with 2′,7′-dichlorofluorescein-diacetate (DCFH-DA) as described previously [18]. The fluorescent dye DCFH-DA is a cell membrane permeable and is converted into cell membrane impermeable nonfluorescent compound DCFH by intracellular esterases. Oxidation of DCFH by reactive oxygen species produces a highly fluorescent DCF. The fluorescence intensity of DCF inside the cells is proportional to the amount of peroxide produced. Briefly HepG2 cells were treated with 40 μM alantolactone for 0, 3, 6, and 12 h. After treatment, cells were further incubated with 10 μmol/L DCFH-DA at 37°C for 30 min. Subsequently cells were harvested, rinsed, resuspended in PBS, filtered with 300 apertures, and analyzed for 2′,7′-dichlorofluorescein (DCF) fluorescence by flow cytometry.

2.7. Measurement of Mitochondrial Membrane Potential (MMP). Rhodamine 123 was used to evaluate the changes in mitochondrial membrane potential as described previously [18]. Briefly HepG2 cells were incubated with 40 μM Alantolactone for 0, 3, 6, and 12 h. Following incubation, cells were collected, resuspended in 1 mL PBS solution containing 10 μg Rhodamine 123, and incubated in the dark for 30 min. After incubation, cells were centrifuged at 500 ×g for 5 min, supernatant was removed, and the pellet was gently rinsed with PBS once and then resuspended in 500 μL PBS. After filtration (300 apertures), the suspension was analyzed by flow cytometry.

2.8. Measurement of GSH and GSSG. The intracellular reduced (GSH) and oxidized (GSSG) glutathione was determined spectrophotometrically using GSH and GSSG assay kit (Beyotime). Briefly, HepG2 cells were treated with 40 μM alantolactone for 0, 3, 6, and 12 h or with 40 μM alantolactone in the presence or absence of 2 mM methionine and 3 mM NAC for 6 h. Following treatment, the intracellular and extracellular (medium) GSH and GSSG were measured according to the instruction of kit. The values were expressed as nmols GSH/mg protein.

2.9. HPLC Analysis. One mM alantolactone was incubated with 0, 5, 15, and 30 mM GSH in DMEM medium without FBS at 37°C for 30 min. Following incubation, the samples were analyzed by HPLC (Waters) using XTerra MS C18

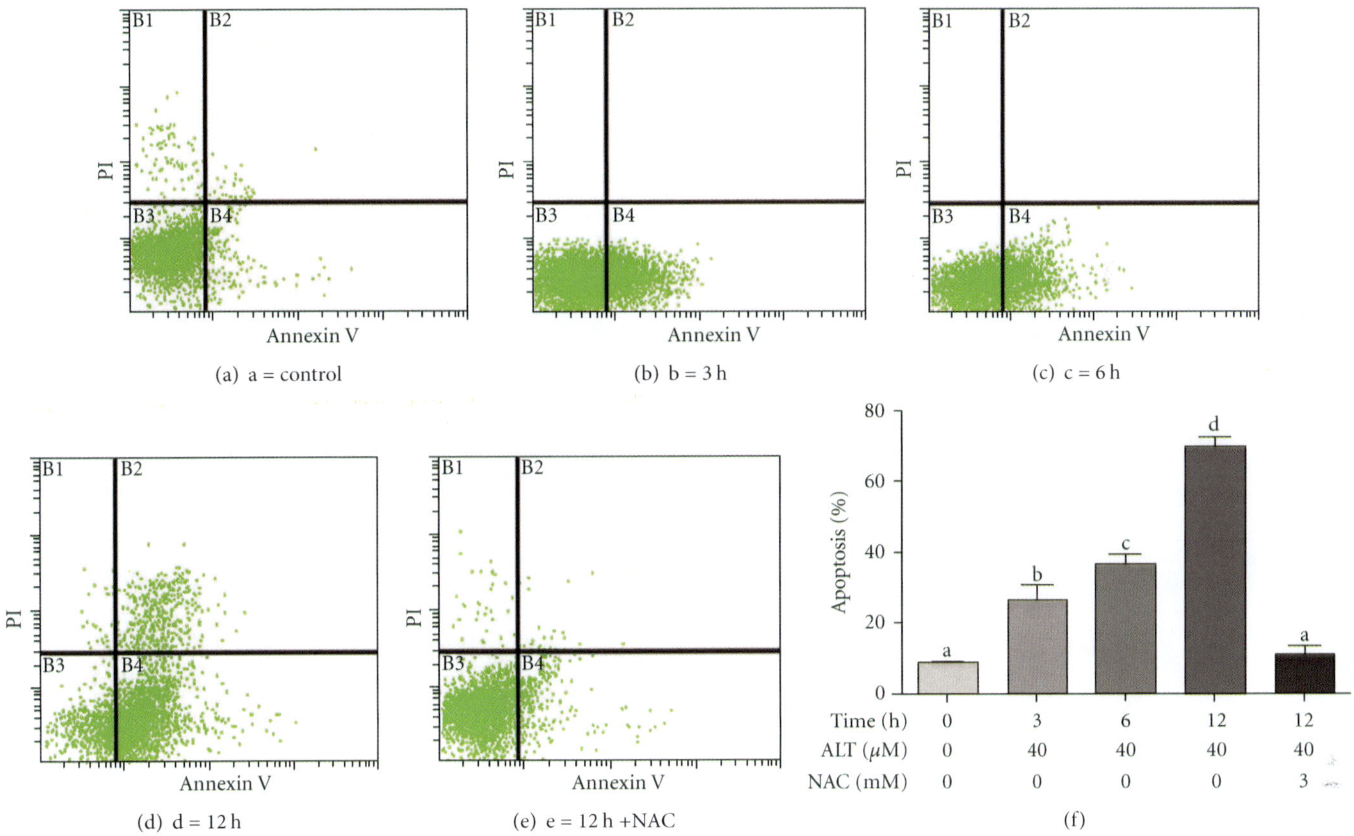

Figure 3: Flow cytometry analysis of apoptosis in HepG2 cells treated with 40 μM alantolactone for various time points. (a) Control, ((b), (c) and (d)) cells were treated with 40 μM alantolactone for 3, 6, and 12 h, respectively. (e) cells were treated with 40 μM alantolactone in the presence of 3 mM NAC for 12 h. (f) Data are expressed as mean ± SD ($n = 3$). Columns not sharing the same superscript letter differ significantly ($P < 0.05$).

(5 μm, 4.6 × 150 mm) column. The mobile phase was composed of acetonitrile (A) and water (B). The gradient program was as follows: 0–30 min, A = 65%, and B = 35%. The elution profile was analyzed at 227 nm by UV detector.

2.10. RNA Isolation and Semiquantitative RT-PCR. Total RNA was isolated from treated and untreated HepG2 cells using AxyPrep Multisource Total RNA Miniprep kit. cDNA was reverse-transcribed from 500 ng of total RNA in a final volume of 10 μL using PrimeScript RT reagent Kit (TakaRa, DRR037A), in accordance with the manufacturer's instructions. This was followed by 35 cycles of 94°C: 1 min; 52°C: 30 sec; 72°C: 1 min) and a final extension of 72°C for 10 min. PCR product was visualized on 1% agarose gel containing ethidium bromide. The primers used were as follows:

γ-GCS, 5′-GGCACAGGTAAAACCAAATAGTAAC-3′ (Forward) and 5′-CAAATTG-TTTAGCAAATGCAGTCA-3′ (Reverse); GAPDH, 5′-ATGACATCAAGAAGGTGG-TG-3′ (Forward) and 5′-CATACCAGGAAATGAGCTTG-3′ (Reverse).

2.11. Immunoblotting. Proteins were isolated from control and alantolactone-treated cells as described previously [18]. 40 μg proteins were electrophoresed on 12% SDS-PAGE and transferred to PVDF membrane. After blocking with 5% (w/v) nonfat milk and washing with Tris-buffered saline-Tween solution (TBST), membranes were incubated for 2 h at room temperature with Bax (1 : 300), Bcl-2 (1 : 1000), Caspase-3, (1 : 500), pTyr^{705} STAT3 (1 : 300), Glutathione Reductase (GR) (1 : 300), and β-actin (1 : 400) antibodies, respectively. After washing, the blots were incubated with horse radish peroxidase conjugated goat antirabbit IgG or goat antimouse IgG secondary antibodies (1 : 5000) for 1 h at room temperature. After washing with TBST, signals were detected using ECL plus chemiluminescence kit (Millipore Corporation) on X-ray film.

2.12. Statistical Analysis. The results are expressed as mean ± SD and statistically compared with control group or within the groups using one-way ANOVA followed by Tukey's multiple comparison test.

3. Results

3.1. Alantolactone Inhibits Growth of HepG2 Cells In Vitro. The effect of alantolactone on the growth of HepG2 cells was evaluated by MTT assay. Treatment with alantolactone

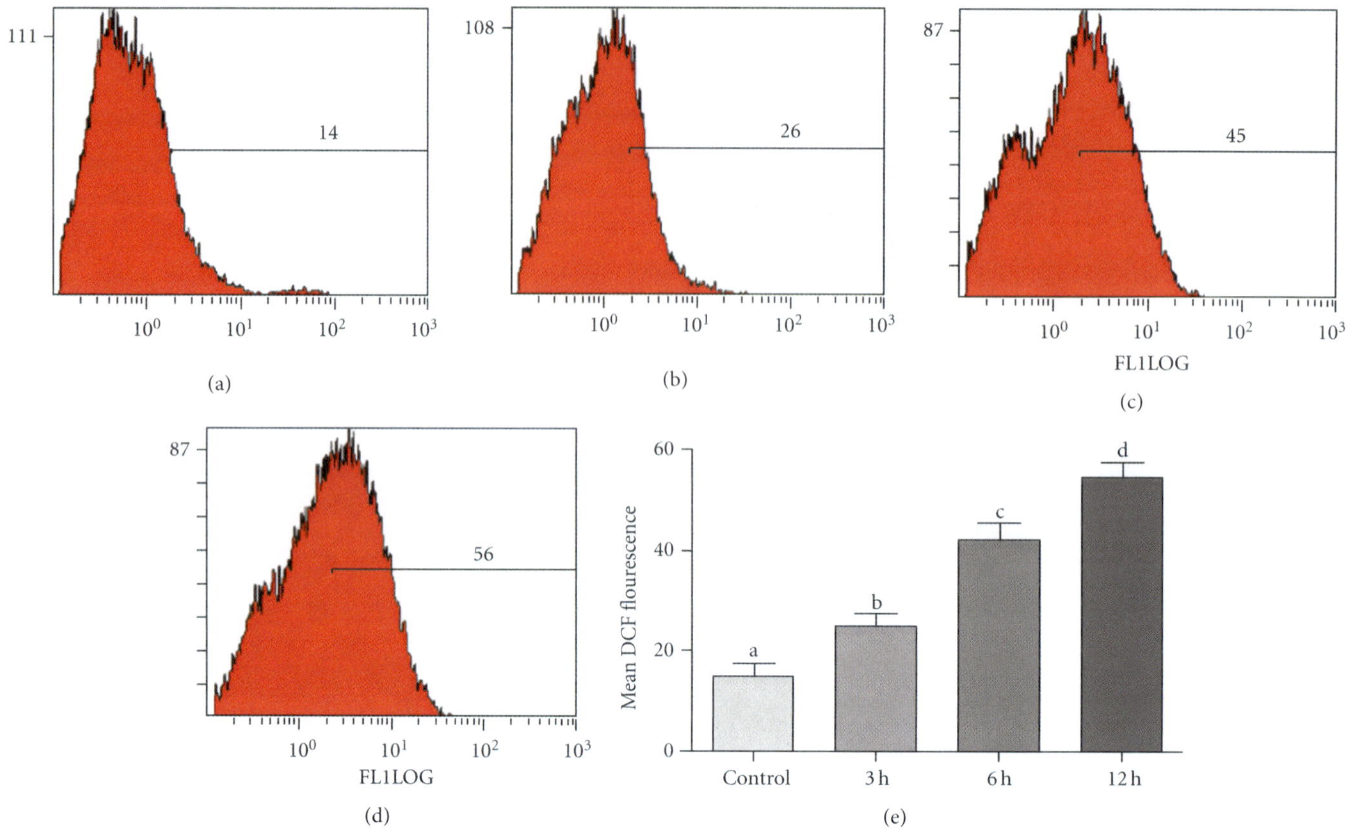

Figure 4: Flow cytometry analysis of ROS generation in control and alantolactone-treated HepG2 cells. (a) Control, ((b), (c) and (d)) cells were treated with 40 μM alantolactone for 3, 6, and 12 h, respectively. After treatment, cells were incubated with DCFH-DA for 30 min at 37°C, washed with PBS, and analyzed for DCF fluorescence by flow cytometry. (e) Data are expressed as mean ± SD ($n = 3$). Columns not sharing the same superscript letter differ significantly ($P < 0.05$).

for 12 h inhibited the growth of cells in a dose-dependent manner (Figure 1). The IC_{50} value of alantolactone was 33 μM after 12 h treatment. 40 μM concentration was selected for the following experiments.

3.2. Microscopic Study of HepG2 Cells. To examine the effect of alantolactone on cell morphology, HepG2 cells were treated with 40 μM alantolactone for various time intervals (3, 6, and 12 h) and morphological changes were observed by phase contrast microscopy. The data showed that alantolactone-induced severe morphological changes of cell death including rounding and shrinkage of cells, in a time-dependent manner (Figure 2). Pretreatment of cells with 3 mM NAC, a specific ROS inhibitor, completely protected the cells from cytotoxic effect of alantolactone. Furthermore, live and dead cells were quantified using fluorescent probes calcein AM and PI. As shown in Figure 2(g), alantolactone treatment reduced the viability of cells in a time-dependent manner. The viability of cells treated with 40 μM alantolactone for 3, 6, and 12 h was 74.33%, 51.6%, and 27%, respectively. These values were significantly lower than those of the control group (98.5%, $P < 0.05$). Pretreatment of cells with 3 mM NAC reversed the cytotoxic effect of alantolactone indicating that alantolactone exerts cytotoxic effect through the generation of ROS. However, NAC alone at this concentration did not affect the viability of cells as shown in Figure 2(g).

3.3. Alantolactone Induces Apoptosis in HepG2 Cells. The effect of alantolactone on cell apoptosis was evaluated by using annexin V-FITC/PI staining and flow cytometry. Translocation of phosphatidylserine (PS) to the outer leaflet of cellular membrane is the key step in the early stages of apoptosis. Annexin V selectively binds to PS and helps to identify cells undergoing apoptosis. When cells are double stained with Annexin V/PI, three different populations of cells can be observed. The cells that do not stain with either annexin V or PI are alive and reside in region B3; the cells that stain with only annexin V are in the stage of early apoptosis and reside in region B4 while the cells that stain with both reagents are nonviable late apoptotic/necrotic cells and scatter in region B2.

Flow cytometric analysis of apoptosis showed that alantolactone-induced apoptosis in HepG2 cells in a time-dependent manner as shown in Figure 3. Moreover, the early and late apoptosis process was also time dependent. Treatment with 40 μM alantolactone for 3 and 6 h only increased the early apoptosis while at 12 h late apoptosis

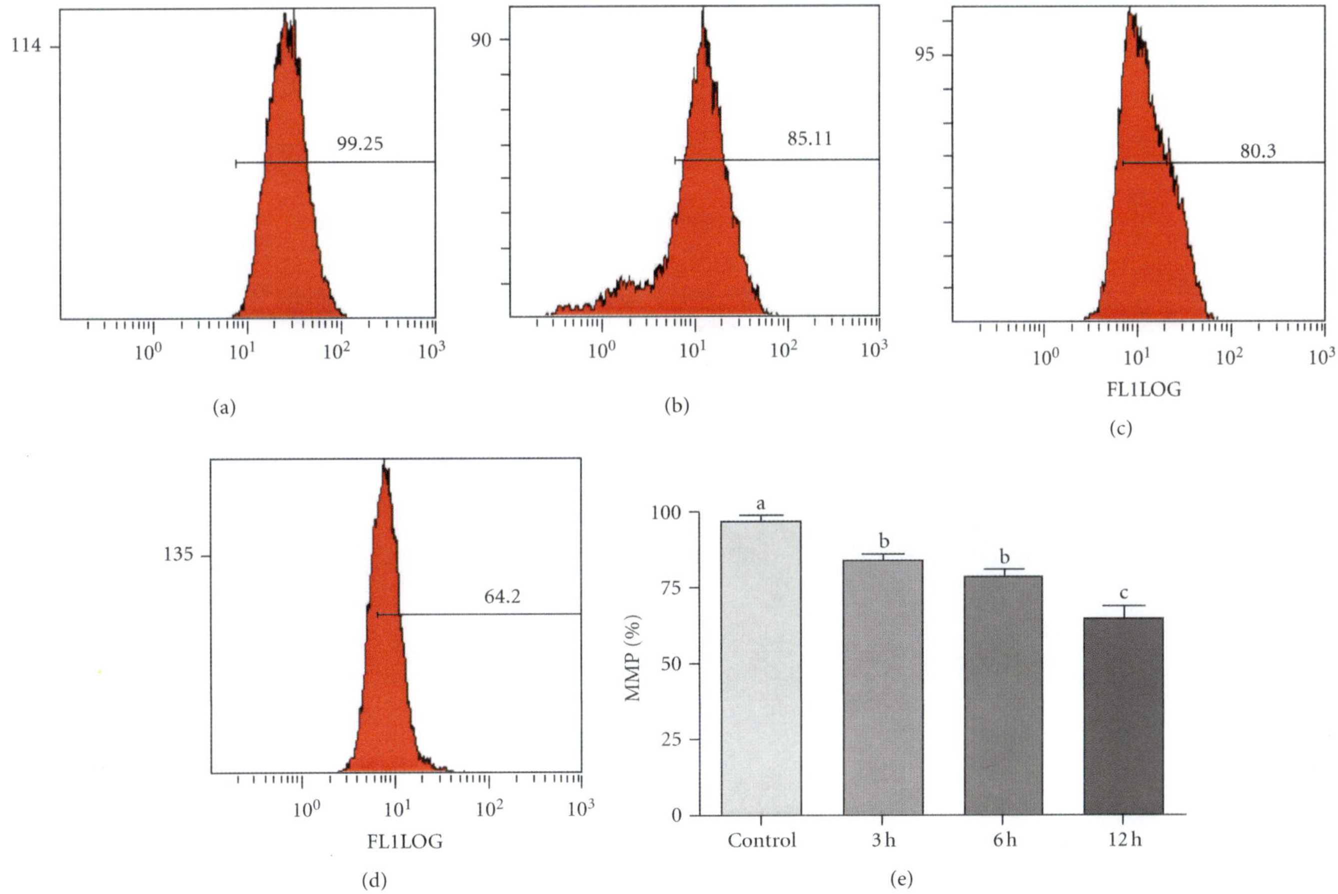

FIGURE 5: Flow cytometry analysis of MMP in control and alantolactone-treated HepG2 cells. (a) Control, (b), (c) and (d) cells were treated with 40 μM alantolactone for 3, 6, and 12 h, respectively. After treatment, cells were incubated with Rhodamine 123 for 30 min in dark, washed with PBS, and analyzed for MMP by flow cytometry. (e) Data are expressed as mean ± SD ($n = 3$). Columns not sharing the same superscript letter differ significantly ($P < 0.05$).

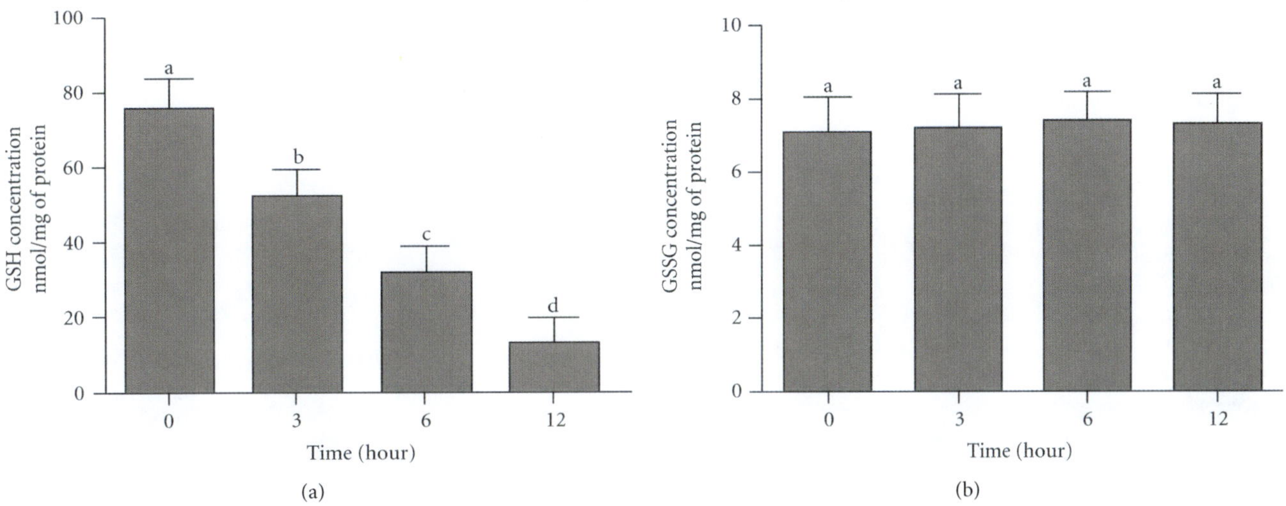

FIGURE 6: Measurement of intracellular GSH and GSSG in control and alantolactone-treated HepG2 cells for various time points. Cells were cultured in 6 well plates and treated with or without 40 μM alantolactone for 3, 6, and 12 h. Intracellular GSH and GSSG were measured according to the instructions of kit. Data are expressed as mean ± SD ($n = 3$). Columns not sharing the same superscript letter differ significantly ($P < 0.0$).

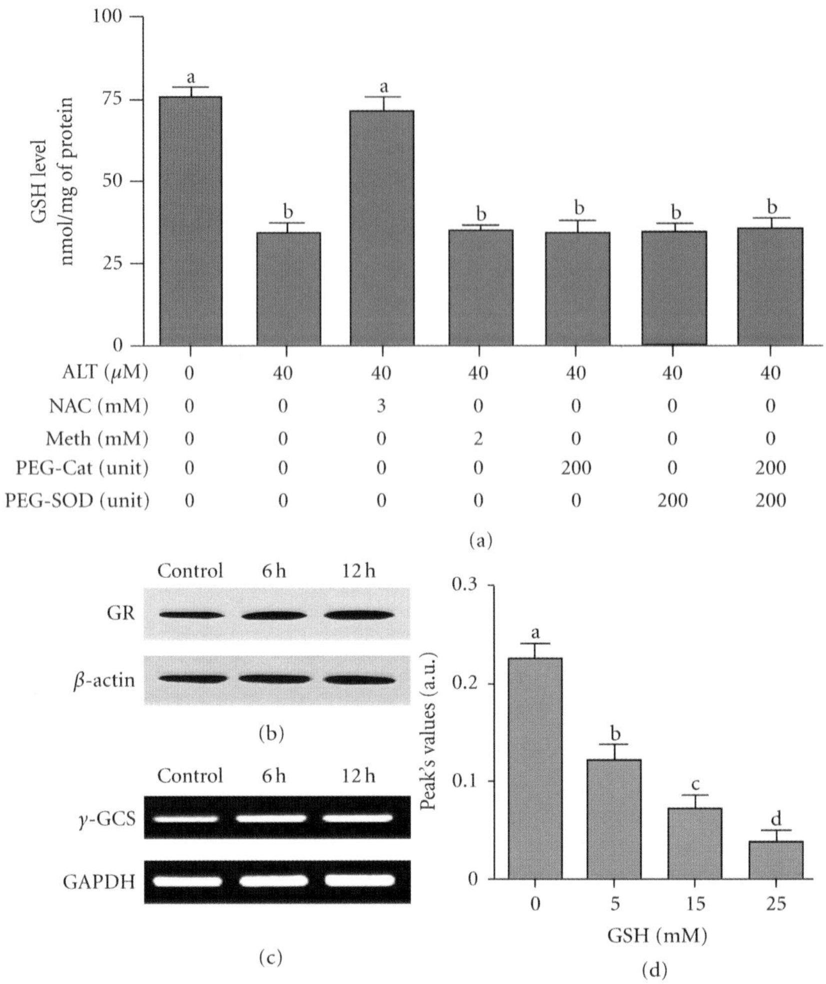

Figure 7: Measurement of GSH in the presence of various inhibitors and expression of genes involved in GSH metabolism. (a) HepG2 cells were treated with 40 μM alantolactone for 6 h in the presence or absence of various inhibitors and concentration of GSH was measured according to kit instructions. Data are expressed as mean ± SD ($n = 3$). Columns not sharing the same superscript letter differ significantly ($P < 0.05$). (b) Cells were treated with 40 μM alantolactone for indicated time points and cell lysates were subjected to Western blot analysis for the expression of glutathione reductase (GR). (c) Cells were treated with 40 μM alantolactone for indicated time points and mRNA expression of γ-glutamyl cysteine synthetase (γ-GCS) was determined by RT-PCR. (d) Alantolactone (1 mM) was incubated with indicated concentrations of GSH in medium for 30 min and amount of alantolactone was assessed using HPLC. The data shows that GSH decreased the amount of alantolactone in a dose-dependent manner. Data are expressed as mean ± SD ($n = 3$). Columns not sharing the same superscript letter differ significantly ($P < 0.05$).

was also observed. The data suggested that alantolactone-induced cell death was through early apoptosis within 6 h; however, with the increase of time, the late apoptotic rate also increased. Next, we treated the cells with 40 μM alantolactone for 12 h in the presence of 3 mM NAC and the apoptosis rate was determined by flow cytometry. The data showed that NAC reversed the apoptotic effect of alantolactone indicating that alantolactone exerts an apoptotic effect in HepG2 cells through generation of ROS (Figure 3(e)).

3.4. Alantolactone Induces Increased Generation of ROS in HepG2 Cells. Intracellular ROS generation in HepG2 cells was measured by flow cytometry using DCFH-DA. The data demonstrated that the level of ROS in cells treated with 40 μM alantolactone for 3, 6, and 12 h was 25%, 42%, and 54%, respectively (Figure 4). These values were significantly higher than those of the control group (15%, $P < 0.05$)

3.5. Alantolactone Disrupts Mitochondrial Membrane Potential (MMP) in HepG2 Cells. Depolarization in MMP is a characteristic feature of apoptosis. Excessive intracellular ROS production has been shown to induce apoptosis by disrupting MMP [19, 20]. To investigate the role of ROS in alantolactone-induced apoptosis, we determined MMP in HepG2 cells using Rhodamine 123 and flow cytometry. The data showed that alantolactone reduced the MMP in HepG2 cells in a time-dependent manner. As shown in Figure 5, MMP in cells treated with 40 μM alantolactone for 3, 6, and 12 h was significantly lower (85%, 79%, and 62% versus 98% in the control group, $P < 0.05$).

3.6. Alantolactone Reduces Intracellular GSH in HepG2 Cells. Intracellular GSH plays major roles in the maintenance of redox status and defense of oxidative stress. GSH depletion is an early hallmark observed in ROS mediated apoptosis. We therefore investigated the status of intracellular GSH in control and alantolactone-treated cells. A time-dependent study revealed that GSH depletion was significant from 3 h of treatment and increased over time (Figure 6(a)). Overproduction of ROS can oxidize GSH into GSSG. We, therefore, measured the level of GSSG in treated and untreated cells. As shown in Figure 6(b), no change in the level of GSSG in control and alantolactone-treated cells was found.

3.7. Alantolactone Depletes Intracellular GSH via Direct Conjugation with GSH. The intracellular GSH depletion might be resulted either from an increased intracellular oxidation of GSH or a stimulated GSH extrusion through a specific carrier or inhibition of GSH synthesis. In addition, sesquiterpene lactones contain α-methylene-β-lactone moiety which is highly reactive with cellular thiols and can deplete GSH by conjugating with sulfhydral group [21]. To shed light on the mechanism accounting alantolactone-mediated GSH depletion in HepG2 cells, we measured the concentration of GSH and GSSG in the culture medium. The concentration of GSH and GSSG in culture medium was not detectable. Overproduction of ROS can oxidize GSH into GSSG. Therefore, we incubated the cells with PEG-catalase and PEG-SOD and measured the level of GSH in cells. Pretreatment of cells with PEG-catalase and PEG-SOD alone or in combination did not prevent GSH depletion indicating that GSH depletion by alantolactone is not due to oxidation of GSH into GSSG (Figure 7(a)). During oxidative stress, GSH is oxidized to GSSG which is catalytically reduced back to GSH by glutathione reductase (GR). Next, we measured the expression of GR by Western blot analysis. The data showed that there was a slight increase in the expression level of GR in alantolactone-treated cell lysates, further confirming that GSH depletion is not linked with its oxidation to GSSG (Figure 7(b)).

Next, we asked if GSH depletion is resulted from GSH extrusion from cells. Therefore, we measured the level of GSH in cells treated with alantolactone for 6 h in the presence of 2 mM methionine, a specific GSH carrier inhibitor. As shown in Figure 7(a), the inhibitor of GSH carrier (methionine) did not prevent GSH depletion, indicating that GSH depletion is not associated with GSH extrusion. To further support this finding, we measured GSH in a culture medium. The level of GSH in a culture medium was not detectable. The data demonstrate clearly that GSH depletion is not due to GSH extrusion.

Next, we treated the cells with 3 mM NAC, a precursor molecule for GSH synthesis for 30 min, followed by treatment with 40 μM alantolactone for 6 h, and intracellular GSH was determined in control and treated cells. As shown in Figure 6(a), pretreatment with NAC completely inhibited the depletion of intracellular GSH. To further exclude the possibility of GSH depletion by inhibition of GSH synthesis, we measured the mRNA expression of γ-glutamylcystein synthetase (γ-GCS) which is a rate limiting enzyme in the synthesis of GSH. As shown in Figure 7(c), no change in the mRNA expression of γ-GCS was observed. The data demonstrate that GSH depletion is not associated with the inhibition of GSH synthesis. Therefore, the depletion of intracellular GSH by alantolactone is most probably the result of rapid binding of exomethylene moiety of alantolactone with intracellular GSH.

Finally, we incubated 1 mM alantolactone with 0, 5, 15, and 30 mM GSH in DMEM medium without FBS at 37°C for 30 min. Following incubation, the samples were analyzed by HPLC (Waters) using XTerra MS C18 (5 μm, 4.6 × 150 mm) column. The mobile phase was composed of acetonitrile (A) and water (B). The gradient program was as follows: 0–30 min, A = 65%, and B = 35%. The elution profile was analyzed at 227 nm by a UV detector. The data showed that the concentration of alantolactone decreased in the presence of increasing concentration of GSH (Figure 7(d)). The data demonstrate clearly the direct interaction of alantolactone with GSH. Taken together, the data demonstrate that alantolactone depletes intracellular GSH in HepG2 cells via direct conjugation with GSH.

3.8. Alantolactone Inhibits STAT3 Activation and its Downstream Target Gene Bcl-2. Recent studies show that under oxidative stress, STAT3 is glutathionylated with a concomitant inhibition of its phosphorylation. In other words, GSH depletion inhibits STAT3 activation [16]. Because alantolactone reduced the intracellular GSH in HepG2 cells, we were interested if alantolactone could inhibit STAT3 activation. Thus we measured the expression of $pTyr^{705}$ STAT3 in cells. As shown in Figure 8, alantolactone treatment decreased the expression of $pTyr^{705}$ STAT3 in a time-dependent manner. After tyrosine phosphorylation (Tyr^{705}) of STAT3, it translocates into the nucleus where it increases the expression of genes implicated in cell proliferation such as Bcl-2 and cyclin D1. Disruption of STAT3 signalling decreases the expression of antiapoptotic proteins and induces apoptosis in tumor cells. Therefore, we measured the expression of Bcl-2 family proteins using Western blot analysis. As expected, alantolactone treatment reduced the expression of antiapoptotic protein Bcl-2 and increased the expression of proapoptotic protein Bax in a time-dependent manner (Figure 8).

3.9. Alantolactone Induces Caspase-3 Activation in HepG2 Cells. Mitochondrial-dependent apoptosis is initiated by recruitment and activation of caspases. Thus we analyzed whether caspase-3 was activated during alantolactone-induced apoptosis of HepG2 cells. As shown in Figure 8, alantolactone stimulated the cleavage of caspase-3 in a time-dependent manner as demonstrated by the appearance of 32 kDa and 17 kDa fragments.

4. Discussion

Currently available chemotherapy remains ineffective to cure hepatoma mainly because of its high hepatotoxicity. Therefore, alternative therapeutic agents that kill cancer cells without or with low hepatotoxicity are highly desirable. Alantolactone, a sesquiterpene lactone, has been reported to possess antibacterial, antifungal, antihelminthic, and anticancer activities. In our previous report, we showed that alantolactone-induced apoptosis in U87 glioblastoma cells via GSH depletion without inducing toxicity in mouse liver and kidneys [15]. However, the molecular mechanism of GSH depletion by alantolactone remained unexplored. The present study was therefore conducted to evaluate whether alantolactone can deplete GSH and induce apoptosis in liver cancer cells. To study the anticancer activity of alantolactone towards liver cancer cells, we used HepG2 cell line as a model cell line. We found that alantolactone inhibited the growth and induced apoptosis in HepG2 cells in a dose- and time-dependent manner as evident by Annexin V positive staining and caspase-3 activation. This alantolactone-induced cell death was completely inhibited when cells were pretreated with NAC, a GSH precursor molecule. The data suggest that GSH depletion might be involved in apoptotic cell death induced by alantolactone. We therefore measured the level of intracellular GSH in control and treated cells. In accordance with our previous study [15], alantolactone reduced the level of GSH in HepG2 cells in a time-dependent manner.

It is well established that intracellular redox status or oxidative stress plays an important role in cancer cells apoptosis [21]. GSH is one of the most abundant intracellular antioxidants involved in the protection of cells against oxidative damage [15, 22]. Depletion of intracellular GSH is an early hallmark in the onset of apoptosis [21, 23]. The intracellular GSH depletion might be resulted either from increased intracellular oxidation of GSH or stimulated GSH extrusion through a specific carrier or the inhibition of GSH synthesis or the direct conjugation of GSH with drug [21]. In the present study, alantolactone-mediated GSH depletion is unlikely to be due to the oxidation of GSH into GSSG since expression of GR is not inhibited and the level of GSSG remained unchanged in cells before and after treatment. Furthermore, GSH and GSSG were not detectable in culture medium and methionine (inhibitor of GSH carrier) did not prevent GSH depletion which excludes the possibility of GSH extrusion as the main mechanism for GSH depletion. The pretreatment of cells with NAC completely inhibited GSH depletion and mRNA expression of γ-GCS remained unchanged in control and alantolactone-treated cells. These sets of data demonstrate clearly that alantolactone-induced GSH depletion in HepG2 cells through a process that does not involve inhibition of GSH synthesis. Therefore, the depletion of intracellular GSH by alantolactone is most probably the result of direct conjugation of alantolactone with GSH. Alantolactone like other sesquiterpene lactones such as parthenolide and helenalin contains α-methylene-γ-lactone moiety which can interact with sulfhydral group of GSH by means of Michael-type conjugation [21]. In order to ascertain the GSH depletion by direct conjugation with alantolactone, we incubated the alantolactone with GSH as described in Section 2 and samples were analyzed by HPLC. The data indicated that the amount of alantolactone decreased with the increasing concentration of GSH demonstrating their direct conjugation.

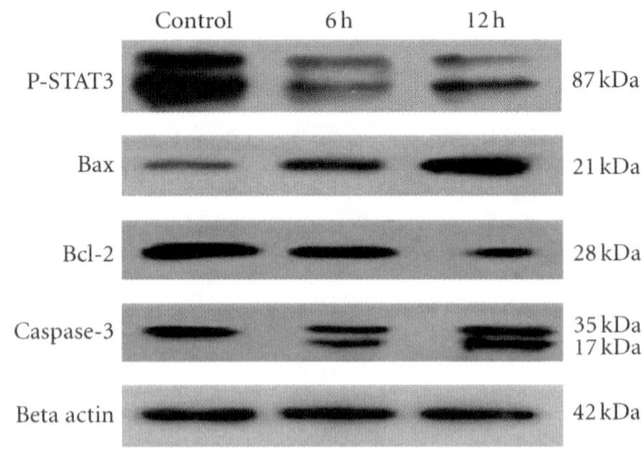

FIGURE 8: Effect of alantolactone on the expressions of apoptosis regulators. HepG2 cells were treated with or without 40 μM alantolactone for 6 and 12 h. The expression of Phospho-STAT3, Bax, Bcl-2, and caspase-3 was measured by Western blot analysis.

An increasing body of literature evidence underlines the critical role of redox reactions in the regulation of various cell functions. Reactive oxygen species are produced inside the cells during normal physiological processes of the cells which are being neutralized by the antioxidant system of the cells [24, 25]. A precise balance between ROS production and antioxidant system's ability to scavenge ROS is critical for normal cellular functions. GSH is one of the most important intracellular antioxidant which plays the major role in protection of cells against oxidative damage. Depletion of GSH results in oxidative stress which is a known inducer of the transcription of specific genes involved in apoptosis [26]. In order to ascertain the mechanism by which alantolactone-induced GSH depletion induces apoptosis in HepG2 cells, we measured the expression of $pTyr^{705}$ STAT3 and its downstream target protein Bcl-2. We found that alantolactone treatment reduced the expression of phosphorylated STAT3 and Bcl-2 in a time-dependent manner. The inhibition of STAT3 by alantolactone is further supported by another recent study that parthenolide a sesquiterpene lactone that depletes GSH in HepG2 cells by direct conjugation with GSH also inhibits STAT3 expression [27]. Both alantolactone and parthenolide share a common α-methylene-γ-lactone moiety which directly conjugates with the self-hydral group of GSH. However, the molecular mechanism by which GSH depletion inhibits STAT3 expression remained unexplored in the present study. Further study is needed to bridge the information link between GSH depletion and STAT3 inhibition.

GSH depletion and ROS generation (oxidative stress) are known to act as second messengers to activate diverse redox-sensitive signalling cascades including mitochondrial intrinsic apoptotic cascade through interaction with Bcl-2 family proteins [20, 28]. Bcl-2 family proteins include a wide variety of antiapoptotic proteins such as Bcl-2 and proapoptotic proteins such as Bax, which are key players of mitochondrial outer membrane permeabilization and apoptosis regulation [20, 29]. GSH depletion and oxidative stress have been reported to activate and translocate proapoptotic protein Bax to outer mitochondrial membrane (OMM) where it forms oligomers which are thought to be important in the formation of permeability transition pores (PTP) and cytochrome c release [20, 22, 30]. Apart from Bax activation, ROS have also been shown to inhibit antiapoptotic protein Bcl-2 [20, 30]. In the present study, the expression of Bax increased while the expression of Bcl-2 decreased in alantolactone-treated cells in a time-dependent manner. The data demonstrated that alantolactone induced apoptosis in HepG2 cells through mitochondrial pathway. This mitochondrial apoptotic pathway was further confirmed by measuring the mitochondrial membrane potential (MMP) using flow cytometry. A significant reduction in MMP has been observed in alantolactone-treated cells, suggesting the opening of mitochondrial permeability transition pore. Therefore, we concluded that alantolactone can promote the opening of mitochondrial permeability transition pore by increasing the Bax/Bcl-2 ratio.

5. Conclusion

In conclusion our data provide evidence for the first time that alantolactone depletes GSH in HepG2 cells by direct conjugation with GSH. The GSH depletion resulted in the inhibition of phosphorylated STAT3 expression and oxidative stress. Consequently, inhibition of STAT3 activation and oxidative stress induced apoptosis in HepG2 cells by modulating mitochondrial Bcl-2 family proteins. Our results suggest that alantolactone may be a promising chemotherapeutic drug candidate for the treatment of liver cancer. Further investigation is needed to validate the contribution of alantolactone to tumor therapy *in vivo*.

Conflict of Interests

The authors have declared that they have no conflict of interests.

Acknowledgments

This work is supported by the Ministry of Education of Pakistan and the Chinese Scholarship Council of China.

References

[1] R. J. Thoppil and A. Bishayee, "Terpenoids as potential chemopreventive and therapeutic agents in liver cancer," *World Journal of Hepatology*, vol. 3, pp. 228–249, 2011.

[2] X. W. Tan, H. Xia, J. H. Xu, and J. G. Cao, "Induction of apoptosis in human liver carcinoma HepG2 cell line by 5-allyl-7-gen-difluoromethylenechrysin," *World Journal of Gastroenterology*, vol. 15, no. 18, pp. 2234–2239, 2009.

[3] L. Andreana, G. Isgro, L. Marelli et al., "Treatment of hepatocellular carcinoma (HCC) by intra-arterial infusion of radio-emitter compounds: trans-arterial radio-embolisation of HCC," *Cancer Treatment Reviews*, vol. 38, pp. 641–649, 2012.

[4] A. Alisi and C. Balsano, "Enhancing the efficacy of hepatocellular carcinoma chemotherapeutics with natural anticancer agents," *Nutrition Reviews*, vol. 65, no. 12, pp. 550–553, 2007.

[5] T. Beppu, K. Sugimoto, K. Shiraki et al., "Clinical significance of tumor markers in detection of recurrent hepatocellular carcinoma after radiofrequency ablation," *International Journal of Molecular Medicine*, vol. 26, no. 3, pp. 425–433, 2010.

[6] P. J. Johnson, "Non-surgical treatment of hepatocellular carcinoma," *HPB*, vol. 7, no. 1, pp. 50–55, 2005.

[7] B. Liu, G. Wang, J. Yang, X. Pan, Z. Yang, and L. Zang, "Berberine inhibits human hepatoma cell invasion without cytotoxicity in healthy Hepatocytes," *PLoS One*, vol. 6, no. 6, Article ID e21416, 2011.

[8] T. W. Chung, Y. C. Lee, and C. H. Kim, "Hepatitis B viral HBx induces matrix metalloproteinase-9 gene expression through activation of ERK and PI-3K/AKT pathways: involvement of invasive potential," *The FASEB Journal*, vol. 18, no. 10, pp. 1123–1125, 2004.

[9] W. Y. Wu, J. Li, Z. S. Wu, C. L. Zhang, and X. L. Meng, "STAT3 activation in monocytes accelerates liver cancer progression," *BMC Cancer*, vol. 11, article 506, 2011.

[10] L. Lin, S. Deangelis, E. Foust et al., "A novel small molecule inhibits STAT3 phosphorylation and DNA binding activity and exhibits potent growth suppressive activity in human cancer cells," *Molecular Cancer*, vol. 9, article 217, 2010.

[11] A. Ghantous, H. Gali-Muhtasib, H. Vuorela, N. A. Saliba, and N. Darwiche, "What made sesquiterpene lactones reach cancer clinical trials?" *Drug Discovery Today*, vol. 15, no. 15-16, pp. 668–678, 2010.

[12] S. Zhang, Y. K. Won, C. N. Ong, and H. M. Shen, "Anti-cancer potential of sesquiterpene lactones: bioactivity and molecular mechanisms," *Current Medicinal Chemistry*, vol. 5, no. 3, pp. 239–249, 2005.

[13] H. C. Pal, I. Sehar, S. Bhushan, B. D. Gupta, and A. K. Saxena, "Activation of caspases and poly (ADP-ribose) polymerase cleavage to induce apoptosis in leukemia HL-60 cells by Inula racemosa," *Toxicology in Vitro*, vol. 24, no. 6, pp. 1599–1609, 2010.

[14] A. Trendafilova, C. Chanev, and M. Todorova, "Ultrasound-assisted extraction of alantolactone and isoalantolactone from Inula helenium roots," *Pharmacognosy Magazine*, vol. 6, no. 23, pp. 234–237, 2010.

[15] M. Khan, F. Yi, A. Rasul et al., "Alantolactone induces apoptosis in glioblastoma cells via GSH depletion, ROS generation, and mitochondrial dysfunction," *IUBMB Life*, vol. 64, no. 9, pp. 783–794, 2012.

[16] E. Butturini, E. Cavalieri, A. C. de Prati et al., "Two naturally occurring terpenes, dehydrocostuslactone and costunolide, decrease intracellular GSH content and inhibit STAT3 activation," *PLoS One*, vol. 6, no. 5, Article ID e20174, 2011.

[17] M. Khan, B. Zheng, F. Yi et al., "Pseudolaric acid B induces caspase-dependent and caspase-independent apoptosis in U87 glioblastoma cells," *Evidence-Based Complementary and Alternative Medicine*, vol. 2012, Article ID 957568, 11 pages, 2012.

[18] M. Khan, B. Yu, A. Rasul et al., "Jaceosidin induces apoptosis in U87 glioblastoma cells through G2/M phase arrest," *Evidence-Based Complementary and Alternative Medicine*, vol. 2012, Article ID 703034, 12 pages, 2012.

[19] X. Ling, Y. Zhou, S. W. Li, B. Yan, and L. Wen, "Modulation of mitochondrial permeability transition pore affects multidrug resistance in human hepatocellular carcinoma cells," *International Journal of Biological Sciences*, vol. 6, no. 7, pp. 773–783, 2010.

[20] Y. B. Ji Yu-Bin, Z. Y. Qu, and X. Zou, "Juglone-induced apoptosis in human gastric cancer SGC-7901 cells via the mitochondrial

pathway," *Experimental and Toxicologic Pathology*, vol. 63, no. 1-2, pp. 69–78, 2011.

[21] S. Zhang, C. N. Ong, and H. M. Shen, "Critical roles of intracellular thiols and calcium in parthenolide-induced apoptosis in human colorectal cancer cells," *Cancer Letters*, vol. 208, no. 2, pp. 143–153, 2004.

[22] P. Guha, A. Dey, R. Sen, M. Chatterjee, S. Chattopadhyay, and S. K. Bandyopadhyay, "Intracellular GSH depletion triggered mitochondrial bax translocation to accomplish resveratrol-induced apoptosis in the U937 cell line," *Journal of Pharmacology and Experimental Therapeutics*, vol. 336, no. 1, pp. 206–214, 2011.

[23] M. L. Circu and T. Y. Aw, "Glutathione and apoptosis," *Free Radical Research*, vol. 42, no. 8, pp. 689–706, 2008.

[24] S. Deng, Y. Yang, Y. Han et al., "UCP2 inhibits ROS-mediated apoptosis in A549 under hypoxic conditions," *PLoS One*, vol. 7, Article ID e30714, 2012.

[25] V. Sharma, C. Joseph, S. Ghosh, A. Agarwal, M. K. Mishra, and E. Sen, "Kaempferol induces apoptosis in glioblastoma cells through oxidative stress," *Molecular Cancer Therapeutics*, vol. 6, no. 9, pp. 2544–2553, 2007.

[26] C. Kretz-Remy and A. P. Arrigo, "Gene expression and thiol redox state," *Methods in Enzymology*, vol. 348, pp. 200–215, 2002.

[27] D. Carlisi, A. D'Anneo, L. Angileri et al., "Parthenolide sensitizes hepatocellular carcinoma cells to trail by inducing the expression of death receptors through inhibition of STAT3 activation," *Journal of Cellular Physiology*, vol. 226, no. 6, pp. 1632–1641, 2011.

[28] Y. Tsujimoto and S. Shimizu, "Role of the mitochondrial membrane permeability transition in cell death," *Apoptosis*, vol. 12, no. 5, pp. 835–840, 2007.

[29] M. L. Circu and T. Y. Aw, "Reactive oxygen species, cellular redox systems, and apoptosis," *Free Radical Biology and Medicine*, vol. 48, no. 6, pp. 749–762, 2010.

[30] E. Mayola, C. Gallerne, D. D. Esposti et al., "Withaferin A induces apoptosis in human melanoma cells through generation of reactive oxygen species and down-regulation of Bcl-2," *Apoptosis*, vol. 16, pp. 1014–1027, 2011.

3

The Protective Effect of Fasudil on the Structure and Function of Cardiac Mitochondria from Rats with Type 2 Diabetes Induced by Streptozotocin with a High-Fat Diet Is Mediated by the Attenuation of Oxidative Stress

Rong Guo, Baoxin Liu, Shunping Zhou, Buchun Zhang, and Yawei Xu

Department of Cardiology, Shanghai Tenth People's Hospital, Tongji University School of Medicine, 301 Yan Chang Zhong Road, Shanghai 200072, China

Correspondence should be addressed to Yawei Xu; xuyawei1960@yahoo.com

Academic Editor: Michael Cunningham

Dysfunction of cardiac mitochondria appears to play a substantial role in cardiomyopathy or myocardial dysfunction and is a promising therapeutic target for many cardiovascular diseases. We investigated the effect of the Rho/Rho-associated protein kinase (ROCK) inhibitor fasudil on cardiac mitochondria from rats in which diabetes was induced by a combination of streptozotocin (STZ) and a sustained high-fat diet. Eight weeks after diabetes was induced by a single intraperitoneal injection of 50 mg/kg STZ followed by a sustained high-fat diet, either fasudil (5 mg/kg bid) or equivalent volumes of saline (control) were administered over four weeks. Fasudil significantly protected against the histopathologic changes of cardiac mitochondria in diabetic rats. Fasudil significantly reduced the abundances of the Rho A, ROCK 1, and ROCK 2 proteins, restored the activities of succinate dehydrogenase (SDH) and monoamine oxidase (MAO) in cardiac mitochondria, inhibited the opening of the mitochondrial permeability transition pore, and decreased the total antioxidant capacity, as well as levels of malonyldialdehyde, hydroxy radical, reduced glutathione, and superoxide dismutase in heart. Fasudil improved the structures of cardiac mitochondria and increased both SDH and MAO activities in cardiac mitochondria. These beneficial effects may be associated with the attenuation of oxidative stress caused by fasudil treatment.

1. Introduction

Mitochondria are recognized as essential cell organelles, which generate most of the cell's energy. In addition, mitochondria are involved in many physiological activities such as cell signaling, proliferation, growth, and death [1]. They have been implicated in cardiac dysfunction and myocardiocyte damage by the loss of metabolic capacity and the production or release of toxic substances [2]. Therefore, mitochondria are regarded as a novel therapeutic target in ischemic heart disease and some cardiomyopathies [3].

Diabetes mellitus (DM) is a major cause of serious microvascular and macrovascular diseases, affecting nearly every system in the body. Elevated oxidative stress in diabetic patients and in animal models of diabetes results from overproduction of reactive oxygen species (ROS) and decreased efficiency of antioxidant defenses [4, 5]. Moreover, diabetes-associated metabolic disorders and glycated or oxidized low-density lipoproteins (ox-LDL) impair the activities of enzymes of the mitochondrial respiratory chain complex [6]. Therefore, oxidative stress is closely related to mitochondrial dysfunction.

Rho-associated kinases (ROCKs) seem to contribute to numerous pathophysiological pathways that are triggered by hyperglycemia and represent promising molecular targets for cardioprotective treatment [7]. Recently, several animal experiments demonstrated that inhibition of either Rho or ROCK (Rho/ROCK) attenuated cardiomyopathy in diabetes and improved myocardial compliance [8–10]. Therefore, a Rho/ROCK inhibitor would be a good candidate for treating diabetes and its complications [7, 11, 12]. The first-generation Rho/ROCK inhibitor fasudil has been studied widely and applied in clinical practice [13]. The safety and efficacy of fasudil in treating pulmonary arterial hypertension and other cardiovascular and cerebrovascular diseases have been identified clearly in clinical trials [14–16]. However, few studies have focused on the effect of Rho/ROCK inhibitors on cardiac mitochondria *in vivo* or *in vitro*.

2. Materials and Methods

2.1. Animals. All experiments were performed according to the Guidelines of Animal Experiments from the Committee of Medical Ethics at the National Health Department of China and were approved by the Laboratory Center of Shanghai Tenth People's Hospital. Male Sprague Dawley rats that weighed 200 g were purchased from the Shanghai Slac Laboratory Animal Co., Ltd., and housed in plastic cages with well-ventilated stainless steel grid tops at room temperature with a 12-hour light/dark cycle.

2.2. Induction of Diabetes and Drug Treatment. Type 2 diabetic (T2DM) rats were induced by a high-fat diet consisting of 42% fat (mainly pork), 19% protein, and 39% carbohydrate as well as a low dose of streptozotocin (STZ) (50 mg/kg intraperitoneally in a 0.1 mol/L citrate buffer, pH 4.5) as described previously [17]. Moreover, an oral glucose tolerance test (OGTT) was performed as described previously to confirm the onset of insulin resistance (IR) after eight weeks of dietary manipulation [17]. Diabetes was induced by a single intraperitoneal injection of STZ (Sigma, St. Louis, MO, USA) given to rats with insulin resistance.

One week after the initial STZ administration, rats with fasting blood glucose (FBG) ≥11.1 mmol/L in two consecutive analyses were considered to qualify as having T2DM. Subsequently, twenty diabetic rats were randomly divided into an untreated diabetic group ($n = 10$) and a fasudil-treated group ($n = 10$). Ten SD rats fed with a normal rat chow were considered as control group. The rats in the fasudil group were treated with fasudil (5 mg/kg bid) by intraperitoneal injection as reported previously [8], whereas untreated diabetic rats and control rats were injected intraperitoneally with equivalent volumes of saline for 4 weeks. All animals remained on the assigned diet until termination of the experiment. Fasudil hydrochloride was obtained from Chase Sun Pharmaceutical Co., Ltd. (Tianjin, China).

After four weeks of high-fat diet initiated at the time of fasudil administration, the FBG level was determined again. The rats were then anaesthetized by using 3% pentobarbital (30 mg/kg intraperitoneally), and plasma (8–10 mL per animal) was immediately collected from the femoral artery and processed into serum. After being washed in ice-cold saline solution, the hearts of the animals were weighed and frozen in liquid nitrogen then stored at −80°C.

2.3. Preparation of Cardiac Mitochondria. Mitochondria were isolated from rat hearts by differential centrifugation using a Tissue Mitochondria Isolation Kit (Thermo Scientific, MA, USA). After removal of the extraventricular tissue, the ventricle was weighed, finely minced in ice-cold buffer (160 mM KCl, 10 mM EGTA, and 0.5% fatty acid-free bovine serum albumin (BSA), pH 7.4), and brought to a final concentration of 1 g/10 mL of buffer. This tissue suspension was homogenized and centrifuged at 1,000 g for 10 min at 2°C. The supernatant was then centrifuged at 8,000 g for 10 min at 2°C to obtain the initial mitochondrial pellet, which was resuspended in suspension buffer (320 mM sucrose, 10 mM Tris-HCl, pH 7.4), and centrifuged again at 8,000 g for 10 min at 2°C to obtain the final mitochondrial pellet.

2.4. Ultrastructural Examination by Transmission Electron Microscopy (TEM). Cardiac tissue was cut into approximately 1 mm^3 pieces, fixed in 2.5% glutaraldehyde in 0.1 mol/L sodium phosphate buffer (pH 7.4) for 3 h at 4°C, and osmicated in 1% osmium tetroxide for 1 h at 4°C. After dehydration with a graded ethanol series, the sample was embedded in Epon812 and sectioned using a Leica EM UC6 (Leica Co., Vienna, Austria) ultramicrotome. Sections were viewed and photographed following TEM using a Tecnai G2 20 (FEI Co., Oregon, USA) at 200 kV.

2.5. Measurements of Succinic Dehydrogenase (SDH) and Monoamine Oxidase (MAO) in Cardiac Mitochondria. Each cardiac tissue sample was weighed to prepare a 10% (w/v) buffered homogenate (100 mg tissue/mL of 50 mM phosphate buffer at pH 7.2). The homogenate was centrifuged, and biochemical analyses were carried out using the supernatant. The protein concentration of the supernatant was determined by the Lowry method, using BSA as a standard. Activities of SDH and MAO in cardiac mitochondria were measured by spectrophotometry-based assays using commercially available kits (Jian Cheng Biological Engineering Institute, Nanjing, China).

2.6. Mitochondrial Permeability Transition Pore (MPTP) Opening in Cardiac Mitochondria. Opening of MPTPs causes mitochondrial swelling [18]. Isolated cardiac mitochondria were resuspended in swelling buffer (120 mM KCl, 10 mM Tris-HCl, 20 mM MOPS 20, 5 mM KH_2PO_4 5, pH 7.4) to a final concentration of 0.25 mg of mitochondrial protein/mL. After a 5 min equilibration period, swelling was induced by the addition of $CaCl_2$ (200 μM). The decrease at A520 was measured spectrophotometrically for 15 min.

2.7. JC-1 Staining and Mitochondrial Membrane Potentials Assay. Loss of mitochondrial membrane potential was assessed using a fluorescence microscope (Leica DMI6000, Leica, Germany) following staining with 5,5′,6,6′-tetrachloro-1,1′,3,3′-tetraethylbenzimidazole-carbocyanide iodine (JC-1; Beyotime, China). Isolated cardiac mitochondria were stained with JC-1 staining solution (5 μg/mL) for 15 min at 37°C and rinsed twice with phosphate buffer solution (PBS).

Mitochondrial membrane potentials were monitored by determining the relative amounts of dual emissions from mitochondrial JC-1 monomers or polymers using the fluorescent microscope. Mitochondrial depolarization was indicated by an increase in the red/green fluorescence intensity ratio. Red emission of the dye represented JC-1 polymers formed after potential-dependent aggregation in the mitochondria, reflecting normal mitochondrial membrane potential. Green fluorescence, which represented the monomeric form of

TABLE 1: Effects of fasudil on body weight, heart weight, blood pressure, blood glucose, serum insulin, glycated hemoglobin, and lipid profiles in diabetic rats either treated with or without fasudil.

	Fasudil-treated diabetic group (n = 10)	Untreated diabetic group (n = 10)	Control group (n = 10)
Start weight (g)	191 ± 7	190 ± 8	192 ± 7
End weight (g)	465 ± 9$^{\#}$	442 ± 10*	465 ± 10
Heart weight (g)	1.72 ± 0.11	1.68 ± 0.09*	1.78 ± 0.06
Mean blood pressure (kpa)	8.21 ± 1.21	9.44 ± 1.59	8.43 ± 1.25
Fasting blood glucose (mmol/L)	20.0 ± 2.6*	19.9 ± 2.4*	6.1 ± 0.2
Serum insulin (ng/mL)	6.17 ± 0.99*	5.97 ± 1.00*	4.78 ± 0.67
Glycated hemoglobin (%)	13.4 ± 1.7*	12.5 ± 1.8*	4.9 ± 0.4
Total cholesterol (mmol/L)	1.41 ± 0.15*	1.40 ± 0.13*	0.95 ± 0.12
Triglyceride (mmol/L)	0.63 ± 0.10	0.61 ± 0.08	0.55 ± 0.06
Free fatty acids (mmol/L)	0.33 ± 0.06	0.40 ± 0.18*	0.28 ± 0.07

Data are presented as the mean ± SD.
$^{*}P < 0.05$ versus control group.
$^{\#}P < 0.05$ versus untreated diabetic group.

JC-1, appeared in the cytosol after depolarization of the mitochondrial membrane.

The fluorescence was detected using a microplate reader (Tecan infinite 200). The wavelengths of excitation and emission used to detect the monomeric form of JC-1 were 514 nm and 529 nm, whereas 585 nm and 590 nm were used to detect polymers of JC-1. The ratio of JC-1 monomers and JC-1 polymers represented the condition of membrane potential of the cardiac mitochondria.

2.8. Protein Extraction and Western Blot Analysis. Cardiac tissues (0.5 cm^3) were homogenized in ice-cold radioimmunoprecipitation assay (RIPA) buffer and centrifuged at 10,000 g for 10 min at 4°C prior to collecting the supernatants. Protein concentrations in the supernatants were measured using the bicinchoninic acid (BCA) protein assay kit (Pierce Chemical Company, Rockford, USA). Proteins (40 μg) were separated with 8% or 10% SDS-polyacrylamide gel electrophoresis and transferred to PVDF membranes, which were then washed with Tris-buffered saline, blocked with 5% skimmed milk powder (except for phosphorylated myosin phosphatase targeting protein (MYPT), which was blocked using 5% BSA) in Tris-buffered saline Tween-20 for 1 h, and incubated with the appropriate primary antibody at dilutions recommended by the supplier. The membrane was then washed, and primary antibodies were detected with secondary antibody conjugated to horseradish peroxidase for 1 h at room temperature. The blots were then developed with SuperSignal-enhanced chemiluminescent substrate solution (Pierce Chemical Company, Rockford, USA). Anti-β-actin, anti-ROCK 1, anti-ROCK 2, anti-RhoA, anti-p-MYPT and anti-MYPT antibodies were purchased from Cell Signaling Technology (Danvers, Massachusetts, USA).

2.9. Measurements of Biomarkers of Oxidative Stress. The supernatant collected after centrifugation of the cardiac tissue homogenate was used to determine the total antioxidant capacity (TAC), as well as malonyldialdehyde (MDA), hydroxy radical, reduced glutathione (GSH), and superoxide dismutase (SOD) levels using commercial kits (Jian Cheng Biological Engineering Institute, Nanjing, China).

2.10. Statistical Analysis. All values were expressed as mean ± SD. Data distributions were examined for normality and homogeneity of variance. Statistical significance was determined by one-way ANOVA with Newman-Keuls post hoc test. For nonparametric analysis, the Mann-Whitney U test with post hoc analysis was used to evaluate the difference among three groups. Values of $P < 0.05$ were considered significant.

3. Results

3.1. Effects of Fasudil on Diabetic Rats. Table 1 details the characteristics of three groups of rats at the end of the experimental period. The final body weights of rats were significantly higher in members of the fasudil-treated and control group compared with members of the diabetes group (all $P < 0.05$). The mean blood pressure (MBP) was a little lower in fasudil-treated rats than in diabetic and control rats, although the difference was not significant. Levels of blood glucose, serum insulin, glycated hemoglobin (HbAlc), and cholesterol were markedly elevated in fasudil-treated and untreated diabetic group compared with the control group (all $P < 0.05$). However, these values have no differences between diabetic rats treated with fasudil and untreated diabetic rats. Although the level of triglyceride was lower in control rats, there were no significant differences among three groups. The untreated diabetic group had significantly higher levels of free fatty acids compared to the other two groups ($P < 0.05$).

3.2. Changes in Mitochondrial Morphology. We examined the mitochondrial morphology by TEM to confirm the cardioprotective effect of fasudil on mitochondrial biogenesis. Analysis using TEM indicated diffuse edema and enlargement in cardiac mitochondria of untreated diabetic rats,

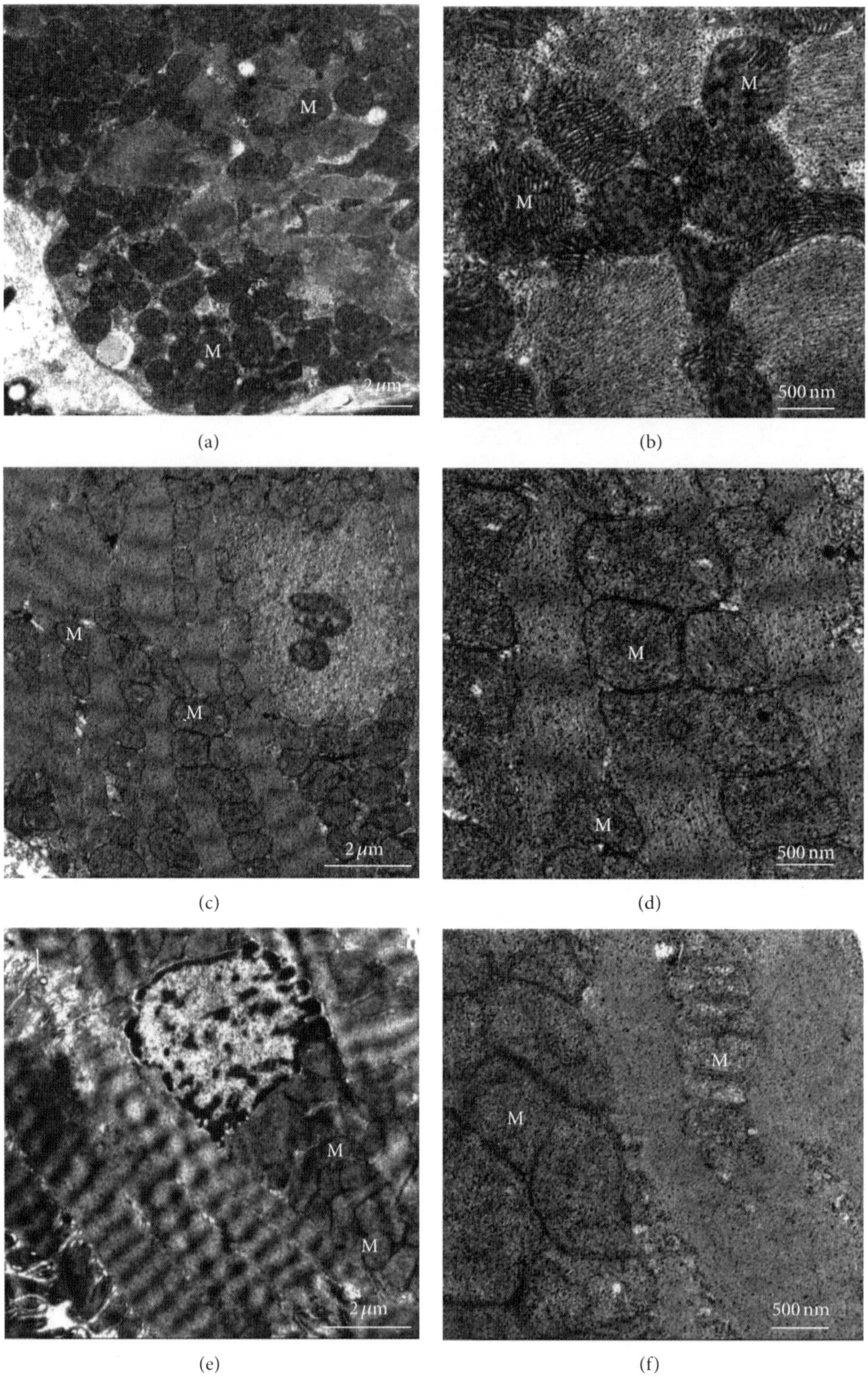

FIGURE 1: Effects of fasudil on the mitochondria of hearts from diabetic rats. The mitochondria of heart tissues were detected by TEM from the left ventricle of the rats. (a) Untreated diabetic group, 2,500x; (b) untreated diabetic group, 6,500x; (c) fasudil-treated diabetic group, 2,500x; (d) fasudil-treated diabetic group, 6,500x; (e) control group, 2,500x; (f) control group, 6,500x. Several mitochondria (M) exhibited swelling, enlargement, and diffuse edema, and disordered and partially disrupted mitochondrial cristae were observed in mitochondria from untreated diabetic rats. The damage to myocardial ultrastructures in fasudil-treated rats was attenuated compared with that of the untreated diabetic group.

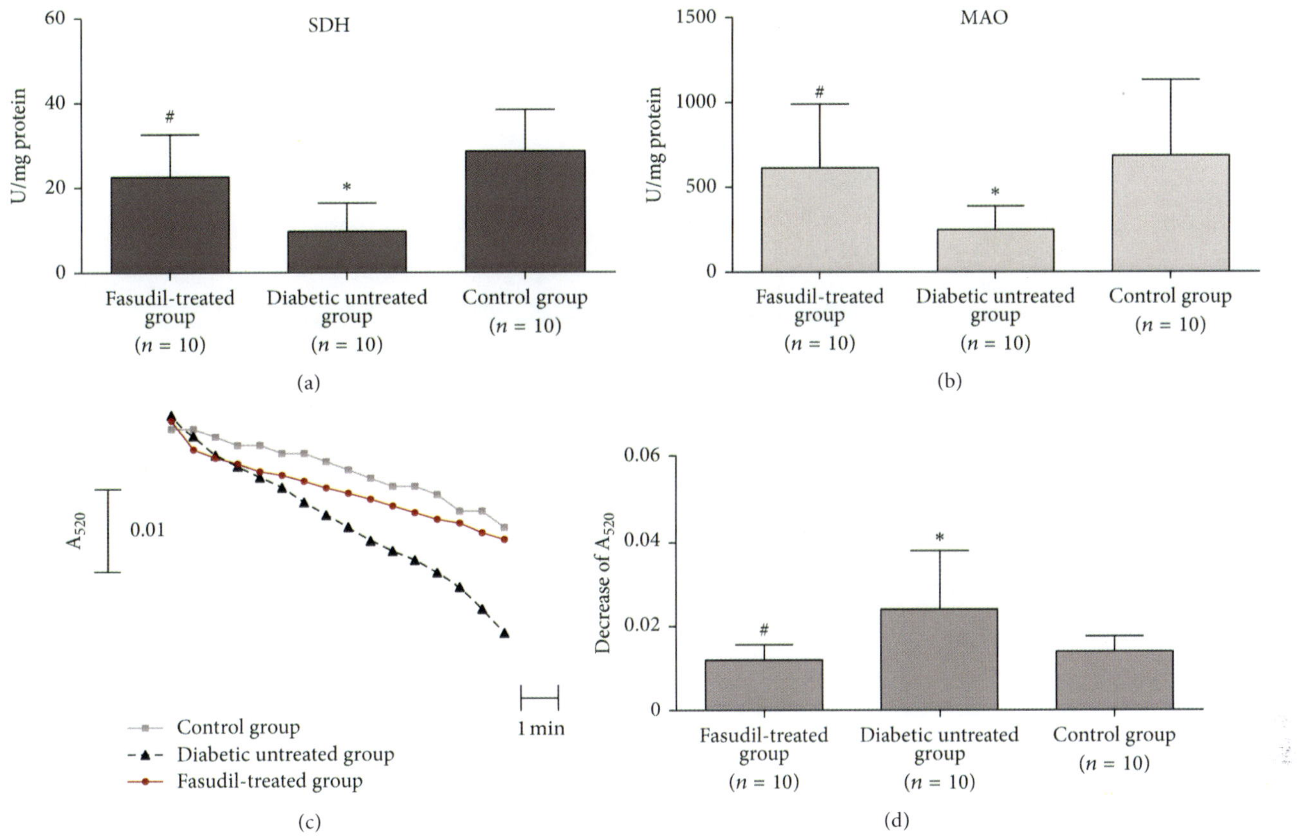

Figure 2: Comparison of SDH and MAO activities, MPTP opening, and decreases in A_{520} for the two groups. (a) Comparison of SDH activities in cardiac mitochondria from fasudil-treated, untreated diabetic, and control rats revealed statistically significant differences. SDH activities in cardiac mitochondria from fasudil-treated group were marked higher than that of untreated diabetic group ($P = 0.003$). (b) Comparison of MAO activities in cardiac mitochondria from fasudil-treated, untreated diabetic, and control rats revealed statistically significant differences. MAO activities in cardiac mitochondria from fasudil-treated group were significantly higher than that of untreated diabetic group ($P = 0.015$). (c) Effects of fasudil on MPTP opening (A_{520}: absorbance at 520 nm). The trace represented the mean of A_{520} from three groups. The top trace represented cardiac mitochondria from SD control rats, the middle trace showed the absorbance in mitochondria from diabetic rats treated with fasudil, and lower traces showed the absorbance in mitochondria from untreated diabetic rats. (d) Comparison of decreases in A_{520} for the three groups. The decreases in A_{520} were significantly lower in diabetic rats treated with fasudil compared to untreated rats ($P < 0.001$).

in which the mitochondrial cristae were disordered and partially disrupted (Figures 1(a) and 1(b)) compared with control group (Figures 1(e) and 1(f)). However, less damage to myocardial ultrastructures was observed in fasudil-treated rats compared with diabetic untreated rats (Figures 1(c) and 1(d)).

3.3. Changes in SDH and MAO Activity in Cardiac Mitochondria. Activities of SDH in fasudil-treated, untreated diabetic, and control rats were 22.8 ± 10.1, 9.8 ± 6.7, and 28.9 ± 9.8 U/mg protein, respectively. Activities of MAO in fasudil-treated group, diabetic-untreated group and control group were 617.9 ± 381.3, 250.4 ± 140.8, and 690.1 ± 451.6 U/mg protein, respectively. Activities of SDH and MAO were significantly higher in the cardiac mitochondria of fasudil-treated diabetic and control rats compared with those from untreated diabetic rats (all $P < 0.05$) (Figures 2(a) and 2(b)). These findings suggest that SDH and MAO activity in cardiac mitochondria could be restored by treatment with fasudil.

3.4. Effect of Fasudil on MPTP. To investigate the degree of mitochondrial swelling, we assessed the opening of MPTP by measuring the absorbance of mitochondrial suspensions at 520 nm (A_{520}) as reported previously [19, 20]. A decrease at A_{520} was considered to indicate swelling of the mitochondrion as a result of opening the pore. The decrease at A_{520} in the mitochondrial suspension was significantly attenuated in fasudil-treated rats compared with that of the mitochondrial suspension prepared from untreated rats (Figure 2(c)). The decrease of A_{520} in the mitochondrial suspension in fasudil-treated group, untreated diabetic group, and control group are 0.012 ± 0.0037, 0.024 ± 0.014, and 0.014 ± 0.0036, respectively. The decrease of A_{520} in fasudil-treated group is significantly lower than that of the untreated diabetic rats ($P = 0.018$) (Figure 2(d)).

3.5. Changes in Mitochondrial Transmembrane Potential. JC-1 could aggregate in normal mitochondria and present red fluorescence. The dissipation of transmembrane potential in

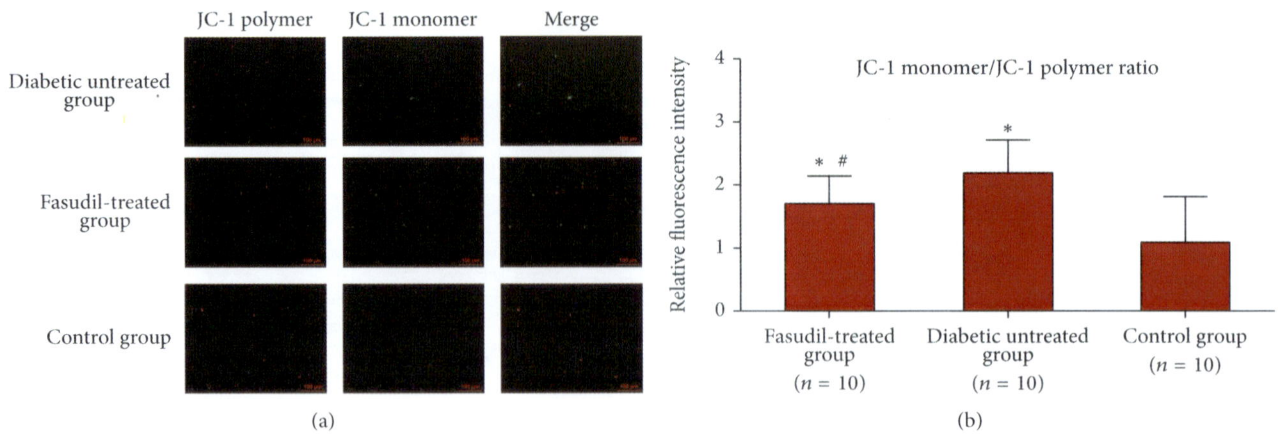

FIGURE 3: Effect of fasudil on transmembrane potential in mitochondria. Red fluorescence represents the mitochondrial aggregate form of JC-1 (JC-1 polymers), which indicates the intact mitochondrial membrane potential. Green fluorescence represents the monomeric form of JC-1 (JC-1 monomers), which indicates the dissipation of mitochondrial transmembrane potential. (a) Representative results of cardiac mitochondria stained with JC-1 and derived from fasudil-treated, untreated diabetic, and control rats. (b) Ratios of JC-1 monomer to JC-1 polymer (red/green fluorescence) for untreated diabetic rats, diabetic rats treated with fasudil, and control rats. Data are expressed as the mean ± SD. The ratio was significantly lower for diabetic rats treated with fasudil than for untreated diabetic rats ($P = 0.037$).

cardiac mitochondria isolated from diabetic-untreated rats was observed as increased green fluorescence (Figure 3(a)) following staining with JC-1. Consistent with its cardioprotective effects, fasudil moderated the dissipation of mitochondrial transmembrane potential. The ratio of red fluorescence to green fluorescence was also used to demonstrate the loss of mitochondrial transmembrane potential and the protective effect of fasudil in mitochondria.

In the fasudil-treated and control group, JC-1 aggregated in mitochondria and the JC-1 monomer/JC-1 polymer ratio were 1.72 ± 0.44 and 1.10 ± 0.73. A higher ratio in the untreated group (2.21 ± 0.53) indicated the dissipation of mitochondrial membrane potential. Diabetic rats treated with fasudil demonstrated attenuated dissipation of mitochondrial membrane potential ($P < 0.05$) (Figure 3(b)).

3.6. Rho/ROCK Activation in Cardiac Tissue and Rho/ROCK Suppression by Fasudil. To investigate the protein expression of ROCK 1, ROCK 2, Rho A, and MYPT, we isolated rat cardiac tissue and performed western blot analysis. These proteins were expressed in the heart tissue of diabetic rats. Moreover, to examine the efficacy of fasudil for Rho/ROCK inhibition in the cardiac tissue, we quantified the amount of phosphorylated MYPT (p-MYPT) and total MYPT. Both phosphorylated and unphosphorylated MYPT are downstream targets of ROCK. As shown in Figure 4(a), levels of ROCK 1, ROCK 2, Rho A, and phosphorylated MYPT were markedly higher in the cardiac tissue of diabetic untreated rats than in the cardiac tissue from fasudil-treated rats (0.95 ± 0.06; 0.57 ± 0.11; 0.69 ± 0.10, $P < 0.05$ versus fasudil-treated group). In comparison, treatment of diabetic rats with fasudil significantly reduced the levels of ROCK 1, ROCK 2, Rho A, and p-MYPT (0.75 ± 0.11; 0.44 ± 0.093; 0.55 ± 0.13) (Figures 4(b), 4(c), and 4(d)).

3.7. Changes in Oxidative Stress Biomarkers. The levels of oxidative stress biomarkers in cardiac tissues of the two groups were significantly different (all $P < 0.05$) (Table 2). Figure 4(e) shows the comparison of TAC, MDA, hydroxy radical, GSH, and SOD levels in cardiac tissues from the two groups of diabetic rats. The levels of TAC, GSH, and SOD were significantly lower in the untreated diabetic rats than in fasudil-treated rats, whereas the levels of MDA and hydroxy radical were significantly higher in diabetic untreated rats compared with diabetic rats treated with fasudil ($P < 0.001$).

4. Discussion

The main aim of this study was to determine whether the Rho/ROCK inhibitor fasudil could protect cardiac mitochondria from diabetic rats fed a combination of a low-dose STZ and a high-fat diet. The effect of fasudil on both the structure and function of cardiac mitochondria were investigated. These data complement findings from our previous study, which suggested that inhibition of Rho/ROCK signaling may have therapeutic potential in preventing diabetes associated with vascular inflammation and atherogenesis [21].

The main function of cardiac mitochondria is to generate adenosine triphosphate (ATP) through oxidative phosphorylation (Ox-Phos). Under normal conditions, the adult heart relies mostly on fatty acids to fuel Ox-Phos, with 10% to 30% of total ATP derived from glucose [22]. It is believed that altered mitochondrial bioenergetics appear to play a substantial role in cardiomyopathy or myocardial dysfunction [23]. T2DM is one of the most common metabolic diseases in the world, and it is associated with an elevated rate of oxidative stress [24]. Reactive oxygen species (ROS) produced by mitochondria have been implicated in the pathogenesis of T2DM and its complications [25–27]. Therefore, mitochondrial defects may play a critical role in pathogens and development of T2DM [28], and the protection of mitochondria could be considered as a potential treatment target for diabetes.

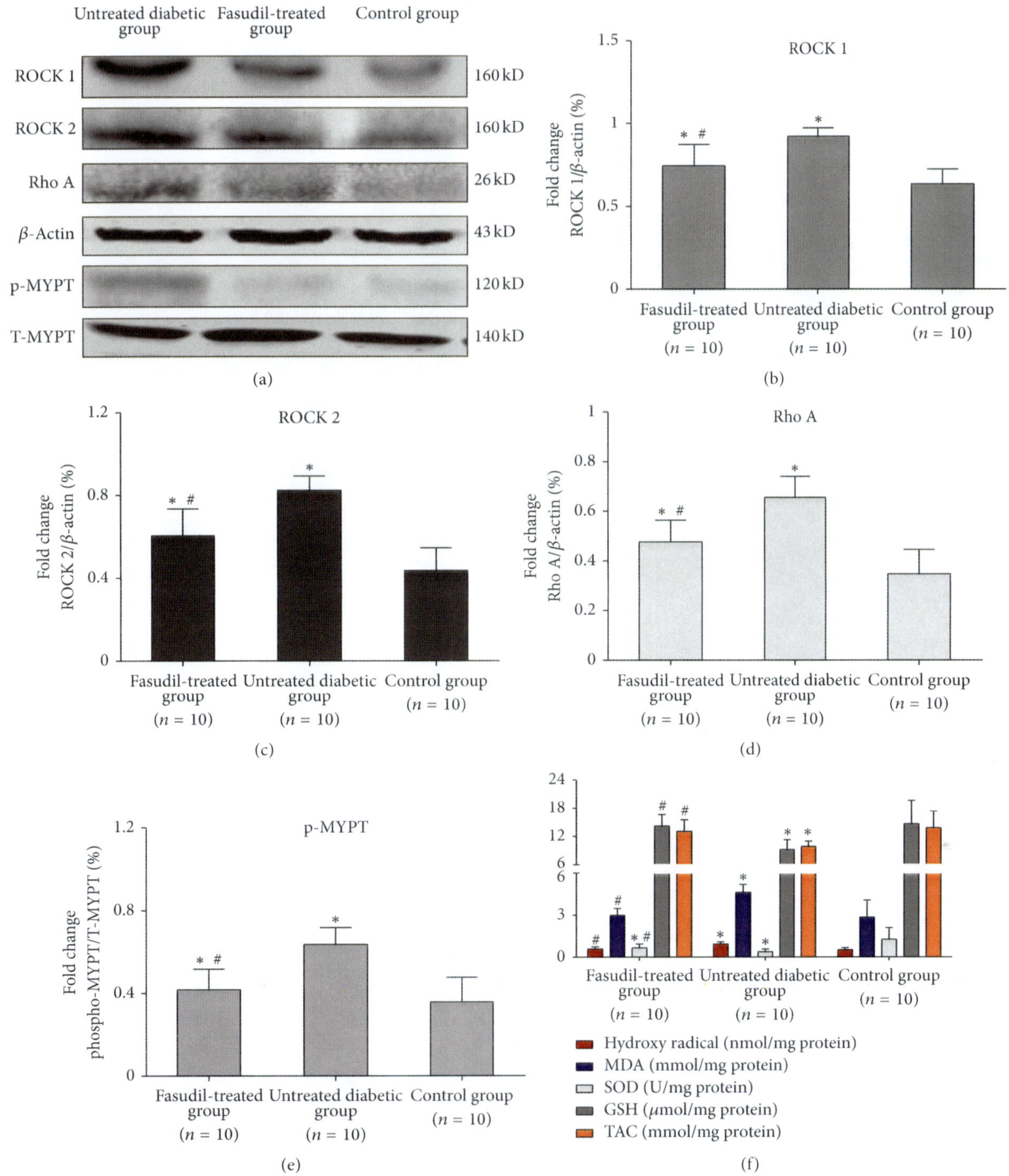

Figure 4: Effect of fasudil on cardiac Rho/ROCK activity. Levels of ROCK 1, ROCK 2, Rho A, and phosphorylated MYPT were detected in rat cardiac tissues using western blot analysis. (a) Representative results of assays of ROCK 1, ROCK 2, Rho A, and phospho-MYPT-1 and beta-actin abundances in rat cardiac tissues. (b) The levels of ROCK 1 protein expression were analyzed by western blot by using a polyclonal antibody to ROCK 1 to quantify its expressions in cardiac tissues. Data are expressed as the mean ± SD ($P < 0.001$ compared with untreated diabetic group). (c) The levels of ROCK 2 protein expression were analyzed by western blot by using a polyclonal antibody to ROCK 2 to quantify its expressions in cardiac tissues. Data are expressed as the mean ± SD ($P < 0.001$ compared with untreated diabetic group). (d) Average signal intensities quantified and expressed as percentage of the ratio of beta-actin to quantify Rho A expressions in cardiac tissues. Data are expressed as mean ± SD. The average signal intensities were significantly lower for diabetic rats treated with fasudil than for untreated diabetic rats ($P = 0.008$). (e) Average signal intensities quantified and expressed as a percentage of the ratio of T-MYPT to quantify levels of phosphorylated MYPT in cardiac tissues. Data are expressed as the mean ± SD. The ratio was significantly lower for diabetic rats treated with fasudil than for untreated diabetic rats ($P = 0.019$). (f) Five oxidative stress biomarkers were measured in heart tissues from diabetic-treated, untreated, and control rats. $^{*}P < 0.05$ versus control group. $^{\#}P < 0.05$ versus untreated diabetic group.

TABLE 2: Comparison of oxidative stress biomarkers in diabetic rats either treated with or without fasudil.

	Fasudil-treated diabetic group ($n = 10$)	Untreated diabetic group ($n = 10$)	Control group ($n = 10$)
TAC (mmol/mg protein)	13.03 ± 2.46#	9.77 ± 1.14*	13.76 ± 3.60
MDA (mmol/mg protein)	3.02 ± 0.49#	4.65 ± 0.57*	2.88 ± 1.21
hydroxy radical (nmol/mg protein)	0.59 ± 0.15#	0.94 ± 0.15*	0.53 ± 0.14
GSH (μmol/mg protein)	14.16 ± 2.47#	9.13 ± 2.06*	14.61 ± 5.07
SOD (U/mg protein)	0.66 ± 0.28#*	0.38 ± 0.20*	1.27 ± 0.83

Data are presented as the mean ± SD.
* $P < 0.05$ versus control group.
# $P < 0.05$ versus untreated diabetic group.

Xie and colleagues [6] reported that diabetes-associated ROS or lipoproteins impair mitochondrial respiration. Reduced activities of SDH and other key mitochondrial enzymes in diabetic animals potentially lead to oxidative stress and the development of diabetic cardiovascular complications. The key respiratory enzyme SDH, which is assembled in mitochondria to form the mitochondrial complex 2, links the Krebs cycle to the electron transport chain. Recent reports have highlighted the relevance of MAO to the formation of mitochondrial ROS formation [29, 30].

The MPTP is a common target of intracellular signal transduction pathways. Opening this pore allows water and solutes to enter the mitochondria, increases the matrix volume, and ruptures the outer mitochondrial membrane, leading to the release of intermembranous cytochrome C. Thus, MPTP was considered to play an important role in cell death and apoptosis [31, 32]. The accumulation of mitochondrial ROS induced by hyperglycemia or diabetes could dissipate mitochondrial transmembrane potential and activate MPTP directly. Dissipation of mitochondrial transmembrane potential also represented mitochondrial dysfunction. Our study showed that the opening of the MPTP was inhibited by fasudil in diabetic rat hearts. In addition, diabetic rats treated with fasudil attenuated the dissipation of mitochondrial transmembrane potential ($P = 0.037$). This indicated that the Rho/ROCK inhibitor fasudil could exert a cardioprotective effect through the inhibition of MPTP and the dissipation of mitochondrial transmembrane potential.

The Rho/ROCK pathway may associate with enhanced oxidative stress by upregulation of NAD(P)H oxidase [33]. Furthermore, it has been reported that fasudil exerted antioxidant effects on hypercholesterolemic rats [34]. We speculate that fasudil has similar effects on cardiac tissue and plays a protective role in cardiac mitochondria. Therefore, several oxidative stress biomarkers (TAC, MDA, hydroxy radical, GSH, and SOD) in cardiac tissue, as well as SDH and MAO activities in cardiac mitochondria were measured in this study. Our study demonstrated that TAC, GSH, and SOD in cardiac tissue and SDH and MAO activities in cardiac mitochondria were significantly higher in fasudil-treated rats than in untreated rats ($P < 0.001$). Additionally, the levels of MDA and hydroxy radicals in cardiac tissue were significantly higher in untreated diabetic rats ($P < 0.001$).

Our findings might have implications regarding the efficacy of the administration of fasudil to treat diabetic cardiomyopathy or diabetic cardiovascular complications. A previous study demonstrated that fasudil might have potential benefits on cardiac function in diabetic rats [8]. Our results further suggest that fasudil is likely to have a cardioprotective effect by protecting cardiac mitochondria, because the structure and function of cardiac mitochondria in fasudil-treated rats were significantly higher than those observed in untreated rats.

5. Conclusions

In summary, we found that not only can the cardiac mitochondrial structure be improved by administration of Rho/ROCK inhibitor fasudil to T2DM rats, but the SDH and MAO activities in cardiac mitochondria were significantly higher in fasudil-treated rats than in untreated rats. These beneficial effects may be associated with the ability of fasudil treatment to attenuate oxidative stress.

Conflict of Interests

The authors declare no conflict of interests.

Acknowledgment

This study is supported by a Grant from the National Natural Science Foundation of China (No. 81070107).

References

[1] H. M. McBride, M. Neuspiel, and S. Wasiak, "Mitochondria: more than just a powerhouse," *Current Biology*, vol. 16, no. 14, pp. R551–R560, 2006.

[2] E. J. Lesnefsky, S. Moghaddas, B. Tandler, J. Kerner, and C. L. Hoppel, "Mitochondrial dysfunction in cardiac disease: ischemia—reperfusion, aging, and heart failure," *Journal of Molecular and Cellular Cardiology*, vol. 33, no. 6, pp. 1065–1089, 2001.

[3] A. M. Walters, G. A. Porter Jr., and P. S. Brookes, "Mitochondria as a drug target in ischemic heart disease and cardiomyopathy," *Circulation Research*, vol. 111, no. 9, pp. 1222–1236, 2012.

[4] G. X. Shen, "Mitochondrial dysfunction, oxidative stress and diabetic cardiovascular disorders," *Cardiovascular & Hematological Disorders—Drug Targets*, vol. 12, no. 2, pp. 106–112, 2012.

[5] G. X. Shen, "Oxidative stress and diabetic cardiovascular disorders: roles of mitochondria and NADPH oxidase," *Canadian Journal of Physiology and Pharmacology*, vol. 88, no. 3, pp. 241–248, 2010.

[6] X. Xie, S. R. Chowdhury, G. Sangle, and G. X. Shen, "Impact of diabetes-associated lipoproteins on oxygen consumption and mitochondrial enzymes in porcine aortic endothelial cells," *Acta Biochimica Polonica*, vol. 57, no. 4, pp. 393–398, 2010.

[7] R. Arita, Y. Hata, S. Nakao et al., "Rho kinase inhibition by fasudil ameliorates diabetes-induced microvascular damage," *Diabetes*, vol. 58, no. 1, pp. 215–226, 2009.

[8] S. J. Guan, Z. H. Ma, Y. L. Wu et al., "Long-term administration of fasudil improves cardiomyopathy in streptozotocin-induced diabetic rats," *Food and Chemical Toxicology*, vol. 50, no. 6, pp. 1874–1882, 2012.

[9] H. Zhou, Y. J. Li, M. Wang et al., "Involvement of RhoA/ROCK in myocardial fibrosis in a rat model of type 2 diabetes," *Acta Pharmacologica Sinica*, vol. 32, no. 8, pp. 999–1008, 2011.

[10] I. Kizub, O. Pavlova, C. Johnson, A. Soloviev, and A. Zholos, "Rho kinase and protein kinase C involvement in vascular smooth muscle myofilament calcium sensitization in arteries from diabetic rats," *British Journal of Pharmacology*, vol. 159, no. 8, pp. 1724–1731, 2010.

[11] L. A. Bach, "Rho kinase inhibition: a new approach for treating diabetic nephropathy?" *Diabetes*, vol. 57, no. 3, pp. 532–533, 2008.

[12] R. Komers, "Rho kinase inhibition in diabetic nephropathy," *Current Opinion in Nephrology and Hypertension*, vol. 20, no. 1, pp. 77–83, 2011.

[13] T. Ishida, Y. Takanashi, and H. Kiwada, "Safe and efficient drug delivery system with liposomes for intrathecal application of an antivasospastic drug, fasudil," *Biological and Pharmaceutical Bulletin*, vol. 29, no. 3, pp. 397–402, 2006.

[14] I. Omeis, N. A. Jayson, R. Murali, and J. M. Abrahams, "Treatment of cerebral vasospasm with biocompatible controlled-release systems for intracranial drug delivery," *Neurosurgery*, vol. 63, no. 6, pp. 1011–1019, 2008.

[15] M. F. Olson, "Applications for ROCK kinase inhibition," *Current Opinion in Cell Biology*, vol. 20, no. 2, pp. 242–248, 2008.

[16] Y. Suzuki, M. Shibuya, S. I. Satoh, Y. Sugimoto, and K. Takakura, "A postmarketing surveillance study of fasudil treatment after aneurysmal subarachnoid hemorrhage," *Surgical Neurology*, vol. 68, no. 2, pp. 126–131, 2007.

[17] M. J. Reed, K. Meszaros, L. J. Entes et al., "A new rat model of type 2 diabetes: the fat-fed, streptozotocin-treated rat," *Metabolism: Clinical and Experimental*, vol. 49, no. 11, pp. 1390–1394, 2000.

[18] C. P. Baines, C. X. Song, Y. T. Zheng et al., "Protein kinase Cε interacts with and inhibits the permeability transition pore in cardiac mitochondria," *Circulation Research*, vol. 92, no. 8, pp. 873–880, 2003.

[19] S. Javadov, M. Karmazyn, and N. Escobales, "Mitochondrial permeability transition pore opening as a promising therapeutic target in cardiac diseases," *Journal of Pharmacology and Experimental Therapeutics*, vol. 330, no. 3, pp. 670–678, 2009.

[20] Q. Gao, S. Z. Zhang, C. M. Cao, I. C. Bruce, and Q. Xia, "The mitochondrial permeability transition pore and the Ca^{2+}-activated K^+ channel contribute to the cardioprotection conferred by tumor necrosis factor-α," *Cytokine*, vol. 32, no. 5, pp. 199–205, 2005.

[21] H. Li, W. Peng, W. Jian et al., "ROCK inhibitor fasudil attenuated high glucose-induced MCP-1 and VCAM-1 expression and monocyte-endothelial cell adhesion," *Cardiovascular Diabetology*, vol. 11, p. 65, 2012.

[22] L. H. Opie, "Substrate utilization and glycolysis in the heart," *Cardiology*, vol. 56, no. 1, pp. 2–21, 1971.

[23] J. M. Huss and D. P. Kelly, "Mitochondrial energy metabolism in heart failure: a question of balance," *The Journal of Clinical Investigation*, vol. 115, no. 3, pp. 547–555, 2005.

[24] F. Piarulli, G. Sartore, and A. Lapolla, "Glyco-oxidation and cardiovascular complications in type 2 diabetes: a clinical update," *Acta Diabetologica*, vol. 50, no. 2, pp. 101–110, 2012.

[25] D. X. Zhang and D. D. Gutterman, "Mitochondrial reactive oxygen species-mediated signaling in endothelial cells," *American Journal of Physiology*, vol. 292, no. 5, pp. H2023–H2031, 2007.

[26] F. Giacco and M. Brownlee, "Oxidative stress and diabetic complications," *Circulation Research*, vol. 107, no. 9, pp. 1058–1070, 2010.

[27] F. Folli, D. Corradi, P. Fanti et al., "The role of oxidative stress in the pathogenesis of type 2 diabetes mellitus micro- and macrovascular complications: avenues for a mechanistic-based therapeutic approach," *Current Diabetes Reviews*, vol. 7, no. 5, pp. 313–324, 2011.

[28] B. B. Lowell and G. I. Shulman, "Mitochondrial dysfunction and type 2 diabetes," *Science*, vol. 307, no. 5708, pp. 384–387, 2005.

[29] F. Di Lisa, N. Kaludercic, A. Carpi, R. Menabò, and M. Giorgio, "Mitochondrial pathways for ROS formation and myocardial injury: the relevance of p66Shc and monoamine oxidase," *Basic Research in Cardiology*, vol. 104, no. 2, pp. 131–139, 2009.

[30] F. Di Lisa, N. Kaludercic, A. Carpi, R. Menabò, and M. Giorgio, "Mitochondria and vascular pathology," *Pharmacological Reports*, vol. 61, no. 1, pp. 123–130, 2009.

[31] A. P. Halestrap, S. J. Clarke, and S. A. Javadov, "Mitochondrial permeability transition pore opening during myocardial reperfusion—a target for cardioprotection," *Cardiovascular Research*, vol. 61, no. 3, pp. 372–385, 2004.

[32] J. N. Weiss, P. Korge, H. M. Honda, and P. Ping, "Role of the mitochondrial permeability transition in myocardial disease," *Circulation Research*, vol. 93, no. 4, pp. 292–301, 2003.

[33] M. Higashi, H. Shimokawa, T. Hattori et al., "Long-term inhibition of Rho-kinase suppresses angiotensin II-induced cardiovascular hypertrophy in rats in vivo: effect on endothelial NAD(P)H oxidase system," *Circulation Research*, vol. 93, no. 8, pp. 767–775, 2003.

[34] Z. Ma, J. Zhang, E. Ji, G. Cao, G. Li, and L. Chu, "Rho kinase inhibition by fasudil exerts antioxidant effects in hypercholesterolemic rats," *Clinical and Experimental Pharmacology and Physiology*, vol. 38, no. 10, pp. 688–694, 2011.

4

Therapeutic Effect of Exendin-4, a Long-Acting Analogue of Glucagon-Like Peptide-1 Receptor Agonist, on Nerve Regeneration after the Crush Nerve Injury

Koji Yamamoto,[1] Masatoshi Amako,[1] Yoritsuna Yamamoto,[2] Toyokazu Tsuchihara,[3] Hitoshi Nukada,[4,5] Yasuo Yoshihara,[1] Hiroshi Arino,[1] Masanori Fujita,[2] Maki Uenoyama,[2] Shoichi Tachibana,[2] and Koichi Nemoto[1]

[1] *Department of Orthopedic Surgery, National Defense Medical College, 3-2 Namiki, Tokorozawa, Saitama 359-8513, Japan*
[2] *Division of Environmental Medicine, National Defense Medical College Research Institute, 3-2 Namiki, Tokorozawa, Saitama 359-8513, Japan*
[3] *Orthopedic Surgery, Japan Self Defense Forces Central Hospital, 1-2-24 Ikejiri, Setagaya-ku, Tokyo 154-0001, Japan*
[4] *Department of Medicine, University of Otago Medical School, P.O. Box 913, Dunedin 9054, New Zealand*
[5] *The Nukada Institute for Medical and Biological Research, 5-18 Inage-cho, Inage-ku, Chiba 263-0035, Japan*

Correspondence should be addressed to Koji Yamamoto; yamagen0610@nifty.com

Academic Editor: Levent Sarıkcıoğlu

Glucagon-like peptide-1 (GLP-1) is glucose-dependent insulinotropic hormone secreted from enteroendocrine L cells. Its long-acting analogue, exendin-4, is equipotent to GLP-1 and is used to treat type 2 diabetes mellitus. In addition, exendin-4 has effects on the central and peripheral nervous system. In this study, we administered repeated intraperitoneal (i.p.) injections of exendin-4 to examine whether exendin-4 is able to facilitate the recovery after the crush nerve injury. Exendin-4 injection was started immediately after crush injury and was repeated every day for subsequent 14 days. Rats subjected to sciatic nerve crush exhibited marked functional loss, electrophysiological dysfunction, and atrophy of the tibialis anterior muscle (TA). All these changes, except for the atrophy of TA, were improved significantly by the administration of exendin-4. Functional, electrophysiological, and morphological parameters indicated significant enhancement of nerve regeneration 4 weeks after nerve crush. These results suggest that exendin-4 is feasible for clinical application to treat peripheral nerve injury.

1. Introduction

Peripheral nerve injury is common in the clinical field and the prevalence is relatively high (2.8% of trauma patients) [1]. However, its prognosis is often unsatisfactory because nerve regeneration is slow and it takes long time to reinnervate the target organs. As a result, some functional and histological changes become irreversible. Therefore, it is important to accelerate nerve regeneration to obtain excellent recovery.

GLP-1 is glucose-dependent insulinotropic hormone secreted from enteroendocrine L cells [2]. However, its therapeutic potential in diabetes is limited by its short biological half-life through degradation by dipeptidyl peptidase IV. Exendin-4 is a GLP-1 analogue derived from the saliva of the glia monster that shares 53% sequence homology with GLP-1 [3, 4]. It is equipotent to GLP-1 and has longer half-life than GLP-1 due to resistance to degradation by dipeptidyl peptidase IV [5]. Therefore, exendin-4 is approved to improve glycemic control in patients with type 2 diabetes mellitus.

GLP-1 and exendin-4 also have effects on the central and peripheral nervous system. GLP-1 and exendin-4 have been shown to have protective effect to the central nervous system from neurodegenerative disease [6–8]. GLP-1 and exendin-4 attenuate the peripheral sensory neuropathy induced by pyridoxine [9]. GLP-1 also promotes neurite outgrowth in PC12 cells *in vitro* [10]. However, to our knowledge, there is no demonstrated data of exendin-4 in the peripheral nerve injury. In this study, we examined whether exendin-4 can enhance functional and histological recovery after crush injury of the rat sciatic nerve.

2. Materials and Methods

2.1. Animals. Forty-eight Wistar rats, 8 weeks old and weighing 175–210 g, were used in all experiments. Animals were obtained from Japan SLC, Inc. (Hamamatsu, Japan). They were housed in a temperature-controlled room with a 12-hour light-dark cycle.

2.2. Design of Animal Experiments. All surgical procedures were carried out as described previously [11]. Rats were divided randomly into 4 equal groups as follows: (1) crush group ($n = 12$), administered 0.5 mL saline/rat/day after a 5 min. nerve crush injury, (2) crush + exendin-4 group ($n = 12$), administered 2.5 μg/rat/day exendin-4 (Sigma-Aldrich, St Louis, MO, USA) in 0.5 mL saline starting after 5 min. of nerve crush injury, (3) exendin-4 group ($n = 12$), administered 2.5 μg/rat/day exendin-4 in 0.5 mL saline only without operation, and (4) sham operation group ($n = 12$), administered 0.5 mL saline/rat/day after sham operation with no crush injury. Injections of exendin-4 or saline were done from 1 to 14 days after the crush.

2.3. Evaluation

2.3.1. Sciatic Functional Index (SFI). For the evaluation of motor function, walking tracks were recorded as previously mentioned [12]. The following measurements were taken: the distance from heel to toe (the print length, PL), the distance between the first and fifth toes (the toe spread, TS), and the distance from the second to the fourth toes (the intermediary toe spread, IT). SFIs were calculated as previously described [13]. Assessments were performed at 11 defined time points and up to 28 days after surgery ($n = 12$ in each group).

2.3.2. Glucose Measurement. Blood samples were obtained from the tail vein, and glucose levels were measured using a blood glucose meter (FreeStyle; Nipro Inc, Osaka, Japan) at 0 (before crush), 1, and 3 days after crush ($n = 6$ in each group).

2.3.3. Electrophysiological Study. At 4 weeks after the crush, the right sciatic nerve was exposed under sodium pentobarbital anesthesia (40–50 mg/kg, i.p.), and the nerve was stimulated at 2 mm distal to the sciatic notch, using a hook-up electrode. Evoked muscle response was recorded from TA using needle electrodes. We kept the distance between the stimulating and recording sites as 42 mm, which was measured on the surface of the fully extended hind limbs. Both compound muscle action potential (CMAP) and distal latency were measured using Neuropack instrumentation (Nihon Kohden inc, Tokyo, Japan) ($n = 6$ in each group).

2.3.4. Assessment of the Wet Weight of TA. At 4 weeks after the crush, both TA were harvested and weighed as previously described [14] ($n = 12$ in each group).

2.3.5. Histological Studies of the Sciatic Nerve. Specimens of the crushed sciatic nerve were taken at 5 mm distal to the crush site after 4 weeks ($n = 6$ in each group). All specimens were fixed in 2.5% glutaraldehyde in 0.1 M phosphate buffer solution (pH 7.4) overnight. Subsequently, they were postfixed with 1% osmium tetroxide, dehydrated, and cut into consecutive 2-3 mm blocks before embedding in Epon resin (EPON 812, TAAB Ltd, Berkshire, England).

Light Microscopic Study. Semi-thin sections (1 μm in thickness) of sciatic nerves were stained with toluidine blue and were examined by light microscope. The area and the number of the myelinated axons were measured as described previously [15–17]. At least, 1400 myelinated fibers were counted in each nerve.

Electron Microscope. Thin sections (60 nm in thickness) of sciatic nerves were stained with uranyl acetate and citrate and were examined by electron microscope. The *g*-ratios of myelinated axons were calculated in 12 different fields of each section and analyzed [18]. In average, we counted 140 myelinated fibers in each nerve.

2.3.6. Statistical Analysis. Statistical analyses were performed using JMP 10 (SAS Institute Inc., Cary, NC, USA). We expressed values for each parameter as means ± SD. P values of <0.05 were considered significant. Two-way analysis of variance (ANOVA) was utilized to examine the main effects of the nerve crush (with crush versus without crush) and exendin-4 administration (exendin-4 injection versus saline injection). Tukey test was run for post hoc analysis.

2.4. Ethics. This experimental study was carried out in accordance with the recommendations in the Guide for the Care and Use of Laboratory Animals published by the National Institutes of Health, and the protocol was approved by the Committee on the Ethics of Animal Experiments of the National Defense Medical College (no. 11102).

3. Results

3.1. Sciatic Functional Index (SFI). In the crush and crush + exendin-4 groups, the SFIs decreased from levels near −10 (representing normal function) to levels near −100 (representing complete loss of function) after surgery. In the crush + exendin-4 group, the SFI recovered rapidly and returned to the precrush levels by 19 days although in the crush group it did not return to the presurgical level at the end of the study. In the sham operation and exendin-4 groups, the SFIs did not alter significantly through this study. At 16, 19, 25, and 28 days after the procedure, two-way ANOVA revealed significant

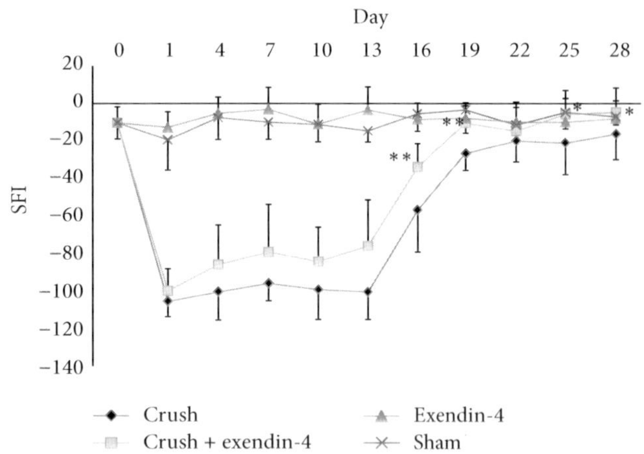

FIGURE 1: Sciatic functional index. SFI was calculated by the following formula [13]: SFI = −38.3(EPL − NPL)/NPL + 109.5(ETS − NTS)/NTS + 13.3(EIT − NIT)/NIT − 8.8. E, and N represent experimental and normal sides, respectively. In the crush + exendin-4 group, the SFI recovered rapidly and returned to the precrush levels by 19 days although in the crush group it did not return to the presurgical level at the end of the study. At 16, 19, 25, and 28 days after the crush injury, the SFIs in the crush + exendin-4 group were significantly higher than those in the crush group ($^{*}P < 0.05$, $^{**}P < 0.01$ compared with crush group).

interaction between the main effects of the nerve crush and exendin-4 administration. The post hoc data indicated that the SFIs in the crush + exendin-4 group were significantly higher than those in the crush group (Figure 1).

3.2. Glucose Measurement. In all groups, the blood glucose levels were normal at 0 (before crush), 1, and 3 days after the nerve crush.

3.3. Electrophysiological Study. The CMAP was increased in the crush + exendin-4 group, compared with that in the crush group at 4 weeks after the crush. However, no interaction ($P = 0.148$) between the main effects of the nerve crush and exendin-4 administration was found. With regard to the distal latency, two-way ANOVA showed that the effects of nerve crush and exendin-4 administration were affected significantly ($P < 0.01$). Interaction between these two factors was significant ($P < 0.01$). The post hoc data showed that the distal latency in the crush group was significantly shorter than that in the crush + exendin-4 group ($P < 0.01$) (Table 1).

3.4. Wet Weight of TA. In the crush and crush + exendin-4 groups, the TAs on the injured side were atrophic, while the TAs on the uninjured side were normal. Two-way ANOVA indicated that the TA ratio (injured side/uninjured side) was affected by the effects of nerve crush ($P < 0.01$) but not affected by exendin-4 administration ($P = 0.23$). There was no interaction ($P = 0.06$) between these two effects (Table 2).

TABLE 1: Electrophysiological study at 4 weeks after crush ($n = 6$ in each group).

Group	CMAP Mean [SD] (mV)	Latency Mean [SD] (ms)
Crush	8.38 [2.43]	3.53 [0.31]
Crush + exendin-4	11.87 [1.56]	2.87 [0.46]**
Exendin-4	15.30 [4.69]	1.46 [0.10]**
Sham operation	16.22 [4.59]	1.45 [0.09]**

$^{**}P < 0.01$ compared with crush group.

TABLE 2: Weight ratio of the TA ($n = 12$ in each group).

Group	Ratio Mean [SD]
Crush	0.79 [0.05]
Crush + exendin-4	0.73 [0.09]
Exendin-4	1.01 [0.05]
Sham operation	1.02 [0.06]

3.5. Histological Studies of the Sciatic Nerve

3.5.1. Light Microscopic Studies. In the crush and crush + exendin-4 groups, degenerating debris and small axons with a thin myelin sheath were prominent at 4 weeks after surgery. In the crush + exendin-4 group, regenerating axons were more mature than those in the crush group. Specimens taken from the sham operation and exendin-4 groups showed dense axon populations with large axons and thick myelin sheaths. In the sham operation and exendin-4 groups, nerve pathology was normal (Figure 2(a)). A histogram of myelinated axon areas in the sham operation group showed a bimodal distribution: small fibers peak at 3.5 μm^2 and large fibers at 12.5 μm^2. In crush and crush + exendin-4 groups, the number of small fibers increased dramatically, resulting from regenerating fibers. Compared with the crush group, the peak of histogram in crush+exendin-4 group shifted to the right which indicates the maturation of regenerating fibers (Figure 2(b)). Analyses to examine the effects of nerve crush and exendin-4 administration on mean axon areas and mean axon numbers were conducted using two-way ANOVA. These results showed that nerve crush has significant effect on both mean axon areas and mean axon numbers ($P < 0.01$) but exendin-4 administration neither has effect on axon areas ($P = 0.849$) nor axon numbers ($P = 0.589$). The interaction between these two effects was significant on both axon areas ($P < 0.05$) and axon numbers ($P < 0.01$) (Table 3).

3.5.2. Electron Microscopic Studies. In both the crush and crush + exendin-4 groups, the thickness of the myelin sheath was thinner than that in the sham operation group. In the crush + exendin-4 group, the thickness of the myelin sheath was slightly greater than that in the crush group (Figure 3). Two-way ANOVA indicated that the g-ratio was affected by the effects of nerve crush ($P < 0.01$) but not affected by exendin-4 administration ($P = 0.71$). Interaction between these two factors was significant ($P < 0.05$) (Table 4).

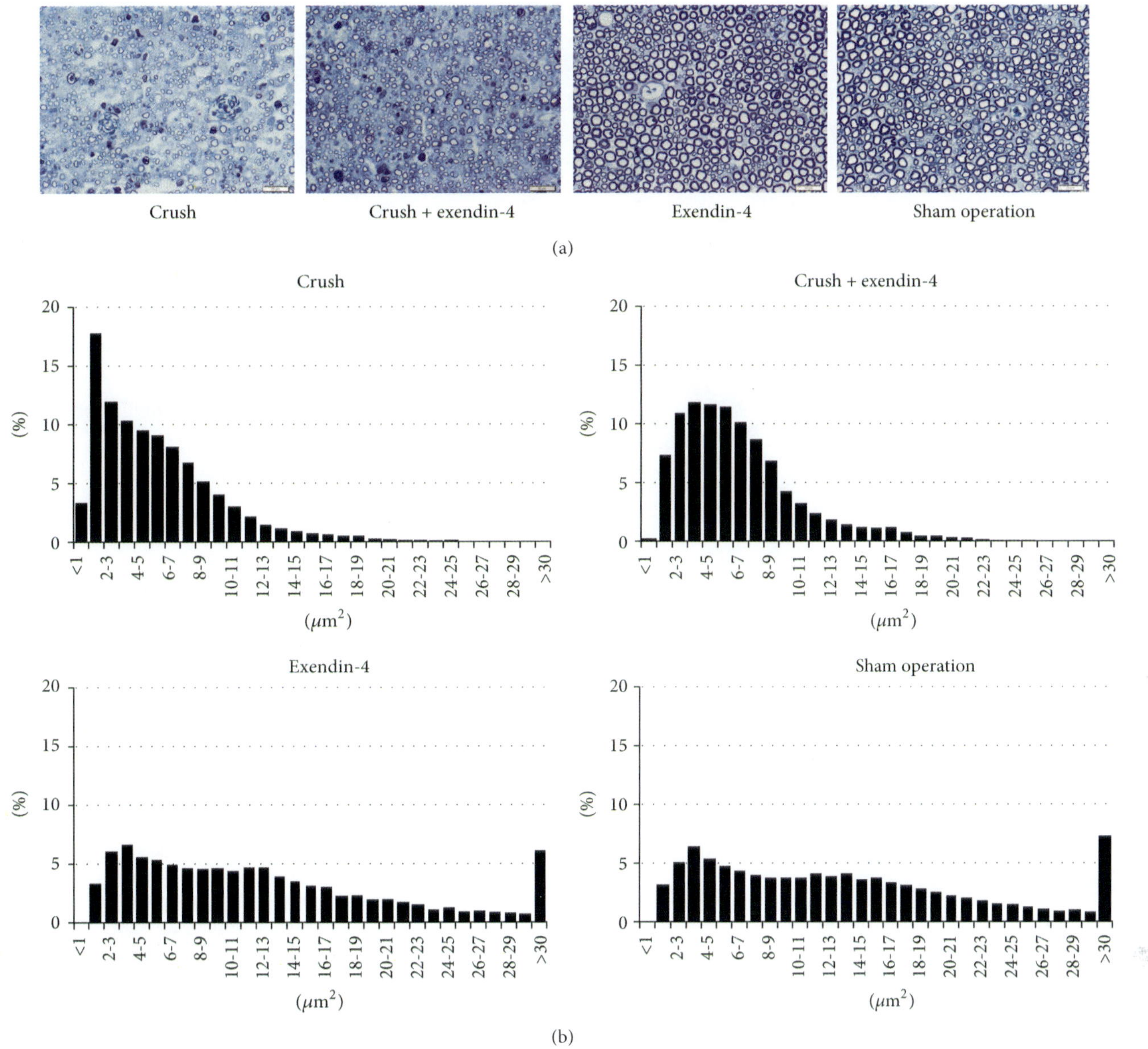

FIGURE 2: Light microscopic findings of the sciatic nerve. (a) Semi-thin transverse sections of myelinated axons of the sciatic nerve at 4 weeks postoperatively. In the crush + exendin-4 group, regenerating axons were more mature than those in the crush group. Scale bar: 20 μm. (b) Histograms of areas of myelinated axons ($n = 6$ in each group). Compared with the crush group, the peak of histogram in crush + exendin-4 group shifted to the right which indicates the maturation of regenerating fibers (Figure 2(b)).

4. Discussion

Exendin-4 is a good candidate as therapeutic agent that facilitates nerve regeneration because of the potency for both the central and peripheral nervous system [6, 8–10, 19] and has been used for patients with type 2 diabetes mellitus in clinical field. In this study, we examined whether exendin-4 can enhance functional and histological recovery after crush injury of the rat sciatic nerve.

We demonstrated that administration of exendin-4 was effective in the crush + exendin-4 group compared with the crush group. (1) The entire SFI curve was shifted to the left, which suggests facilitation of nerve regeneration. (2) In the electrophysiological study, shortening of the mean latency was demonstrated. (3) In light microscopic findings, nerve regeneration was enhanced by the administration of exendin-4 (4) The morphometrical findings of light microscopic study showed enhancement of nerve regeneration. (5) The g-ratio was significantly lower. Together, these results suggest that the administration of exendin-4 accelerated regeneration of the injured nerve and final functional recovery.

In the current study, we adopted the nerve crush model to evaluate the effectiveness of exendin-4. Since it represents an axonotmesis-type injury [20–22] in which the basal membrane of Schwann cells is maintained, it prevents misdirection, and functional recovery occurs relatively quickly.

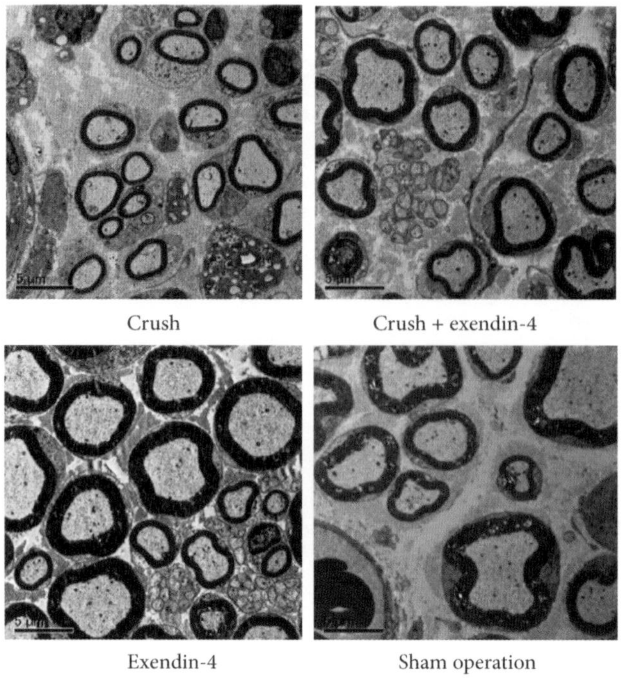

Figure 3: Electron microscopic findings of the sciatic nerve. Thin sections (60 nm in thickness) of sciatic nerve at 4 weeks postoperatively, stained with uranyl acetate and citrate. In the crush + exendin-4 group, the thickness of the myelin sheath was slightly greater than that in the crush group. Scale bar: 5 μm.

Table 3: Mean axon areas and numbers of myelinated axon at 4 weeks after nerve crush ($n = 6$ in each group).

Group	Axon area Mean [SD] (μm^2)	Axon number Mean [SD]
Crush	5.67 [0.72]	1950.6 [162.6]
Crush + exendin-4	6.57 [0.86]	1736.1 [203.1]
Exendin-4	12.77 [1.09]	1774.6 [114.2]
Sham operation	13.84 [1.22]	1611.5 [125.9]

Table 4: g-ratio of the right sciatic nerves ($n = 6$ in each group).

Group	g-ratio Mean [SD]
Crush	0.71 [0.01]
Crush + exendin-4	0.69 [0.02]
Exendin-4	0.64 [0.01]
Sham operation	0.63 [0.02]

In nerve transection models, it is difficult to obtain sufficient functional recovery within a year because of misdirection and chronic joint contracture [23].

The doses of exendin-4 vary among animal studies: 10 μg/mouse to reduce the size of cerebral infarction [24] and, 3.5 pM/kg/min for neuroprotection of peripheral nerves [5, 9, 10]. In this study, we administered 2.5 μg/rat/day exendin-4 for 14 days, which is the highest total dose compared with previous studies. Low-dose administrations of exendin-4 are effective mainly for chronic conditions such as Alzheimer's disease or DM neuropathy, while high-dose administration of exendin-4 is required in acute injury.

Exendin-4, a long-acting analogue of GLP-1, can improve hyperglycemic states [7] and can inhibit major complications of diabetes mellitus, such as neuropathy, nephropathy, or retinopathy [25–27]. In the present study, the levels of blood glucose were normal in all groups. Studies showed that the administration of exendin-4 exerted neuroprotection for peripheral sensory neuropathy induced by pyridoxine [9] and transient cerebral focal cerebral ischemia [24]. Jolivalt et al. [28] mentioned that exendin-4 could protect peripheral nerves by the GLP-1 receptor (GLP-1R) activation mediated by ERK signaling independent of glycemic control. Liu et al. [25] also noted that exendin-4 may prevent peripheral nerve degeneration by the activation of GLP-1R, antiapoptotic effects, and restoration of cyclic adenosine monophosphate content rather than an improvement of blood glucose.

In peripheral nerve regeneration, remyelination of the regenerated axons is required [29], and Schwann cells are responsible for the remyelination [30]. Previous studies demonstrated that GLP-1Rs were expressed in the Schwann cells of the sciatic nerve and activated by exendin-4 [25, 28]. These results suggest that, in the crushed nerve, exendin-4 encourages peripheral nerve regeneration through activation of Schwann cells mediated by GLP-1Rs.

In conclusion, repeated i.p. injections of exendin-4 can promote nerve regeneration and functional recovery after nerve crush injury. Therefore, exendin-4 is feasible for clinical application to treat peripheral nerve injury.

Abbreviations

GLP-1:	Glucagon-like peptide-1
GLP-1R:	Glucagon-like peptide-1 receptor
i.p.:	Intraperitoneal
TA:	Tibialis anterior muscle
SFI:	Sciatic functional index
CMAP:	Compound muscle action potential
ANOVA:	Analysis of variance.

Conflict of Interests

The authors declare that they have no conflict of interests.

Acknowledgments

The authors thank Ms. Y. Ichiki and Mr. H. Kasamatsu for their excellent technical assistance.

References

[1] J. Noble, C. A. Munro, V. S. S. V. Prasad, and R. Midha, "Analysis of upper and lower extremity peripheral nerve injuries in a population of patients with multiple injuries," *Journal of Trauma*, vol. 45, no. 1, pp. 116–122, 1998.

[2] T. J. Kieffer and J. F. Habener, "The glucagon-like peptides," *Endocrine Reviews*, vol. 20, no. 6, pp. 876–913, 1999.

[3] J. Eng, "Exendin peptides," *Mount Sinai Journal of Medicine*, vol. 59, no. 2, pp. 147–149, 1992.

[4] R. Goke, H.-C. Fehmann, T. Linn et al., "Exendin-4 is a high potency agonist and truncated exendin-(9–39)-amide an antagonist at the glucagon-like peptide 1-(7–36)-amide receptor of insulin-secreting β-cells," *The Journal of Biological Chemistry*, vol. 268, no. 26, pp. 19650–19655, 1993.

[5] T. Perry and N. H. Greig, "The glucagon-like peptides: a double-edged therapeutic sword?" *Trends in Pharmacological Sciences*, vol. 24, no. 7, pp. 377–383, 2003.

[6] G. Bertilsson, C. Patrone, O. Zachrisson et al., "Peptide hormone exendin-4 stimulates subventricular zone neurogenesis in the adult rodent brain and induces recovery in an animal model of Parkinson's disease," *Journal of Neuroscience Research*, vol. 86, no. 2, pp. 326–338, 2008.

[7] J. J. Holst, "Glucagon-like peptide-1: from extract to agent. The Claude Bernard Lecture, 2005," *Diabetologia*, vol. 49, no. 2, pp. 253–260, 2006.

[8] B. Martin, E. Golden, O. D. Carlson et al., "Exendin-4 improves glycemic control, ameliorates brain and pancreatic pathologies, and extends survival in a mouse model of huntington's disease," *Diabetes*, vol. 58, no. 2, pp. 318–328, 2009.

[9] T. Perry, H. W. Holloway, A. Weerasuriya et al., "Evidence of GLP-1-mediated neuroprotection in an animal model of pyridoxine-induced peripheral sensory neuropathy," *Experimental Neurology*, vol. 203, no. 2, pp. 293–301, 2007.

[10] T. Perry, D. K. Lahiri, D. Chen et al., "A novel neurotrophic property of glucagon-like peptide 1: a promoter of nerve growth factor-mediated differentiation in PC12 cells," *Journal of Pharmacology and Experimental Therapeutics*, vol. 300, no. 3, pp. 958–966, 2002.

[11] N. Kato, K. Nemoto, K. Nakanishi et al., "Nonviral HVJ (hemagglutinating virus of Japan) liposome-mediated retrograde gene transfer of human hepatocyte growth factor into rat nervous system promotes functional and histological recovery of the crushed nerve," *Neuroscience Research*, vol. 52, no. 4, pp. 299–310, 2005.

[12] M. Amako and K. Nemoto, "Influence of water immersion stress on peripheral nerve recovery in the rat," *Journal of Orthopaedic Science*, vol. 3, no. 1, pp. 32–41, 1998.

[13] J. R. Bain, S. E. Mackinnon, and D. A. Hunter, "Functional evaluation of complete sciatic, peroneal, and posterior tibial nerve lesions in the rat," *Plastic and Reconstructive Surgery*, vol. 83, no. 1, pp. 129–136, 1989.

[14] M. Ochi, M. Noda, K. Nakamitsu et al., "Promotion of sciatic nerve regeneration in rats by a new neurotrophic pyrimidine derivative MS-430," *General Pharmacology*, vol. 26, no. 1, pp. 59–64, 1995.

[15] S. Canan, H. H. Bozkurt, M. Acar et al., "An efficient stereological sampling approach for quantitative assessment of nerve regeneration," *Neuropathology and Applied Neurobiology*, vol. 34, no. 6, pp. 638–649, 2008.

[16] S. Kaplan, S. Geuna, G. Ronchi, M. B. Ulkay, and C. S. von Bartheld, "Calibration of the stereological estimation of the number of myelinated axons in the rat sciatic nerve: a multicenter study," *Journal of Neuroscience Methods*, vol. 187, no. 1, pp. 90–99, 2010.

[17] S. Kaplan, A. Pişkin, M. Ayyildiz et al., "The effect of melatonin and platelet gel on sciatic nerve repair: an electrophysiological and stereological study," *Microsurgery*, vol. 31, no. 4, pp. 306–313, 2011.

[18] J. Makoukji, M. Belle, D. Meffre et al., "Lithium enhances remyelination of peripheral nerves," *Proceedings of the National Academy of Sciences of the United States of America*, vol. 109, no. 10, pp. 3973–3978, 2012.

[19] C. Holscher, "Incretin analogues that have been developed to treat type 2 diabetes hold promise as a novel treatment strategy for Alzheimer's disease," *Recent Patents on CNS Drug Discovery*, vol. 5, no. 2, pp. 109–117, 2010.

[20] M. J. Buehler, A. V. Seaber, and J. R. Urbaniak, "The relationship of functional return to varying methods of nerve repair," *Journal of Reconstructive Microsurgery*, vol. 6, no. 1, pp. 61–69, 1990.

[21] L. De Medinaceli, W. J. Freed, and R. J. Wyatt, "An index of the functional condition of rat sciatic nerve based on measurements made from walking tracks," *Experimental Neurology*, vol. 77, no. 3, pp. 634–643, 1982.

[22] J. K. Terzis and K. J. Smith, "Repair of severed peripheral nerves: comparison of the 'de Medinaceli' and standard microsuture methods," *Experimental Neurology*, vol. 96, no. 3, pp. 672–680, 1987.

[23] G. M. T. Hare, P. J. Evans, S. E. Mackinnon et al., "Walking track analysis: a long-term assessment of peripheral nerve recovery," *Plastic and Reconstructive Surgery*, vol. 89, no. 2, pp. 251–258, 1992.

[24] S. Teramoto, N. Miyamoto, K. Yatomi et al., "Exendin-4, a glucagon-like peptide-1 receptor agonist, provides neuroprotection in mice transient focal cerebral ischemia," *Journal of Cerebral Blood Flow and Metabolism*, vol. 31, no. 8, pp. 1696–1705, 2011.

[25] W. J. Liu, H. Y. Jin, K. A. Lee, S. H. Xie, H. S. Baek, and T. S. Park, "Neuroprotective effect of the glucagon-like peptide-1 receptor agonist, synthetic exendin-4, in streptozotocin-induced diabetic rats," *British Journal of Pharmacology*, vol. 164, no. 5, pp. 1410–1420, 2011.

[26] C. W. Park, H. W. Kim, S. H. Ko et al., "Long-term treatment of glucagon-like peptide-1 analog exendin-4 ameliorates diabetic nephropathy through improving metabolic anomalies in *db/db* mice," *Journal of the American Society of Nephrology*, vol. 18, no. 4, pp. 1227–1238, 2007.

[27] Y. Zhang, Q. Wang, J. Zhang, X. Lei, G. Xu, and W. Ye, "Protection of exendin-4 analogue in early experimental diabetic retinopathy," *Graefe's Archive for Clinical and Experimental Ophthalmology*, vol. 247, no. 5, pp. 699–706, 2009.

[28] C. G. Jolivalt, M. Fineman, C. F. Deacon, R. D. Carr, and N. A. Calcutt, "GLP-1 signals via ERK in peripheral nerve and prevents nerve dysfunction in diabetic mice," *Diabetes, Obesity and Metabolism*, vol. 13, no. 11, pp. 990–1000, 2011.

[29] Z. Chen, W. Yu, and S. Strickland, "Peripheral regeneration," *Annual Review of Neuroscience*, vol. 30, pp. 209–233, 2007.

[30] B. Garbay, A. M. Heape, F. Sargueil, and C. Cassagne, "Myelin synthesis in the peripheral nervous system," *Progress in Neurobiology*, vol. 61, no. 3, pp. 267–304, 2000.

5

Protective Effect of Egyptian Propolis against Rabbit Pasteurellosis

Somia A. Nassar,[1] Amira H. Mohamed,[2] Hamdy Soufy,[1] and Soad M. Nasr[1]

[1] *Department of Parasitology and Animal Diseases, National Research Center, El-Behouse Street, Dokki, P.O. Box 12622, Giza, Egypt*
[2] *Department of Clinical Pathology, Faculty of Veterinary Medicine, Cairo University, P.O. Box 12211, Giza, Egypt*

Correspondence should be addressed to Soad M. Nasr; soadnasr@yahoo.com

Academic Editor: Stelvio M. Bandiera

The present study was conducted to study the protective effect of ethanolic extract of propolis given subcutaneously (S/C) either alone or in combination with inactivated formalized *Pasteurella multocida* (*P. multocida*) vaccine in rabbits challenged with virulent *P. multocida* strain. Twenty-eight New-Zealand rabbits, 6–8 weeks old and not vaccinated against pasteurellosis, were randomly divided into four equal groups. Group (1) was kept as nonvaccinated control. Group (2) was injected S/C with propolis. Group (3) was vaccinated (S/C) with *P. multocida* vaccine only. Group (4) was injected with vaccine mixed with propolis as adjuvant. Groups (2, 3, and 4) received the same doses of propolis and vaccine after 4 weeks as a booster dose. The experiment continued for six weeks during which clinical signs, body weight, and mortality rate were recorded. Blood samples were collected every 2 weeks of treatment for evaluating the erythrogram and biochemical parameters. At the end of six weeks, all groups were subjected to challenge with a virulent strain of *P. multocida*. Two weeks later, tissue specimens were collected from different organs for histopathological investigation. Results showed that before challenge all rabbits of different groups were apparently healthy and had good appetite. After challenge, control group (1) showed acute form of the disease, 100% mortality rate, and severe histopathological changes. Rabbits of groups (2 and 3) showed less severe clinical signs, mortality rate, and histopathological changes than control. Rabbits of group (4) were apparently healthy with normal histological picture. In conclusion, an ethanolic extract of propolis injected alone or combined with formalized inactivated *P. multocida* vaccine improved general health conditions, liver and kidney functions in addition to reduction of the severity of adverse clinical signs, mortality rates, and histopathological changes associated with challenge of rabbits with *P. multocida* strain.

1. Introduction

One of the most important health problems in rabbit is pasteurellosis, which is considered as a common bacterial disease caused by *Pasteurella multocida* (*P. multocida*) and has been reported as a constant serious and highly contagious disease of domestic rabbits [1].

Rabbit pasteurellosis causes symptoms that range from fatal septicemia, severe pleuritis, and pneumonia to less severe sequelae such as multiple abscesses, chronic rhinitis, and otitis media [2]. It mostly affects rabbits at 4–8 weeks of age. Rabbits older than 8 months to 1 year of age showed lower incidence [3].

Pasteurellosis exhibited 3 forms in rabbits. The first one is snuffles or nasal catarrhal inflammation which is characterized by acute, subacute, and chronic inflammation of the air passages and lungs. This form of the disease often ends with death and the cured animals became carriers. The second form is characterized by abscess formation at any part of the body and the case is terminated with septicemia. The last form is characterized by genital infection, which manifests as acute and subacute inflammation of uterus and testicles. Also, rhinitis is the most common clinical manifestation in rabbit pasteurellosis [4–6].

Propolis is a resinous hive product collected by honey bees from exudates and buds of plants and mixed with wax and bee enzymes [7]. Hegazi et al. [8] recorded that the chemical composition of raw Egyptian propolis sample (collected from Dakahlia Governorate) as investigated by GC/MS, 65 compounds were identified, such as aromatic acids: benzoic, cinnamic, trans-p-coumaric, 3,4-dimethoxycinnamic, ferulic, and caffeic acids. Of the 19 esters identified, Egyptian propolis contained 11 caffeate esters including two new to propolis, tetradecenyl caffeate (isomer) and tetradecanyl caffeate. Egyptian propolis contained some new triterpenoids including lupeol and alpha-amyrin. It also contained flavonoids, sugar, and aliphatic acids. The investigators stated that Dakahlia propolis sample was a typical popular propolis. The composition of the propolis depends upon the time, vegetation, and the area of collection [9].

Propolis has several biological and pharmacological properties, as antimicrobial [10], anti-inflammatory [11], antioxidant [12–15], antiparasitic [16], immune modularity and immune stimulant effects and it increased the percentage of protected animals suggesting its use in vaccines as an adjuvant [17, 18].

A reasonable approach to control and eliminate pasteurellosis in rabbits is to develop an improved vaccine as the current experimental vaccines do not provide a complete protection [19].

Therefore, the present work was adopted to evaluate the protective effect of an ethanolic extract of Egyptian propolis when injected S/C alone or in combination with inactivated *P. multocida* vaccine against experimental challenge of rabbits with *P. multocida* strain. The study was based on hematological, biochemical, and histopathological investigations.

2. Materials and Methods

This study was carried out according to guidelines for animal experimentation and approved by the Institutional Animal Care and Use Committee, National Research Centre Animal Care Unit, Dokki, Giza, Egypt.

2.1. Animal Used. Twenty-eight male New-Zealand rabbits of 1.5–2 kg body weight and 6–8 weeks old were used in this experiment. Rabbits were not previously vaccinated against pasteurellosis, and bacteriological examination of nasopharyngeal swabs proved that they were free from Pasteurella infection.

2.2. Extraction of Propolis. One hundred grams of the resinous material of Egyptian propolis (obtained from Dakahlia Governorate, Egypt) was cut into small pieces and extracted at room temperature with 50 mL of 70% ethanol. Extraction was performed twice with 24 hours interval. The alcoholic extract was evaporated under vacuum at 50°C until dryness. Obtained dried ethanolic extract of propolis (28 g) was suspended in phosphate buffered saline (PBS) (pH 7.2) [8]. The dose of propolis used in this experiment was 50 mg/kg BW [20].

2.3. Experimental Design. The experiment was carried out at the Experimental Rabbit Unit of Lab Animal House, National Research Center, Dokki, Giza, Egypt. Rabbits were housed in separate cages, fed on a balanced commercial ration, and water was available *ad libitum*. The animals were assigned into four equal groups which were treated with alcoholic extract of propolis alone or in combination with *P. multocida* inactivated vaccine (obtained from Veterinary Serum and Vaccine Research Institute, Abbasia, Cairo). Propolis was administrated subcutaneously (S/C) (a single dose of 50 mg/kg B.W.). The vaccine was given as a single S/C dose of 2 mL. Treatment of different rabbit groups was as follows: group (1) was injected S/C with 2 mL sterile phosphate buffer saline solution (PBS) and was kept as normal control, group (2) was injected S/C with a single dose of propolis, group (3) was vaccinated with *P. multocida* vaccine only, and group (4) was injected S/C with the vaccine mixed with propolis as an adjuvant. Treatments of propolis and vaccine were repeated as a booster dose after four weeks in all groups. The experiment continued for 6 weeks, at the end of which challenge was performed by injection with virulent strain of *P. multocida*. The strain was obtained from Veterinary Serum and Vaccine Research Institute, Abbasia, Cairo, in the form of lyophilized ampoules. It was activated by culturing in nutrient broth, inoculation in Swiss mice, and reisolation of the organism from heart blood of mice on nutrient agar plates (Difco). Pasteurella colonies were suspended in sterile saline, and the density was adjusted to contain 5×10^9 bacterial cell/mL. The suspension was used for S/C inoculation of rabbits in the challenge test [21].

2.4. Erythrogram and Biochemical Analysis. During the 6 weeks experimentation time, rabbits were weighed and blood samples were collected every 2 weeks. Two blood samples were obtained from the ear vein of each rabbit. The first sample was anticoagulated and used for the determination of the erythrocytes count, packed cell volume, hemoglobin concentration, and red cell indices by using Coulter (MEDONIC CA620). The second sample was collected for serum separation and determination of serum biochemical constituents. The activities of aspartate aminotransferase (AST) and alanine aminotransferase (ALT) [22] and alkaline phosphatase [23] were determined. The concentration of urea [24] and creatinine [25] was estimated. Test kits supplied by bioMérieux-France were used.

2.5. Challenge Test and Pathological Studies. At the end of the experiment (6th week), experimental rabbits were challenged by S/C injection of 0.2 mL/rabbit of broth culture of virulent *P. multocida*. Re isolation and identification of *Pasteurella* organisms were done from the heart blood of rabbits died after challenge [21]. Two weeks later after challenge, *Postmortem* findings were detected, and tissue specimens from heart, trachea, lungs, liver, kidneys, and spleen were collected from dead and sacrificed animals, fixed in 10% formol saline, dehydrated, cleared, and embedded in paraffin blocks. Paraffin sections of $5\,\mu$ thickness were prepared, stained by H&E, and examined microscopically for detection of histopathological alterations [26].

2.6. Statistical Analysis. All data were subjected to statistical analysis including the calculation of the mean and standard error. Differences between control and treated groups were tested for significance using a one-way analysis of variance followed by Duncan's multiple range test. Differences were

Table 1: Erythrogram in different experimental groups of rabbits before and after treatment for six weeks (Mean ± SE, $N = 5$).

Parameters	Periods (week)	G1 Control	G2 Propolis S/C	G3 Vaccine S/C only	G4 Propolis + Vaccine S/C	Sig.
RBCs count ($\times 10^6/\mu L$)	0	5.73 ± 0.31	5.73 ± 0.31	5.47 ± 0.35	5.27 ± 0.21	NS
	2	5.38 ± 0.16	5.56 ± 0.17	5.16 ± 0.14	5.46 ± 0.34	NS
	4	5.84 ± 0.33	5.75 ± 0.28	5.04 ± 0.16	5.81 ± 0.33	NS
	6	6.35 ± 0.18^a	5.42 ± 0.25^{ab}	4.93 ± 0.45^b	5.42 ± 0.20^{ab}	*
Packed cell volume (PCV) (%)	0	34.24 ± 1.82	34.24 ± 1.82	33.84 ± 1.89	30.17 ± 0.90	NS
	2	32.30 ± 0.90	33.12 ± 0.52	30.48 ± 0.78	30.92 ± 1.63	NS
	4	32.54 ± 1.54	34.36 ± 1.68	31.25 ± 1.27	33.84 ± 1.69	NS
	6	34.55 ± 0.53^a	33.45 ± 1.16^a	29.64 ± 2.51^c	31.28 ± 1.37^b	*
Hemoglobin (g/dL)	0	11.78 ± 0.67	11.78 ± 0.67	10.92 ± 0.56	10.37 ± 0.31	NS
	2	11.24 ± 0.30	11.32 ± 0.15	10.58 ± 0.30	10.84 ± 0.60	NS
	4	10.88 ± 0.47	11.46 ± 0.60	10.40 ± 0.46	11.26 ± 0.41	NS
	6	11.60 ± 0.18	11.33 ± 0.34	10.24 ± 0.91	11.74 ± 0.57	NS
Mean corpuscular volume (MCV) (fl)	0	59.80 ± 0.82	59.80 ± 0.82	63.80 ± 3.36	57.47 ± 0.72	NS
	2	60.12 ± 0.95	59.66 ± 1.58	59.13 ± 1.23	56.78 ± 1.10	NS
	4	59.94 ± 0.92^b	59.74 ± 0.77^b	61.98 ± 1.04^a	58.32 ± 1.20^b	*
	6	58.63 ± 2.20^b	59.28 ± 1.41^b	62.18 ± 0.78^a	60.08 ± 1.37^b	*
Mean corpuscular hemoglobin (MCH) (pg)	0	20.52 ± 0.15	20.52 ± 0.15	20.60 ± 0.56	19.73 ± 0.21	NS
	2	20.90 ± 0.26	20.38 ± 0.32	20.55 ± 0.40	19.94 ± 0.37	NS
	4	20.10 ± 0.46	19.96 ± 0.33	20.60 ± 0.31	19.48 ± 0.85	NS
	6	19.35 ± 0.35	20.08 ± 0.55	20.88 ± 0.24	20.71 ± 0.84	NS
Mean corpuscular hemoglobin concentration (MCHC) (g/dL)	0	34.36 ± 0.37	34.36 ± 0.37	32.46 ± 1.00	34.30 ± 0.22	NS
	2	34.82 ± 0.36	36.04 ± 1.86	34.73 ± 0.14	35.08 ± 0.17	NS
	4	33.52 ± 0.33	33.38 ± 0.21	33.25 ± 0.47	33.38 ± 0.84	NS
	6	33.57 ± 0.07	33.88 ± 0.22	34.49 ± 0.18	34.24± 0.40^a	NS

Means with different superscripts in the same row are significantly different at $P < 0.05$. $^*P < 0.05$, NS: non-significant.

considered significant at $P < 0.05$ level [27] using SPSS version 10 computer programme.

3. Results

3.1. Clinical Signs. Along the experimental period before challenge, all rabbits of different groups were apparently healthy and had good appetite. During the 1st day after challenge of rabbits with *P. multocida* strain, rabbits of control group (1) showed acute form of the disease (depression, sneezing, and respiratory manifestations), while some of them showed nervous symptoms and sudden death. Rabbits of groups (2) and (3) showed less severe clinical signs than control group. Some rabbits of group (3) showed superficial multiple abscesses as a chronic form of the disease. Rabbits of group (4) were apparently healthy till time of scarification at the end of the experimental (15 days after challenge (dpc)).

3.2. Mortality Rate. No mortalities were observed in group (4) that administrated propolis with vaccine. Mortalities in group (3) (vaccinated only) represented 28.57% after challenge, but in group (2) (administrated propolis only), mortalities were about 57.14%, while mortalities in control group (1) were about 100%. Most of the mortalities occurred during the 2 dpc.

3.3. Body Weight. No significant changes were demonstrated in the values of body weight of different experimental rabbit groups along the period of the treatment.

3.4. Erythrogram. At the 6th week of treatment, there was a significant decrease in RBCs count and PCV% values, while MCV values exhibited increase in rabbits given vaccine only (group 3) compared to control group (1). Along the period of treatment, no significant changes were demonstrated in the values of Hb content, MCH, and MCHC (Table 1).

3.5. Serum Biochemistry. Compared to control group, the activity of AST and ALT significantly increased at the 2nd and 4th weeks in group (3), while markedly decreased in the other treated groups all over the experimental period. Changes in ALP activity were less marked in different experimental groups (Table 2).

Table 2: Serum enzymes activities and serum creatinine and urea levels in different experimental groups of rabbits before and after treatment for six weeks (Mean ± SE, $N = 5$).

Parameters	Periods (week)	Groups G1 Control	G2 Propolis S/C	G3 Vaccine S/C only	G4 Propolis + vaccine S/C	Sig.
Aspartate amino transferase (IU/L)	0	48.46 ± 2.40	48.69 ± 0.36	47.39 ± 1.20	49.42 ± 2.90	NS
	2	49.71 ± 2.94^{b}	40.96 ± 0.46^{c}	60.73 ± 2.29^{a}	49.11 ± 0.74^{b}	*
	4	48.90 ± 0.01^{b}	44.41 ± 1.00^{c}	66.86 ± 2.40^{a}	43.45 ± 0.49^{c}	*
	6	51.26 ± 1.87^{a}	43.13 ± 1.47^{c}	50.35 ± 1.90^{ab}	41.16 ± 0.83^{c}	*
Alanine amino transferase (IU/L)	0	54.79 ± 0.82	54.90 ± 3.36	55.70 ± 1.68	56.37 ± 3.26	NS
	2	51.91 ± 0.46^{b}	47.60 ± 4.23^{c}	60.45 ± 0.57^{a}	45.40 ± 3.80^{c}	*
	4	41.24 ± 3.94^{c}	47.47 ± 3.09^{b}	55.68 ± 1.24^{a}	39.28 ± 1.50^{c}	*
	6	53.07 ± 1.23^{a}	40.27 ± 1.91^{c}	47.25 ± 2.75^{b}	39.28 ± 1.50^{c}	*
Alkaline phosphatase (IU/L)	0	15.74 ± 1.23	15.59 ± 2.06	16.67 ± 1.09	16.46 ± 0.17	NS
	2	16.87 ± 1.02^{a}	15.03 ± 0.29^{ab}	17.59 ± 0.70^{a}	16.39 ± 1.11^{a}	NS
	4	15.55 ± 1.35^{b}	14.87 ± 1.55^{b}	20.14 ± 1.17^{a}	15.91 ± 0.90^{b}	*
	6	15.15 ± 0.83	13.43 ± 0.94	15.83 ± 1.00	14.49 ± 0.52	NS
Creatinine (mg/dL)	0	1.37 ± 0.05	1.68 ± 0.04	1.80 ± 0.12	1.68 ± 0.07	NS
	2	1.17 ± 0.08^{b}	0.91 ± 0.04^{b}	1.42 ± 0.01^{a}	0.87 ± 0.04^{b}	*
	4	1.07 ± 0.03^{b}	0.76 ± 0.03^{c}	1.39 ± 0.04^{a}	0.76 ± 0.05^{c}	*
	6	1.22 ± 0.27^{a}	0.61 ± 0.03^{b}	1.24 ± 0.02^{a}	0.60 ± 0.03^{b}	*
Urea (mg/dL)	0	35.56 ± 1.86	35.60 ± 1.81	33.22 ± 1.47	36.13 ± 2.09	NS
	2	39.02 ± 1.54^{a}	27.14 ± 1.54^{d}	35.37 ± 0.97^{b}	31.11 ± 1.42^{c}	*
	4	39.85 ± 2.21^{a}	24.29 ± 1.06^{c}	32.75 ± 1.67^{b}	29.94 ± 1.22^{b}	*
	6	38.15 ± 1.49^{a}	24.23 ± 1.05^{c}	40.14 ± 0.82^{a}	33.25 ± 1.43^{b}	*

Means with different superscripts in the same row are significantly different at $P < 0.05$. $^{*}P < 0.05$. NS: nonsignificant.

Serum creatinine and urea levels showed significant decrease throughout the experiment in groups (2) and (4). While group (3) demonstrated significant increase in creatinine level all over the experimental time compared to control group (Table 2).

3.6. Pathological Findings

3.6.1. Postmortem Examination. Rabbits of control group (1) challenged with *P. multocida* strain showed severe acute form of pasteurellosis. After challenge, rabbits demonstrated severe rhinitis with nasal discharge, congested blood vessels with S/C hemorrhage, presence of blood in thorax and abdomen with severe congestion of trachea, lungs and heart. After 40 hours post challenge rabbits showed congested heart accompanied with enlarged and congested S/C blood vessels, necrotic foci in the liver, brown peritoneum, congested friable kidneys, and dark brown with normal size spleen. Trachea, lungs, and heart were congested, hyperemic and filled with blood. Rabbits administrated propolis only (group 2) showed first deaths after 24 hours after challenge and characterized by sneezing, S/C hyperemic patches, congested heart, trachea and lungs with patches, enlarged and patched liver with necrotic foci, and congested and enlarged spleen. Rabbits administered the vaccine only (group 3) showed less incidence of the disease after challenge represented by presence of multiple lung abscesses, congestion and darkness of the lung and when cut oozing blood, enlarged aorta, and urinary bladder was distended and filled with urine and salts.

Rabbits administered propolis and vaccine (group 4) resisted challenge and were apparently healthy with normal liver, spleen, and heart when scarified at 15 dpc, but some of them showed multiple S/C abscesses in front leg and neck.

3.6.2. Histopathological Findings. Heart of rabbits from different experimental groups, before challenge, showed normal cardiac tissue. Heart of rabbit from group (1) challenged with *P. multocida* strain, that died within one dpc, showed edema in the pericardium which was infiltrated with inflammatory cells that extended to the myocardium (Figure 1(a)). Heart of rabbit from group (2) that died within 2 dpc showed hydropericardium and hemorrhage between the myocardium muscles (Figure 1(b)). Sections of heart from group (3) and (4) of rabbits, which were sacrificed 15 dpc, showed normal myocardial muscle (Figure 1(c)).

Sections of trachea from rabbits of group (1) which died within 1 dpc showed hyperplasia in the lamina epithelialis and leukocytic infiltration in the lamina propia and submucosa (Figure 2(a)), in addition to marked submucosal edema accompanied with marked congestion of vessels. Trachea from rabbits of group (2), that died 2 dpc, showed

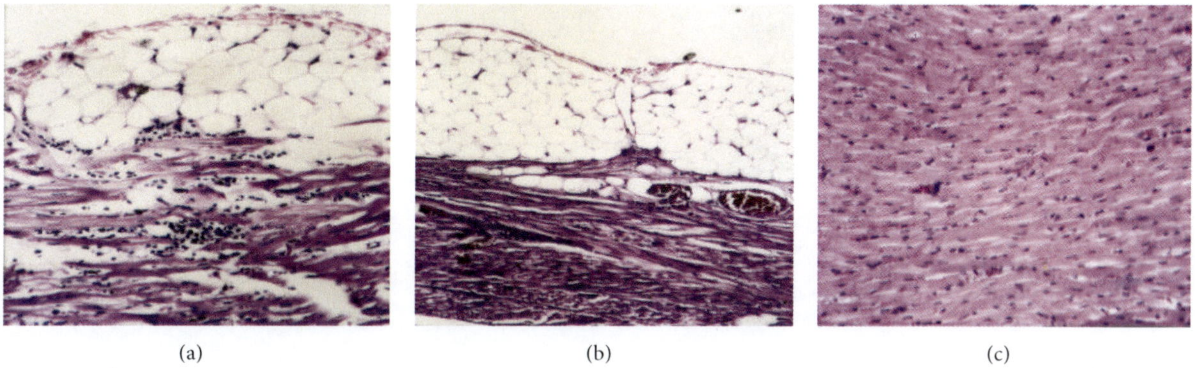

FIGURE 1: Histopathological changes in the heart of rabbits from different experimental groups. (a) Heart from group (1) rabbits (36 hr pc) showing edema in the pericardium infiltrated with inflammatory cells that extend to the myocardium (H & E ×200). (b) Heart from group (2) rabbits (2 dpc) showing hydropericardium and hemorrhage between the myocardium muscles (H & E ×100). (c) Heart from group (3) rabbits (15 dpc) showing normal myocardial muscle (H & E ×200).

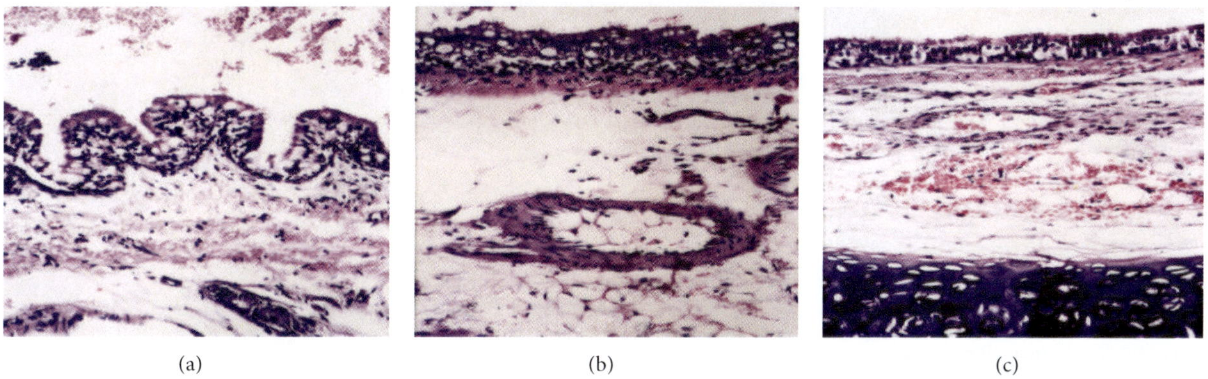

FIGURE 2: Histopathological changes in the trachea from different experimental groups. (a) Trachea from group (1) rabbits (1 dpc) showing hyperplasia in the lamina epithelialis and leukocytic infiltration in the lamina propia and submucosa. (b) Trachea from group (2) rabbits (2 dpc) showing degenerated mucosa infiltrated with inflammatory cells and edemated submucosa with congestion. (c) Trachea from group (3) rabbits (15 dpc) showing normal mucosa and submucosal edema, hemorrhage, and mononuclear cell infiltration (H & E ×200).

degenerated mucosa infiltrated with inflammatory cells and edemated submucosa with congestion (Figure 2(b)). Trachea of rabbits from group (3), which were sacrificed 15 dpc, showed normal mucosa and submucosal edema, hemorrhage, and mononuclear cell infiltration (Figure 2(c)). Trachea of rabbits from group (4), which were sacrificed 15dpc showed normal mucosa with mild edema in the submucosa.

Microscopical examination of lung from group (1) before challenge showed normal histological structure. After challenge, the lungs showed peribronchitis, severely congested vessels with vasculitis, and marked alveolar collapse. Moreover, diffused interstitial inflammatory reaction and giant alveoli were observed (Figure 3(a)). Also edema in the plural sac was noticed. Lung of group (2) after challenge showed chronic venous congestion in the lung tissue (Figure 3(b)), while lungs of group (3) showed vasculitis and mild interstitial inflammatory reaction (Figure 3(c)). Sections from lungs of group (4) which were sacrificed 15dpc showed normal lung tissue.

Microscopical examination of liver from group (1) before challenge revealed normal histology of hepatic lobules. After challenge, the liver showed marked portal tract changes in the form of hyperplasia, congested vessels, newly formed bile ductules, and leukocytic infiltration (Figure 4(a)). Liver of rabbits from group (2), which died after challenge, showed focal scattered necrotic nodules infiltrated with leukocytes (Figure 4(b)) and mild bile duct hyperplasia, mild congestion, and mild inflammatory reaction (Figure 4(c)), but liver of rabbits from group (3) 15 dpc showed normal portal area. Sections from liver of group (4) which were sacrificed 15 dpc showed normal hepatic tissue.

Microscopical examination of kidney from group (1) before challenge showed normal renal tissue, while after challenge the kidney showed congestion in the interstitial blood vessels and glomerular capillaries (Figure 5(a)), in addition to degenerated tubules with formation of renal hyaline cast (Figure 5(b)). Kidneys from group (2) after challenge showed severe vacuolation in the tubules and glomerular tuft (Figure 5(c)). Kidneys from group (3) showed mild vacculation in the tubules and glomerular tafft (Figure 5(d)). Kidneys from group (4) which were sacrificed 15 dpc showed normal renal tissue.

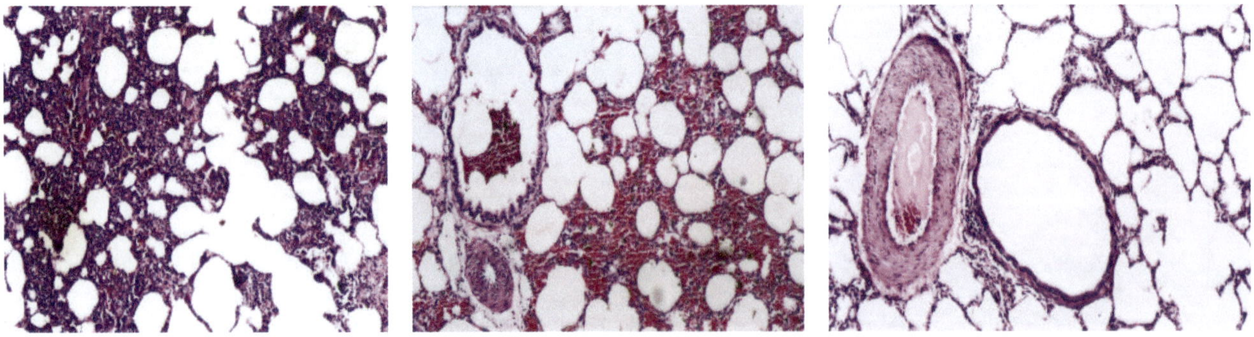

(a) (b) (c)

Figure 3: Histopathological changes in the lung from different experimental groups (a) Lung from group (1) rabbits (1 dpc) showing diffused interstitial inflammatory reaction and giant alveoli. (b) Lung from group (2) rabbits (15 dpc) showing chronic venous congestion in the lung tissue. (c) Lung from group (3) rabbits (15 dpc) showing vasculitis and mild interstitial inflammatory reaction (H & E ×100).

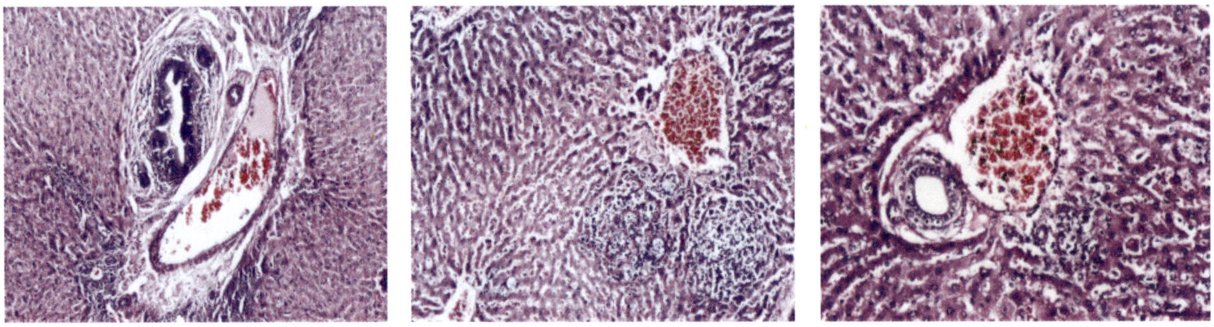

(a) (b) (c)

Figure 4: Histopathological changes in the liver from different experimental groups (a) Liver from group (1) rabbits (2 dpc) showing marked portal tract changes in the form of hyperplastic bile duct, congested vessels, newly formed bile ductules, and leukocytic infiltration (H & E ×100). (b) Liver from group (2) rabbits (7 dpc) showing focal scattered necrotic nodules infiltrated with leukocytes (H & E ×100). (c) Liver from group (2) rabbits (15 dpc) showing mild bile duct hyperplasia, mild congestion, and mild inflammatory reaction (H & E ×200).

Microscopical examination of spleen from group (1) before challenge showed normal lymphoid follicles; in contrast after challenge spleen showed depletion in the lymphoid follicles (Figure 6(a)). In group (2), there was hemorrhage in between the lymphoid follicles at 2 dpc (Figure 6(b)). Spleen from group (3) showed atrophied follicles (Figure 6(c)). Spleen from group (4) which was sacrificed 15 dpc showed normal splenic follicles.

4. Discussion

The present experiment was conducted to study the effect of an ethanolic extract of propolis given by S/C injection either alone or in combination with inactivated formalized *P. multocida* vaccine on general performance, erythrogram, biochemical parameters, and pathological lesions induced by challenge of rabbits with virulent *P. multocida* strain at the end of the experiment.

The symptoms which were observed within one dpc of group (1) with *P. multocida* strain ranged from severe acute to subacute forms of the disease. Signs of septicemia, acute rhinitis, sneezing, bronchopneumonia, and conjunctivitis and abscess formation agreed with that reported by [1, 2, 28]. These signs were confirmed by macroscopic and microscopic examination of different organs of rabbits of group (1) after challenge. Less severe symptoms observed in group (2) may be due to the effect of propolis as antibacterial, anti-inflammatory, and immunomodularity agent and increase the antibody production [19, 29, 30]. In addition, propolis has broad activities against *P. multocida in vitro* and *in vivo* (in the tracheal region of the rabbits) [31]. The chronic form of pasteurellosis, superficial multiple abscesses observed in group (3) may be due to that inactivated vaccine enhance mainly humeral immunity response and immunoglobulins (Ig) level specially IgG [19, 32, 33]. These results were confirmed by the normal microscopic structure of spleen tissue after challenge. Absence of clinical signs in group (4) may be attributed to the synergetic protective effect of both propolis and vaccine. These results agreed with the normal histological structure of different organs in this group.

Mortality rate was 100% in group (1), 57.14% in group (2), and about 28.57% in group (3). Mortality in group (1) may be due to severe septicemia and bronchopneumonia [5, 34], while lower mortalities in group (2) may be attributed to the antibacterial, anti-inflammatory, immune stimulant, and immune modularity effects of propolis [19, 35]. Good

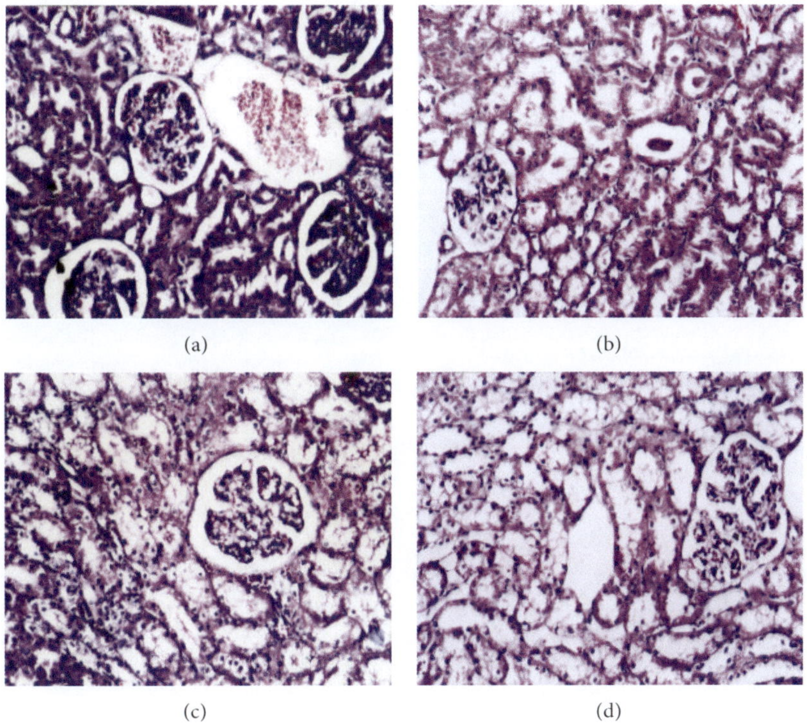

FIGURE 5: Histopathological changes in the kidney from different experimental groups. (a) Kidney from group (1) rabbits (1 dpc) showing congestion in the interstitial blood vessels and glomerular capillaries. (b) Kidney from group (1) rabbits (2 dpc) showing degenerated tubules with formation of renal hyaline casts. (c) Kidney from group (2) rabbits (15 dpc) showing severe vacuolation in the tubules and glomerular tuft. (d) Kidney from group (3) rabbits (15 dpc) showing mild vacuolation in the tubules and glomerular tuft (H & E ×200).

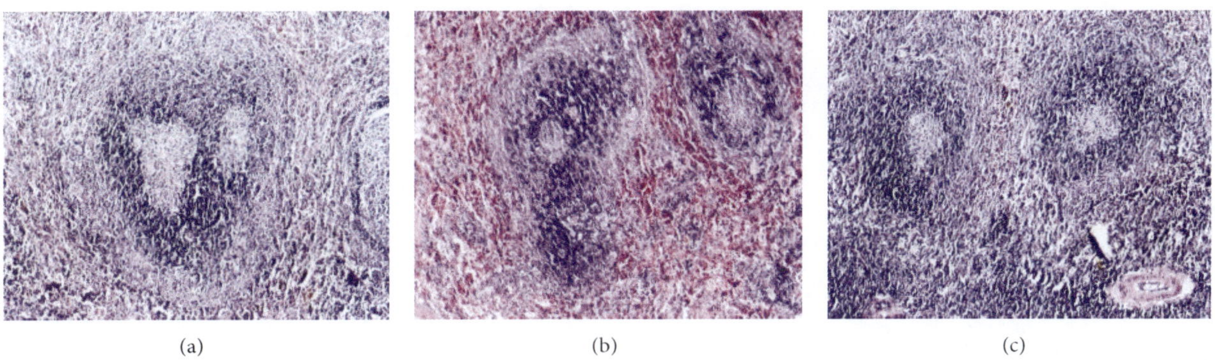

FIGURE 6: Histopathological changes in the spleen from different experimental groups. (a) Spleen from group (1) rabbits (2 dpc) showing depletion in the lymphoid follicles. (b) Spleen from group (2) rabbits (2 dpc) showing hemorrhage between the lymphoid follicles. (c) Spleen from group (3) rabbits (15 dpc) showing atrophied follicles (H & E ×100).

protection in group (3) may be attributed to good antibody response and protection induced by the vaccine against experimental challenge with *P. multocida* [19, 36, 37].

Results of body weight showed no significant difference between all groups along the experimental period.

Results of erythrogram revealed significant decrease in RBCs count, PCV in group (3) which may be due to the cytotoxic effect of vaccine causing inhibition of erythropoiesis [38]. These results agreed with [39].

Regarding serum enzyme activities, AST showed significant gradual decrease in different groups along the period of experiment except group (3) in comparison with control group. This result agreed with Talas and Gulhan [40]. Administration of propolis to rats at a dose of 150–1500 mg/kg BW caused slight inhibition in the activity of aminotransferase enzymes [41]. The demonstrated result in the present study revealed that administration of propolis had no toxic effect on rabbit. A significant decrease in serum ALT level was observed in propolis-treated groups; similar result was observed by Eraslan et al. [42]. No alterations in the activity of AST and ALT in serum of rabbits treated with crude propolis extract [43]. The level of ALP was decreased in group administrated propolis compared to the control group. This decrease may be due to the action of propolis as reducing agent to ALP. These results agreed with Eraslan et al. [42]. Results of liver enzymes activities support that propolis is able to induce hepatoprotective effects which are similar to those of the previous work on propolis that act as hepatoprotective against d-galactosamine, and paracetamol induced liver damage in rats and mice, respectively [44, 45]. The present results were confirmed by absence of histopathological changes in livers of groups (2) and (4) in comparison with liver of control group.

Results of serum creatinine and urea revealed significant decrease in groups (2 and 4) compared to control group. Similar results were recorded by Sforcin et al. [46]. They found that propolis did not induce kidney damage in rats as demonstrated by normal levels of urea and creatinine.

5. Conclusion

ethanolic extract of propolis injected S/C alone or combined with formalized inactivated *P. multocida* vaccine improved general health conditions, liver and kidney functions in addition to reduction of the severity of adverse clinical signs, mortality rates, and histopathological changes associated with challenge of rabbits with *P. multocida strain*.

Conflict of Interests

The authors have declared that there is no conflict of interests and there is not any fund for their research.

Acknowledgment

The authors would like to thank Dr. Emad H. Mohamed for his cooperation and help during this work.

References

[1] J. F. Gracy, "Infection of rabbits and horses," in *Meat Hygiene*, pp. 482–486, Bailliere Tindall, East Sussex, UK, 8th edition, 1986.

[2] D. H. Percy, J. F. Prescott, and J. L. Bhasin, "Inactivated bacterial antigen were complemented with adjuvents in order to increase the immunogenicity of the vaccines," *Journal of Complementary Medicine*, vol. 46, pp. 227–229, 1985.

[3] M. El-Ghawy, *The bacteriological flora of respiratory tract of rabbits in health and disease [M.S. thesis Bacteriology]*, Faculty Veterinary Medicine, Cairo University, 1972.

[4] A. Y. E. Elham, *Bacteriological studies on Pasteurella infection in rabbits in Kalubia Governorate [M.S. thesis]*, Faculty Veterinary Medicine, Banha Branch, Zgzig University, 1972.

[5] T. E. Zimmerman, B. J. Deeb, and R. F. DiGiacomo, "Polypeptides associated with *Pasteurella multocida* infection in rabbits," *The American Journal of Veterinary Research*, vol. 53, no. 7, pp. 1108–1112, 1992.

[6] J. Sandford, *Domestic Rabbit*, Granada Publishing, London, UK, 5th edition, 1996.

[7] G. A. Burdock, "Review of the biological properties and toxicity of bee propolis (propolis)," *Food and Chemical Toxicology*, vol. 36, no. 4, pp. 347–363, 1998.

[8] A. G. Hegazi, F. K. Abd El Hady, F. A. El Menway, and H. Al Mehdar, "Egyptian propolis: 5 influence of propolis adminestration on some chicken biochemical parameters," *Journal of Applied Veterinary Science NRC*, vol. 1, pp. 43–58, 2004.

[9] A. H. Banskota, Y. Tezuka, I. K. Adnyana et al., "Cytotoxic, hepatoprotective and free radical scavenging effects of propolis from Brazil, Peru, the Netherlands and China," *Journal of Ethnopharmacology*, vol. 72, no. 1-2, pp. 239–246, 2000.

[10] F. K. Abd El Hady and A. G. Hegazi, "Egyptian propolis: 2. Chemical composition, antiviral and antimicrobial activities of East Nile Delta propolis," *Zeitschrift fur Naturforschung C*, vol. 57, no. 3-4, pp. 386–394, 2002.

[11] E. H. Park and J. H. Kahng, "Suppressive effects of propolis in rat adjuvant arthritis," *Archives of Pharmacal Research*, vol. 22, no. 6, pp. 554–558, 1999.

[12] F. D. Marquele, V. M. Di Mambro, S. R. Georgetti, R. Casagrande, Y. M. L. Valim, and M. J. V. Fonseca, "Assessment of the antioxidant activities of Brazilian extracts of propolis alone and in topical pharmaceutical formulations," *Journal of Pharmaceutical and Biomedical Analysis*, vol. 39, no. 3-4, pp. 455–462, 2005.

[13] L. Pari and M. Gnanasoundari, "Influence of naringenin on oxytetracycline mediated oxidative damage in rat liver," *Basic and Clinical Pharmacology and Toxicology*, vol. 98, no. 5, pp. 456–461, 2006.

[14] K. B. H. Salah, M. A. Mahjoub, J. P. Chaumont et al., "Chemical composition and in vitro antifungal and antioxidant activity of the essential oil and methanolic extract of *Teucrium sauvagei* Le Houerou," *Natural Product Research*, vol. 20, no. 12, pp. 1089–1097, 2006.

[15] M. Kanbur, G. Eraslan, and S. Silici, "Antioxidant effect of propolis against exposure to propetamphos in rats," *Ecotoxicology and Environmental Safety*, vol. 72, no. 3, pp. 909–915, 2009.

[16] A. G. Hegazi, F. K. Abd El Hady, and H. A. Shalaby, "An in vitro effect of propolis on adult worms of *Fasciola gigantica*," *Veterinary Parasitology*, vol. 144, no. 3-4, pp. 279–286, 2007.

[17] G. Fischer, M. B. Cleff, L. A. Dummer et al., "Adjuvant effect of green propolis on humoral immune response of bovines immunized with bovine herpesvirus type 5," *Veterinary Immunology and Immunopathology*, vol. 116, no. 1-2, pp. 79–84, 2007.

[18] S. A. Nassar, A. H. Mohamed, H. Soufy, S. M. Nasr, and K. M. Mahran, "Effect of propolis as an immunostimulant in rabbits," *The Scientific World Journal*, vol. 2012, Article ID 901516, 9 pages, 2012.

[19] Y. S. Lu and S. P. Pakes, "Protection of rabbits against experimental pasteurellosis by a streptomycin-dependent *Pasteurella multocida* serotype 3:A live mutant vaccine," *Infection and Immunity*, vol. 34, no. 3, pp. 1018–1024, 1981.

[20] H. Türkez, M. I. Yousef, and F. Geyikoglu, "Propolis prevents aluminium-induced genetic and hepatic damages in rat liver," *Food and Chemical Toxicology*, vol. 48, no. 10, pp. 2741–2746, 2010.

[21] R. Cruickshank, J. P. Duguid, B. P. Marmion, and R. H. A. Swain, *Medical Microbiology*, vol. 2, Churchill Livingstone, Edinburgh, UK, 12th edition, 1975.

[22] S. M. D. Reitman and S. Frankel, "A colorimetric method for the determination of serum glutamic oxalacetic and glutamic pyruvic transaminases," *The American Journal of Clinical Pathology*, vol. 28, no. 1, pp. 56–63, 1957.

[23] N. W. Tietz, *Clinical Guide to Laboratory Tests*, WB Saunders, Philadelphia, Pa, USA, 3rd edition, 1995.

[24] C. J. Patton and S. R. Crouch, "Spectrophotometric and kinetics investigation of the berthelot reaction for the determination of ammonia," *Analytical Chemistry*, vol. 49, no. 3, pp. 465–469, 1977.

[25] O. Houot, *Interpretation of Clinical Laboratory Tests*, edited by G. Siest, J. Henny, F. Schiele and D. S. Young, Biochemical Publications, 1985.

[26] J. D. Banchroft, A. Stevens, and D. R. Turner, *Theory and Practice of Histological Techniques*, Churchill Livingstone, New York, NY, USA, 4th edition, 1996.

[27] G. W. Snedecor and W. G. Cochran, *Statistical Methods*, Iowa State University Press, Ames, Iowa, USA, 8th edition, 1989.

[28] A. Y. E. Elham, *Bacteriological studies on Pasteurella infection in rabbits in Kalubia Governorate [M.S. thesis]*, Faculty of Veterinary Medicine, Zagazig University , Banha Branch, 1992.

[29] F. Hu, H. R. Hepburn, Y. Li, M. Chen, S. E. Radloff, and S. Daya, "Effects of ethanol and water extracts of propolis (bee glue) on acute inflammatory animal models," *Journal of Ethnopharmacology*, vol. 100, no. 3, pp. 276–283, 2005.

[30] N. Orsolic and I. Basic, "Immuno-modulation by water-soluble derivatives of propolis: a factor of anti-tumour reactivity," *Journal of Ethnopharmacology*, vol. 84, no. 2-3, pp. 265–273, 2003.

[31] R. C. Garcia, M. E. P. de Sá, H. Langoni, and S. R. C. Funari, "Effect of alcohol extract of propolis on *Pasteurella multocida* in vitro and in rabbits," *Acta Scientiarum—Animal Sciences*, vol. 26, no. 1, pp. 69–77, 2004.

[32] B. Borkowska-Opacka, A. Kędrak, and M. Truszczyński, "*Pasteurella multocida* serum level in rabbits vaccinated against pasteruellosis," *Bulletin of the Veterinary Institute in Pulawy*, vol. 40, no. 2, pp. 97–104, 1996.

[33] B. Borkowska-Opacka, A. Kędrak, and M. Truszczyński, "Application of the ELISA for determination of anti-*Pasteurella multocida* IgG in the sera of rabbits vaccinated against pasteurellosis under field conditions," *Bulletin of the Veterinary Institute in Pulawy*, vol. 41, no. 1, pp. 17–24, 1997.

[34] R. F. DiGiacomo, B. J. Deeb, W. E. Giddens Jr., B. L. Bernard, and M. M. Chengappa, "Atrophic rhinitis in New Zealand white rabbits infected with *Pasteurella multocida*," *The American Journal of Veterinary Research*, vol. 50, no. 9, pp. 1460–1465, 1989.

[35] G. Fischer, F. R. Conceição, F. P. L. Leite et al., "Immunomodulation produced by a green propolis extract on humoral and cellular responses of mice immunized with SuHV-1," *Vaccine*, vol. 25, no. 7, pp. 1250–1256, 2007.

[36] L. Okerman and L. Spanoghe, "Protective effects of inactivated pasteurella vaccines in specific pathogen free rabbits," *Comparative Immunology, Microbiology and Infectious Diseases*, vol. 4, no. 2, pp. 223–228, 1981.

[37] S. K. Cho, J. M. Park, J. Y. Kim, and Y. D. Yoon, "Studies on the development of combined vaccine for control of snuffles (*Pasteurella multocida, Bordetella bronchiseptica* infection) in rabbits," *The Research Reports of the Rural Development Administration*, vol. 31, no. 3, pp. 29–37, 1989.

[38] Z. Kleinrok, Z. Borzecki, S. Scheller, and W. Matuga, "Biological properties and clinical application of propolis. X. Preliminary pharmacological evaluation of ethanol extract of propolis (EEP)," *Arzneimittel-Forschung*, vol. 28, no. 2, pp. 291–292, 1978.

[39] I. Jasprica, A. Mornar, Z. Debeljak et al., "In vivo study of propolis supplementation effects on antioxidative status and red blood cells," *Journal of Ethnopharmacology*, vol. 110, no. 3, pp. 548–554, 2007.

[40] Z. S. Talas and M. F. Gulhan, "Effects of various propolis concentrations on biochemical and hematological parameters of rainbow trout (*Oncorhynchus mykiss*)," *Ecotoxicology and Environmental Safety*, vol. 72, no. 7, pp. 1994–1998, 2009.

[41] A. M. Badawi, *Some biochemical effects of the propolis under the normal conditions in rats [M.S. thesis]*, Faculty of Agriculture, Cairo University, Giza, Egypt, 1990.

[42] G. Eraslan, M. Kanbur, and S. Silici, "Evaluation of propolis effects on some biochemical parameters in rats treated with sodium fluoride," *Pesticide Biochemistry and Physiology*, vol. 88, no. 3, pp. 273–283, 2007.

[43] T. T. Oliveira, T. J. Nagem, and J. N. Ribeiro, "Serum activities of aspartate aminotransferase, alanine aminotransferase and gamma glutamyl transpeptidase enzymes in rabbits treated with crude extract of propolis," *Revista de Ciencias Farmaceuticas Basica e Aplicada*, vol. 26, no. 1, pp. 25–28, 2005.

[44] Y. Sugimoto, T. Tarumi, Y. Kaneko et al., "Effect of propolis extract on D-galactosamine-induced hepatic injury in rats," *Biological and Pharmaceutical Bulletin*, vol. 22, no. 11, pp. 1237–1239, 1999.

[45] S. K. Nirala, M. S. Bhadauria, S. Shukla et al., "Pharmacological intervention of tiferron and propolis to alleviate beryllium-induced hepatorenal toxicity," *Fundamental and Clinical Pharmacology*, vol. 22, no. 4, pp. 403–415, 2008.

[46] J. M. Sforcin, E. L. B. Novell, and S. R. C. Funarl, "Seasonal effect of Brazilian propolis on seric biochemical variables," *Journal of Venomous Animals and Toxins*, vol. 8, pp. 1–6, 2002.

6

Antiproliferative Activity of Xanthones Isolated from *Artocarpus obtusus*

Najihah Mohd Hashim,[1] Mawardi Rahmani,[1] Gwendoline Cheng Lian Ee,[1] Mohd Aspollah Sukari,[1] Maizatulakmal Yahayu,[1] Winda Oktima,[1] Abd Manaf Ali,[2] and Rusea Go[3]

[1] *Department of Chemistry, Universiti Putra Malaysia, Selangor, 43400 Serdang, Malaysia*
[2] *Faculty of Agriculture and Biotechnology, Universiti Sultan Zainal Abidin, 20400 Kuala Terengganu, Malaysia*
[3] *Department of Biology, Universiti Putra Malaysia, Selangor, 43400 Serdang, Malaysia*

Correspondence should be addressed to Mawardi Rahmani, mawardi@science.upm.edu.my

Academic Editor: Masa-Aki Shibata

An investigation of the chemical constituents in *Artocarpus obtusus* species led to the isolation of three new xanthones, pyranocycloartobiloxanthone A (**1**), dihydroartoindonesianin C (**2**), and pyranocycloartobiloxanthone B (**3**). The compounds were subjected to antiproliferative assay against human promyelocytic leukemia (HL60), human chronic myeloid leukemia (K562), and human estrogen receptor (ER+) positive breast cancer (MCF7) cell lines. Pyranocycloartobiloxanthone A (**1**) consistently showed strong cytotoxic activity against the three cell lines compared to the other two with IC_{50} values of 0.5, 2.0 and 5.0 μg/mL, respectively. Compound (**1**) was also observed to exert antiproliferative activity and apoptotic promoter towards HL60 and MCF7 cell lines at respective IC_{50} values. The compound (**1**) was not toxic towards normal cell lines human nontumorigenic breast cell line (MCF10A) and human peripheral blood mononuclear cells (PBMCs) with IC_{50} values of more than 30 μg/mL.

1. Introduction

Tropical rain forests contain a lot of interesting pharmacologically active constituents and many more are still waiting to be discovered as they still offer undoubtedly valuable and amazing chemical entities. The World Health Organization (WHO) reported that 11% of the 252 drugs considered as basic and essential in this century were exclusively origin from flowering plants [1]. Many impressive modern drugs available in the market were derived from plants source and most of them were based on their ethnomedicinal uses. Hence, many works on tropical plants from Malaysia are being and have been extensively studied as well as their biological activity. One of them is *Artocarpus* species. The *Artocarpus* species is one of the genus in the Moraceae family [2] and is made of about 55 species. The genus is widely distributed throughout subtropical and tropical region of the Indian subcontinent south of the Himalayas, Sri Lanka, Burma, Thailand, Indo-China, Southern China, Taiwan, Hainan, Malesia, and Melanesia [2, 3]. Some parts of the plants are also used in traditional medicine preparations for the treatment of various diseases such as diarrhea, fever, liver cirrhosis, hypertension, diabetes, inflammation, malaria, ulcers, wound, and for tapeworm infection [4–8]. Many interesting biological activities and phytochemical work have been carried out on the plants with the identification of various classes of interesting phenolic compounds [9–18]. Our previous works on the stem bark of *A. altilis* and *A. obtusus* have led to the isolation of prenylated flavonoids and xanthones [19, 20].

In preliminary screening for cytotoxic, antioxidant and antimicrobial activity of thirteen Malaysian *Artocarpus* species has resulted in the potential of a few species for further examination in particular *A. obtusus* Jarret [13]. The plant is endemic to Sarawak, and, in continuation of our investigation on Malaysian plants, we now described the antiproliferative activity of three new xanthones isolated from the stem bark of *A. obtusus*. The cytotoxic activity was tested using MTT assay against human promyelocytic leukemia (HL60), human chronic myeloid leukemia (K562), and human estrogen receptor (ER+) positive breast cancer (MCF7). The most active xanthone was further tested against mouse embryo fibroblast (3T3), human cervical cancer (HeLa), human estrogen receptor (ER−) negative (MDA-MB 231), human colon cancer (HT29) and human hepatocarcinoma (HepG2), human nontumorigenic breast cell line (MCF10A), and human peripheral blood mononuclear cells (PBMCs). The potential compound was also analyzed for its antiproliferative activity and effect on cell morphology of HL60 and MCF7 cell lines at selected concentrations using BrdU and acridine orange and propium iodide staining, respectively. Currently, there is no recognized ethnomedicinal data and reported biological activity for *A. obtusus*; thus, this is the first report on antiproliferative activity studies of the isolated xanthones from the plant as well as the isolation and structural elucidation of compound (**3**).

2. Materials and Methods

2.1. General Experimental Procedures. All melting points (m.p.) were determined using a hot stage melting point apparatus model Leica GALEN III equipped with microscope and are uncorrected. UV and IR spectra were measured with Shimadzu UV 2100 and Perkin Elmer FTIR (model 1725X) spectrophotometers, respectively. The ^{1}H-NMR and ^{13}C-NMR spectra were obtained with JEOL ECA-400 spectrometer operating at 400 and 100 MHz with tetramethylsilane (TMS) as an internal standard, respectively. The MS were obtained with Shimadzu GCMS-QP5050 spectrometer with Direct Induction Probe (DIP) using ionization induced by electron impact at 70 eV. Column chromatography was carried out using Merck Si gel 60 No. 1.07734, Darmstadt, Germany. Analytical thin layer chromatography (TLC) was performed on commercially available Merck TLC plastic sheet precoated Kieselgel 60 F_{254}, 0.2 mm thickness, and the chromatotron plates were coated with Kieselgel 60 F_{254} and scrapped to 1 mm thickness.

2.2. Plant Material. Sample of the air-dried stem bark of *Artocarpus obtusus* was collected from Sarawak in 2004, identified by Dr. Rusea Go, and a voucher specimen (S94402) has been deposited at the Herbarium, Department of Biology, Faculty of Science, Universiti Putra Malaysia.

2.3. Preparation of Plant Extracts and Isolation Procedure. The dried ground stem bark (640 g) of *Artocarpus obtusus* was sequentially extracted with *n*-hexane, chloroform and methanol at room temperature. The extracts were concentrated *in vacuo* to give 3 g (0.47%), 9 g (1.4%), and 6 g (0.94%) of dark viscous *n*-hexane, chloroform, and methanol extracts, respectively. The chromatographic isolation procedure to obtain pyranocycloartobiloxanthone A (**1**) and dihydroartoindonesianin C (**2**) from the chloroform extract has been described previously [20]. Similarly, the dark viscous methanol extract (6 g) was separated by gravity column chromatography and eluted with mixture of solvents of increasing polarity consisting of *n*-hexane, *n*-hexane/$CHCl_3$, $CHCl_3$, $CHCl_3$/MeOH, and MeOH to afford 45 fractions of 200 mL each. Another batch of compounds (**1**) and (**2**) were obtained from fractions 11–19 after a series of silica gel column chromatographic separation. Fractions 26–32 were combined and applied on column chromatography of Sephadex LH20 and eluted with methanol to give 45 fractions of 100 mL each. The combined fractions 18–28 were further chromatographed by a series of column chromatography using silica gel and eluted with solvent mixture of *n*-hexane, *n*-hexane/$CHCl_3$, $CHCl_3$, $CHCl_3$/MeOH, and MeOH to afford yellow solid (25.0 mg). The solid was recrystallized with chloroform as needle-shaped pyranocycloartobiloxanthone B (**3**) with R_f value of 0.5 (EtOAc : $CHCl_3$;,4 : 1) and m.p. 218–220°C.

2.4. Spectral Data. Pyranocycloartobiloxanthone A (**1**); $C_{25}H_{22}O_8$, yellow needle-shaped crystals, and m.p. 288–290°C. The spectral data of the compound are identical to literature values [20].

Dihydroartoindonesianin C (**2**); $C_{25}H_{24}O_6$, yellow needle-shaped crystals, and m.p. 210–212°C. The spectral data of the compound are identical to literature values [20].

Pyranocycloartobiloxanthone B (**3**), $C_{25}H_{22}O_8$, yellow needle-shaped crystal with m.p. 218–220°C; UV (Acetone) λ_{max} nm (log ε): 381 (0.57), 256 (4.00), and 229 (0.32); IR ν_{max} cm^{-1} (KBr): 3390 (OH), 1642 (C = O), 1474, 1270, 1160, 982; EIMS m/z (% intensity): 450 (26.50), 436 (28.00), 435 (100), 377 (60.00), 378 (18.00), 349 (6.00), 331 (4.50), 188 (14.00), and 166 (6.00); HREIMS m/z 450.1329 $[M]^+$ (calcd for $C_{25}H_{22}O_8$, 450.1314). ^{1}H-NMR (400 MHz, Acetone-d_6): 1.19 (3H, *d*, J = 6.4 Hz, H-15), 1.45 (6H, s, H-19, H-20), 1.91 (1H, *m*, H-11), 2.25 (1H, *dd*, J = 15.6, 7.7 Hz, H-13), 2.76 (1H, *m*, H-12), 3.32 (1H, *m*, H-11), 5.47 (1H, *s*, H-14), 5.65 (1H, *d*, J = 10.0 Hz, H-17), 6.12 (1H, *s*, H-6), 6.49 (1H, *s*, H-3′), 6.93 (1H, *d*, J = 10.0 Hz, H-16), 7.96 (1H, *brs*, OH-13), 8.44 (1H, *brs*, OH-2′), 8.84 (1H, *brs*, OH-4′), 13.37 (1H, *brs*, OH-5); ^{13}C-NMR (100 MHz Acetone-d_6): 16.5 (C-15), 24.2 (C-11), 29.8 (C-19), 30.0 (C-20), 33.9 (C-12), 38.8 (C-13), 80.2 (C-18), 96.5 (C-14), 101.3 (C-6), 103.6 (C-3), 105.5 (C-3′), 105.8 (C-10), 107.1 (C-8), 114.3 (C-1′), 117.6 (C-16), 127.3 (C-6′), 129.4 (C-17), 135.0 (C-5′), 153.2 (C-4′), 153.6 (C-2′), 153.8 (C-5), 161.0 (C-9), 163.1 (C-2), 164.1 (C-7), and 182.3 (C-4) (Figure 1).

2.5. In Vitro Assay for Antiproliferative Activity

2.5.1. Cell Lines. The cancerous and noncancerous cell lines (suspension and anchorage-dependent cells) were obtained from the American Type Culture Collection (ATCC) and the RIKEN Cell Bank (RCB). The cancerous cell lines used were HL-60 (human acute promyelocytic leukemia) (RCB), K562 (human chronic myeloid leukemia) (ATCC), MCF7 (human estrogen receptor (ER+) positive breast cancer) (ATCC), HeLa (human cervical cancer) (ATCC), HepG2 (human hepatocarcinoma) (ATCC), HT29 (human colon cancer) (RCI), and MDA-MB 231 (human estrogen receptor (ER−) negative) (ATCC). The noncancerous cell line and normal cells were 3T3 (Mouse embryo fibroblast) (ATCC),

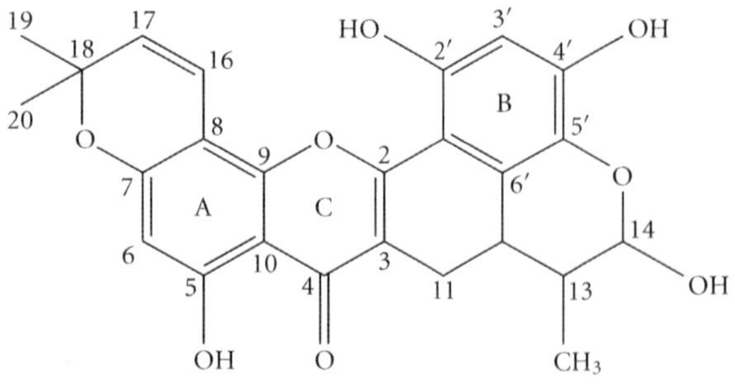

(1)

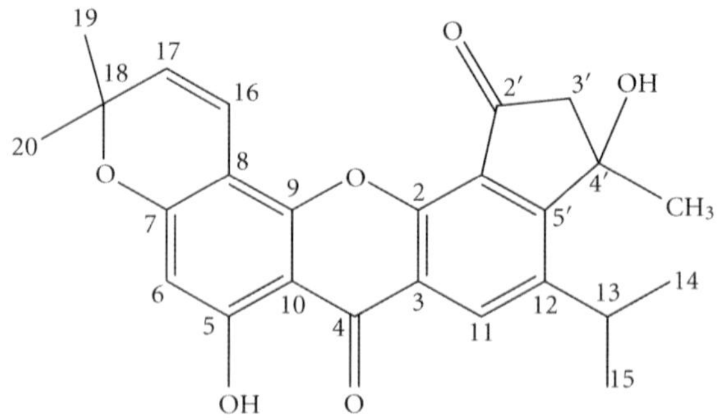

(2)

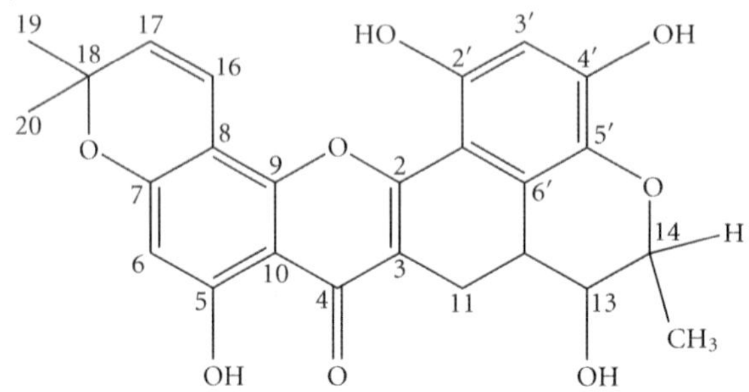

(3)

Figure 1: The chemical structure of the three isolated compounds tested for antiproliferative activity, pyranocycloartobiloxanthone A (**1**), dihydroartoindonesianin C (**2**), and pyranocycloartobiloxanthone B (**3**).

MCF10A (human nontumorigenic breast cell line) (ATCC) and PBMC (human peripheral blood mononuclear cells). PBMCs were obtained from one of the authors herself. Blood (10–12 mL) was taken from the donor by using the 25 mL syringe. The blood sample was diluted with same volume of PBS. The diluted blood sample was carefully layered on Ficoll-Paque Plus (Amersham Biosciences, USA) the ratio of 2 : 1. The mixture was centrifuged at 1500× g for 40 minutes at 18–20°C. The undisturbed lymphocyte layer was carefully transferred into centrifuge tube. The lymphocyte was washed and spun down three times by adding 10 mL sterile PBS and to get the pellet and resuspended in RPMI 1640 (Sigma, USA) with 100 IU/mL of penicillin, 100 μg/mL of streptomycin (Flowlab, Australia), and 10% v/v Fetal Bovine Serum (FBS) (PAA, Austria). Cell counting was performed to determine the PBMC number in equal volume of trypan blue.

2.5.2. Cytotoxic Analysis by the MTT Assay. The colorimetric assay was performed on the isolated compounds using a modified microculture tetrazolium salt (MTT) assay (Sigma, USA) [21]. Varying concentrations of 0.46, 0.93, 1.87, 3.75, 7.5, 15, and 30 μg/mL of pyranocycloartobiloxanthone A (**1**), dihydroartoindonesianin C (**2**), and pyranocycloartobiloxanthone B (**3**) were prepared from the substock solutions by serial dilution in RPMI 1640 to give a volume of 100 μL in each microtitre plate well (96-flat bottom microwell plates). Each well was then added with 100 μL of cell lines in complete growth media (RPMI 1640) 5×10^5 cells/mL. Untreated cells were used as control and included for each sample. The assay for each concentration of compounds was performed in triplicate. The culture plates were incubated for 72 hour at 37°C in a humidified (90%) incubator with 5% CO_2. After incubation, the fractions of surviving cells were determined relative to the untreated cell population using the colorimetric MTT assay. In this method, the viabilities of the cells were determined by measuring the amount of blue formazan crystals formed after 20 mL of freshly prepared MTT solution (5 mg in 1 mL PBS) was added to each well followed by four hours of incubation at 37°C. Then, 170 μL of the remaining supernatant was removed, 100 μL of DMSO was added to each well, and the mixture was stirred thoroughly to dissolve the blue crystal formazan. The plate was then incubated for 30 minutes to ensure that all the crystals were dissolved. Finally, the absorbance (OD) of each well at 570 nm of wavelength was read using the microplate reader (ELISA reader, EL340 Biokinetic Reader, Bio-Tek Instrumentation). Doxorubicin was used as a positive control. A graph was plotted for the percentage of cell viability against concentration of the extract, and the cytoxicity index used was IC_{50}, the concentration that yields 50% inhibition of the cell compared with untreated control. The percentage of cell viability was determined as follows:

$$\%\ \text{Viability} = \frac{\text{OD}_{\text{sample}}}{\text{OD}_{\text{control}}} \times 100\%. \quad (1)$$

2.6. Cell Proliferation ELISA BrdU (5-bromo-2′-deoxyuridine) Assay (Colorimetric). This assay was conducted to determine the antiproliferative effects of the tested compound. In this assay, three different concentrations of

TABLE 1: ^{1}H-NMR (400 MHz) and ^{13}C-NMR (100 MHz) spectral data of pyranocycloartobiloxanthone B (3) and pyranocycloartobiloxanthone A (1).

H/C	(3) In acetone-d_6			(1) In DMSO [13]	
	δ_H (in ppm, J in Hz)	δ_C (in ppm)	HMBC	δ_H (in ppm)	δ_C (in ppm)
2	—	163.1	—	—	160.7
3	—	103.6	—	—	100.8
4	—	182.3	—	—	179.1
5	—	153.8	—	—	151.2
6	6.12 (1H, s)	101.3	C-5, 7, 8	6.17	98.7
7	—	164.1	—	—	160.7
8	—	107.1	—	—	104.3
9	—	161.0	—	—	157.9
10	—	105.8	—	—	103.6
11	1.91 (1H, *m*)	24.2	C-3, 6′	1.88	21.5
	3.32 (1H, *m*)		C-3, 4, C-12	3.32	
12	2.76 (1H, *m*)	33.9	C-13, 1′, 5′, 6′	2.55	31.2
13	2.25 (1H, *dd*, J = 15.6, 7.7)	38.8	C-12, 14, 6′	1.82	35.7
14	5.47 (1H, *s*)	96.5	C-13, 15	5.32	93.1
15	1.19 (3H, *d*, J = 6.4, CH_3)	16.5	C-12, 13, 14	1.08	14.6
16	6.93 (1H, *d*, J = 10.0)	117.6	C-7, 9, 18	6.86	114.8
17	5.65 (1H, *d*, J = 10.0)	129.4	C-16, 18, 19	5.74	127.3
18	—	80.2	—	—	78.0
19	1.45 (3H, *s*, CH_3)	29.8	C-17, 18	1.44	27.7
20	1.45 (3H, *s*, CH_3)	30.0	C-17, 18	1.42	27.9
1′	—	114.3	—	—	111.0
2′	—	153.6	—	—	151.2
3′	6.49 (1H, s)	105.5	C-2′, 4′, 5′	6.43	103.1
4′	—	153.2	—	—	151.1
5′	—	135.0	—	—	132.5
6′	—	127.3	—	—	124.6
OH-5	13.37 (1H, *brs*)	—	C-6, 7, 10	13.36	—
OH-13	7.96 (1H, *brs*)	—	—	—	—
OH-14	—	—	—	6.93	—
OH-2′	8.44 (1H, *brs*)	—	—	9.91	—
OH-4′	8.84 (1H, *brs*)	—	C-3′	9.81	—

compound or test sample were prepared together with control. The concentration chosen were 1 μg/mL, the IC_{50} concentration, and 20 μg/mL. Two types of cells were selected: HL-60 (suspension) and MCF7 (adherent) cells, since they gave the most significant results for the cytotoxic activity. The procedures are according to the instruction manual from Roche. Each sample was assayed in triplicate, and control samples include a blank (no cells) and background (without BrdU). The cells were treated by pyranocycloartobiloxanthone A (**1**) for 24, 48, and 72 hours. The cells were cultured together with various dilutions of test substance (tested compound) in 96-well MP flat bottom in a final volume of 100 μL/well, and 10 μL BrdU label (diluted by 1/2000 in media) was added to each well and incubated for 24 hour at 37°C. BrdU label was then replaced with 200 μL of fix/denaturing solution for 30 min at room temperature (25°C) and removed by inverting the plate. The anti-BrdU-POD working solution (100 μL/well) (diluted by 1/100 in dilution buffer) was added and incubated for one hour at room temperature. The cells were washed three times with wash buffer and once with dH_2O. Then, removed dH_2O and 100 μL of substrate solution was added to each well and incubated for 15 min at room temperature in the dark. The stop solution (100 μL/well) was added, and the absorbance was measured using ELISA reader at 450 nm, (reference wavelength 690). The activity was observed by the optical density (OD) of the absorbance at 450 nm, and graphs were plotted from the optical density obtained against time of exposure for each cell lines.

2.7. Acridine Orange (AO) and Propodium Iodide (PI) Staining. Cell suspensions were mixed with an equal volume of staining solution (1 : 1) containing 10 μg/mL acridine orange and 10 μg/mL propium iodide (dissolved in PBS) and observed under fluorescence microscope within 30 minutes. The viable (green intact cells), apoptotic (green

Table 2: The IC_{50} values of isolated compounds towards various cell lines.

Cell line	IC_{50} (μg/mL)			
	(**1**)	(**2**)	(**3**)	Doxorubicin
HL60	2 ± 0.7	26 ± 0.8	17 ± 0.8	0.2 ± 0.03
K562	0.5 ± 0.05	>30	>30	nt
MCF7	5 ± 1.2	27 ± 1.9	23 ± 1.3	0.2 ± 0.06
HeLa	8 ± 3.3	nt	nt	nt
MDA-MB 231	12 ± 1.1	nt	nt	nt
HT29	14 ± 1.5	nt	nt	nt
HepG2	20 ± 2.0	nt	nt	nt
3T3	7 ± 1.6	nt	nt	nt
MCF10	>30	nt	nt	nt
PBMC	>30	nt	nt	>30

Note: (nt)-not tested, (**1**)-pyranocycloartobiloxanthone A, (**2**)-dihydroartoindonesianin C, and (**3**)-pyranocycloartobiloxanthone B. Data represent mean ± SD of triplicate determinations from three independent experiments.

shrinking cells with condensed of fragmented nucleus), and necrotic (red cells) were the morphological changes that were examined under fluorescence microscope.

3. Results and Discussion

Based on the biological screening test results on 39 extracts from thirteen species of *Artocarpus* species, the three extracts of *Artocarpus obtusus* exhibited excellent cytotoxic activity against HL60 cells with IC_{50} values from 1.4 to 8.4 μg/mL [13]. However, only chloroform extract of *A. obtusus* exhibited cytotoxic activity towards MCF7 cells with IC_{50} values 22.60 μg/mL, while the other extracts were inactive towards the cell. These extracts were further phytochemically investigated with the isolation and identification of three new xanthones, pyranocycloartobiloxanthone A (**1**), dihydroartoindonesianin C (**2**), and pyranocycloartobiloxanthone B (**3**). The structural elucidation of two of xanthones, (**1**) and (**2**) isolated from the chloroform extract, has already been published recently [20], and the structure determination of the third xanthone (**3**) is included in this presentation. After chromatographic separation of the methanol extract, pyranocycloartobiloxanthone B (**3**) was obtained as yellow needle-shaped crystals with m.p. 218–220°C. The UV spectrum exhibited absorption bands at λ_{max} 381, 256, and 229 nm for a typical xanthone skeleton. Broad and strong absorptions were noted at 3390 and 1642 cm^{-1} in the IR spectrum due to the presence of hydroxyl and carbonyl functionalities. The EIMS gave molecular ion peak at m/z 450 which is consistent with molecular formula $C_{25}H_{22}O_8$. The high-resolution EIMS exhibited molecular ion peak at m/z 450.1329 (calculated $C_{25}H_{22}O_8$ for m/z 450.1314). The ^{1}H-NMR displayed characteristic signals for chelated phenolic hydroxyl group at δ 13.37 and a 2,2-dimethylchromene ring substituent with the observation of a pair of olefinic protons at δ 6.93 and 5.65 with identical coupling constant of 10.0 Hz and a sharp singlet of two overlapped methyl groups at δ 1.45. The aromatic region also revealed the occurrence of two

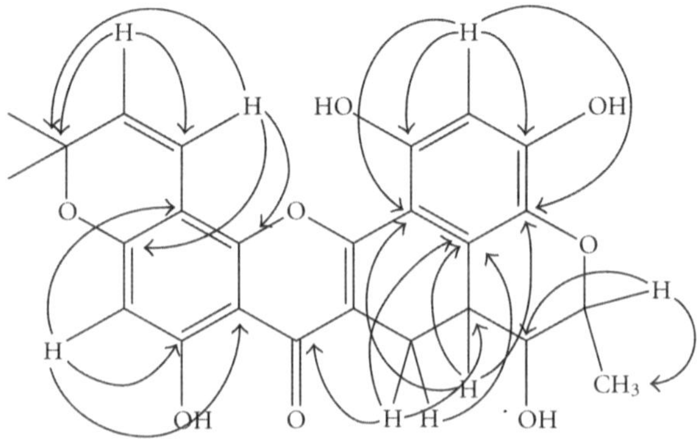

Figure 2: Selected HMBC of pyranocycloartobiloxanthone B (**3**).

singlets at δ 6.12 (H-6) and 6.49 (H-3′), and another high field resonance at δ 1.19 assigned to methyl group at C-15. The two broad chemical shifts noted at δ 8.44 and 8.84 were due to the hydroxyl groups attached to aromatic ring at C-2′ and C-4′.

The ^{13}C-NMR and DEPT spectra indicated the existence of twenty-five signals contributed by fourteen quaternary carbons including a conjugated carbonyl (δ 182.3), seven methine, one methylene (δ 24.2), and three methyl (δ 16.5, 29.8, and 30.0) carbon atoms. These ^{1}H-NMR and ^{13}C-NMR spectral data were quite similar to pyranocycloartobiloxanthone A (**1**) but with some obvious differences especially the location of one the hydroxyl groups at C-14 now shifted to C-13 which occurred at δ 38.8. The methyl group at C-13 shifted to C-14 and the chemical shift of this carbon now shifted upfield at δ 96.5 (Table 1). On the basis of HMQC and HMBC spectral analysis, the chemical shifts were fully assigned, and the positions of the substituents on the pyran and aromatic rings were determined. The ^2J and ^3J correlations of both protons at H-6 to -5, C-7, and C-8, H-3′ to C-2′, C-4′, and C-5′ confirmed the position of each respective aromatic protons. The two-bond and three-bond correlations were also used to locate the positions of both methyl and hydroxyl groups in the pyran ring (Figure 2). In (**1**), the methyl protons at C-15 exhibited correlations with C-12, -13, and -14 [20]. However, the methyl protons only showed correlations to C-13 and 14 in compound (**3**) which supported the attachment of this methyl group at C-14. Similarly, the methine proton at C-12 do not indicate any correlation to the methyl group. Based on these spectral data, the structure of this new xanthone was assigned and given trivial name pyranocycloartobiloxanthone B (**3**).

By using three tumor cell lines (HL60, K562, and MCF7), a comparison was made between the three new xanthones to establish which has greater cytotoxicity. The cytotoxic activity was assayed at various concentrations, expressed in IC_{50} values (μg/mL) under continuous exposure for 72 hours, and is summarized in Table 2. The estimated IC_{50} values were obtained from the plotted graphs of percentage cell viability (%) against various concentrations of the compounds (μg/mL) (Figures 3 and 4). The study showed pyranocycloartobiloxanthone A (**1**) exhibited potent cytotoxic activity against the three cell lines with IC_{50} ranged from

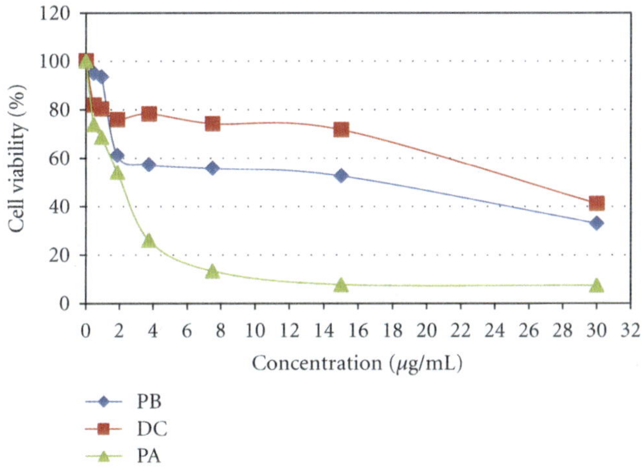

Figure 3: Percentage viability of HL60 cells treated with different concentration of pyranocycloartobiloxanthone A (**1**) (PA), dihydroartoindonesianin C (**2**) (DC), and pyranocycloartobiloxanthone B (**3**) (PB) measured after 72 hours using MTT assay.

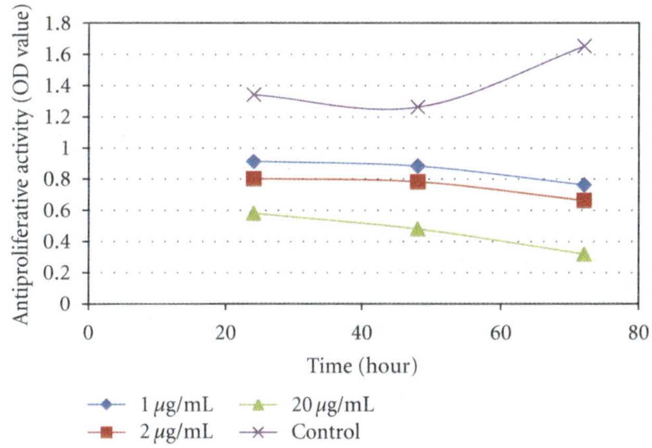

Figure 5: Effect of pyranocycloartobiloxanthone A (**1**) on the proliferation of HL60 cells *in vitro*. After treatment with 1 μg/mL, 2 μg/mL (IC_{50} based on MTT results) and 20 μg/mL for 24, 48, and 72 hours cellular proliferation of HL60 cells was assayed using BrdU incorporation ELISA.

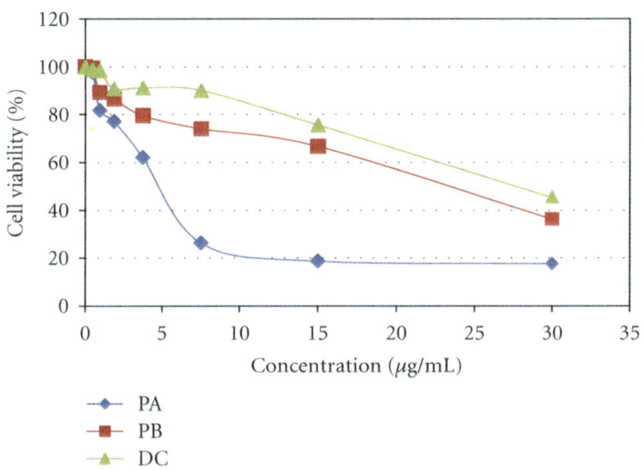

Figure 4: Percentage viability of MCF7 cells treated with different concentration of pyranocycloartobiloxanthone A (**1**) (PA), dihydroartoindonesianin C (**2**) (DC), and pyranocycloartobiloxanthone B (**3**) (PB) measured after 72 hours using MTT assay.

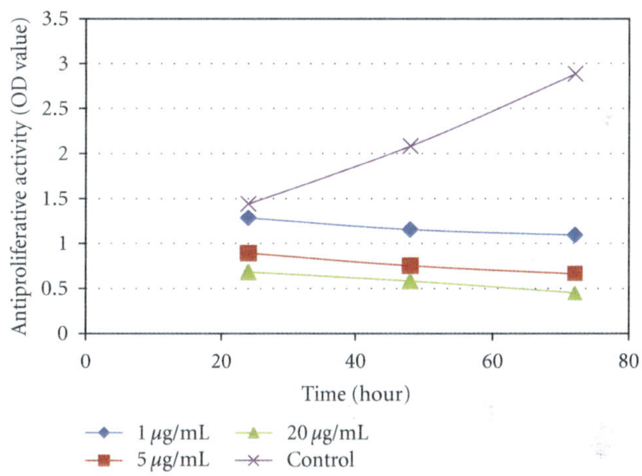

Figure 6: Effect of pyranocycloartobiloxanthone A (**1**) on the proliferation of MCF7 cells *in vitro*. After treatment with 1 μg/mL, 5 μg/mL (IC_{50} based on MTT results) and 20 μg/mL for 24, 48, and 72 hours cellular proliferation of MCF7 cells was assayed using BrdU incorporation ELISA.

0.5–5.0 μg/mL in comparison with the other two compounds which only displayed moderate cytotoxic activities towards HL60 and MCF7 cell lines. Both compounds also failed to inhibit the growth of K562 cell line. In order to establish the potential of pyranocycloartobiloxanthone A (**1**) as a good cytotoxic agent, the compound was further tested against seven other cell lines (HeLa, MDA-MB 231, HT29, HepG2, 3T3, MCF10A, and PBMC). Due to insufficient amount of samples, compounds (**2**) and (**3**) were not further tested against these cell lines. The IC_{50} values on the sensitivity of MDA-MB 231, HT29, and HepG2 cell lines towards pyranocycloartobiloxanthone A (**1**) were obtained at 12.0, 14.0, and 20.0 μg/mL, respectively. However, the compound was not toxic towards normal cell lines, MCF10A and PBMC except for 3T3. The toxic effect of the compound displayed against 3T3 may be due to genetic changes occurred in the cell, or the compound was toxic to mouse cells. However further tests are needed to be carried out to underline the effect. The sensitivity of the compound towards the cell lines were comparable to doxorubicin used in the test.

The investigation on the potential cell proliferation inhibition activity of pyranocycloartobiloxanthone A (**1**) on HL60 and MCF7 cells was conducted due to their significant sensitivity (based from MTT assay) towards the compound. The results showed that at high and IC_{50} concentrations of pyranocycloartobiloxanthone A (**1**) on treated HL60 and MCF7 populations, the degree of cell killing or antiproliferative activity was significant, denoted by slight declined of OD value of absorbance over prolonged exposures in comparison to the untreated control population (Figures 5 and 6). The OD values for the IC_{50-} treated HL60 populations were 0.8, 0.78, and 0.66 for 24, 48, and 72 hours, respectively. On the other hand, OD values of the untreated

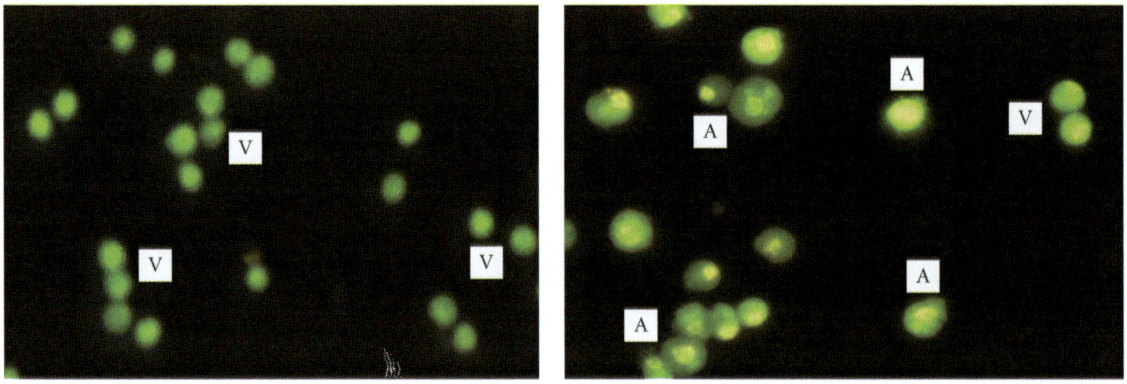

FIGURE 7: Morphology features of HL60 cells incubated with pyranocycloartobiloxanthone A (**1**) after being stained with acridine orange and propidium iodide were observed under fluorescence microscope (magnification 200x) (a) untreated HL60 cells (b) treated with pyranocycloartobiloxanthone A (**1**) at 2 μg/mL (IC_{50} value), after 72 hours. Note: V: viable, A: apoptosis, and N: necrosis.

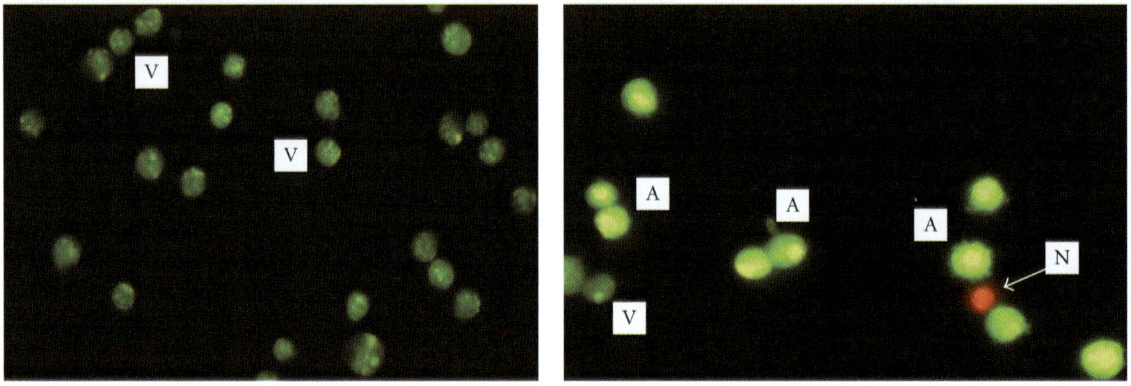

FIGURE 8: Morphology features of MCF7 cells incubated with pyranocycloartobiloxanthone A (**1**) were observed under fluorescence microscope (magnification 200x) (a) untreated MCF7cells (b) treated with pyranocycloartobiloxanthone A (**1**) at 5 μg/mL (IC_{50} value), after 72 hours. Note: V: viable, A: apoptosis, and N: necrosis.

HL60 populations were 1.34, 1.26, and 1.65 for 24, 48, and 72 hours, respectively. Therefore, the exposure of HL60 cells to pyranocycloartobiloxanthone A (**1**) at IC_{50} concentration for 24, 48, and 72 hours resulted in a reduction from 60 to 40% of BrdU incorporation in comparison with the untreated population. A slight decline of OD values for IC_{50}-treated MCF7 populations was observed from 0.89, 0.75, and 0.66 at 24, 48, and 72 hours, respectively. In the untreated populations, the OD values were 1.44, 2.08, and 2.88 for 24, 48, and 72 hours, respectively. The exposure has resulted in reduction from 61.8 to 23% of BrdU incorporation in comparison with untreated population. As indicated above, the data exhibited the exposure time remarkably influenced on the growth of HL60 and MCF7 cells in the ELISA BrdU assay. Both cells experienced a noteworthy decline in cell proliferations compared to the control populations at any concentration as the time of exposure increased. The time course studies indicated that pyranocycloartobiloxanthone A (**1**) was sensitive to HL60 and MCF7 cells by inhibiting the cell proliferation. Hence, the inhibition of cellular proliferation for both cells treated with pyranocycloartobiloxanthone A (**1**) was consistent with the decline in cell viability from the MTT assay evaluation. Hence, the reduction of OD or viability which is observed in MTT assay may reflect cell death and/or reduced rate of proliferation.

In contrast, by utilizing AO/PI staining, we were able to determine the percentage and mode of cell death by uptake of different fluorescence dyes and morphological changes of individual cell in the treatment group. In the morphological study, pyranocycloartobiloxanthone A (**1**) was chosen for further study as it has shown significant activity against selected cancer cell lines compared to other isolated compounds. The cells, HL60 and MCF7, were treated with respective IC_{50} values, 2 μg/mL, and 5 μg/mL of pyranocycloartobiloxanthone A (**1**) after 72 hours of incubation. The cells were observed under fluorescence microscope prior AOPI staining. Both apoptotic and necrotic features were observed in HL60 and MCF7 cells population after treatment with pyranocycloartobiloxanthone A (**1**) at their respective IC_{50} dose (Figures 7 and 8). However, the compound seemed to kill both cells in apoptotic manner at IC_{50} dose, whereby upon swelling of the cells, little buds started to appear around the cells. The buds disintegrate from the mother cell to form apoptotic bodies while the mother cell will shrunk. Cell rupture was observed after the prolonged exposure (72 hours) and resulted in the formation of cellular debris. There are several genes involved with apoptosis in mammalian cells, and the apoptotic response is determined by a balance between antiapoptotic genes (Bcl-2 and p53) and proapoptotic genes (C-myc and Bax proteins) [22]. In cancer, there is a lack of equilibrium between the rate of cell division and cell death (apoptosis), therefore, any compounds or agents that are able to promote or suppress apoptosis are potential to be developed as anticancer drugs.

The current study showed that the compounds were sensitive or toxic towards the selected cell lines, and the response of each cell lines towards the compounds was different. Differential antiproliferative activity of the compounds indicated that the cells may have different particular molecular site or receptor for selected compounds to interact, which may influence the response of the activity [22]. Pyranocycloartobiloxanthone A (**1**) exhibited poor toxicity with high IC_{50} values (>30 μg/mL) against PBMC and MCF10A cells which is a good indication that normal human cell lines may be resistant to the compound. The suggested effective doses for a 50% inhibition in cell viability for plant extracts and pure compound to be considered active according to National Cancer Institute (NCI) guidelines should be less than 20 and 4 μg/mL, respectively [23]. It is interesting to note that, pyranocycloartobiloxanthone A (**1**), at low concentration, exhibited its antiproliferative effect against most of the selected cancer cell lines. On the other hand, the other two compounds, dihydroartoindonesianin C (**2**) and pyranocycloartobiloxanthone B (**3**) require high concentrations to exert their antiproliferative effect towards HL60, K562, and MCF7 cells. This finding is possibly due to the presence of active sites in the structure of the compounds, whereby the presence of the resorcinol moiety in ring B and isoprenyl substituent at C-3 of the flavones skeleton may contribute to the interesting activity [9, 24]. Therefore, by having the above two features together in the chemical structure of pyranocycloartobiloxanthone A (**1**), they have substantiated the remarkable antiproliferative activity displayed. Surprisingly, in spite of having both active features together and also an isomer to compound (**1**), pyranocycloartobiloxanthone B (**3**) displayed lower antiproliferative activity towards the target cell lines. This may be due to the migration of the hydroxyl group from C-14 to C-13 and methyl group in the opposite direction in compound (**3**). As for dihydroartoindonesianin C (**2**), position C-3 is also substituted with isoprenyl group but without the resorcinol skeleton in the chemical structure, and this may be caused much lower antiproliferative effect than compound (**1**). These findings indicated that both resorcinol moiety in ring B and isoprenyl substituent at C-3 position must be the most important features for revealing the potent activity. Thus, the continuing phytochemical investigation of Malaysian *Artocarpus* species cannot only identify new lead compounds as anticancer agents but also provide a pool of chemicals for future biological target studies.

4. Conclusion

The extracts *of A. obtusus* were found to exhibit good cytotoxic and potential antiproliferative activity against some cell lines and further isolation work on the extracts resulted in the isolate ion of three new xanthones. The structures of the compounds were established by spectroscopic method and comparison with literature values. One of the xanthones, pyranocycloartobiloxanthone A (**1**), showed potent antiproliferative activity towards various cell lines and inactive when tested on normal cell lines. The compound (**1**) was able to induce apoptosis against HL60 and MCF7 cell lines at its respective IC_{50} values.

Acknowledgment

The authors wish to thank Universiti Putra Malaysia for providing facilities to carry out this work, Malaysian Government for providing research grant under IRPA Program, and N. M. Hashim wishes to thank Universiti Sains Malaysia for granting study leave.

References

[1] I. Raskin, D. M. Ribnicky, S. Komarnytsky et al., "Plants and human health in the twenty-first century," *Trends in Biotechnology*, vol. 20, no. 12, pp. 522–531, 2002.

[2] K. M. Kochummen and R. G. Moraceae, in *Tree Flora Sabah and Sarawak*, pp. 181–212, Ampang Press, Kuala Lumpur, Malaysia, 2000.

[3] S. Jamil, H. M. Sirat, I. Jantan, N. Aimi, and M. Kitajima, "A new prenylated dihydrochalcone from the leaves of *Artocarpus lowii*," *Journal of Natural Medicines*, vol. 62, no. 3, pp. 321–324, 2008.

[4] M. R. Khan, A. D. Omoloso, and M. Kihara, "Antibacterial activity of *Artocarpus heterophyllus*," *Fitoterapia*, vol. 74, no. 5, pp. 501–505, 2003.

[5] B. N. Su, M. Cuendet, M. E. Hawthorne et al., "Constituents of the bark and twigs of *Artocarpus dadah* with cyclooxygenase inhibitory activity," *Journal of Natural Products*, vol. 65, no. 2, pp. 163–169, 2002.

[6] A. D. Patil, A. J. Freyer, L. Killmer et al., "A new dimeric dihydrochalcone and a new prenylated flavone from the bud covers of *Artocarpus altilis*: potent inhibitors of cathepsin K," *Journal of Natural Products*, vol. 65, no. 4, pp. 624–627, 2002.

[7] C. Boonlaksiri, W. Oonanant, P. Kongsaeree, P. Kittakoop, M. Tanticharoen, and Y. Thebtaranonth, "An antimalarial stilbene from *Artocarpus integer*," *Phytochemistry*, vol. 54, no. 4, pp. 415–417, 2000.

[8] T. T. Jong, C. N. Lin, and W. L. Shieh, "A pyranodihydrobenzoxanthone epoxide from *Artocarpus communis*," *Phytochemistry*, vol. 31, no. 7, pp. 2563–2564, 1992.

[9] E. H. Hakim, S. A. Achmad, L. D. Juliawaty et al., "Prenylated flavonoids and related compounds of the Indonesian *Artocarpus* (Moraceae)," *Journal of Natural Medicines*, vol. 60, no. 3, pp. 161–184, 2006.

[10] K. Shimizu, R. Kondo, K. Sakai, S. Buabarn, and U. Dilokkunanant, "A geranylated chalcone with 5α-reductase inhibitory properties from *Artocarpus incisus*," *Phytochemistry*, vol. 54, no. 8, pp. 737–739, 2000.

[11] L. Makmur, Syamsurizal, Tukiran et al., "Artoindonesianin C, a new xanthone derivative from *Artocarpus teysmanii*," *Journal of Natural Products*, vol. 63, no. 2, pp. 243–244, 2000.

[12] U. B. Jagtap and V. A. Bapat, "*Artocarpus*: a review of its traditional uses, phytochemistry and pharmacology," *Journal of Ethnopharmacology*, vol. 129, no. 2, pp. 142–166, 2010.

[13] M. Rahmani, H. M. Hashim, M. A. Sukari et al., "Antioxidant, cytotoxic and antibacterial activities of thirteen species of *Artocarpus* (Moraceae)," *Journal of Medicinal and Aromatic Plant Sciences*, vol. 31, no. 2, pp. 142–146, 2009.

[14] E. T. Arung, S. Muladi, E. Sukaton, K. Shimizu, and R. Kondo, "Artocarpin, a promosing compound as whitening agent and anti-skin cancer," *Journal of Tropical Wood Science and Technology*, vol. 6, no. 1, pp. 33–36, 2008.

[15] K. Likhitwitayawuid, B. Sritularak, and W. de-Eknamkul, "Tyrosinase inhibitors from *Artocarpus gomezianus*," *Planta Medica*, vol. 66, no. 3, pp. 275–277, 2000.

[16] E. H. Hakim, A. Fahriyati, M. S. Kau et al., "Artoindonesianins A and B, two new prenylated flavones from the root of *Artocarpus champeden*," *Journal of Natural Products*, vol. 62, no. 4, pp. 613–615, 1999.

[17] L. Jayasinghe, B. A. I. S. Balasooriya, W. C. Padmini, N. Hara, and Y. Fujimoto, "Geranyl chalcone derivatives with antifungal and radical scavenging properties from the leaves of *Artocarpus nobilis*," *Phytochemistry*, vol. 65, no. 9, pp. 1287–1290, 2004.

[18] M. Sato, S. Fujiwara, H. Tsuchiya et al., "Flavones with antibacterial activity against cariogenic bacteria," *Journal of Ethnopharmacology*, vol. 54, no. 2-3, pp. 171–176, 1996.

[19] S. S. Shamaun, M. Rahmani, N. M. Hashim et al., "Prenylated flavones from *Artocarpus altilis*," *Journal of Natural Medicines*, vol. 64, no. 4, pp. 478–481, 2010.

[20] N. M. Hashim, M. Rahmani, M. A. Sukari et al., "Two new xanthones from *Artocarpus obtusus*," *Journal of Asian Natural Products Research*, vol. 12, no. 2, pp. 106–112, 2010.

[21] T. R. Mosmann, "Rapid colorimetric assay for cellular growth and survival: application to proliferation and cytotoxicity assays," *Journal of Immunological Methods*, vol. 65, no. 1-2, pp. 55–68, 1983.

[22] A. Lupulescu, "Cancer cell metabolism and multidrug resistance (MDR)," in *Cancer Cell Metabolism and Cancer Treatment*, pp. 85–108, Hartwood Academic Publisher, 2001.

[23] R. I. Geran, N. H. Greenberg, M. M. McDonald, A. M. Scumaker, and B. J. Abbot, "Protocols for screening chemical agents and natural products against animal tumours and other biological systems," *Cancer Chemotherapy Reports*, no. 3, pp. 1–61, 1972.

[24] K. Shimizu, R. Kondo, and K. Sakai, "Inhibition of tyrosinase by flavonoids, stilbenes and related 4-substituted resorcinols: structure-activity investigations," *Planta Medica*, vol. 66, no. 1, pp. 11–15, 2000.

7

Antilipogenic and Anti-Inflammatory Activities of *Codonopsis lanceolata* in Mice Hepatic Tissues after Chronic Ethanol Feeding

Areum Cha,[1] Youngshim Choi,[1] Yoojeong Jin,[1] Mi-Kyung Sung,[2] Yun-Chang Koo,[3] Kwang-Won Lee,[3] and Taesun Park[1]

[1] *Department of Food and Nutrition, Yonsei University, 262 Seongsanno, Seodaemun-gu, Seoul 120-749, Republic of Korea*
[2] *Department of Food and Nutrition, Sookmyung Women's University, 52 Hyochangwon-gil, Yongsan-gu, Seoul 140-742, Republic of Korea*
[3] *Department of Food Science, College of Life Sciences and Biotechnology, Korea University, 1, 5-ga, Anam-dong, Sungbuk-ku, Seoul 136-701, Republic of Korea*

Correspondence should be addressed to Taesun Park, tspark@yonsei.ac.kr

Academic Editor: Masa-Aki Shibata

This study evaluated the antilipogenic and anti-inflammatory effects of *Codonopsis lanceolata (C. lanceolata)* root extract in mice with alcohol-induced fatty liver and elucidated its underlying molecular mechanisms. Ethanol was introduced into the liquid diet by mixing it with distilled water at 5% (wt/v), providing 36% of the energy, for nine weeks. Among the three different fractions prepared from the *C. lanceolata* root, the *C. lanceolata* methanol extract (CME) exhibited the most remarkable attenuation of alcohol-induced fatty liver with respect to various parameters such as hepatic free fatty acid concentration, body weight loss, and hepatic accumulations of triglyceride and cholesterol. The hepatic gene and protein expression levels were analysed via RT-PCR and Western blotting, respectively. CME feeding significantly restored the ethanol-induced downregulation of the adiponectin receptor (adipoR) 1 and of adipoR2, along with their downstream molecules. Furthermore, the study data showed that CME feeding dramatically reversed ethanol-induced hepatic upregulation of toll-like receptor- (TLR-) mediated signaling cascade molecules. These results indicate that the beneficial effects of CME against alcoholic fatty livers of mice appear to be with adenosine- and adiponectin-mediated regulation of hepatic steatosis and TLR-mediated modulation of hepatic proinflammatory responses.

1. Introduction

Fatty liver is the most common and earliest response of the liver to heavy alcohol consumption and may develop into alcoholic hepatitis and fibrosis [1]. It has been traditionally held that, during alcohol metabolism, the increase in the cellular NADH concentration generated by alcohol and aldehyde dehydrogenases impairs β-oxidation and tricarboxylic acid cycle activity in the liver, which in turn leads to severe FFA overload and enhanced synthesis of triacylglycerol in the liver [2]. More recently, two transcription factors, the peroxisome proliferator-activated receptor (PPAR) α and PPARγ, have been discovered as new mechanisms that control hepatic fatty acid oxidation and synthesis, respectively [3, 4]. Ethanol feeding impairs fatty acid catabolism in the liver partly by blocking PPARα-mediated responses in C57BL/6J mice. In the meantime, dietary supplementation of ethanol-fed animals with a PPARα agonist induces the expression of PPARα target genes and stimulates the rate of fatty acid β-oxidation, which prevents alcoholic fatty liver [5]. In contrast to PPARα, hepatic PPARγ contributes to triglyceride homeostasis, which regulates both triglyceride clearance from the circulation and the lipogenic program [6]. Ethanol increases the mRNA expressions of PPARγ and lipid synthetic enzymes, ATP citrate lyase (ACL), and fatty acid synthase (FAS) in mice liver [1].

Ethanol is well known to stimulate increased extracellular adenosine concentration through its action on the nucleoside transporter. Ethanol ingestion increases purine release into the bloodstream and urine in normal volunteers [7–9] and into the extracellular space in liver slices obtained from mice [10, 11]. Extracellular adenosine regulates various physical processes [12], including hepatic fibrosis [10, 11], ureagenesis [13, 14], and glycogen metabolism [15, 16], as well as peripheral lipid metabolism [17, 18]. These physiological effects of adenosine are mediated by a family of four G-protein-coupled receptors: A_1, A_{2A}, A_{2B}, and A_3 (A1R, A2AR, A2BR, and A3R), each of which has a unique pharmacological profile, tissue distribution, and effector coupling [19]. Recently, Peng et al. reported that ethanol-mediated increases in extracellular adenosine, which act via adenosine A1R and A2BR, link the ingestion and metabolism of ethanol to the development of hepatic steatosis. Thus, they suggested that targeting adenosine receptors may be effective in the prevention of alcohol-induced fatty liver [1].

Although fatty liver was thought to be relatively benign, more recent studies show that fat accumulation makes the liver more susceptible to injury from other agents such as drugs and toxins, especially endotoxins [20], which are believed to be involved in the pathogenesis of alcoholic hepatitis and fibrosis [21, 22]. Alcohol consumption induces a state of a "leaky gut" that increases plasma and liver endotoxin levels and leads to the production of the tumor necrosis factor α (TNFα) by Kupffer cells via the toll-like receptor (TLR) 4, which is known to mediate lipopolysaccharide- (LPS-) induced signal transduction and to eventually contribute to liver injury [23]. Ethanol-fed mice exhibited an oxidative stress that was dependent on the upregulation of multiple TLRs (TLR1, 2, 4, 6, 7, 8, and 9) in the liver and was sensitive to liver inflammation induced by multiple bacterial products recognized by the TLRs [24].

Codonopsis lanceolata (*C. lanceolata*), which belongs to the Campanulaceae family, is a perennial herb that grows naturally in moist places in woods, low mountains, and hills [25]. It is commonly found in East Asia, particularly in China [25]. *C. lanceolata*, which is composed of various active components including tannins, saponins, polyphenolics, alkaloids, essential oils, and steroids, has long been prescribed in traditional folk medicine in Korea, Japan, and China [26–28]. The dried roots of *C. lanceolata* have been used as a traditional remedy for lung inflammatory diseases such as asthma, tonsillitis, and pharyngitis. The total methanol extracts of the fresh leaves or roots of *C. lanceolata* significantly suppress the production of TNFα and nitric oxide, the expression of interleukin (IL)-3 and IL-6, and LPS-mediated phagocytic uptake in RAW 264.7 cells [28]. In a rat model, *C. lanceolata* water extract significantly improved the hepatic accumulation of triglyceride and cholesterol induced by a high-fat diet [29]. Although the lipid-lowering effect of *C. lanceolata* extract has been demonstrated in a rodent model with diet-induced obesity, the protective effects of this plant against alcoholic fatty liver diseases have not yet been explored. In this study, the potent bioactivities of the *C. lanceolata* methanol extract that can be used as natural compound or pharmaceutical supplements for the prevention and/or treatment of alcoholic fatty liver were demonstrated. The mechanisms by which the *C. lanceolata* methanol extract performs its antilipogenic and anti-inflammatory actions were investigated in the hepatic tissues of mice with chronic ethanol consumption.

2. Materials and Methods

2.1. Preparation of C. lanceolata Extract. *C. lanceolata*, which is cultivated in Gangwon-do, Korea, was purchased and freeze dried. Freshly dried material was ground into fine powder in an electric grinder and stored in dessicator. 200 g plant powder was refluxed with 95% methyl alcohol (MeOH) in a round bottom flask on a water bath for 3 h. Crude MeOH extract was filtered out and evaporated to dryness for the preparation of the *C. lanceolata* methanol extract (CME). The residual methanol extract was again refluxed with distilled water for 5 h and filtered. The filtrate, thus obtained, was again added with ethanol at the ratio of 1 : 4 and then stirred for 1 h at 4°C. Following their centrifugation at 5,000 ×g for 30 min at 4°C, the supernatant was concentrated in a rotary vacuum evaporator and freeze dried for the preparation of the *C. lanceolata* ethanol supernatant (CES), and the pellets were air dried and freeze dried for the preparation of the *C. lanceolata* ethanol precipitate (CEP). The yields of these three extracts were 3.84% (CME), 5.05% (CES), and 3.30% (CEP) of the wet *C. lanceolata* root, respectively.

2.2. Animals and Diets. Specific pathogen-free male C57BL/6N mice (eight weeks old) were purchased (Orient, Gyeonggi-do, Korea) and acclimatized to the authors' animal facility for one week prior to the experimentation. The mice were kept individually in sterilized animal quarters with controlled temperature (at 21 ± 2°C) and humidity (at 50 ± 5%) and with 12 h light and dark cycles and were allowed free access to standard chow and tap water during the acclimatization period. The animals were then randomly divided into five groups ($n = 8$) and fed the normal diet (ND), the ethanol diet (ED), the CME-supplemented ethanol diet (MED), the CES-supplemented ethanol diet (ESD), or the CEP-supplemented ethanol diet (EPD) for nine weeks. The mice in the ED group consumed a liquid diet wherein ethanol provided 36% of the energy, as described by Lieber et al. [30]. Ethanol was introduced into the diet by gradually mixing it with distilled water, from 0% (wt/v) to 5% (wt/v), over a one-week period for adaptation, and was provided at 5% (wt/v) for the next eight weeks. The ND mice received the same diet but with isocaloric amounts of dextrin-maltose instead of ethanol, and the MED, ESD, and EPD mice were fed the ethanol diet that contained 0.091% (wt/v) CME, CES, and CEP, respectively. The compositions of the experimental diets are given in Table 1. The ND, MED, DES, and EPD mice were pair fed so that their consumption would be isocalorically equivalent to the consumption on the previous day of the ED mice that were individually paired with them. The animals that were used in this study were treated in accordance with the Guide for the Care and Use of Laboratory Animals (Institute of Laboratory Animal Resources, Commission on Life Sciences, National Research Council, 1996), as approved by the Institutional Animal Care and Use Committee of Yonsei University.

2.3. Histological Examination. The liver tissue specimens were fixed in 10% buffered formalin and embedded in

TABLE 1: Compositions of experimental diets.

Ingredient	ND	ED	MED	ESD	EPD
			g/L		
Casein	41.4	41.40	41.40	41.40	41.40
L-cystine	0.50	0.50	0.50	0.50	0.50
DL-methionine	0.30	0.30	0.30	0.30	0.30
Corn oil	8.50	8.50	8.50	8.50	8.50
Olive oil	28.40	28.40	28.40	28.40	28.40
Safflower oil	2.70	2.70	2.70	2.70	2.70
Dextrine-maltose[1]	115.20	25.60	25.60	25.60	25.60
Vitamin mix (AIN-76G)[2]	2.50	2.50	2.50	2.50	2.50
Mineral mix (AIN-76G)[3]	8.75	8.75	8.75	8.75	8.75
Choline bitartrate	0.53	0.53	0.53	0.53	0.53
Cellulose	10.00	10.00	10.00	10.00	10.00
Xanthan gum	3.00	3.00	3.00	3.00	3.00
Ethanol		50.00	50.00	50.00	50.00
CME			0.91		
CES				0.91	
CEP					0.91
Water	778.22	817.82	816.91	816.91	816.91
Total	1000	1000	1000	1000	1000

[1]Dextrin : maltose = 80 : 20.

[2]Vitamin mixture (g/kg mix); thiamin · HCl 0.6; riboflavin 0.6; nicotinamide 25; pyridoxine· HCl 0.7; nicotinic acid 3; D-calcium pantothenate 1.6; folic acid 0.2; D-biotin 0.02; cyanocobalamin (vitamin B_{12}) 0.001; retinyl palmitate (250,000 IU/gm) 1.6; DL-α-tocopherol acetate (250 IU/gm) 20; cholecalciferol (vitamin D_3) 0.25; menaquinone (vitamin K_2) 0.05; sucrose, finely powdered 972.9.

[3]AIN-76 Mineral mixture (g/kg mix); $CaHPO_4$ 500; NaCl 74; $K_2H_6O_7H_2O$ 220; $K_2SO_4$52; MgO 24; $MnCO_3$ 3.57; Fe $(C_6H_5O_7)\cdot 6H_2O$ 6; $ZnCO_3$ 1.6; $CuCO_3$ 0.3; KIO_3 0.01; $Na_2SeO_3\cdot 5H_2O$ 0.01; CrK $(SO_4)_2$ 0.55; sucrose, finely powdered 118.

paraffin, cut at thicknesses of 5 μm, and later stained with hematoxylin and eosin (H&E) for the histological examination of fat droplets.

2.4. Biochemical Assays. The serum concentrations of total cholesterol, HDL cholesterol, triglyceride, and free fatty acid were determined using commercial kits (BioClinical System, Gyeonggi-do, Korea). Hepatic lipids were extracted through the procedure developed by Folch et al. [31], using a chloroform-methanol mixture (2 : 1, v/v). The dried lipid residues were dissolved in 1 mL of ethanol for the cholesterol and triglyceride measurements. The hepatic cholesterol, triglyceride, and free fatty acid concentrations were analyzed using the same enzymatic kit that was used in the serum analyses. The serum alanine aminotransferase (ALT) and aspartate aminotransferase (AST) activities were measured using commercial reagents (Bayer, USA).

2.5. Isolation of Total RNA and Semiquantitative RT-PCR. The total RNA was extracted from the liver using a Trizol reagent (Invitrogen, USA) and was reverse transcribed using the Superscript II kit (Invitrogen, USA) according to the manufacturer's recommendations. The primers for the PCR analysis were synthesized by Bioneer (Korea). The forward (F) and reverse (R) primer sequences for the genes that were involved in the experiment are shown in the Supplementary Material available online at doi: 10.1155/2012/141395. The PCR for the glyceraldehyde-3-phosphate dehydrogenase (GAPDH) was performed on each sample as an internal positive-control standard. The number of cycles and the annealing temperature were optimized for each primer pair. Amplification of the GAPDH, A1R, A2AR, A2BR, A3R, PPARα, carnitine palmitoyltransferase (CPT-1), microsomal triglyceride transfer protein (MTP), long-chain acyl-CoA dehydrogenase (LCAD), medium-chain acyl-CoA dehydrogenase (MCAD), PPARγ, retinoid X receptor (RXR), CCAAT-enhancer-binding protein-α (C/EBPα), lipoprotein lipase (LPL), adipocyte protein 2 or fatty acid binding protein 4 (aP2), FAS, TLRs, LPS binding protein (LBP), cluster of differentiation 14 (CD14), myeloid differentiation primary response gene 88 (MyD88), myelin and lymphocyte protein (MAL), TLR adaptor molecule (TRIF), TNF-receptor-associated factor 6 (TRAF6), interferon regulatory factors (IRFs), nuclear factor kappa B-p50 (p50), p65, interferon α (IFNα), IFNβ, IL-12-p40, chemokine (C-X-C motif) ligand 2 (CXCL2), adiponectin receptor 1 (adipoR1), adipoR2, silent-mating-type information regulation 2 homolog 1 (SIRT1), peroxisome proliferative activated receptor gamma coactivator 1 alpha (PGC1α), and sterol regulatory element binding transcription factor 1 (SREBP-1c) was initiated via 5 min of denaturation at 94°C for 1 cycle, followed by 30 or 35 cycles at 94°C for 30 s, 55 or 60°C for 30 s, and 72°C for 1 min and via 10 min of incubation at 72°C. The sequences of the primer pairs and PCR conditions (annealing temperatures, cycles, and product sizes) that were used in the RT-PCR experiments are shown in the Supplementary Material. The PCR products were then separated in a 2% agarose gel and visualized in a gel documentation system (Alpha Innotech, USA). The intensity of the bands on the gels was converted into a digital image with a gel analyzer.

2.6. Western Blot Analysis. For the Western blot studies, protein extracts were obtained from the mice livers using a commercial lysis buffer (Intron, USA) that contained a protease inhibitor cocktail (Roche, USA). The protein concentrations were determined with the Bio-rad protein assay kit (Bio-rad, USA). The Western blot analysis was performed with antibodies that were specific to AMP-activated protein kinase (AMPK), phospho-AMPK (Thr 72), Acetyl-CoA carboxylase (ACC), phospho-ACC (Ser 79) (Cell Signaling, USA), and β-actin (Santa Cruz, USA). After the SDS-PAGE at 10% acrylamide concentrations, the proteins were transferred to the nitrocellulose membrane, blocked with 5% skim milk in a Tris-buffered saline/Tween buffer (10 mM Tris-HCl, pH 7.5, 150 mM NaCl, and 0.05% Tween 20), and incubated with appropriate antibodies overnight. The blots were washed extensively, incubated with a horseradish-peroxidase-linked

Table 2: Body weight gain and serum biochemistries of mice fed experimental diets.

	ND	ED	MED	ESD	EPD
Body weight gain (g/9 weeks)	10.9 ± 0.4^{a}[1]	5.3 ± 0.8^{c}	7.6 ± 0.7^{b}	7.5 ± 0.6^{b}	4.6 ± 0.6^{c}
Triglyceride (mmol/L)	0.78 ± 0.01^{b}	0.81 ± 0.02^{ab}	0.74 ± 0.03^{b}	0.86 ± 0.02^{a}	0.75 ± 0.02^{b}
Total cholesterol (mmol/L)	2.17 ± 0.19^{b}	2.15 ± 0.13^{b}	1.96 ± 0.13^{b}	2.65 ± 0.18^{a}	2.23 ± 0.10^{a}
HDL cholesterol (mmol/L)	0.88 ± 0.04^{b}	1.10 ± 0.10^{a}	1.17 ± 0.06^{a}	1.04 ± 0.08^{ab}	1.09 ± 0.06^{ab}
VLDL + LDL cholesterol (mmol/L)[2]	1.29 ± 0.19^{ab}	1.06 ± 0.15^{b}	0.79 ± 0.12^{b}	1.60 ± 0.21^{a}	1.14 ± 0.15^{ab}
Atherogenic index[3]	1.52 ± 0.25^{a}	1.07 ± 0.21^{ab}	0.70 ± 0.13^{b}	1.65 ± 0.21^{a}	1.12 ± 0.10^{ab}
Free fatty acid (μEq/L)	808 ± 31^{b}	990 ± 27^{a}	848 ± 36^{b}	1074 ± 52^{a}	883 ± 32^{b}
ALT (IU/ml)	6.87 ± 0.42^{c}	21.2 ± 0.89^{a}	17.5 ± 0.53^{b}	21.3 ± 0.78^{a}	21.2 ± 1.04^{a}
AST (IU/ml)	17.63 ± 1.63^{b}	22.3 ± 2.05^{a}	17.4 ± 1.05^{b}	24.6 ± 1.04^{a}	24.9 ± 0.98^{a}

[1]Each value is expressed as mean ± SEM ($n = 8$). Means with different letters within a row are significantly different ($P < 0.05$).
[2]VLDL + LDL cholesterol (mmol/L) = Total cholesterol − HDL cholesterol.
[3]Atherogenic index = (Total cholesterol − HDL cholesterol)/ HDL cholesterol.

anti-rabbit or -mouse Ig (Santa Cruz, USA), and washed again. The detection was carried out with the ECL Western blotting kit (Animal Genetics, Korea), after which the blots were exposed to an X-ray film (Agfa, Belgium).

2.7. Statistical Analysis. The results of the body weight gain, liver weight, and serum and hepatic biochemistries were expressed as the mean values ± SEM of the eight mice in each group. The results of the semiquantitative RT-PCR and Western blot were expressed as the mean values ± SEM of the three independent experiments in which the RNA and protein samples from the eight mice were used, respectively. The analysis of the variance (ANOVA) and the Duncan's multiple range method were used to compare significant differences among the groups. The level of significance was set at $P < 0.05$ for all the statistical tests.

3. Results

3.1. Body Weight Gain and Blood Biochemistries. The nine-week body weight gain of the mice in the ED group was 51% lower than the value for the pair fed ND mice. The animals that were fed the MED (43% greater) or the ESD (41% greater) exhibited significantly greater body weight gains than the ED mice, whereas the mice that were fed the EPD did not recover the weight they lost from ethanol consumption (Table 2).

Compared to the values for the ED mice, the mice that were fed the MED exhibited significantly lower levels of serum FFA (17% reduction) and lower activities of serum ALT (17% reduction) and AST (22% reduction). They also demonstrated a tendency towards decreasing serum triglyceride, total cholesterol, VLDL + LDL cholesterol, and atherogenic indices, albeit at statistically insignificant levels than those for the mice that were fed the ED. In contrast, the ESD or EPD failed to improve both the lipid levels and enzyme activities in the blood of the mice with chronic ethanol consumption (Table 2).

3.2. Liver Weight and Hepatic Lipid Levels. Histological analysis of the livers with H&E staining revealed prominent lipid accumulation in the livers of the ED fed mice whereas lipid droplets were rare in the livers of the MED, ESD, and EPD-fed mice (Figure 1). ED feeding of the mice for nine weeks resulted in more significant increases in the relative weight of their livers (by 8%) and in the hepatic levels of their triglycerides (43% increase), cholesterol (36% increase), and FFA (52% increase) than in the ND group (Figure 1). The MED or ESD significantly improved the ethanol-induced enlargement of the liver (the relative liver weight was 7% or 6% lower, resp.). The MED, ESD, or EPD significantly reversed the ethanol-induced hepatic accumulations of triglycerides (18%, 11%, and 18% reductions, resp.), cholesterol (22%, 12%, and 18% reductions, resp.), and FFA (29%, 14%, and 22% reductions, resp.). The triglyceride and cholesterol levels in the liver were lowest after the MED consumption among the diets that were supplemented with different fractions of the *C. lanceolata* root, but the differences between the diets were not statistically significant. The MED group exhibited the most prominent and the most significant improvement in the reduction of the hepatic FFA accumulation, better than did the ESD and EPD groups ($P < 0.05$) (Figure 1).

3.3. Regulation of Adenosine Receptor-Mediated Signaling Molecules. MED feeding significantly reversed the ethanol-induced upregulation of the A1R and A2BR genes in the livers of the mice and restored the ethanol-induced downregulation of the PPARα, CPT-1, MTP, LCAD, and MCAD genes in the livers of the mice (Figures 2(a) and 2(b)). The supplementation of the ethanol diet with CME significantly blunted the upregulation of these transcription factors and of their target genes due to ethanol.

3.4. Regulation of Adiponectin Receptor-Mediated Signaling Molecules. Chronic ethanol ingestion led to more significant decreases in the hepatic expression of the adipoR1 and adipoR2 genes than in the ND mice, and MED feeding significantly restored these ethanol-induced changes in the adiponectin receptor genes. Similarly, the MED feeding significantly reversed the marked decreases in the mRNA levels of the hepatic SIRT1 and PGC1α, which were induced

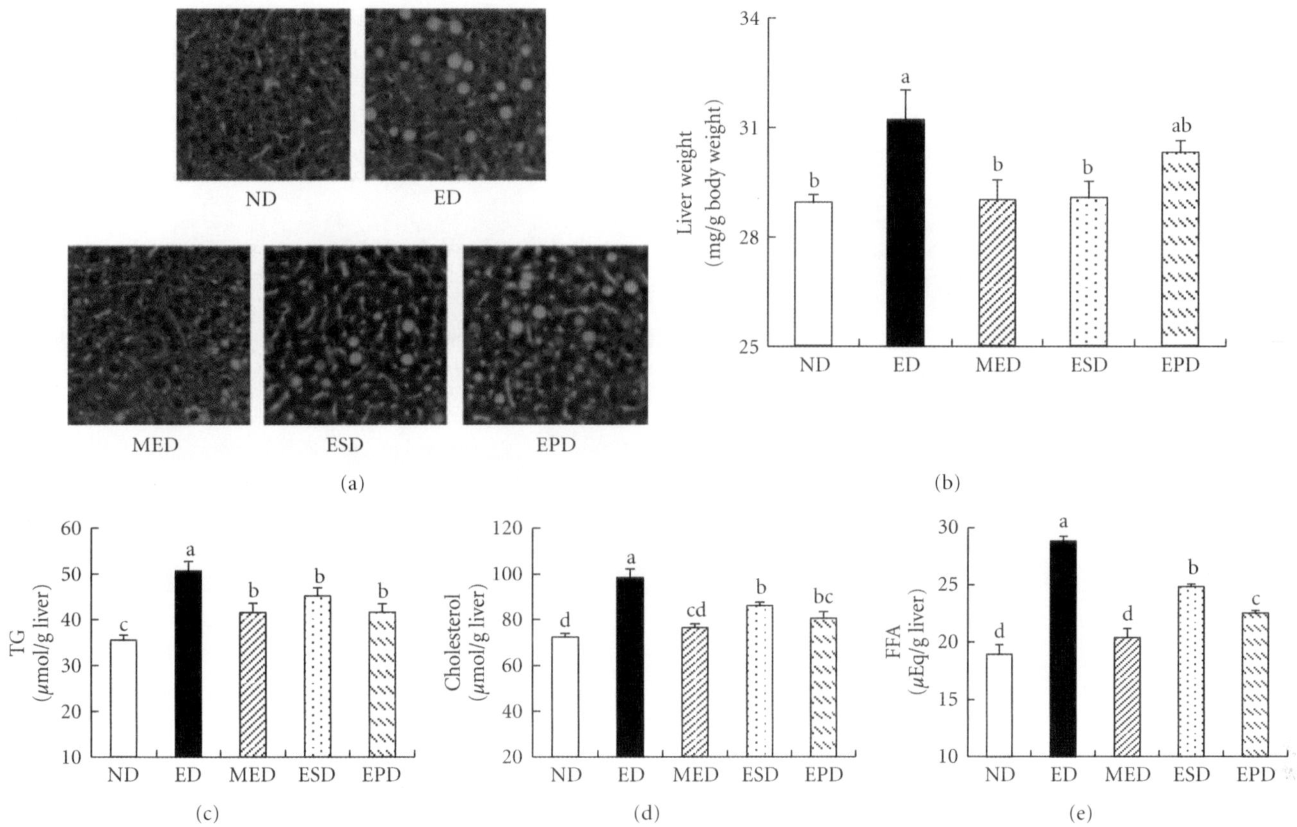

Figure 1: *Codonopsis lanceolata* extracts substantially reduces alcohol-induced liver steatosis. (a) Hematoxylin and eosin-stained sections of representative liver samples of the treated groups (100×). (b) Changes in the liver-to-body weight ratio. Hepatic triglyceride, free fatty acid, and cholesterol levels are shown in (c, d, and e). The data are expressed as means ± SEM (n = 8). [a,b,c,d]Means not sharing a common letter are significantly different ($P < 0.05$).

by ethanol feeding. In addition, the MED efficiently counteracted the ethanol-induced upregulation of the SREBP-1c gene (higher 57% reduction than in the ED mice, $P < 0.05$) (Figure 3). The MED significantly blunted the downregulation of the phospho-AMPK/total AMPK (146% increase) ratio and of the phospho-ACC/total ACC ratio (700% increase), which were caused by chronic ethanol ingestion, in the livers of the mice (Figures 3(b) and 3(c)).

3.5. Regulation of TLRs-Mediated Signaling Molecules. The hepatic expression of the TLR mRNAs was measured after nine weeks of ethanol exposure. More significant increases in the TLR1, TLR2, TLR3, TLR4, TLR6, TLR7, TLR8, TLR9, TLR12, and TLR13 mRNA levels were observed in the livers of the ethanol-fed control mice than of the pair fed ND mice. The MED significantly alleviated the ethanol-induced upregulation of the hepatic TLR1, TLR2, TLR4, TLR6, TLR7, TLR8, TLR9, TLR12, and TLR13 gene expressions. The hepatic TLR3, which was upregulated by the ethanol feeding, and the hepatic TLR5, which was unaffected by the ethanol feeding, did not respond to the MED feeding (Figure 4).

After endotoxin bound itself to the LPS-binding protein (LBP), it associates in the portal blood with the CD14 prior to its binding to TLR4 and all the TLRs that were recruited by MyD88, MAL, TRIF, and TRAF6 for their proinflammatory signaling. The mRNA levels of the LBP and CD14, as well as of the adaptor molecules of the TLRs (MyD88, MAL, TRIF, and TRAF6), all more significantly increased in the livers of the ED mice than of the ND mice, whereas the MED feeding led to more significant decreases in the hepatic mRNA levels of the LBP, CD14, MyD88, MAL, TRIF, and TRAF6 than in the ED mice (Figure 5(a)). Among the extremely significant recent discoveries on TLR signaling is that the MyD88-dependent pathway also activates some IRFs, such as IRF1, 3, 5, and 7. In this study, the mRNA levels of the IRF1, 3, 5, and 7 genes more significantly increased in the livers of the ED mice than of the ND mice and these ethanol-induced upregulations of the hepatic IRFs were significantly reversed by the MED feeding (Figure 5(b)). The RT-PCR analysis of the hepatic mRNAs of NFκB (p50 and p65) and of its target cytokine genes such as TNFα, IL-6, IFNα, IFNβ, IL-12-p40, and CXCL2 was performed next. The MED feeding significantly downregulated the expressions of the p50, p65, TNFα, IL-6, IFNα, IFNβ, IL-12-p40, and CXCL2 genes compared to the ED mice (Figure 5(c)).

4. Discussion

The authors' previous study showed that the supplementation of the Lieber-DeCarli ethanol diet with *C. lanceolata*

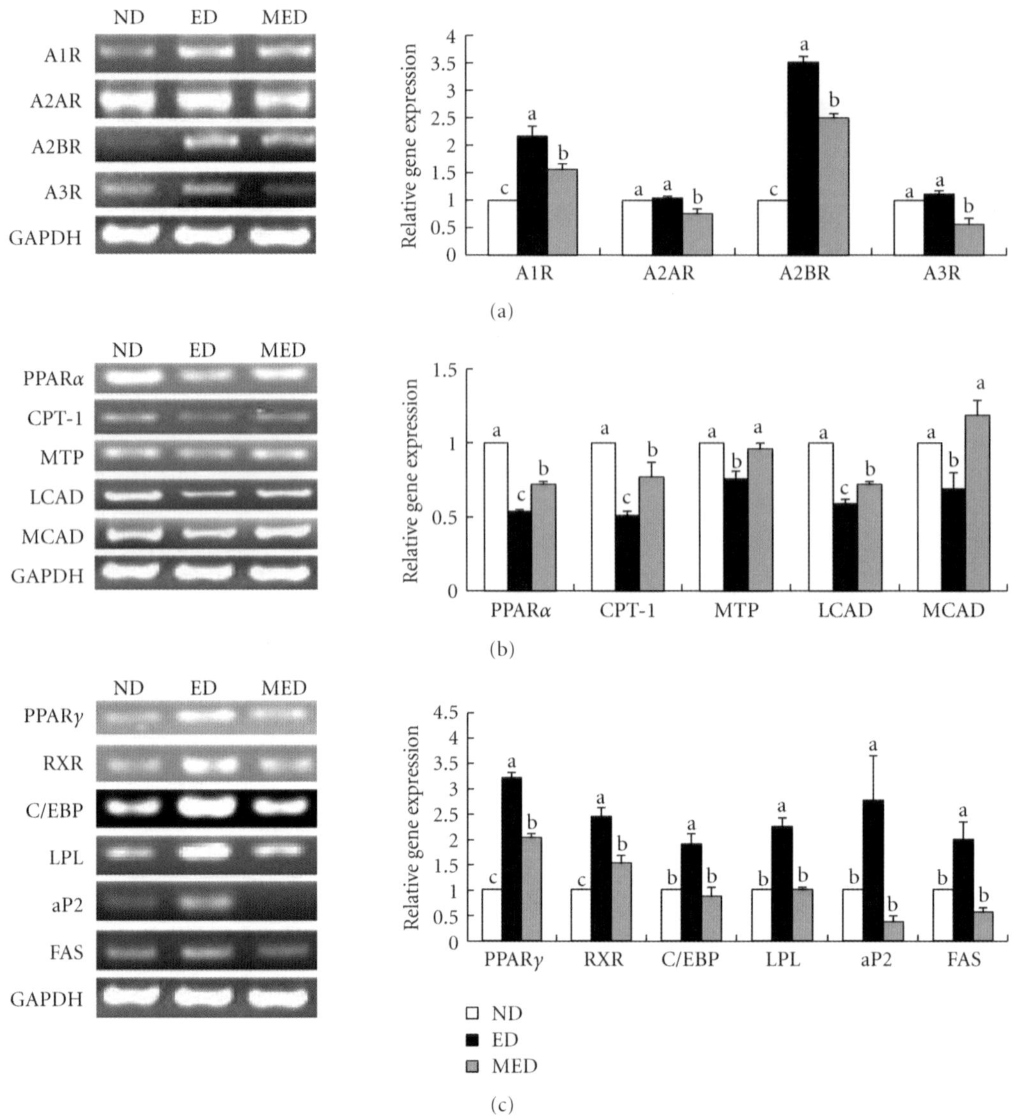

Figure 2: mRNA expression of the hepatic genes that are involved in fatty acid oxidation or adipogenesis. The left panel shows an RT-PCR analysis of (a) A1R, A2AR, A2BR, and A3R (b) PPARα, CPT-1, MTP, LCAD, and MCAD and (c) PPARγ, RXR, C/EBPα, LPL, aP2, and FAS expression. The images show the representative agarose gel electrophoresis of the PCR products. The right panel shows the relative expressions of (a) A1R, A2AR, A2BR, and A3R (b) PPARα, CPT-1, MTP, LCAD, and MCAD and (c) PPARγ, RXR, C/EBPα, LPL, aP2, and FAS levels. The data were normalized to the GAPDH levels, and all the expression levels that are displayed are relative to the ND. The results that are shown represent the means ± SEM of the three independent experiments in which RNA samples from eight mice were used. [a,b,c]Means not sharing a common letter are significantly different ($P < 0.05$).

water extract (5 mg/L of a liquid diet) showed a significant improvement in the amount of weight that was gained and in the hepatic lipid levels (in the press). In this study, the effects of three different fractions of *C. lanceolata* roots, which were prepared using different solvents, on the protection from alcoholic fatty liver were tested. Several studies have demonstrated that the protective effects of various plant extracts from alcoholic liver injury in animals, such as of fenugreek seed (*Trigonella foenum fraecum*) methanol extract [32], and hot water extracts of avaram leaves (*Cassia auriculata*) [33] and green tea (*Camellia sinensis*) [34] were manifested at dosages of between 200 and 500 mg/kg of body weight. Based on these studies, *C. lanceolata* root fractions were added to a liquid diet at 0.091% (wt/v), which is equivalent to a daily intake of 300 mg/kg of body weight, assuming that a mouse weighs 30 g and consumes 10 ml of a liquid diet per day.

Among the three different fractions that were prepared from the *C. lanceolata* root, CME exhibited the most remarkable attenuation of alcohol-induced fatty liver in terms of various parameters. For example, CME more significantly reduced the serum ALT and AST activities and the hepatic FFA concentration in the mice that were fed ethanol than did CES or CEP. Besides, alcohol-induced body weight loss and

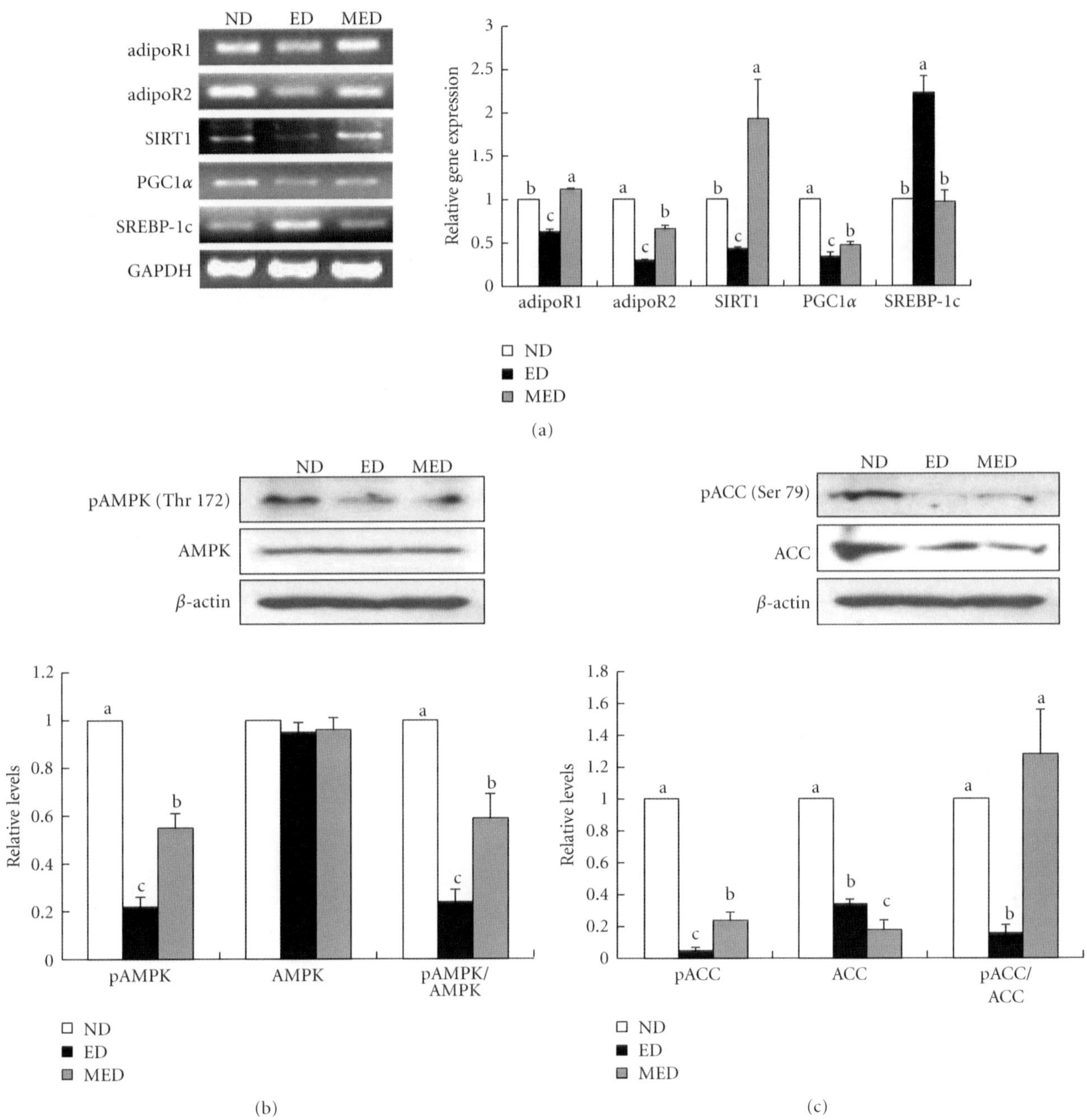

Figure 3: Alcohol-induced liver adiponectin receptors and involved genes in mRNA or protein expression. (a) The left panel shows the results of the RT-PCR analysis of adipoR1, adipoR2, SRIT1, PGC1α, and SREBP-1c expressions. The images show the representative agarose gel electrophoresis of the PCR products. The right panel shows the relative expressions of the adipoR1, adipoR2, SRIT1, PGC1α, and SREBP-1c levels. The data were normalized to the GAPDH levels, and all the expression levels that are shown are relative to the ND. (b) The upper panel shows the results of the Western blot analysis of the phosphorylated and total AMPK. The images show representative Western blotting images. The bottom panel shows the relative expressions of those levels and the ratios of the phosphorylated protein level to the total protein level. (c) The upper panel shows the results of the Western blot analysis of the phosphorylated and total ACC. The images show representative Western blotting images. The bottom panel shows the relative expressions of those levels and the ratios of the phosphorylated protein level to the total protein level. These results represent the means ± SEM of the three independent experiments in which RNA or protein samples from eight mice were used. [a, b, c]Means not sharing a common letter are significantly different ($P < 0.05$).

hepatic accumulations of triglycerides and cholesterol more significantly improved in mice that were supplemented with CME than in animals that were supplemented with ESD or EPD, although the difference was statistically insignificant. Therefore, CME appeared to be the most potent, among the fractions that were obtained from the *C. lanceolata* root, in protecting animals from alcohol-induced hepatic accumulation of lipids. Further investigated were the underlying mechanisms of CME against hepatic steatosis induced by chronic ethanol administration. The ethanol-induced

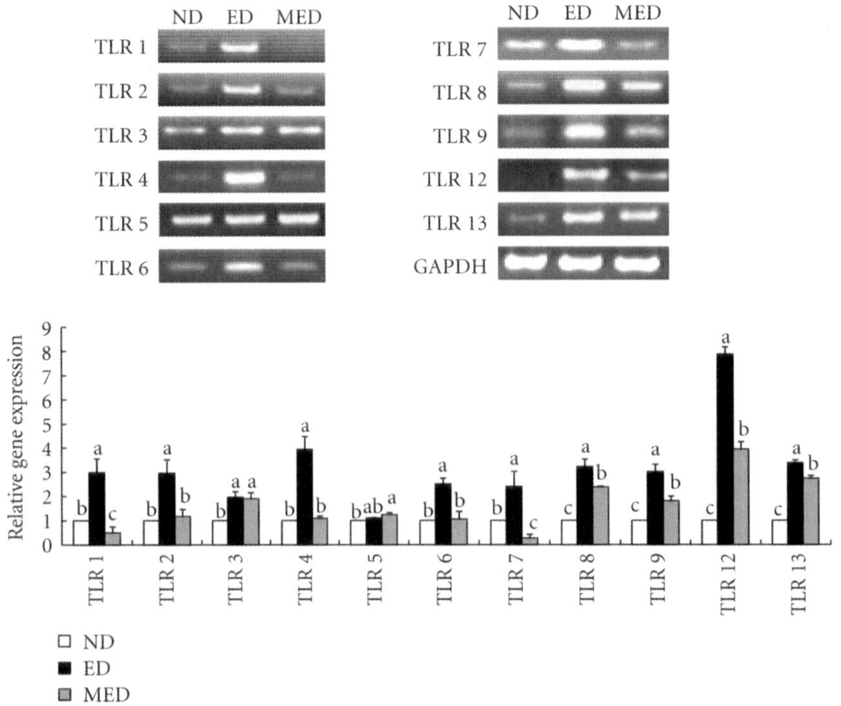

FIGURE 4: Alcohol-induced liver TLR mRNA expression. The upper panel shows the results of the RT-PCR analysis of the TLR1~9, 12, and 13 expressions. The images show the representative agarose gel electrophoresis of the PCR products. The bottom panel shows the relative expressions of the TLR1~9, 12, and 13 levels. The data were normalized to the GAPDH levels, and all the expression levels that are shown are relative to the ND. The results that are shown represent the means ± SEM of the three independent experiments in which RNA samples from eight mice were used. [a, b, c]Means not sharing a common letter are significantly different ($P < 0.05$).

elevation of the plasma HDL cholesterol concentration, as observed in the current study, has been suggested as a cardioprotective response in animals chronically loaded with ethanol [35]. The elevated HDL concentration and the reduced LDL concentration, which are characteristic of the lipoprotein pattern in chronic alcoholics, could well explain the reduced risk of coronary heart disease in alcoholics [36].

In this present study, the mRNA expression of the hepatic A2BR and A1R was markedly elevated by chronic ethanol feeding. Furthermore, the expression of PPARα and of its target genes, such as CPT-1, MTP, LCAD, and MCAD, all significantly decreased, whereas the expression of PPARγ and of its target genes, such as RXR, C/EBP, LPL, aP2, and FAS, all significantly increased in the livers of the ethanol-fed ED mice than of the ND mice (Figure 6). These results are in accordance with recent findings from experiments with mice that adenosine generated by ethanol metabolism plays an important role in ethanol-induced hepatic steatosis via A1R and A2BR, which leads to the upregulation of PPARγ and the downregulation of PPARα, respectively [1]. It was observed that CME supplementation reversed ethanol-induced elevation of the expressions of A2BR, A1R, PPARγ, and their target genes in the liver tissues of mice. These results suggest that CME ameliorates hepatic steatosis in mice, at least partly by modulating adenosine-receptor-mediated signaling molecules that are responsible for fatty acid oxidation and lipogenesis.

Adiponectin stimulates hepatic AMPK, which, in turn, phosphorylates ACC on Ser-79 and attenuates ACC activity. Inhibition of ACC directly reduces lipid synthesis and indirectly enhances fatty acid oxidation by blocking the production of malonyl-CoA, an allosteric inhibitor of CPT-1 [37]. Activation of AMPK by adiponectin in the liver also leads to decreased mRNA and protein expression of SREBP-1c [38–41], which results in decreased hepatic lipid synthesis. Adiponectin is also known to stimulate the activities of both PGC1α and PPARα, which mainly control the transcription of a panel of genes that encode fatty acid oxidation enzymes [42, 43]. As a result, adiponectin-mediated AMPK activation favors lipid catabolism and opposes lipid deposition in the liver [44–49]. Chronic ethanol administration is known to significantly decrease the plasma adiponectin level in mice [50]. In this study, more significant decreases in the mRNA levels of AdipoR1 and AdipoR2 were observed in the livers of the ED mice than of the pair fed ND mice. These alcohol-induced reductions in the hepatic AdipoRs expression appear to have been associated with the subsequent decreases in the phosphorylation of AMPK and ACC as their phosphorylations in the liver more significantly decreased in the ED mice than in the ND mice (Figure 6).

Besides, the hepatic mRNA levels of SIRT1, PGC1α, SREBP-1c, PPARα, and CPT1 were also more significantly reduced in the ED mice than in the ND mice (Figure 6). SIRT1 has been gaining recognition as one of the critical agents in the mediation of adiponectin signaling to AMPK [37], which is the central mechanism in the regulation of lipid metabolism [52–55]. Although PGC1α was initially identified as a coactivator of PPARγ, it has subsequently

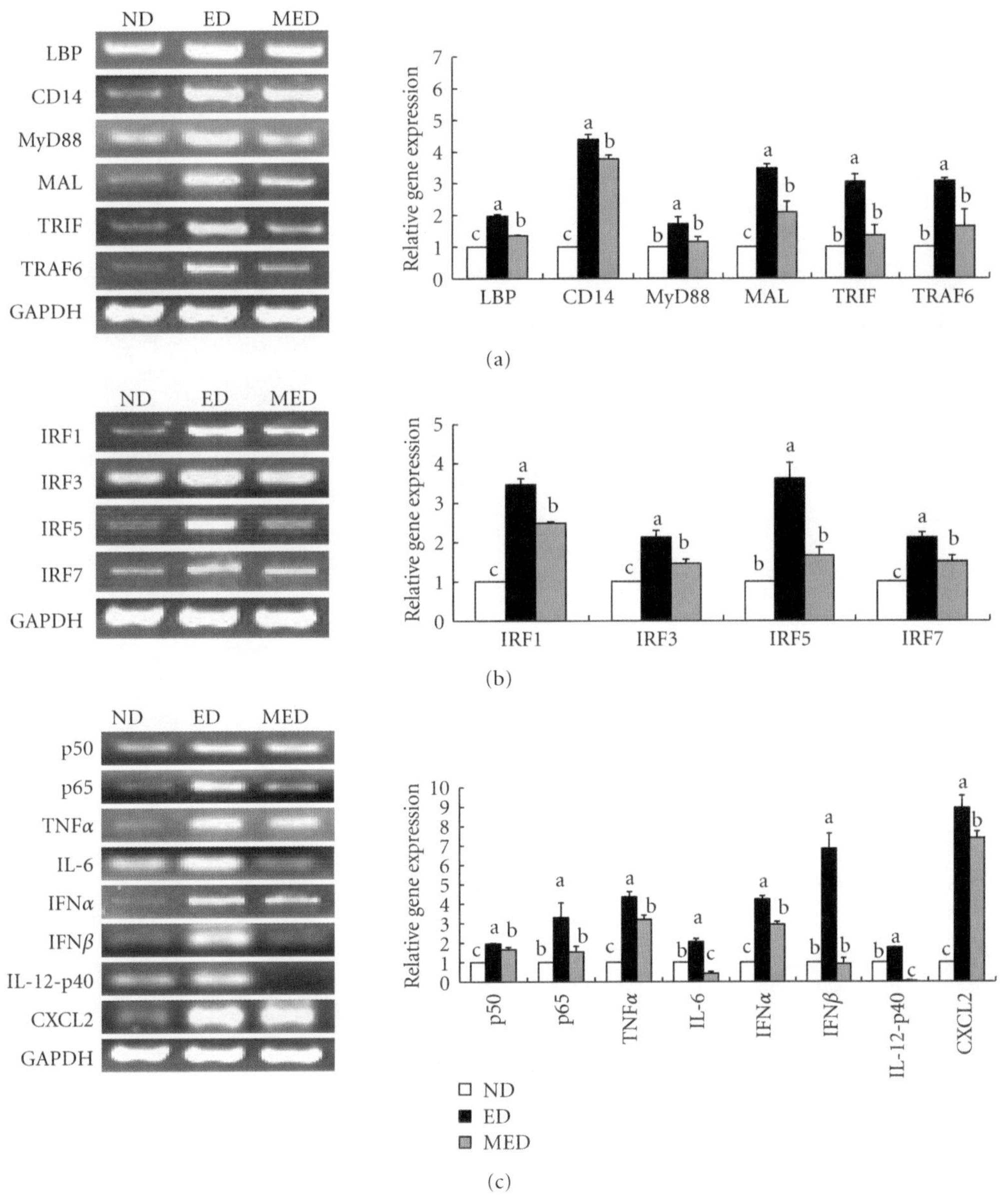

FIGURE 5: mRNA expressions of the hepatic genes that were involved in the inflammation. The left panel shows the results of the RT-PCR analysis of the (a) LBP, CD14, MyD88, MAL, TRIF, and TRAF6, (b) IRF1, IRF3, IRF5, and IRF7, and (c) p50, p65, TNFα, IL-6, IFNα, IFNβ, IL-12-p40, and CXCL2 expressions. The images show the representative agarose gel electrophoresis of the PCR products. The right panel shows the relative expressions of the (a) LBP, CD14, MyD88, MAL, TRIF, and TRAF6, (b) IRF1, IRF3, IRF5, and IRF7, and (c) p50, p65, TNFα, IL-6, IFNα, IFNβ, IL-12-p40, and CXCL2 levels. The data were normalized to the GAPDH levels, and all the expression levels that are shown are relative to the ND. The results that are shown represent the means ± SEM of the three independent experiments in which RNA samples from eight mice were used. [a,b,c]Means not sharing a common letter are significantly different ($P < 0.05$).

been shown to serve as a cofactor of several other transcription factors, including PPARα [56, 57]. Treatment with adiponectin restored the ethanol-inhibited PGC1α/PPARα activity in cultured hepatic cells and in animal livers, which suggests that the stimulation of adiponectin-SIRT1 signaling may serve as an effective therapeutic strategy for treating or preventing human alcoholic fatty liver [38–40]. In this study, CME significantly restored the ethanol-induced downregulation of adiponectin-mediated signaling molecules, including adipoR1, adipoR2, pAMPK/AMPK, pACC/ACC, SIRT1, and PGC1α, which led to increased fatty acid oxidation and decreased lipogenesis in the livers of the mice.

It was recently shown that innate immune cells recognize conserved pathogen-associated molecular patterns through pattern recognition receptors, among which the family of TLRs occupies an important place [24]. LBP, which is present in normal serum, recognizes and binds to LPS with high affinity through its lipid moiety [58, 59]. LPS-LBP complexes

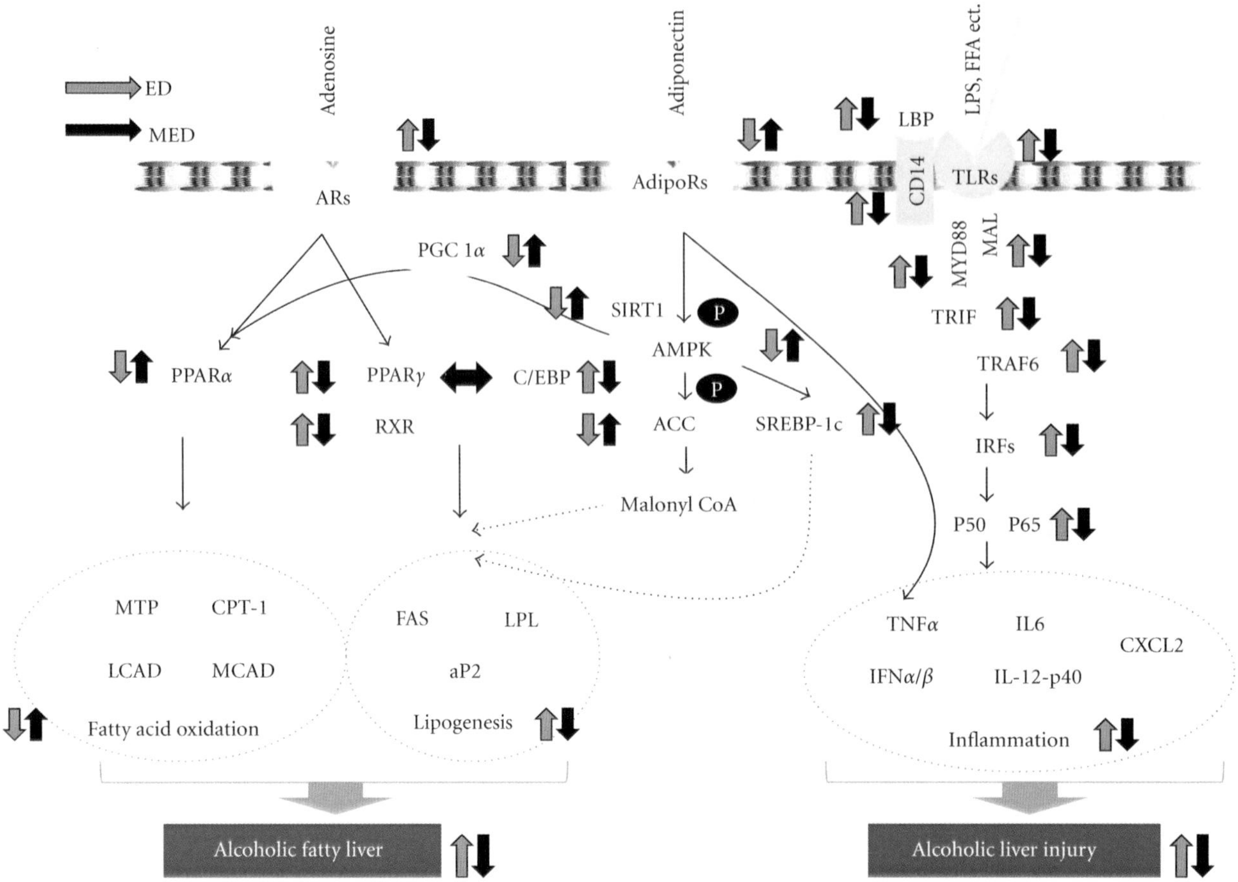

FIGURE 6: Schematic diagram illustrating the antilipogenic and anti-inflammatory activities of *Codonopsis lanceolata* in the liver of mice with chronic ethanol consumption. Adapted from Peng [1], You and Rogers [37, 51]. The arrows denote the direction of the responses to altered conditions with ED feeding relative to ND feeding (gray arrows), and with MED feeding relative to ED feeding (black arrows).

then activate cells through the second glycoprotein, the membrane-bound CD14, to produce inflammatory mediators [60–62] in the presence of only a functional TLR4 [63]. Although LPS was not detected in the blood, more significant increases in the mRNA levels of LBP and CD14 were observed in the livers of the ED mice than of the ND mice (Figure 6). TLRs have a TIR domain that initiates the signaling cascade through TIR adapters, such as MyD88 [64], Mal [65, 66], and TRIF, which interact with TRAF6, the downstream adaptor. TRAF6 activates the IRFs, which leads to NF-κB activation and induction of the expressions of proinflammatory cytokines [67], such as of TNFα, IL-6, IFNα, and IFNβ.

It was demonstrated that chronic ethanol feeding induces hepatic steatosis and clear upregulation of TLR1, 2, 3, 4, 6, 7, 8, 9, 12, and 13 in the liver. These findings are supported by previous reports that ethanol-fed mice exhibited hepatic inflammation that was dependent on the upregulation of multiple TLRs in the liver [24]. The expressions of the MyD88, MAL, TRIF, TRAF6, IRF1, 3, 5, and 7 genes, along with the mRNA levels of NFκB and proinflammatory cytokines, were all more significantly elevated in the livers of the ED mice than of the ND mice (Figure 6). These results are also in accordance with previous observations that MyD88 is required for the development of fibrosis [68], a predisposing condition for hepatocellular cancer development, and that IRF7 expression more significantly increased in the livers of alcohol-fed MyD88-deficient mice than of pair fed control mice [69]. These results suggest that chronic ethanol intake may activate TLR-mediated proinflammatory signaling cascades. The study data show that these hepatic inductions of TLR-mediated signaling cascade molecules, which involve both MyD88-dependent and -independent pathways, along with their target proinflammatory cytokine genes, such as TNFα, IL-6, IFNα, IFNβ, IL-12-p40, and CSCL2, due to ethanol feeding were all dramatically reversed with CME supplementation.

Taken together, these beneficial effects of CME against alcoholic fatty livers in mice appear to have occurred with adenosine- and adiponectin-mediated regulations of hepatic steatosis and TLR-mediated modulation of hepatic proinflammatory responses, since ethanol-induced changes in the expression of the molecules that are involved in these three signaling pathways were all significantly reversed with CME feeding. Although alcoholic fatty liver is a major risk factor for advanced liver injuries such as steatohepatitis, fibrosis, and cirrhosis [51], previous studies have mostly focused on the antilipogenic or -inflammatory activity alone, but not in combination, of a compound and extracts. For example, Kumar et al. evaluated the effect of the *Cassia auriculata* leaf extract on lipid metabolism in alcohol-induced hepatic steatosis [33]. Resveratrol prevents the development of hepatic steatosis induced by alcohol, by restoring the inhibited hepatic SIRT1-AMPK signaling system [70]. This study demonstrated that both lipogenesis and inflammation are associated with the development of alcoholic fatty liver and that CME has both antilipogenic and anti-inflammatory effects through coordinated multiple signaling pathways. Although much further study is required concerning the exact identities of the chemical constituents of the *C. lanceolata* methanol extract that are responsible for the findings described herein, the results of this study provide some insights on the basic mechanism that underlies the therapeutic effect of the extract on mice hepatic tissues after chronic ethanol feeding.

Acknowledgments

This study was supported by a grant from the BioGreen 21 Program of the Rural Development Administration (Code no. 20080401034049) and in part by a grant of the Korea Healthcare Technology R&D Project, Ministry for Health & Welfare Affairs (Code no. A085136) of the Republic of Korea.

References

[1] Z. Peng, P. A. Borea, K. Varani et al., "Adenosine signaling contributes to ethanol-induced fatty liver in mice," *Journal of Clinical Investigation*, vol. 119, no. 3, pp. 582–594, 2009.

[2] D. W. Crabb, "Recent developments in alcoholism: the liver," *Recent Developments in Alcoholism*, vol. 11, pp. 207–230, 1993.

[3] D. W. Crabb and S. Liangpunsakul, "Alcohol and lipid metabolism," *Journal of Gastroenterology and Hepatology*, vol. 21, supplement 3, pp. S56–S60, 2006.

[4] H. Tsukamoto, H. She, S. Hazra, J. Cheng, and J. Wang, "Fat paradox of steatohepatitis," *Journal of Gastroenterology and Hepatology*, vol. 23, supplement 1, pp. S104–S107, 2008.

[5] M. Fischer, M. You, M. Matsumoto, and D.W. Crabb, "Peroxisome proliferator-activated receptor α (PPARα) agonist treatment reverses PPARα dysfunction and abnormalities in hepatic lipid metabolism in ethanol-fed mice," *Journal of Biological Chemistry*, vol. 278, no. 30, pp. 7997–8004, 2003.

[6] O. Gavrilova, M. Haluzik, K. Matsusue et al., "Liver peroxisome proliferator-activated receptor γ contributes to hepatic steatosis, triglyceride clearance, and regulation of body fat mass," *Journal of Biological Chemistry*, vol. 278, no. 36, pp. 34268–34276, 2003.

[7] L. E. Nagy, I. Diamond, D. J. Casso, C. Franklin, and A. S. Gordon, "Ethanol increases extracellular adenosine by inhibiting adenosine uptake via the nucleoside transporter," *Journal of Biological Chemistry*, vol. 265, no. 4, pp. 1946–1951, 1990.

[8] J. G. Puig and I. H. Fox, "Ethanol-induced activation of adenine nucleotide turnover. Evidence for a role of acetate," *Journal of Clinical Investigation*, vol. 74, no. 3, pp. 936–941, 1984.

[9] L. E. Nagy, "Ethanol metabolism and inhibition of nucleoside uptake lead to increased extracellular adenosine in hepatocytes," *American Journal of Physiology*, vol. 262, no. 5, pp. C1175–C1180, 1992.

[10] E. S. Chan, M. C. Montesinos, P. Fernandez et al., "Adenosine A_{2A} receptors play a role in the pathogenesis of hepatic cirrhosis," *British Journal of Pharmacology*, vol. 148, no. 8, pp. 1144–1155, 2006.

[11] Z. Peng, P. Fernandez, T. Wilder et al., "Ecto-5′-nucleotidase (CD73) -mediated extracellular adenosine production plays a critical role in hepatic fibrosis," *FASEB Journal*, vol. 22, no. 7, pp. 2263–2272, 2008.

[12] B. B. Fredholm, "Adenosine, an endogenous distress signal, modulates tissue damage and repair," *Cell Death and Differentiation*, vol. 14, no. 7, pp. 1315–1323, 2007.

[13] R. Guinzberg, I. Laguna, A. Zentella, R. Guzman, and E. Piña, "Effect of adenosine and inosine on ureagenesis in hepatocytes," *Biochemical Journal*, vol. 245, no. 2, pp. 371–374, 1987.

[14] R. Guinzberg, A. Diaz-Cruz, S. Uribe, and E. Pina, "Inhibition of adenosine mediated responses in isolated hepatocytes by depolarizing concentrations of K^+ ," *Biochemical and Biophysical Research Communications*, vol. 197, no. 1, pp. 229–234, 1993.

[15] S. A. Tinton, V. H. Lefebvre, O. C. Cousin, and P. M. Buc-Calderon, "Cytolytic effects and biochemical changes induced by extracellular ATP to isolated hepatocytes," *Biochimica et Biophysica Acta*, vol. 1176, no. 1-2, pp. 1–6, 1993.

[16] E. Gonzalez-Benitez, R. Guinzberg, A. Diaz-Cruz, and E. Pina, "Regulation of glycogen metabolism in hepatocytes through adenosine receptors. Role of Ca^{2+} and cAMP," *European Journal of Pharmacology*, vol. 437, no. 3, pp. 105–111, 2002.

[17] A. K. Dhalla, M. Santikul, M. Smith, M. Y. Wong, J. C. Shryock, and L. Belardinelli, "Antilipolytic activity of a novel partial A1 adenosine receptor agonist devoid of cardiovascular effects: comparison with nicotinic acid," *Journal of Pharmacology and Experimental Therapeutics*, vol. 321, no. 1, pp. 327–333, 2007.

[18] A. K. Dhalla, M. Y. Wong, P. J. Voshol, L. Belardinelli, and G. M. Reaven, "A_1 adenosine receptor partial agonist lowers plasma FFA and improves insulin resistance induced by high-fat diet in rodents," *American Journal of Physiology*, vol. 292, no. 5, pp. E1358–E1363, 2007.

[19] E. C. Klaasse, A. P. Ijzerman, W. J. de Grip, and M. W. Beukers, "Internalization and desensitization of adenosine receptors," *Purinergic Signalling*, vol. 4, no. 1, pp. 21–37, 2008.

[20] B. S. Bhagwandeen, M. Apte, L. Manwarring, and J. Dickeson, "Endotoxin induced hepatic necrosis in rats on an alcohol diet," *Journal of Pathology*, vol. 152, no. 1, pp. 47–53, 1987.

[21] S. Q. Yang, H. Z. Lin, M. D. Lane, M. Clemens, and A. M. Diehl, "Obesity increases sensitivity to endotoxin liver injury: implications for the pathogenesis of steatohepatitis," *Proceedings of the National Academy of Sciences of the United States of America*, vol. 94, no. 6, pp. 2557–2562, 1997.

[22] A. M. Diehl, "Nonalcoholic fatty liver disease: implications for alcoholic liver disease pathogenesis," *Alcoholism: Clinical and Experimental Research*, vol. 25, no. 5, supplement ISBRA, pp. 8S–14S, 2001.

[23] F. J. Cubero and N. Nieto, "Kupffer cells and alcoholic liver disease," *Revista Espanola de Enfermedades Digestivas*, vol. 98, no. 6, pp. 460–472, 2006.

[24] T. Gustot, A. Lemmers, C. Moreno et al., "Differential liver sensitization to Toll-like receptor pathways in mice with alcoholic fatty liver," *Hepatology*, vol. 43, no. 5, pp. 989–1000, 2006.

[25] W. L. Guo, L. Gong, Z. F. Ding et al., "Genomic instability in phenotypically normal regenerants of medicinal plant *Codonopsis lanceolata* benth. et hook. f., as revealed by ISSR and RAPD markers," *Plant Cell Reports*, vol. 25, no. 9, pp. 896–906, 2006.

[26] K. T. Lee, J. Choi, W. T. Jung, J. H. Nam, H. J. Jung, and H. J. Park, "Structure of a new echinocystic acid bisdesmoside isolated from *Codonopsis lanceolata* roots and the cytotoxic activity of prosapogenins," *Journal of Agricultural and Food Chemistry*, vol. 50, no. 15, pp. 4190–4193, 2002.

[27] K. W. Lee, H. J. Jung, H. J. Park, D. G. Kim, J. Y. Lee, and K. T. Lee, "β-D-xylopyranosyl-(1 $\rightarrow$ 3)-β-D-glucuronopyranosyl echinocystic acid isolated from the roots of *Codonopsis lanceolata* induces caspase-dependent apoptosis in human acute promyelocytic leukemia HL-60 cells," *Biological and Pharmaceutical Bulletin*, vol. 28, no. 5, pp. 854–859, 2005.

[28] Y. G. Lee, J. Y. Kim, J. Y. Lee et al., "Regulatory effects of *Codonopsis lanceolata* on macrophage-mediated immune responses," *Journal of Ethnopharmacology*, vol. 112, no. 1, pp. 180–188, 2007.

[29] E. G. Han, H. G. Moon, and S. Y. Cho, "Effect of *Codonopsis lanceolata* water extract on the levels of lipid in rats fed high fat diet," *Journal of the Korean Society of Food Science and Nutrition*, vol. 27, pp. 940–944, 1998.

[30] C. S. Lieber, L. M. DeCarli, and M. F. Sorrell, "Experimental methods of ethanol administration," *Hepatology*, vol. 10, no. 4, pp. 501–510, 1989.

[31] J. Folch, M. Lees, and G. H. S. Stanley, "A simple method for the isolation and purification of total lipides from animal tissues," *The Journal of Biological Chemistry*, vol. 226, no. 1, pp. 497–509, 1957.

[32] S. Kaviarasan, P. Viswanathan, and C. V. Anuradha, "Fenugreek seed (*Trigonella foenum graecum*) polyphenols inhibit ethanol-induced collagen and lipid accumulation in rat liver," *Cell Biology and Toxicology*, vol. 23, no. 6, pp. 373–383, 2007.

[33] R. S. Kumar, M. Ponmozhi, P. Viswanathan, and N. Nalini, "Effect of *Cassia auriculata* leaf extract on lipids in rats with alcoholic liver injury," *Asia Pacific Journal of Clinical Nutrition*, vol. 11, no. 2, pp. 157–163, 2002.

[34] G. E. Arteel, T. Uesugi, L. N. Bevan et al., "Green tea extract protects against early alcohol-induced liver injury in rats," *Biological Chemistry*, vol. 383, no. 3-4, pp. 663–670, 2002.

[35] E. E. Emeson, M. Vlasios, S. Todd, and T. Majid, "Chronic alcohol feeding inhibits atherogenesis in C57BL/6 hyperlipidemic mice," *American Journal of Pathology*, vol. 147, no. 6, pp. 1749–1758, 1995.

[36] G. Szabo, "Consequences of alcohol consumption on host defence," *Alcohol and Alcoholism*, vol. 34, no. 6, pp. 830–841, 1999.

[37] C. Q. Rogers, J. M. Ajmo, and M. You, "Adiponectin and alcoholic fatty liver disease," *IUBMB Life*, vol. 60, no. 12, pp. 790–797, 2008.

[38] S. Shklyaev, G. Aslanidi, M. Tennant et al., "Sustained peripheral expression of transgene adiponectin offsets the development of diet-induced obesity in rats," *Proceedings of the National Academy of Sciences of the United States of America*, vol. 100, no. 2, pp. 14217–14222, 2003.

[39] T. Yamauchi, Y. Nio, T. Maki et al., "Targeted disruption of AdipoR1 and AdipoR2 causes abrogation of adiponectin binding and metabolic actions," *Nature Medicine*, vol. 13, no. 3, pp. 332–339, 2007.

[40] T. Yamauchi, J. Kamon, Y. Ito et al., "Cloning of adiponectin receptors that mediate antidiabetic metabolic effects," *Nature*, vol. 423, no. 6941, pp. 762–769, 2003.

[41] X. Mao, C. K. Kikani, R. A. Riojas et al., "APPL1 binds to adiponectin receptors and mediates adiponectin signalling and function," *Nature Cell Biology*, vol. 8, no. 5, pp. 516–523, 2006.

[42] M. You, R. V. Considine, T. C. Leone, D. P. Kelly, and D. W. Crabb, "Role of adiponectin in the protective action of dietary saturated fat against alcoholic fatty liver in mice," *Hepatology*, vol. 42, no. 3, pp. 568–577, 2005.

[43] M. A. Jay and J. Ren, "Peroxisome proliferator-activated receptor (PPAR) in metabolic syndrome and type 2 diabetes mellitus," *Current Diabetes Reviews*, vol. 3, no. 1, pp. 33–39, 2007.

[44] T. Kadowaki, T. Yamauchi, and N. Kubota, "The physiological and pathophysiological role of adiponectin and adiponectin receptors in the peripheral tissues and CNS," *FEBS Letters*, vol. 582, no. 1, pp. 74–80, 2008.

[45] T. Kadowaki, T. Yamauchi, N. Kubota, K. Hara, K. Ueki, and K. Tobe, "Adiponectin and adiponectin receptors in insulin resistance, diabetes, and the metabolic syndrome," *Journal of Clinical Investigation*, vol. 116, no. 7, pp. 1784–1792, 2006.

[46] T. Kadowaki and T. Yamauchi, "Adiponectin and adiponectin receptors," *Endocrine Reviews*, vol. 26, no. 3, pp. 439–451, 2005.

[47] N. Méndez-Sánchez, N. C. Chavez-Tapia, D. Zamora-Valdés, and M. Uribe, "Adiponectin, structure, function and pathophysiological implications in non-alcoholic fatty liver disease," *Mini-Reviews in Medicinal Chemistry*, vol. 6, no. 6, pp. 651–656, 2006.

[48] P. Misra, "AMP activated protein kinase: a next generation target for total metabolic control," *Expert Opinion on Therapeutic Targets*, vol. 12, no. 1, pp. 91–100, 2008.

[49] J. D. Browning and J. D. Horton, "Molecular mediators of hepatic steatosis and liver injury," *Journal of Clinical Investigation*, vol. 114, no. 2, pp. 147–152, 2004.

[50] A. Xu, Y. Wang, H. Keshaw, L. Y. Xu, K. S. Lam, and G. J. Cooper, "The fat-derived hormone adiponectin alleviates alcoholic and nonalcoholic fatty liver diseases in mice," *Journal of Clinical Investigation*, vol. 112, no. 1, pp. 91–100, 2003.

[51] M. You and C. Q. Rogers, "Adiponectin: a key adipokine in alcoholic fatty liver," *Experimental Biology and Medicine*, vol. 234, no. 8, pp. 850–859, 2009.

[52] X. Hou, S. Xu, K. A. Maitland-Toolan et al., "SIRT1 regulates hepatocyte lipid metabolism through activating AMP-activated protein kinase," *Journal of Biological Chemistry*, vol. 283, no. 29, pp. 20015–20026, 2008.

[53] F. Lan, J. M. Cacicedo, N. Ruderman, and Y. Ido, "SIRT1 modulation of the acetylation status, cytosolic localization, and activity of LKB1: possible role in AMP-activated protein kinase activation," *Journal of Biological Chemistry*, vol. 283, no. 41, pp. 27628–27635, 2008.

[54] G. Suchankova, L. E. Nelson, Z. Gerhart-Hines et al., "Concurrent regulation of AMP-activated protein kinase and SIRT1 in mammalian cells," *Biochemical and Biophysical Research Communications*, vol. 378, no. 4, pp. 836–841, 2009.

[55] M. Fulco and V. Sartorelli, "Comparing and contrasting the roles of AMPK and SIRT1 in metabolic tissues," *Cell Cycle*, vol. 7, no. 23, pp. 3669–3679, 2008.

[56] P. Puigserver and B. M. Spiegelman, "Peroxisome proliferator-activated receptor-γ coactivator 1α (PGC-1 α): transcriptional coactivator and metabolic regulator," *Endocrine Reviews*, vol. 24, no. 1, pp. 78–90, 2003.

[57] R. B. Vega, J. M. Huss, and D. P. Kelly, "The coactivator PGC-1 cooperates with peroxisome proliferator-activated receptor α in transcriptional control of nuclear genes encoding

mitochondrial fatty acid oxidation enzymes," *Molecular and Cellular Biology*, vol. 20, no. 5, pp. 1868–1876, 2000.

[58] R. R. Schumann, S. R. Leong, G. W. Flaggs et al., "Structure and function of lipopolysaccharide binding protein," *Science*, vol. 249, no. 4975, pp. 1429–1431, 1990.

[59] G. L. Su, R. L. Simmons, and S. C. Wang, "Lipopolysaccharide binding protein participation in cellular activation by LPS," *Critical Reviews in Immunology*, vol. 15, no. 3-4, pp. 201–214, 1995.

[60] R. J. Ulevitch and P. S. Tobias, "Receptor-dependent mechanisms of cell stimulation by bacterial endotoxin," *Annual Review of Immunology*, vol. 13, pp. 437–457, 1995.

[61] T. R. Martin, S. M. Mongovin, P. S. Tobias et al., "The CD14 differentiation antigen mediates the development of endotoxin responsiveness during differentiation of mononuclear phagocytes," *Journal of Leukocyte Biology*, vol. 56, no. 1, pp. 1–9, 1994.

[62] S. D. Wright, R. A. Ramos, P. S. Tobias, R. J. Ulevitch, and J. C. Mathison, "CD14, a receptor for complexes of lipopolysaccharide (LPS) and LPS binding protein," *Science*, vol. 249, no. 4975, pp. 1431–1433, 1990.

[63] G. L. Su, R. D. Klein, A. Aminlari et al., "Kupffer cell activation by lipopolysaccharide in rats: role for lipopolysaccharide binding protein and Toll-like receptor 4," *Hepatology*, vol. 31, no. 4, pp. 932–936, 2000.

[64] R. Medzhitov, P. Preston-Hurlburt, E. Kopp et al., "MyD88 is an adaptor protein in the hToll/IL-1 receptor family signaling pathways," *Molecular Cell*, vol. 2, no. 2, pp. 253–258, 1998.

[65] K. A. Fitzgerald, E. M. Palsson-Mcdermott, A. G. Bowie et al., "Mal (MyD88-adapter-like) is required for Toll-like recepfor-4 signal transduction," *Nature*, vol. 413, no. 6851, pp. 78–83, 2001.

[66] T. Horng, G. M. Barton, and R. Medzhitov, "TIRAP: an adapter molecule in the Toll signaling pathway," *Nature Immunology*, vol. 2, no. 9, pp. 835–841, 2001.

[67] A. Takaoka, H. Yanai, S. Kondo et al., "Integral role of IRF-5 in the gene induction programme activated by Toll-like receptors," *Nature*, vol. 434, no. 2, pp. 243–249, 2005.

[68] E. Seki, S. de Minicis, C. H. Österreicher et al., "TLR4 enhances TGF-β signaling and hepatic fibrosis," *Nature Medicine*, vol. 13, no. 11, pp. 1324–1332, 2007.

[69] I. Hritz, P. Mandrekar, A. Velayudham et al., "The critical role of Toll-like receptor (TLR) 4 in alcoholic liver disease is independent of the common TLR adapter MyD88," *Hepatology*, vol. 48, no. 4, pp. 1224–1231, 2008.

[70] J. M. Ajmo, X. Liang, C. Q. Rogers, B. Pennock, and M. You, "Resveratrol alleviates alcoholic fatty liver in mice," *American Journal of Physiology*, vol. 295, no. 4, pp. G833–G842, 2008.

8

Trace Level Determination of Polyether Ionophores in Feed

Mervi Rokka,[1] Marika Jestoi,[2] and Kimmo Peltonen[1]

[1] *Chemistry and Toxicology Unit, Research and Laboratory Department, Finnish Food Safety Authority Evira, Mustialankatu 3, 00790 Helsinki, Finland*
[2] *Product Safety Unit, Control Department, Finnish Food Safety Authority Evira, Mustialankatu 3, 00790 Helsinki, Finland*

Correspondence should be addressed to Mervi Rokka; mervi.rokka@evira.fi

Academic Editor: Adam Huczynski

A liquid chromatography-mass spectrometric method was developed and validated to determine six polyether ionophores (lasalocid sodium, monensin sodium, salinomycin sodium, narasin, maduramicin ammonium alpha, and semduramicin sodium) in feed samples. The method developed was very straightforward, involving extraction with 84% acetonitrile of the coccidiostats from the feed samples and filtration of the raw extract prior to chromatographic analysis. Method validation included the determination of selectivity, linearity, specificity, repeatability, the limit of detection, limit of quantification, decision limit (CCα), detection capability (CCβ), and recovery. Feed samples from the Finnish national feed control programme and suspected carry-over samples from a feed manufacturer were analysed in parallel with an existing liquid chromatography method coupled with ultraviolet detection. All feed control samples were negative in LC-UV, but with the developed MS method, monensin, salinomycin, and narasin were detected at concentrations of <0.025–0.73 mg/kg, <0.025–0.027 mg/kg, and <0.025–1.6 mg/kg, respectively. In suspected carry-over samples after an output of 2.0 tonnes of unmedicated feed in the pelletizer line, the concentrations of monensin, salinomycin, and narasin varied from undetected to 16 mg/kg. In the mixer line, after 3.2 tonnes of unmedicated feed output, the concentrations of monensin, salinomycin, and narasin varied from undetected to 2.4 mg/kg.

1. Introduction

The polyether ionophores lasalocid, monensin, salinomycin, narasin, maduramicin, and semduramicin (Figure 1) are widely used feed additives in the poultry industry to prevent and control coccidiosis caused by the genus *Eimeria*. They are added to feeds as their sodium salts at levels of 75–125 mg/kg (lasalocid), 60–125 mg/kg (monensin), 20–70 mg/kg (salinomycin), 60–70 mg/kg (narasin), 5 mg/kg (maduramicin), and 20–25 mg/kg (semduramicin). Broiler chickens receive coccidiostats via feed during their entire lifespan, whereas for egg-laying birds the use of coccidiostats is forbidden. Anticoccidial drugs can also be administered, for example, to cattle to improve feed efficacy, that is, to increase their body mass. Due to the extensive use of coccidiostats, the safety of these compounds has been tested in many animal experiments (in both target and nontarget animal species). Although monensin, salinomycin, narasin, and maduramicin are forbidden for laying hens, these compounds were not found to have significant effects, for instance, on egg production or shell thickness when used at the permitted levels [1]. The safe dose levels of coccidiostats for cattle have been noted to be lower than the feeding levels for poultry, for example, monensin 30–45 mg/kg [2], lasalocid 10–35 mg/kg, [3] and narasin 25 mg/kg [4]. Although maduramicin 0–10 mg/kg and semduramicin 0–25 mg/kg were reported to have no effects on horses [5, 6], in a feeding trial on horses with narasin at the level of 80 mg/kg, some reduction in feed intake was observed [4]. Coccidiostats are not used in human medicine because of their cardiovascular effects [7], and indeed lasalocid (<1.0 μM) has been found to cause contraction of the human heart in test systems [8]. However, the residues of coccidiostats in food have not induced any short-term clinical symptoms in humans [9].

A withdrawal period of 5 days is required for lasalocid, salinomycin, narasin, maduramicin, and semduramicin, and 3 days for monensin in order to avoid coccidiostat residues in edible tissues, although there is no risk to consumers' health

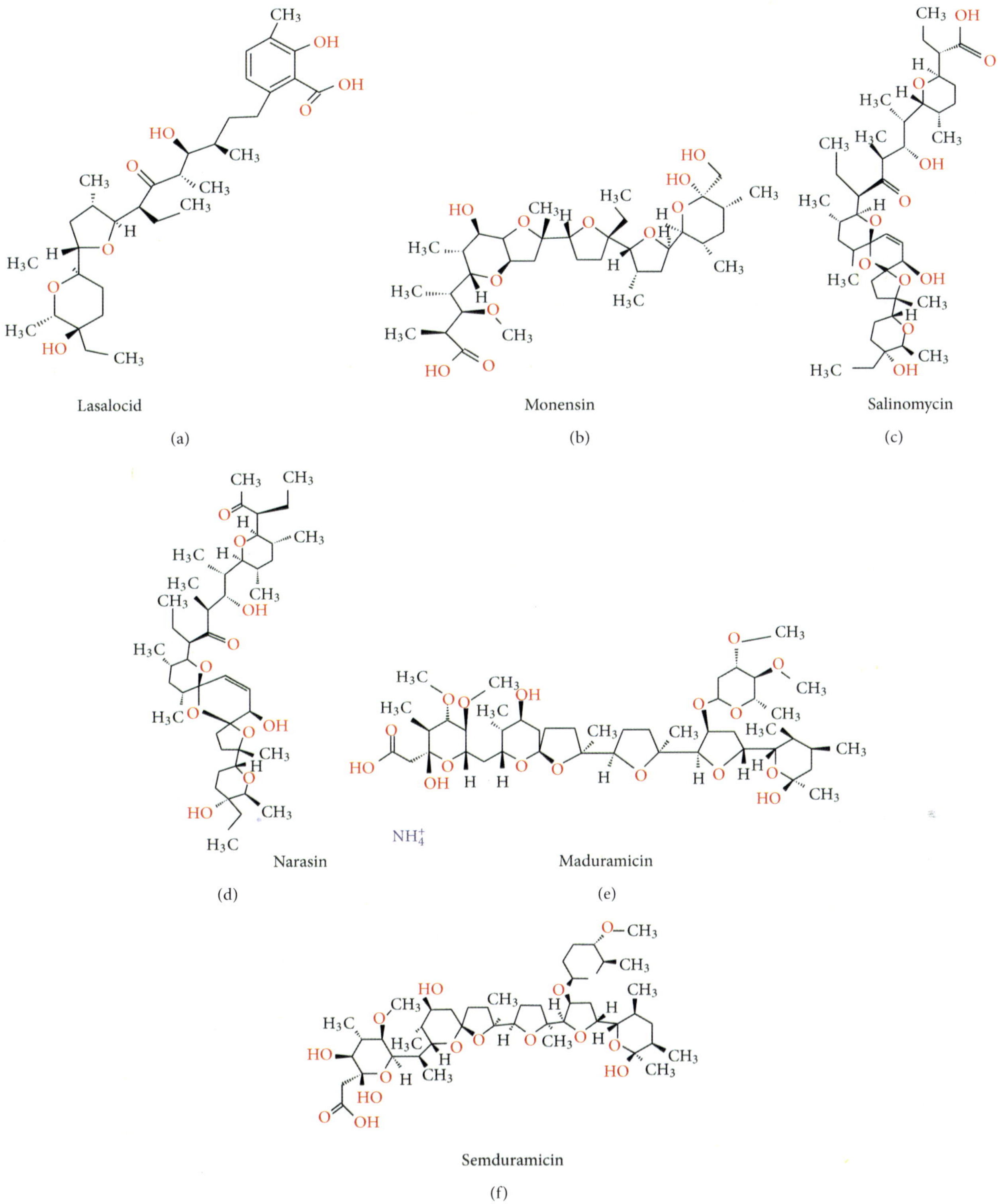

FIGURE 1: The structures of polyether ionophores.

from ingestion of coccidiostats residues in tissues of animals exposed to feed cross-contaminated up to a level of 10%. [e.g., 4-6] Lasalocid, monensin, and salinomycin are used for laying birds up to the age of 12–16 weeks, depending on the additive. None of the coccidiostats are licensed for the use in egg-laying birds and therefore eggs should be free from coccidiostats contamination. Nonetheless, residues of polyether ionophores have been detected in European eggs at levels from 0.3 to <40 μg/kg [10–14]. In addition, traces of polyether ionophores have found in different European poultry tissues at levels of 0.04–4.2 μg/kg [12, 15, 16]. However, in most samples the concentrations of these compounds have been below the limits of quantification.

Several methods used to determine polyether ionophores in feed are based on high performance liquid chromatography (HPLC) with fluorescence detection [17, 18] or UV detection [19–23]. In these methods, sample preparation includes precolumn or postcolumn derivatization or solid phase extraction. The limits of quantification (LOQ) in HPLC-based methods are mainly higher than 1 mg/kg, with some exceptions for lasalocid and narasin (LOQ 0.5 mg/kg) [17, 20]. Liquid chromatography-mass spectrometry (LC-MS) was also used to determine polyether ionophores in feed [24–29]. The use of a mass spectrometer detector enables sample preparation to be minimized and also increases the sensitivity of the method in the analysis of complex sample matrices, since it can be used for either selected ion monitoring or multiple reaction monitoring to detect only the desired ions produced by the analytes. However, in these MS methods, apart from the study of Huang et al. [29], solid phase extraction has been used in sample preparation. With the methods mentioned above, polyether ionophores can be detected at levels of 0.001–50 mg/kg. Although the limits of quantification are low (μg/kg), most of the methods have been validated at the mg/kg level. In addition, apart from the study of Delahaut et al. [30], the validated methods have only been tested with medicated feeds, not with real samples from the feed industry. Delahaut et al. [30] analysed feed samples in which the concentrations of monensin, salinomycin, and narasin were above 2.1 mg/kg. The reported findings of polyether ionophores residues in eggs and tissues have been attributed to the contamination of unmedicated feed at the feed manufacturer [11, 14]. For instance, lasalocid is known to be a very dusty compound that can easily contaminate feed during the manufacturing process. For this reason, a suitable method is needed for analysing polyether ionophores at the trace level in feed.

The European Commission has established official maximum contents of polyether ionophores in feed (lasalocid 1.25 mg/kg; narasin 0.7 mg/kg; salinomycin 0.7 mg/kg; monensin 1.25 mg/kg; semduramicin 0.25 mg/kg; maduramicin 0.05 mg/kg) [31]. Based on this regulation, the aims of our study were to (i) develop and validate an LC-MS/MS method for analysing lasalocid, monensin, salinomycin, narasin, maduramicin, and semduramicin at the required performance levels in feed; (ii) apply the validated method in the analysis of both medicated and contaminated feed; and (iii) compare the results determined with LC-MS/MS and the existing LC-UV method.

2. Materials and Methods

2.1. Samples. A cereal mixture (wheat/rye/barley, 1 : 1 : 1, w/w/w) was used in the validation study. The validated method was used in analysis of poultry feed from the Finnish national feed control programme (2008: 8 samples) and suspected carry-over samples from a European feed manufacturer (2006: 12 samples; 2008: 12 samples). The carry-over of monensin, salinomycin, and narasin from medicated feed to unmedicated feed was investigated. Three batches of unmedicated feed were collected after one batch of medicated feed. Unmedicated feed samples from the mixer line were collected after 1 min (0.8 tonnes output), 2.5 min (2.0 tonnes), and 4 min (3.2 tonnes). In proportion, unmedicated feed samples from the pelletizer line were collected after 3 min (0.6 tonnes output), 5 min (1.0 tonnes), and 10 min (2.0 tonnes).

2.2. Chemicals and Reagents. Standards of monensin (sodium salt, ~90–95%), salinomycin (~96%), and narasin (~97%) were purchased from Sigma (St. Louis, MO, USA), lasalocid (sodium salt) from Fluka Chemie (Buchs, Switzerland), maduramicin (ammonium, ~96.5%) from Alpharma (Willow Island, NE, USA), and semduramicin from BVL (Braunschweig, Germany). Standard stock solutions (1 mg/mL) and working standard solutions for LC-MS/MS analysis (monensin, salinomycin, narasin, maduramicin: 1 μg/mL & 10 μg/mL; lasalocid, semduramicin; 8 μg/mL & 80 μg/mL) were prepared in methanol. Standard stock solutions for HPLC (0.5 mg/mL) were prepared in methanol. Working standard solutions for HPLC were prepared in methanol : water (90 : 10, v/v). Methanol, acetonitrile, acetic acid (analytical grade), ammonium acetate, and sulphuric acid were purchased from J. T. Baker (Deventer, Holland). Vanillin (99%) was purchased from Fluka Chemie (Buchs, Switzerland). A vanillin postcolumn reagent was freshly prepared daily by dissolving 30 g vanillin in 970 mL methanol/sulphuric acid (20 mL sulphuric acid added to 950 mL methanol, with the solution then cooled in an ice bath). The water used was purified with a Millipore Milli-Q Plus System (Millipore, Espoo, Finland).

2.3. LC-MS/MS: Sample Preparation and Analysis. Samples were ground with a laboratory mill (Bamix, Mettlen, Switzerland). Then, 25 g of ground sample was extracted with 100 mL of 84% acetonitrile in water for two hours using a VKS-75 horizontal shaker (Edmund Bühler, Bodelshansen, Germany) at room temperature. Samples in the validation study were spiked with different concentrations of polyether ionophores standard solutions just before extraction. As the matrix of carry-over samples was different than matrix used in the validation, the samples were also spiked before extraction to ensure suitability of the method for these samples. The extracted samples were filtered through S&S 602 H 1/2 filter paper (Schleicher & Schuell, Dassal, Germany), and the filtered extracts were stored at +4°C until analysis. One millilitre of extract was evaporated to dryness under nitrogen at 40°C. The sample was dissolved in 1 mL of mobile phase (acetonitrile: 2 mM ammonium acetate containing 2% acetic acid (95 : 5 v/v)) and filtered using a 0.2-μm syringe filter (Pall Gelamn Sciences, Ann Arbor, MI, USA) into an autosampler vial.

Polyether ionophores were analysed with a Waters Alliance 2695 liquid chromatograph (Waters, Milford, MA, USA) connected to a MicroMass Quattro Micro triple-quadrupole mass spectrometer (Micromass, Manchester,

TABLE 1: LC-MS/MS acquisition for polyether ionophores. The product ions (in bold) were used for the quantification.

Compound	Precursor ion (m/z)	Product ions	Cone Voltage (kV)	Collision gas energy (eV)
Lasalocid	613.6 $[M + Na]^+$	359.4; **377.4**	50	40
Semduramicin	911.4 $[M + K]^+$	**849.6**; 867.0	34	40
Monensin	693.7 $[M + Na]^+$	461.4; **675.7**	60	40
Salinomycin	773.8 $[M + Na]^+$	**431.4**; 531.5	70	45
Narasin	787.8 $[M + Na]^+$	**431.4**; 531.5	60	50
Maduramicin	954.8 $[M + K]^+$	**893.3**; 911.3	34	40

UK). The separation of polyether ionophores was conducted as described by Jestoi et al. [16]. The analytical column was a Luna $C_{18}(2)$ (5 μm), 3.0 × 150 mm (Phenomenex, Cheshire, UK). The flow rate of the mobile phase was 0.5 mL/min and the injection volume was 10 μL. A positive ionisation mode was used with an ESI probe. The parameters of the MS were optimized using a standard solution. The best response was recorded with the following parameters: capillary voltage 3.75 kV, source temperature 130°C and desolvation temperature 250°C. The optimized cone voltages and collision gas energies for each of the analysed coccidiostats are presented in Table 1. Argon (AGA, Finland) was used as a collision gas. Coccidiostats were detected as either their sodium or potassium adducts.

2.4. LC-UV: Sample Preparation and Analysis. The LC-UV method for polyether ionophores was modified from the method AM-AA-CR-J424-AC-791 [32]. Briefly, 5 g of ground sample was extracted with 50 mL of 90% methanol in water for one hour at room temperature. After extraction, 50 mL of extraction solution was added and sample solids were allowed to settle. The sample solution was filtered using a 0.45 μm syringe filter (Pall Gelamn Sciences, Ann Arbor, MI, USA) into an autosampler vial.

Monensin, salinomycin, and narasin were analysed using an Agilent 1100 liquid chromatograph (Agilent, Waldbron, Germany) and postcolumn reagent pump (Shimadzu Instruments, Maryland, USA). Coccidiostats were detected at 520 nm. The analytical column was a Shandon 250 × 4.6 mm Hypersil ODS (5 μm). The flow rate was 0.8 mL/min for the mobile phase (methanol : water : acetic acid, 94 : 6 : 1, v/v/v) and 0.7 mL/min for the vanillin reagent. The injection volume was 50 μL. In this method, the limit of detection (LOD) for monensin, salinomycin, and narasin was 2 mg/kg, 2 mg/kg, and 3 mg/kg, respectively, and the respective limits of quantification (LOQ) for these analytes were 4 mg/kg, 4 mg/kg, and 5 mg/kg.

2.5. Validation of the LC-MS/MS Method. Method validation included the determination of selectivity, linearity, specificity, reproducibility, recovery, the decision limit (CCα), detection capability (CCβ), limit of detection (LOD), and limit of quantification (LOQ). Six replicates of samples spiked at three concentrations (spiking level 1: monensin, salinomycin, narasin, and maduramicin 0.025 mg/kg, lasalocid and semduramicin 0.20 mg/kg; spiking level 2: monensin, salinomycin, narasin, and maduramicin 0.05 mg/kg, lasalocid and semduramicin 0.40 mg/kg; spiking level 3: monensin, salinomycin, narasin, and maduramicin 0.10 mg/kg, lasalocid and semduramicin 0.80 mg/kg) and calibration curves with and without the matrix were analysed on three separate days. The calibration curves were constructed with external standards by injecting standards prepared in the mobile phase and matrix at five different concentrations (monensin, salinomycin, narasin, and maduramicin 0.010–2.0 mg/kg; lasalocid and semduramicin 0.080–2.0 mg/kg). The blank matrix was spiked with corresponding amounts of standards and prepared as regular samples.

3. Results

3.1. LC-MS/MS Method Development. The LC-MS/MS method was developed to provide confirmatory data for the analysis of six polyether ionophores in feed. Sample preparation was simple, involving the extraction of coccidiostats from feed samples and filtration of the extract prior to chromatographic analysis. As the chemical structures and particularly the mode of action of coccidiostats and emerging *Fusarium*-mycotoxins are closely related, we utilized earlier published sample extraction method for beauvericin and enniatins [33]. The MS/MS fragmentation conditions and collision energies were optimised for each individual compound to give the best response. The compounds were separated with an earlier-developed LC method for separating lasalocid, monensin, salinomycin, narasin, and maduramicin in eggs and tissues [16]. In this method development, the sixth compound, semduramicin could be added as such to the already existing LC method.

3.2. LC-MS/MS Method Validation. The selectivity of the developed method was tested by comparing (two-sided t-test) the slopes of the five-point calibration curves obtained with and without the matrix (for calibration curve ranges, see section Validation of the LC-MS/MS method). Due to the presence of significant matrix effects ($P < 0.05$), the calibration curves for all compounds were prepared in the matrix. The matrix effect, calculated as the ratio of signal suppression to enhancement (SSE%) as described in Sulyok et al. [34], was 3.0%, 4.1%, 2.8%, 4.2%, 19%, and 43% for lasalocid, monensin, salinomycin, narasin, maduramicin, and semduramicin, respectively. This further demonstrated the suppressive effect of the matrix components on the signal

TABLE 2: CCα (mg/kg) and CCβ (mg/kg) values obtained for polyether ionophores in feed.

	Lasalocid	Monensin	Salinomycin	Narasin	Maduramicin	Semduramicin
CCα (mg/kg)	0.37	0.025	0.025	0.027	0.027	0.24
CCβ (mg/kg)	0.50	0.030	0.029	0.031	0.033	0.29

TABLE 3: The mean recoveries with the corresponding standard deviations of the polyether ionophores analysed at three spiking levels ($n = 18$).

	Spiking level (mg/kg)	Mean concentration (mg/kg)	Recovery %	Relative standard deviation (%)
Lasalocid	0.20	0.19	95	35
	0.40	0.45	112	5.0
	0.80	0.76	95	6.0
Monensin	0.025	0.019	75	13
	0.05	0.050	100	26
	0.10	0.10	100	9.2
Salinomycin	0.025	0.19	77	13
	0.05	0.054	108	12
	0.10	0.097	97	9.8
Narasin	0.025	0.020	81	112
	0.05	0.054	109	9.5
	0.10	0.096	96	5.9
Maduramicin	0.025	0.019	74	18
	0.05	0.055	109	9.5
	0.10	0.095	95	7.4
Semduramicin	0.20	0.15	77	20
	0.40	0.43	106	17
	0.80	0.74	92	16

intensity. The acceptability of linearity of each point of the matrix-assisted calibration curves was tested by using the least-square method [35]. The maximum response/mass ratio of ±10% for each calibration point was accepted. On this basis, it can be stated that the measurement of polyether ionophores in the matrix was linear over the actual studied ranges (0.010–2.0 mg/kg). The specificity of the method was tested using by analysing 20 different blank samples separately and no interference signals close to the retention times of polyether ionophores were detected in any blank samples analysed. Chromatograms of a blank sample, a spiked sample, and a positive sample are presented in Figures 2, 3, and 4, respectively.

LOD and LOQ values for polyether ionophores were calculated using the responses of blank samples ($n = 20$). LODs (blank sample mean response + 3 × standard deviation) for lasalocid, monensin, salinomycin, narasin, maduramicin, and semduramicin were 0.0029 mg/kg, 0.0042 mg/kg, 0.0047 mg/kg, 0.0026 mg/kg, 0.0011 mg/kg, and 0.0022 mg/kg, respectively. The corresponding LOQs (blank sample mean response + 10 × standard deviation) for the compounds analysed were 0.0075 mg/kg, 0.011 mg/kg, 0.012 mg/kg, 0.0071 mg/kg, 0.0029 mg/kg, and 0.0060 mg/kg, respectively. Although lower concentrations of the analytes could be quantified with the method, for practical reasons the LOQs used for the analytes were the lowest spiking level of 0.025 mg/kg for monensin, salinomycin, narasin, and maduramicin, and 0.080 mg/kg for lasalocid and semduramicin. CCα and CCβ values were calculated using data on within-laboratory reproducibility from this study (data not shown). CCα and CCβ values for monensin, salinomycin, narasin, and maduramicin were 0.025–0.027 mg/kg and 0.029–0.033 mg/kg, respectively. CCα values for lasalocid and semduramicin were 0.37 mg/kg and 0.24 mg/kg, respectively, and the corresponding CCβ values, in turn, were 0.50 mg/kg and 0.29 mg/kg (Table 2).

The mean recoveries of six replicates on three separate days at three different spiking levels of the analytes are presented in Table 3. The recoveries of coccidiostats in feed varied between 74–112%, which was acceptable for monitoring purposes. In addition, the method was repeatable, as demonstrated by the relative standard deviations of the mean recoveries (Table 3).

3.3. Sample Analysis with LC-MS/MS. To ensure the usefulness of the LC-MS/MS method for the detection of polyether ionophores, especially at trace levels, feed samples from the Finnish national feed control programme and suspected carry-over samples from a European feed manufacturer were analysed with the developed method. For the analyses of medicated feed there was a need for a wider calibration curve (10–100 mg/kg), which was also tested to be linear over the range. For that reason, carry-over samples could be analysed with any dilution. The carry-over samples were also spiked and the result was corrected

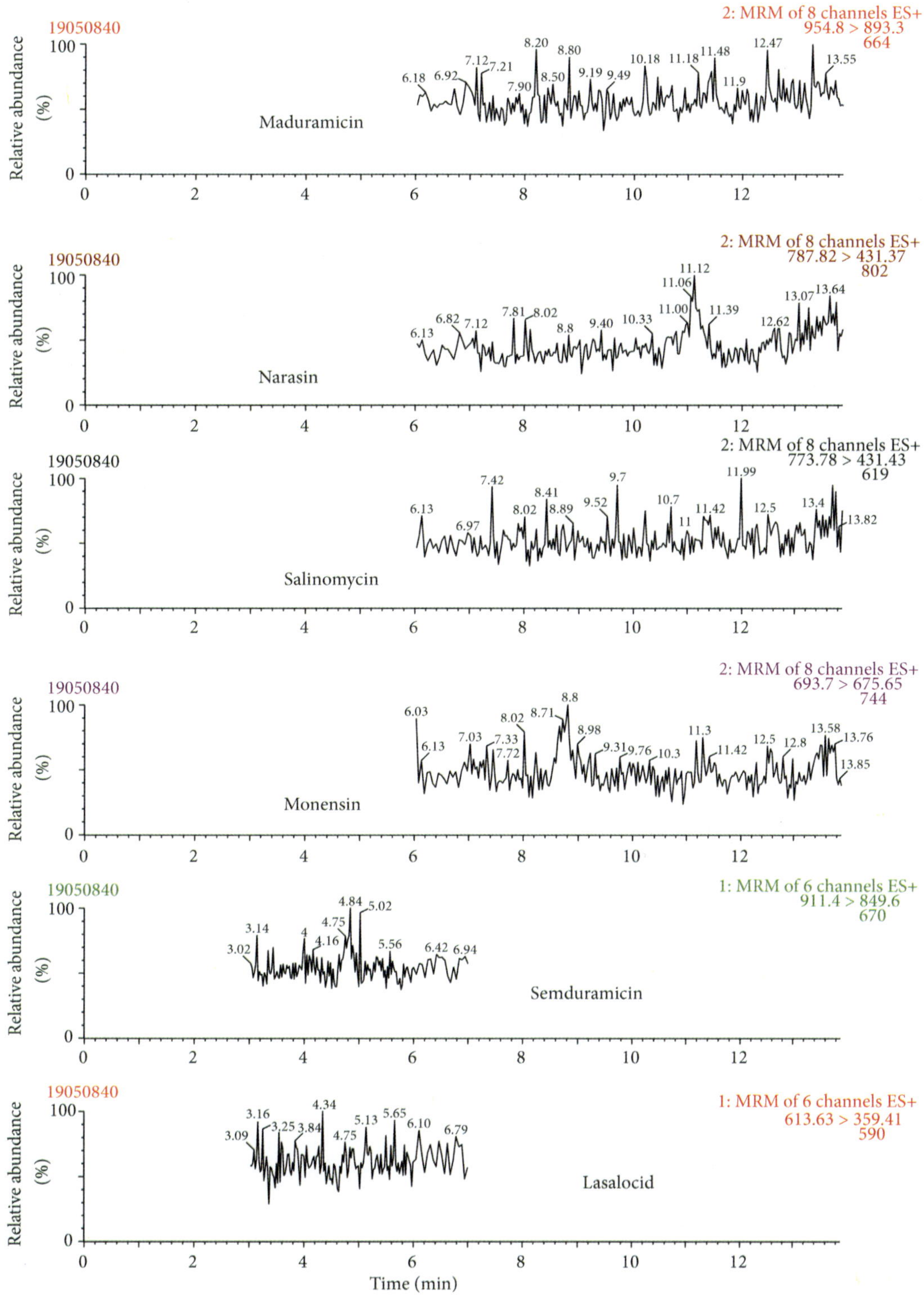

FIGURE 2: LC-MS/MS chromatogram of a blank feed sample.

by recovery, if the recovery % was over the range recoveries obtained during the validation. Lasalocid, maduramicin, and semduramicin were not detected in any samples analysed with LC-MS/MS. In samples from the feed control programme the concentrations of monensin and narasin were <0.025–0.73 mg/kg and <0.025–1.6 mg/kg, respectively (Table 4). Salinomycin was not detected in any feed control samples.

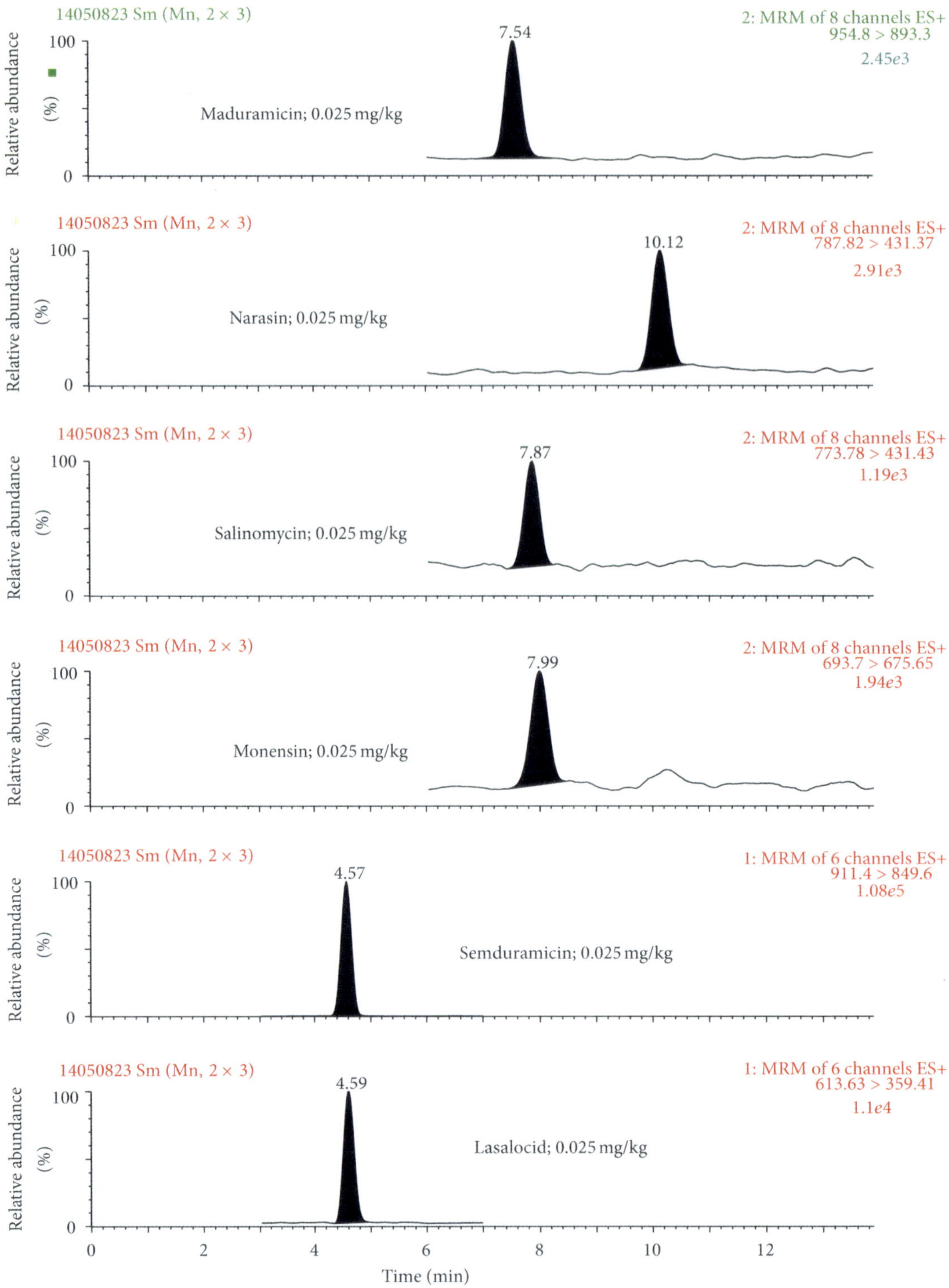

Figure 3: LC-MS/MS chromatogram of a spiked feed sample at the levels of 0.025 for monensin, salinomycin, narasin, and maduramicin and 0.20 mg/kg for lasalocid and semduramicin.

In the suspected carry-over samples from the pelletizer line, after an output of 2.0 tonnes of unmedicated feed, the level of monensin was 8 mg/kg and 16 mg/kg in two turkey feeds. In two broiler feeds, the concentration of narasin after 2.0 tonnes of unmedicated feed output was 16 mg/kg and 17 mg/kg. Carry-over was also detected in the mixer line, but it was minor compared to the pelletizer line. After 3.2 tonnes of unmedicated feed output, the concentration of monensin in feed for turkey and broiler was 0.58–2.4 mg/kg and <0.025–0.27 mg/kg, respectively.

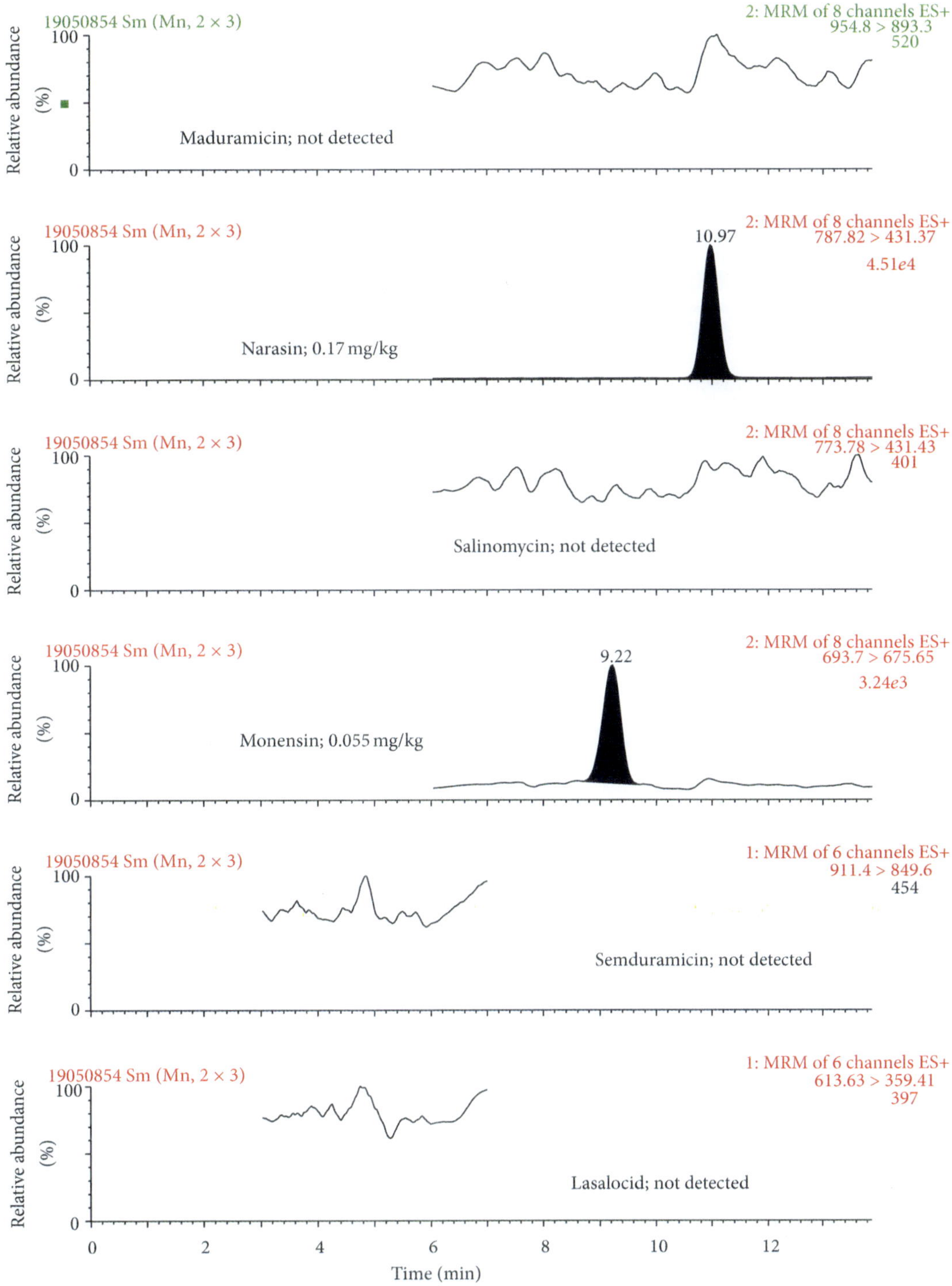

Figure 4: LC-MS/MS chromatogram of a positive feed sample; monensin at the level of 0.055 mg/kg, narasin at the level of 0.17 mg/kg.

The concentration of narasin was 0.16–0.28 mg/kg in turkey feed and 0.094–1.5 mg/kg in broiler feed. Salinomycin was detected in nine samples (<0.025–0.027 mg/kg) from both the pelletizer and mixer lines. All the results for these suspected carry-over samples are presented in Table 5.

3.4. Sample Analysis with LC-UV. The samples mentioned in Section 3.3 were also analysed for their content of monensin, salinomycin, and narasin with the already existing LC-UV method to compare the results with those determined with LC-MS/MS. The samples from the feed control programme

TABLE 4: Samples from the Finnish national feed control programme from 2008 analysed by LC-MS/MS.

	Monensin (mg/kg)	Narasin (mg/kg)
Feed 1	0.046	<0.025
Feed 2	0.73	<0.025
Feed 3	<0.025	0.26
Feed 4	0.059	0.47
Feed 5	<0.025	0.12
Feed 6	0.080	1.6
Feed 7	0.036	0.26
Feed 8	0.055	0.17

Lasalocid, maduramicin, and semduramicin were not detected with LC-MS/MS. All samples analysed with HPLC-UV were negative. Lasalocid, maduramicin, and semduramicin were not measured with HPLC-UV.

were all negative in LC-UV. In carry-over samples, salinomycin was also not found using LC-UV. The concentration of monensin in six feed samples for turkey varied between 6.9 mg/kg and 36 mg/kg, which was slightly lower than determined using LC-MS/MS (8–39 mg/kg). In addition, the content of narasin in six broiler feed samples was lower when analysed with LC-UV (8.3–39 mg/kg) than with LC-MS/MS (16–70 mg/kg). In other carry-over samples, the concentrations of monensin and narasin ranged from undetected to <5 mg/kg when analysed with LC-UV (Table 5).

4. Discussion

The developed LC-MS/MS method proved to be sensitive and repeatable in the analysis of six polyether ionophores, as shown in the validation results. The obtained LOD, LOQ, CCα, and CCβ values demonstrated that the method is capable of quantifying polyether ionophores in feed below the maximum concentrations stated in Commission Directive 2009/8/EC [30].

The European Union has not set any recommendation concerning the performance of analytical methods or the interpretation of results for contaminants in feed. Accordingly, the developed LC-MS/MS method was validated according to Commission Decision 2002/657/EC [36], which has been set for residues in food of animal origin. It sets criteria, for example, for the accuracy and precision of quantitative methods. As no CRM (certified reference material) sample was available for polyether ionophores at the trace level, the accuracy of the LC-MS/MS method was determined through the recovery of known amounts of the analytes added to a blank matrix. Although the recovery was under 80% for monensin, salinomycin, maduramicin, and semduramicin at the lowest spiking level, the recoveries were generally repeatable between different days and the method was therefore considered acceptable for analysing polyether ionophores in feed at low levels. The precision of the method was determined from intralaboratory reproducibility. According to Commission Decision 2002/657/EC [36], the coefficient of variation (CV) of intralaboratory reproducibility for concentrations lower 0.10 mg/kg should be as low as possible. The precision of the LC-MS/MS method was in accordance with the criterion. For concentrations over 0.10 mg/kg, the intralaboratory CV would typically be between 12% and 15%. In a few cases this was not met, but overall the method can be considered reproducible for analysing polyether ionophores.

As with other ionophoric compounds, coccidiostats can also form electrically neutral pseudo-macrocyclic complexes with several metal cations, such as Na^+ and K^+. Complex formation occurs by intramolecular hydrogen bonding between a carboxylic group at one end of the molecule and a terminal alcohol group at the other [37]. Polyether ionophores are usually detected as their sodium adducts in tissues and eggs samples [38–40]. Sodium adducts of polyether ionophores have also been detected in feed [26, 27]. In this study, during method testing, both sodium and potassium adducts were found. Without any control of the MS parameters, the occurrences of these adducts were variable, and thus there were problems in quantification. By optimizing the cone voltages for each of the analysed coccidiostats, the potassium adducts of semduramicin and maduramicin gave a more intensive response than their sodium adducts and were used for both detection and quantification.

The most widely used method to compensate for matrix effects in LC-MS methods is the use of an internal standard, since this allows the response of an analyte of interest to be normalized, for example, compensating for possible variations during sample preparation, injection, chromatography, and matrix effects. The best choice for an internal standard would be the isotope-labelled analogues of coccidiostats, which would have identical chemical and structural properties to those of the analyte [41]. We observed remarkable increase in the intensity of the compounds when proceeding the sequence. As no internal standards are available for coccidiostats, to solve the problem of increasing intensity, the matrix-assisted calibration curve was run two times before the samples were analysed in order to stabilize the instrument. Moreover, if large numbers of samples were to be analysed, the calibration curve was run after every ten samples and was used to quantify the samples run after the curve, although the increasing of intensity reached a plateau during the analysing run.

As the operator control samples from the feed mill demonstrated, cross-contamination is possible during manufacture. Unfortunately, the levels of monensin and narasin in medicated feed were not available. According to the legislation, monensin can be added at concentrations of between 100 and 125 mg/kg to feed for broilers and between 60 and 100 mg/kg to feed for turkeys. Narasin can be added at concentrations of between 60 and 70 mg/kg to feed for broilers. Based on these addition levels, 10–20% of the added monensin was still left after three unmedicated feed batches (2.0 tonnes) in the pelletizer line (Figure 5). In addition, about 20% of the added narasin was left in the same pelletizer line. When unmedicated feed was run in the mixer line, about 2% of the added levels of monensin and narasin were left after three batches. When comparing the concentrations of monensin and narasin in unmedicated feed with the maximum content, the concentrations in feed were much higher than the permitted levels. As the analysed feeds were

TABLE 5: Levels (mg/kg) of polyether ionophores in carry-over samples (turkey and broiler feed) from pelletizer and mixer lines analysed by both LC-MSMS and LC-UV.

Feed	Tonnes of feed	Monensin		Salinomycin		Narasin	
		LC-MSMS	LC-UV	LC-MSMS	LC-UV	LC-MSMS	LC-UV
Turkey A	0.6	29	17	<0.025	n.d.	1.9	n.d.
pelletizer	1.0	17	11	<0.025	n.d.	1.2	n.d.
line	2.0	8.0	6.9	<0.025	n.d.	0.74	n.d.
Turkey B	0.6	39	36	n.d.	n.d.	1.3	n.d.
pelletizer	1.0	18	16	n.d.	n.d.	0.60	n.d.
line	2.0	16	16	n.d.	n.d.	0.52	n.d.
Turkey C	0.8	0.60	n.d.	n.d.	n.d.	0.16	n.d.
mixer	2.0	0.73	n.d.	n.d.	n.d.	0.14	n.d.
line	3.2	0.58	n.d.	n.d.	n.d.	0.16	n.d.
Turkey D	0.8	5.3	4.3	n.d.	n.d.	0.35	n.d.
mixer	2.0	6.0	<4.0	n.d.	n.d.	0.24	n.d.
line	3.2	2.4	<4.0	n.d.	n.d.	0.28	n.d.
Broiler A	0.6	3.6	<4.0	n.d.	n.d.	70	39
pelletizer	1.0	3.6	4.3	n.d.	n.d.	51	32
line	2.0	3.3	4.1	n.d.	n.d.	16	14
Broiler B	0.6	0.070	n.d.	0.027	n.d.	47	30
pelletizer	1.0	0.066	n.d.	<0.025	n.d.	33	20
line	2.0	0.031	n.d.	<0.025	n.d.	17	8.3
Broiler C	0.8	<0.025	n.d.	<0.025	n.d.	6.0	4.0
mixer	2.0	<0.025	n.d.	<0.025	n.d.	0.54	n.d.
line	3.2	<0.025	n.d.	<0.025	n.d.	0.094	n.d.
Broiler D	0.8	0.35	n.d.	n.d.	n.d.	1.9	<5.0
mixer	2.0	0.33	<4.0	n.d.	n.d.	2.1	n.d.
line	3.2	0.27	n.d.	n.d.	n.d.	1.5	n.d.

n.d.: not detected
Lasalocid, maduramicin, and semduramicin were not detected with LC-MS/MS. Lasalocid, maduramicin, and semduramicin were not measured with LC-UV.

not fed to poultry, no data were available on the transfer of these contaminants to eggs or tissues. Kennedy et al. [11] reported the carry-over of lasalocid from medicated feed to unmedicated batches of feed during manufacture. Lasalocid was found at levels as high as 0.5–1.0 mg/kg in the ninth batch of unmedicated feed, a level high enough to result in residues in eggs.

The results determined with the developed LC-MS/MS method and the existing LC-UV method were compared. In those carry-over samples in which the concentrations of coccidiostats were more than 10 mg/kg, the results determined with both methods were similar. As expected, significant differences between the results of two analytical methods were observed at trace levels of coccidiostats, since the LOQ values of the LC-MS/MS method (0.025–0.080 mg/kg) were much lower than those of the LC-UV method (4-5 mg/kg). Samples from the national feed control programme were collected from feed batches that should not contain any polyether ionophores. With the LC-UV method, samples were previously found to be negative for monensin, salinomycin, and narasin. However, with the LC-MS/MS method, both monensin and narasin were detected at concentrations ranging from <0.025–0.73 mg/kg and <0.025–1.6 mg/kg, respectively. It is notable that narasin was found in one sample at the concentration of 1.6 mg/kg, which exceeded the permissible content (0.7 mg/kg). Moreover, in those carry-over samples that were found to be negative for monensin and narasin with the LC-UV method, both compounds were detected with the LC-MS/MS method. Thus, the developed LC-MS/MS method proved to be suitable for detecting trace amounts of polyether ionophores in feed.

5. Conclusion

In conclusion, a new LC-MS/MS method was developed for the determination of six polyether ionophores at trace levels. Sample preparation was minimized, because the raw extracts were only filtered before the LC run. The use of mass spectrometry enabled polyether ionophores to be analysed without precolumn or postcolumn derivatization. The validation data indicate that the developed method is reliable

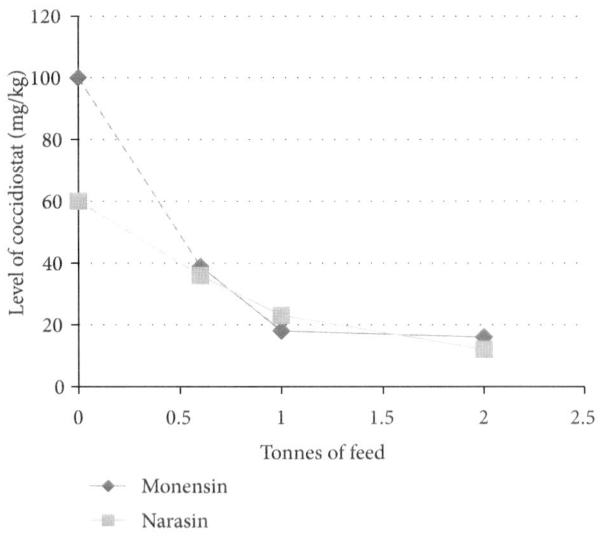

Figure 5: Carry-over of monensin and narasin in the pelletizer line during feed manufacturing.

in the determination of coccidiostats in feed at the existing contamination levels. The LC-MS/MS method demonstrated its efficiency in the analysis of coccidiostats at trace levels against the conventional LC method. In feed samples that tested negative with the LC-UV method, concentrations of coccidiostats of up to 2.10 mg/kg were detected with LC-MS/MS. The suspected carry-over of coccidiostats during the manufacture of feed was tested by analysing unmedicated feed batches produced after medicated feed. Coccidiostats could be still detected after 3.2 tonnes of unmedicated feed output.

Acknowledgments

The authors thank the laboratory technicians Kristiina Kuitunen and Pirjo Kuusjärvi for their technical assistance with the coccidiostat analyses.

References

[1] J. E. Jones, J. Solis, B. L. Hughes, D. J. Castaldo, and J. E. Toler, "Production and egg-quality responses of White Leghorn layers to anticoccidial agents," *Poultry Science*, vol. 69, no. 3, pp. 378–387, 1990.

[2] EFSA (European Food Safety Authority), "Opinion of the Scientific Panel on Additives and Products or Substances used in Animal Feed on the safety and efficacy of the coccidiostat Elancoban (monensin sodium) as a feed additive for calves for rearing and cattle for fattening in accordance with Regulation (EC) No 1831/2003," *The European Food Safety Authority Journal*, vol. 387, pp. 1–33, 2006.

[3] "Report of Scientific Committee for Animal Nutrition on the use of lasalocid sodium in feedingstuffs for finishing cattle," Opinion expressed, 27 July 1990.

[4] EFSA (European Food Safety Authority), "Cross-contamination of non-target feedingstuffs by narasin authorised for use as a feed additive," *The European Food Safety Authority Journal*, vol. 552, pp. 1–35, 2007.

[5] EFSA (European Food Safety Authority), "Cross-contamination of non-target feedingstuffs by maduramicin authorised for use as a feed additive," *The European Food Safety Authority Journal*, vol. 594, pp. 1–30, 2008.

[6] EFSA (European Food Safety Authority), "Cross-contamination of non-target feedingstuffs by semduramicin authorised for use as a feed additive," *The European Food Safety Authority Journal*, vol. 593, pp. 1–27, 2008.

[7] G. Kabell, R. K. Saini, P. Somani, and B. C. Pressman, "Effects of the carboxylic ionophore monensin on regional blood flow in normal and ischemic myocardium in anesthetized dogs," *Journal of Pharmacology and Experimental Therapeutics*, vol. 211, no. 1, pp. 231–237, 1979.

[8] J. V. Levy and G. Inesi, "Positive inotropic effect on isolated human atrial muscle produced by the ionophore X 537A: preliminary report," *Journal of Clinical Pharmacology*, vol. 14, no. 1, pp. 32–34, 1974.

[9] G. Weiss, "The integration of pharmacological and toxicological testing of tissue residues in the evaluation of their human food safety," *Drug Metabolism Reviews*, vol. 22, no. 6-8, pp. 829–848, 1990.

[10] D. G. Kennedy, P. J. Hughes, and W. J. Blanchflower, "Ionophore residues in eggs in Northern Ireland: incidence and cause," *Food Additives and Contaminants*, vol. 15, no. 5, pp. 535–541, 1998.

[11] D. G. Kennedy, W. J. Blanchflower, P. J. Hughes, and W. J. McCaughey, "The incidence and cause of lasalocid residues in eggs in Northern Ireland," *Food Additives and Contaminants*, vol. 13, no. 7, pp. 787–794, 1996.

[12] J. Rosén, "Efficient and sensitive screening and confirmation of residues of selected polyether ionophore antibiotics in liver and eggs by liquid chromatography-electrospray tandem mass spectrometry," *The Analyst*, vol. 126, no. 11, pp. 1990–1995, 2001.

[13] "Results of residue examination of products of animal origin in Finland 2003," National Food Agency (NFA), National Veterinary and Food Research Institute (EELA) and Ministry of Agriculture and Forestry (MAF), Helsinki, Finland, pp. 1–69, 2004.

[14] M. Rokka, S. Eerola, U. Perttilä et al., "The residue levels of narasin in eggs of laying hens fed with unmedicated and medicated feed," *Molecular Nutrition and Food Research*, vol. 49, no. 1, pp. 38–42, 2005.

[15] "Results of residue examinations of products of animal origin in Finland 2003," National Food Agency (NFA), National Veterinary and Food Research Institute (EELA) and Ministry of Agriculture and Forestry (MAF), Helsinki, Finland, pp. 1–69, 2004.

[16] M. Jestoi, M. Rokka, and K. Peltonen, "An integrated sample preparation to determine coccidiostats and emerging Fusarium-mycotoxins in various poultry tissues with LC-MS/MS," *Molecular Nutrition and Food Research*, vol. 51, no. 5, pp. 625–637, 2007.

[17] D. K. Matabudul, N. T. Crosby, I. Lumley, and S. Sumara, "The optimisation of a rapid method for the determination of lasalocid in poultry feed using supercritical fluid extraction and high performance liquid chromatography," *Food Chemistry*, vol. 75, no. 4, pp. 465–471, 2001.

[18] C. Focht, H. Campbell, J. Dalgleish et al., "Determination of lasalocid sodium in animal feeds and premixes by reversed-phase liquid chromatography: collaborative study," *Journal of AOAC International*, vol. 91, no. 3, pp. 479–488, 2008.

[19] G. Dusi and V. Gamba, "Liquid chromatography with ultraviolet detection of lasalocid, monensin, salinomycin and narasin in poultry feeds using pre-column derivatization," *Journal of Chromatography A*, vol. 835, no. 1-2, pp. 243–246, 1999.

[20] A. Thalmann, K. Wagner, M. Tomassen, J. Driessen, and J. de Jong, "Liquid chromatographic method to determine narasin in feedingstuffs and premixtures: development, validation, and interlaboratory study," *Journal of AOAC International*, vol. 87, no. 6, pp. 1278–1286, 2004.

[21] J. de Jong, B. Stoisser, K. Wagner et al., "Determination of maduramicin in feedingstuffs and premixtures by liquid chromatography: development, validation, and interlaboratory study," *Journal of AOAC International*, vol. 87, no. 5, pp. 1033–1041, 2004.

[22] H. Campbell, G. Nayeri, J. M. Costa et al., "Determination of monensin, narasin, and salinomycin in mineral premixes, supplements, and animal feeds by liquid chromatography and post-column derivatization: collaborative study," *Journal of AOAC International*, vol. 89, no. 5, pp. 1229–1242, 2006.

[23] G. Tavcar-Kalcher, K. Pavsic-Vrtac, and A. Vengust, "Validation of the procedure for the determination of maduramicin in concentrates, premixes, and feeds by liquid chromatography," *Food Additives and Contaminants*, vol. 22, pp. 1–5, 2008.

[24] J. Wang and P. Sporns, "MALDI-TOF MS quantification of coccidiostats in poultry feeds," *Journal of Agricultural and Food Chemistry*, vol. 48, no. 7, pp. 2807–2811, 2000.

[25] V. Hormazábal, Ø. Østensvik, and M. Kaldhusdal, "An improved LC-MS method for the determination of lasalocid, monensin, narasin, and salinomycin in feed," *Journal of Liquid Chromatography & Related Technologies*, vol. 28, no. 17, pp. 2769–2776, 2005.

[26] J. G. Ebel, T. Wachs, and J. D. Henion, "Rapid forensic selected reaction monitoring liquid chromatography/mass spectrometry determination of ionophore antibiotics found at toxic levels in animal feeds," *Journal of AOAC International*, vol. 87, no. 1, pp. 25–30, 2004.

[27] U. Vincent, M. Chedin, S. Yasar, and C. von Holst, "Determination of ionophore coccidiostats in feedingstuffs by liquid chromatography-tandem mass spectrometry. Part I. Application to targeted feed," *Journal of Pharmaceutical and Biomedical Analysis*, vol. 47, no. 4-5, pp. 750–757, 2008.

[28] S. B. Turnipseed, J. E. Roybal, A. P. Pfenning, S. A. Gonzales, J. A. Hurlbut, and M. R. Madson, "LC/MS confirmation of ionophores in animal feeds," *Journal of AOAC International*, vol. 84, no. 3, pp. 640–647, 2001.

[29] M. Huang, W. K. Rumbeiha, W. Emmett Braselton, and M. Johnson, "Rapid and reliable identification of ionophore antibiotics in feeds by liquid chromatography-tandem mass spectrometry," *Journal of Veterinary Diagnostic Investigation*, vol. 23, no. 2, pp. 358–363, 2011.

[30] P. Delahaut, G. Pierret, N. Ralet, M. Dubois, and N. Gillard, "Multi-residue method for detecting coccidiostats at carry-over level in feed by HPLC-MS/MS," *Food Additives and Contaminants A*, vol. 27, no. 6, pp. 801–809, 2010.

[31] "Commission Directive 2009/8/EC amending Annex I to Directive 2002/32/EC of the European Parliament and of the Council as regards maximum levels of unavoidable carry-over of coccidiostats or histomonostats in non-target feed," *Official Journal of the European Union*, vol. 40, pp. 19–25, 2009.

[32] AM-AA-CR-J424-AC-791, *Determination of Narasin in Raw Material, Premix and Poultry and Cattle Rations by HPLC Using Post-Column Derivatization*, Animal Science Chemical Research Lilly Research Laboratories A Division of Eli Lilly and Company Greenfield, Indiana, USA.

[33] M. Jestoi, M. Rokka, A. Rizzo, K. Peltonen, and S. Aurasaari, "Determination of Fusarium-mycotoxins beauvericin and enniatins with liquid chromatography-tandem mass spectrometry (LC-MS/MS)," *Journal of Liquid Chromatography & Related Technologies*, vol. 28, no. 3, pp. 369–381, 2005.

[34] M. Sulyok, F. Berthiller, R. Krska, and R. Schuhmacher, "Development and validation of a liquid chromatography/tandem mass spectrometric method for the determination of 39 mycotoxins in wheat and maize," *Rapid Communications in Mass Spectrometry*, vol. 20, no. 18, pp. 2649–2659, 2006.

[35] J. M. P. van Trijp and A. H. Roos, "Model for the calculation of calibration curves," RIKILT Report 91.02, 1991.

[36] "Commission Decision 2002/657/EC of 12 August 2002," *Official Journal of the European Communities L*, vol. 221, p. 8, 2002.

[37] D. A. Volmer and C. M. Lock, "Electrospray ionization and collision-induced dissociation of antibiotic polyether ionophores," *Rapid Communications in Mass Spectrometry*, vol. 12, pp. 157–164, 1998.

[38] M. Rokka and K. Peltonen, "Simultaneous determination of four coccidiostats in eggs and broiler meat: validation of an LC-MS/MS method," *Food Additives and Contaminants*, vol. 23, no. 5, pp. 470–478, 2006.

[39] L. Mortier, E. Daeseleire, and C. van Peteghem, "Determination of the ionophoric coccidiostats narasin, monensin, lasalocid and salinomycin in eggs by liquid chromatography/tandem mass spectrometry," *Rapid Communications in Mass Spectrometry*, vol. 19, no. 4, pp. 533–539, 2005.

[40] D. K. Matabudul, I. D. Lumley, and J. S. Points, "The determination of 5 anticoccidial drugs (nicarbazin, lasalocid, monensin, salinomycin and narasin) in animal livers and eggs by liquid chromatography linked with tandem mass spectrometry (LC-MS-MS)," *The Analyst*, vol. 127, no. 6, pp. 760–768, 2002.

[41] L. L. Jessome and D. A. Volmer, "Ion suppression: a major concern in mass spectrometry," *LC-GC North America*, vol. 24, no. 5, pp. 498–510, 2006.

9

Management of Cosmetic Embarrassment Caused by *Malassezia* spp. with Fruticose Lichen *Cladia* Using Phylogenetic Approach

Anand Pandey,[1] Rohit K. Mishra,[1] Amit K. Tiwari,[1] Awadhesh Kumar,[2] A. K. Bajaj,[3] and Anupam Dikshit[1]

[1] *Biological Product Laboratory, Department of Botany, University of Allahabad, Allahabad 211002, India*
[2] *Department of Horticulture and Medicinal Plants, Mizoram University, Aizawl 796004, India*
[3] *Department of Dermatology, Moti Lal Nehru Medical College, Allahabad 211002, India*

Correspondence should be addressed to Anupam Dikshit; anupambplau@rediffmail.com

Academic Editor: Marco Bazzicalupo

During anti-*Malassezia* screening of plants by CLSI broth microdilution method, *Cladia aggregata* (Swartz) Nyl. (family Cladoniaceae), a fruticose lichen from Sikkim (northeast Himalayan region), has been found effective at minimum inhibitory concentrations (mg/mL) of 2.72, 0.63, and 1.28 against yeast-like fungi namely, *M. furfur, M. globosa* and *M. sympodialis,* respectively. These test pathogens are responsible for pityriasis versicolor (PV) and seborrheic dermatitis (SD) in humans. We tried to establish the reason for variable MICs against various *Malassezia* spp. using bioinformatical tools, thereby reducing the cost of the experimentation. This is the first report on anti-*Malassezia* activity of *C. aggregata* and thus can serve as a potential source for the development of cosmaceuticals.

1. Introduction

Unicellular yeast like fungus *Malassezia* is responsible for causing pityriasis versicolor (PV) and dandruff, which manifests as seborrheic dermatitis (SD) in its severe form in humans (as well as animals) causing physical discomfort and cosmetic embarrassment globally. Hypo- or hyper-pigmented skin on the seborrheic areas of the body characterizes the onset of PV. The symptoms of dandruff can range from mild scaling to fine patchy scales attributed to hyperproliferation of the scalp epidermis, as judged by cell turnover studies and the presence of parakeratotic nuclei present in the shed flakes and the stratum corneum [1, 2]. The widespread occurrence of dandruff can be considered physiological because of the critical maturation processes owing to desquamation of the skin surface arising from the continuous separation of scaly layers of the stratum corneum [3, 4].

French scientist Malassez [5] originally identified *Malassezia*. Later on, Raymond Sabouraud [6] identified a dandruff causing organism in 1904 and named the fungus as "Pityrosporum malassez" in honour of the pioneering work of the French scientist. Further research revealed the strains to be the same at species level and name *Malassezia* was given to the fungus and classified the taxa. Lipophilic *Malassezia* is a common mycoflora of human skin, especially the upper sebaceous parts such as hair which has high sebum excretion [7, 8]. Dandruff is a very common problem worldwide, but in temperate and tropical countries, temperatures are high and people sweat a lot in the summer, providing favourable conditions to the pathogen. As teenagers generally perspire more in comparison to older persons, there is a high chance of proliferation of *Malassezia* in teenagers during summer [9]. Presently, about 14 spp. of *Malassezia* are known [10]. Classical *Malassezia furfur* in scales from the disease PV consists of spherical yeasts, 2.5–8 μm in diameter, producing buds from a narrow base, associated with short filaments which are often distorted and angular [11]. Biochemical investigations showed that azelaic acid produced by *Malassezia* spp. is repressive to neutrophils [12] and is a competitive inhibitor of tyrosinase, a key enzyme in melanogenesis [13], suggesting that azelaic acid may play an important role in abnormal skin pigmentation associated with PV.

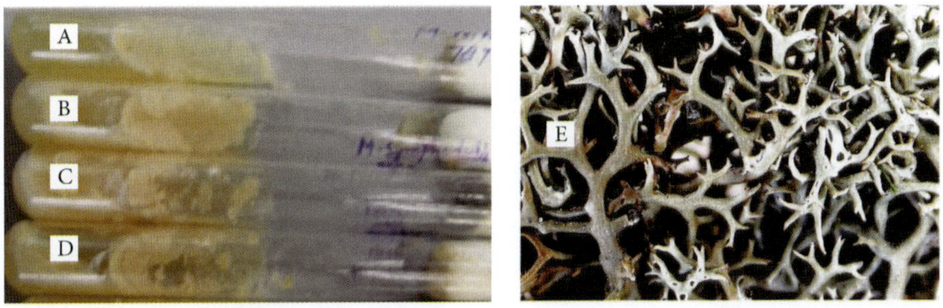

(a) (b)

FIGURE 1: Cultures of *Malassezia* spp.: (A) *Malassezia furfur*, (B) *M. sympodialis*, (C) *M. globosa*, (D) *M. restricta*, and (E) lichen *Cladia aggregata* collected from Sikkim.

All these findings have opened the pathway for understanding disease development in human beings with baseline information about *Malassezia* spp. The use of traditional medicines for curing skin ailments in the world of dermatology has a long historical backdrop. Recent researches have revealed that herbal products have better antifungal efficacy and less or negligible undesirable effects on human beings as compared to chemotherapeutic agents [14]. The changing environmental setting and its prejudicial impact on human health have also stirred scientists to search for nonconventional methods of treatment of various maladies.

Lichens are composite organism consisting of two distinct and dissimilar components: the photobiont and the mycobiont. Later one, being the dominant partner, lichens are taxonomically treated as a class of fungi. The diversity of lichens is maintained by approximately 18,800 recognized species [15]. In comparison with the higher taxa of medicinal and aromatic plants (mainly angiosperms), they have been less explored in the medicinal world, and this portends a very wide scope for a novel search among them for potential agents against *Malassezia*.

Cladia aggregata (Swartz) Nyl., a fruticose lichen spp. belonging to the family Cladoniaceae, exhibits good growth in mesic habitats of temperate Himalayas with their following taxonomic characteristics. The primary squamulose thallus bears podetia with elliptical perforations in cortex, 3–7 mm long up to 2 mm in diameter. The podetia have yellow to pale brownish younger parts and dichotomous or sympodial branching in older parts with shiny brown texture. Barbatic acid is the main active compound in addition to other substances such as the stictic, norstictic, and fumarprotocetraric acids, whose occurrence and percentage depend on the area where the lichen is found. Barbatic acid and usnic acid are reported as efficient against microorganisms, cancer cells, and tumors [16, 17].

2. Materials and Methods

2.1. Test Pathogens. 10 cultures of unicellular yeast like fungus *Malassezia* spp., namely, *M. furfur, M. globosa, M. restricta, M. sympodialis, M. obtusa, M. sloffiae, M. dermatis, M. yamatoensis, M. nana, and M. japonica,* were obtained from Centraal bureau voor Schimmelcultures (CBS) Fungal Biodiversity Centre, Institute of the Royal Netherlands Academy of Arts and Sciences (KNAW), The Netherlands. *M. furfur* 1878, *M. restricta* 7877, *M. globosa* 7966 and *M. sympodialis* 7222 (Figure 1 (A), (B), (C), and (D)) were selected for this study due to their strong prevalence in causing PV and dandruff in the defined climatic conditions. These cultures were maintained in solid media BPL5 M (patent application number DEL/546/2012) supplemented with powdered milk [18, 19].

2.2. Collection of Lichen Material and Preparation of Ethanolic (50% v/v) Extract. The lichen *Cladia aggregata* (Swartz) Nyl. was collected from Sikkim (Figure 1 (E)) and the adjoining areas [20]. The lichen was identified according to the key provided in the Macrolichens of India by Awasthi [21] and further verified by Dr. G. P. Sinha, Scientist, Botanical Survey of India, Central Zone, Allahabad, India. The voucher specimen of air dried lichen material was submitted to the Duthie Herbarium of Department of Botany, University of Allahabad. The air-dried lichen material was washed thoroughly with tap water and then continuous flow of distilled water. After pat drying the sample, 5 grams of lichen sample was weighed and crushed in pestle mortar. It was subjected for cold extraction in 50 mL of ethanolic (50% v/v) solution followed by incubation at 37°C for 24 hours. Subsequently, the extract solution was filtered by Whatman No. 1 filter paper, and filtrate was evaporated in rotary evaporator apparatus at 45–60°C to obtain crude extract. The extract was dried completely and weighed for obtaining percentage yield (0.756 gram, approx. 15%).

2.3. Antifungal Susceptibility Testing. The susceptibility of the *Malassezia* spp. was assayed against lichen crude extract using the broth microdilution method recommended by the Clinical and Laboratory Standards Institute (CLSI) [22]. Freshly prepared broth medium BPL5O supplemented with cottonseed oil was used for the assay [18, 19]. Stock solution (50 mg/mL) of extract was prepared in DMSO. In brief, the initial fungal inocula suspension, prepared as per 0.5 McFarland standard (corresponding to a CFU of 1.5×10^7 cell/mL), was inoculated in two-fold serially diluted candidate extract to be tested. Fluconazole, as a synthetic standard, was also subjected to the antifungal assay. The

Table 1: Antifungal activity of 50% ethanolic extract of *Cladia aggregata* (Swartz) Nyl. compared with synthetic fluconazole against the *Malassezia* spp.

Selected pathogens	Antifungal activity: Ethanolic extract *Cladia aggregata* (Swartz) Nyl.		Fluconazole	
	IC_{50} (mg/mL)	MIC (mg/mL)	IC_{50} (mg/mL)	MIC (mg/mL)
M. furfur	2.51	2.72	0.021	0.034
M. globosa	0.31	0.63	0.0004	0.006
M. sympodialis	0.04	1.28	0.047	0.051
M. restricta	No activity	No activity	0.026	0.051

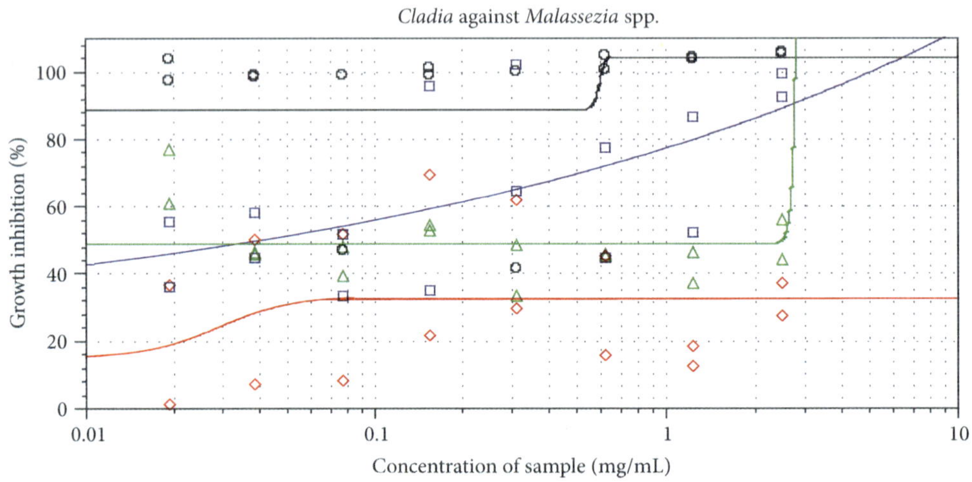

4-P fit: $y = (A - D)/(1 + (x/C)^B) + D$:	A	B	C	D	R^2
△ *Cladia* versus Mf (group 1: concentration versus inhibition (%))	48.5	36.7	3.32	$4.88e + 04$	0.00226
○ *Cladia* versus Mg (group 2: concentration versus inhibition (%))	88.3	44.1	0.598	105	0.157
□ *Cladia* versus Msy (group 3: concentration versus inhibition (%))	21.8	0.212	$9.57e + 22$	$4.22e + 06$	0.36
◇ *Cladia* versus Mr (group 4: concentration versus inhibition (%))	14.9	3.45	0.0291	33.2	0.0593

Curve fit option – Fixed weight value

Figure 2: % inhibition curve of *Cladia aggregata* against *Malassezia* spp. (generated by SoftMax Pro using model SpectraMax Plus^{384}).

MICs and IC_{50} were obtained by measuring absorbance using spectrophotometer (SpectraMax Plus^{384}, Molecular Devices Corporation, USA) at 530 nm, after an incubation of 48 hrs at 35 ± 2°C.

2.4. Phylogenetic Treatment of Malassezia spp. Studied for Antifungal Assay. Chitin synthase gene (*chs* and/or *chs*-2) responsible for synthesis of chitin (building block of fungal cell wall) was selected for phylogenetic study. This was done because phenolic acids cause initial disruption of cell wall to further act at molecular level. Gene sequences procured from GenBank NCBI database were blasted in the *blastx* programme of NCBI, and amino acid sequences were obtained for the strains (CBS 1878, CBS 7966, CBS 7222, and CBS 7877) used for study [23, 24]. The alignment of the gene sequence (Figure 4) was done by ClustalW analysis, and further phylogeny was constructed (Figure 4) in form of N-J bootstrapped phylogenetic tree [25–27] by MEGA4 software version 4.0 [28]. Some homologous sequences obtained in *blastx* run were also selected randomly for further phylogenetic studies in relation to antifungal susceptibility of *Malassezia* spp. against the extract of *Cladia aggregata* lichen. The phylogenetic tree (Figure 5) was constructed for the *chs* gene along with the translated protein alignment (Figure 6) of the strains studied.

3. Results and Discussion

The ethanolic extract of lichen *C. aggregata* (Figure 1 (E)) exhibited an IC_{50} (mg/mL) of 2.51, 0.31, and 0.04 and MIC (mg/mL) of 2.72, 0.63, and 1.28 against *M. furfur, M. globosa,* and *M. sympodialis,* respectively, while no activity was recorded against *M. restricta* (Table 1).

Fluconazole used as the standard in our study has an IC_{50} (mg/mL) of 0.021, 0.0004, 0.047, and 0.026 and MIC (mg/mL) of 0.034, 0.006, 0.051, and 0.051 against *M. furfur, M. globosa,*

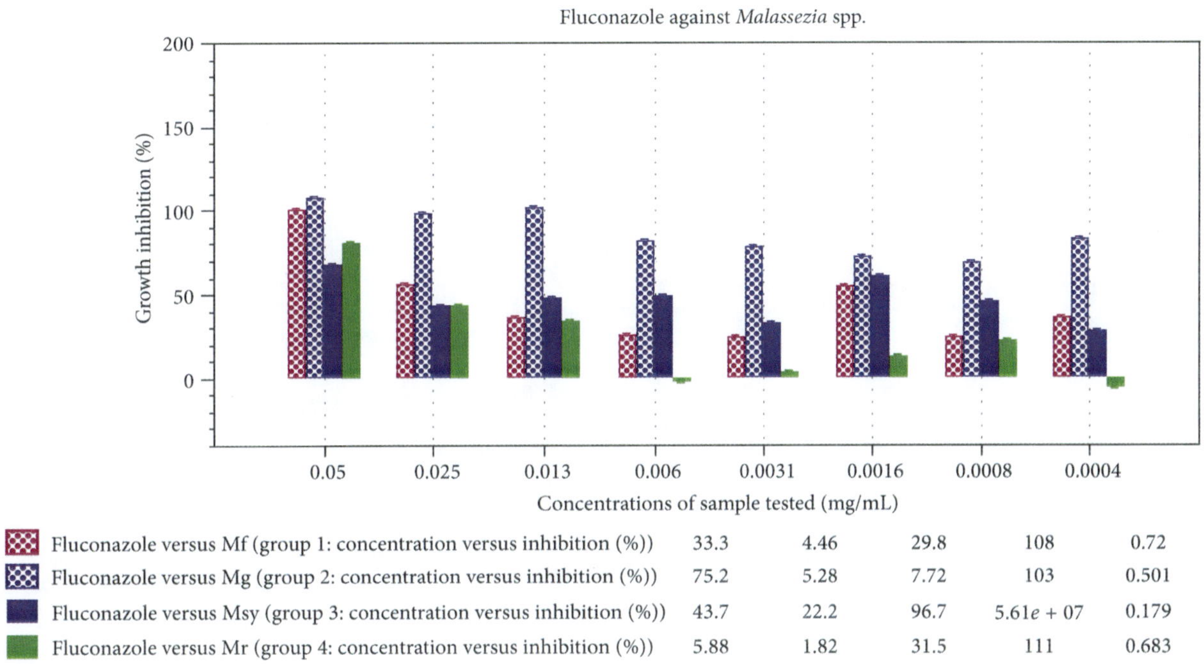

FIGURE 3: % inhibition curve of fluconazole against *Malassezia* spp. (generated by SoftMax Pro using model SpectraMax Plus^{384}).

M. sympodialis and *M. restricta,* respectively (Table 1). The standard error plot of mean standard deviation (±SD) has been given in the graph calculated by the SoftMax Pro ELISA reader software (Figures 2 and 3).

With the point of view of reducing the cost of experimentation for analyzing the variability in MICs against the lichen, *Malassezia* spp. were exposed to phylogenetic analysis by ClustalW analysis and bootstrapping NJ plotting by MEGA 4 (version 4.0). The gene alignment and protein sequences of the *chs* gene obtained from NCBI blast have shown homology in the sequences (Figure 4) and greater confidence level in 1000 bootstrapped N-J plot. The phylogenetic plot also reflected strong susceptibility of *M. globosa* and *M. sympodialis* to *Cladia* extract. It may be considered that more complex species, that is, *M. globosa* and *M. sympodialis,* have more susceptibility to herbal extracts, which was evident from the MICs obtained, that is, 0.63 mg/mL against *M. globosa* and 1.28 mg/mL against *M. sympodialis,* respectively. On the other hand, inhibition of growth of *M. furfur*, which is more primitive, was obtained at 2.72 mg/mL, indicating some resistivity to the herbal extracts. It is noteworthy that *M. globosa* and *M. sympodialis* are frequently isolated pathogenic species from human scalp [29, 30].

This might be due to the homology in the chitin synthase enzyme translated by *chs* gene (Figure 6). The wall structure of the fungi can be considered as one factor. The more primitive *M. furfur* has a stouter wall, which restricts the action of antifungal agent, whereas *M. globosa* and *M. sympodialis* have shown more susceptibility to the agent. Moreover, on the basis of molecular phylogeny of various available strains of *Malassezia* along with CBS standard strains used for our study (Figure 5), the effectiveness of the extract was in strict accordance to the closely related *Malassezia* spp.; it can be conceived that the *Cladia* extract will also be effective against other anthropophilic and zoophilic spp., namely, *M. pachydermatis, M. japonica, M. yamatoensis* and *M. equii.* The *C. aggregata*, along with *Usnea baileyi* and *Everniastrum nepalense*, has been found active against multidrug resistant *Staphylococcus aureus* [31, 32]. Established results on the antifungal activity of *Everniastrum cirrhatum* with minimum fungicidal concentration (MFC) of as low as 60 μL/mL against human pathogenic fungi (dermatophytes), namely, *Epidermophyton floccosum, Microsporum gypseum, M. canis, M. audounii, Trichophyton rubrum, T. mentagrophytes, T. violaceum,* and *T. tonsurans,* have also been reported in the past [33]. *Heterodermia leucomelos* was also found effective against human as well as plant pathogenic fungi [34]. Some macrolichens extracts, namely, *Parmelia tinctorum, Ramalina* sp., *Teloschistes flavicans,* and *Usnea undulata*, were tested and found effective against some pathogenic fungi [35]. Broad spectrum antifungal properties at 80 μL/mL were evident in the aqueous extract of *Parmelia cirrhatum* against some human and plant pathogens [36]. The phenolic compounds and their derivatives in lichen have been proved to be detrimental for pathogenic microbial fauna. These substances generally acidify the microbial cell wall and consequently, cause cytoplasm membrane rupture, inactivate or immobilize the enzymes, and interfere with physiological functions such as electrons transport and oxidative phosphorylation [37–39]. A number of higher plants have been reported effective against dandruff causing *Malassezia* [40], but none have comparable potentiality with lichens against *Malassezia.* To the best of our knowledge, the activity of lichen *C. aggregata* against *Malassezia furfur, M. globosa* and *M. sympodialis* is reported for the

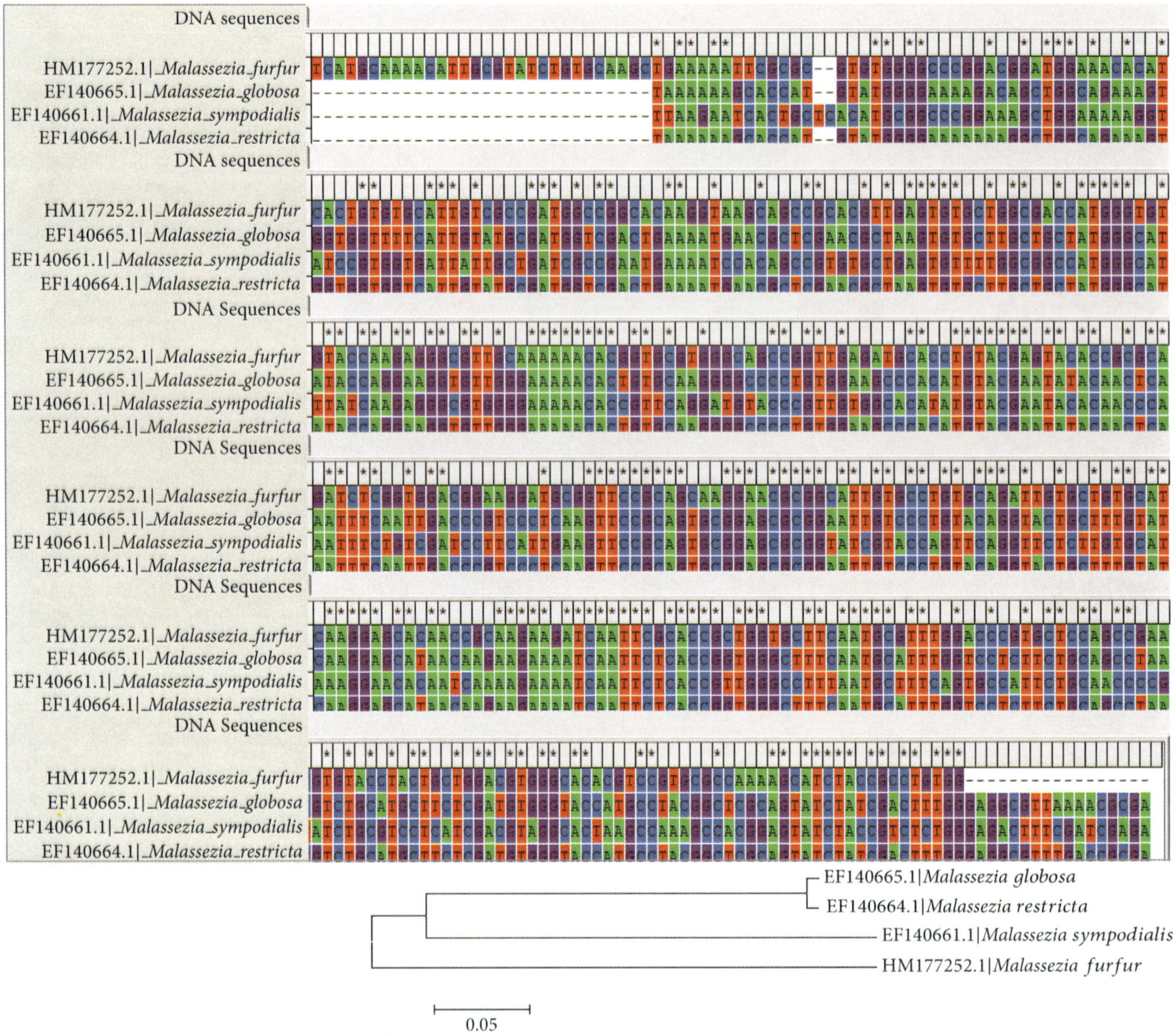

FIGURE 4: Alignment of the chitin synthase (*chs* gene) of *Malassezia furfur, M. globosa, M. sympodialis* and *M. restricta* by bootstrapped ClustalW program in MEGA 4 (version 4.0) and its phylogenetic tree constructed using the sequences of (*chs* gene) by bootstrapped N-J plot used for the antifungal susceptibility test (sequences of the strains were obtained from NCBI database).

first time and will have potential for the development of cosmaceuticals.

4. Conclusion

The present finding creates an interest in the exploration of lichens for novel antimicrobials. The nontoxic nature of herbal medicines complements conventional treatment and excels over the synthetic drugs such as fluconazole, which are effective but come with considerable side effects and have high disease reoccurrence rate. Moreover, the bioprospection should not be limited to mere exploration of the novel antimicrobials but should lead to development of the formulation after successful multicentral topical testing, pharmacological, and toxicological investigations. To the best of our knowledge, this is the first report for the anti-*Malassezia* property of lichen *Cladia aggregata* (Swartz) Nyl. against the three most prevalent PV and dandruff causing mycoflora, namely, *M. globosa, M. furfur* and *M. sympodialis.* The prediction of the susceptibility of the pathogenic fungus towards active compounds based on their phylogenetic position is a novel approach. Thus, the present findings strongly support the potentiality of the lichen *C. aggregata* as a useful herbal cosmaceutical after successful topical testing, which is in progress.

Acknowledgments

Thanks are due to the Head of Department of Botany, University of Allahabad for laboratory facilities, to Professor

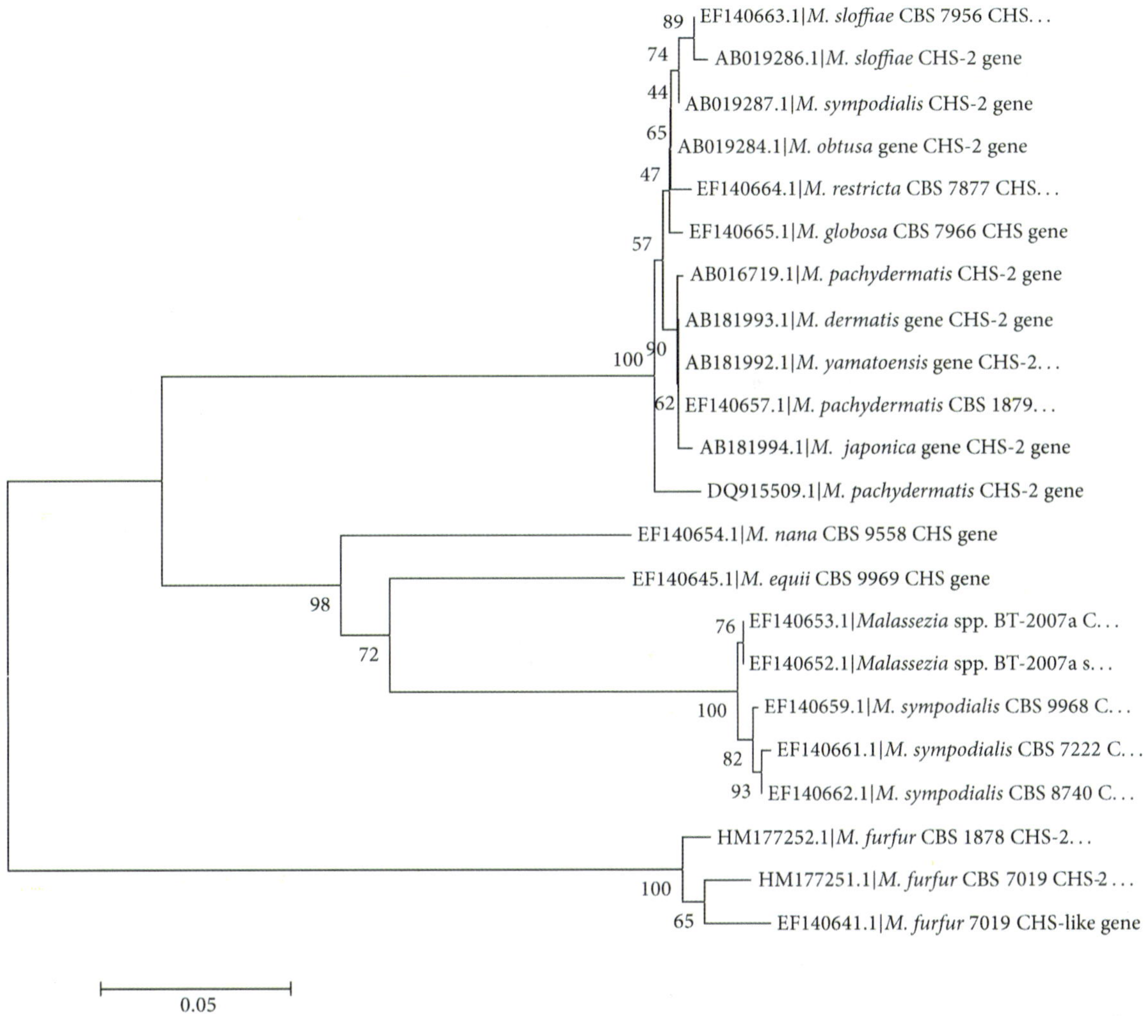

FIGURE 5: Molecular phylogenetic tree constructed using the sequences of *chs* (chitin synthase) gene of available strains of the genus *Malassezia* with CBS strains used for study (CBS 1878, CBS 7966, CBS 7222 and CBS 7877). The number of branch points represents the percentage of 1000 bootstrapped datasheets showing specific internal branches (sequences of the strains were obtained from NCBI database-accession number given) (constructed by MEGA 4 version 4.0).

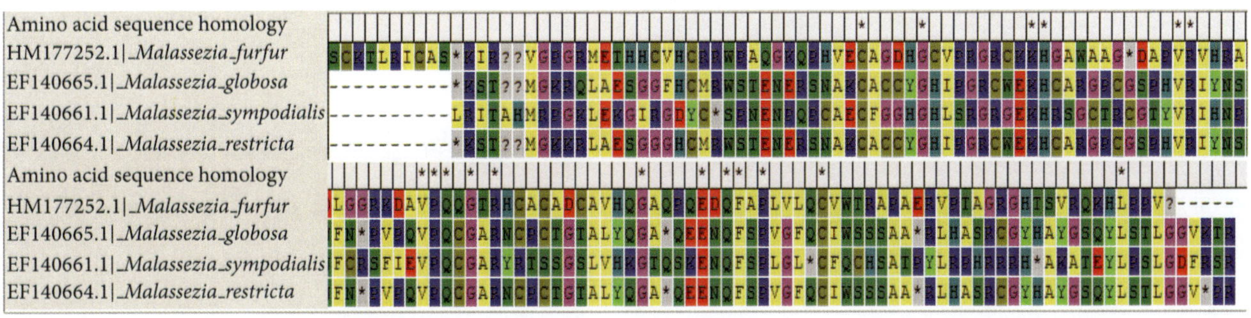

FIGURE 6: Alignment of the amino acid sequences of *Malassezia furfur* (CBS 1878), *M. globosa* (CBS 7966), *M. sympodialis* (CBS 7222) and *M. restricta* (CBS 7877) (constructed by MEGA 4 version 4.0).

V. P. Singh and Zeeshan- ur- Rehman, Department of Botany, Delhi University for fruitful discussion on bioinformatical studies, Professor V. C. Pandey, University of Allahabad for critically reviewing the paper and the Department of Science and Technology (DST), New Delhi, India, for financial assistance.

References

[1] A. Prohic and L. Ozegovic, "*Malassezia* species isolated from lesional and non-lesional skin in patients with pityriasis versicolor," *Mycoses*, vol. 50, no. 1, pp. 58–63, 2007.

[2] C. E. Orfanos and R. Happle, *Hair and Hair Diseases*, Springer, Berlin, Germany, 1st edition, 1989.

[3] A. K. Tiwari, R. K. Mishra, A. Kumar et al., "A comparative novel method of antifungal susceptibility for *Malassezia furfur* and modification of culture medium by adding lipid supplement," *Journal of Phytology*, vol. 3, no. 3, pp. 44–52, 2011.

[4] C. R. Harding, A. Watkinson, A. V. Rawlings, and I. R. Scott, "Dry skin, moisturization and corneodesmolysis," *International Journal of Cosmetic Science*, vol. 22, no. 1, pp. 21–52, 2000.

[5] L. Malassez, "Note sur le champignon du pityriasis simple," *Archives de Physiologie*, vol. 1, article 451, 1874.

[6] A. C. Inamadar and A. Palit, "The genus *Malassezia* and human disease," *Indian Journal of Dermatology, Venereology and Leprology*, vol. 69, no. 4, pp. 265–270, 2003.

[7] M. J. Marcon and D. A. Powell, "Human infections due to *Malassezia* spp.," *Clinical Microbiology Reviews*, vol. 5, no. 2, pp. 101–119, 1992.

[8] J. P. Leeming and F. H. Notman, "Improved methods for isolation and enumeration of *Malassezia furfur* from human skin," *Journal of Clinical Microbiology*, vol. 25, no. 10, pp. 2017–2019, 1987.

[9] J. W. Rippon, *Medical Mycology: The Pathogenic Fungi and the Pathogenic Actinomycetes*, W. B. Saunders, Philadelphia, Pa, USA, 2nd edition, 1982.

[10] G. Gaitanis, P. Magiatis, M. Hantschke, I. D. Bassukas, and A. Velegraki, "The *Malassezia* genus in skin and systemic diseases," *Clinical Microbiology Reviews*, vol. 25, no. 1, pp. 106–141, 2012.

[11] G. Midgley, "The diversity of *Pityrosporum* (*Malassezia*) yeasts *in vivo* and *in vitro*," *Mycopathologia*, vol. 106, no. 3, pp. 143–153, 1989.

[12] M. Nazzaro-Porro and S. Passi, "Identification of tyrosinase inhibitors in cultures of *Pityrosporum*," *Journal of Investigative Dermatology*, vol. 71, no. 3, pp. 205–208, 1978.

[13] H. Akamatsu, J. Komura, Y. Asada, Y. Miyachi, and Y. Niwa, "Inhibitory effect of azelaic acid on neutrophil functions: a possible cause for its efficacy in treating pathogenetically unrelated diseases," *Archives of Dermatological Research*, vol. 283, no. 3, pp. 162–166, 1991.

[14] A. C. Shukla, K. P. Pandey, R. K. Mishra, A. Dikshit, and N. Shukla, "Broad spectrum antimycotic plant as a potential source of therapeutic agent," *Journal of Natural Products*, vol. 4, pp. 42–50, 2011.

[15] T. Feuerer and D. L. Hawksworth, "Biodiversity of lichens, including a world-wide analysis of checklist data based on Takhtajan's floristic regions," *Biodiversity and Conservation*, vol. 16, no. 1, pp. 85–98, 2007.

[16] E. C. Pereira, N. H. Silva, G. M. Campos-Takaki, L. Xavier-Filho, M. E. Legaz, and C. Vicente, "Antimicrobial activity of biologically-active compounds from lichen *Cladonia crispatula*," *Boletin Ecotropica*, vol. 31, pp. 09–19, 1997.

[17] E. C. Pereira, S. C. Nascimento, R. C. Lima et al., "Analysis of *Usnea fasciata* crude extracts with antineoplastic activity," *Tokai Journal of Experimental and Clinical Medicine*, vol. 19, no. 1-2, pp. 47–52, 1994.

[18] A. Dikshit, A. K. Tiwari, and R. K. Mishra, "New medium for rapid diagnosis and determination of antifungal testing against *Malassezia* spp.: a potential candidate for industries," *National Academy Science Letters*, vol. 36, no. 1, pp. 61–66, 2013.

[19] A. Dikshit, A. K. Tiwari, and R. K. Mishra, "A culture medium for the growth of *Malassezia* spp.," Filed for patent App. No. 546/DEL/2012, 2012.

[20] A. Pandey, R. Kumar, A. Pathak, R. Tandon, and A. Dikshit, "An eco-taxonomic study of some lichens of Sikkim and adjoining areas," in *Medicinal Plants: Various Perspectives*, pp. 228–253, 2012.

[21] D. D. Awasthi, "A key to the macro lichens of India and Nepal," *Hattori Botanical Laboratory*, vol. 65, pp. 207–302, 1988.

[22] CLSI, "Reference method for broth dilution antifungal susceptibility testing of yeasts, approved standard," CLSI Document M27-A3, CLSI, Wayne, Pa, USA, 2008, 3rd edition.

[23] C. Cafarchia, M. S. Latrofa, L. A. Figueredo et al., "Physiological and molecular characterization of atypical lipid-dependent *Malassezia* yeasts from a dog with skin lesions: adaptation to a new host?" *Medical Mycology*, vol. 49, no. 4, pp. 365–374, 2011.

[24] F. J. Cabañes, B. Theelen, G. Castellá, and T. Boekhout, "Two new lipid-dependent *Malassezia* species from domestic animals," *FEMS Yeast Research*, vol. 7, no. 6, pp. 1064–1076, 2007.

[25] N. Saitou and M. Nei, "The neighbor-joining method: a new method for reconstructing phylogenetic trees," *Molecular biology and evolution*, vol. 4, no. 4, pp. 406–425, 1987.

[26] J. Felsenstein, "Confidence limits on phylogenies: an approach using the bootstrap," *Evolution*, vol. 39, pp. 783–791, 1985.

[27] K. Tamura, M. Nei, and S. Kumar, "Prospects for inferring very large phylogenies by using the neighbor-joining method," *Proceedings of the National Academy of Sciences of the United States of America*, vol. 101, no. 30, pp. 11030–11035, 2004.

[28] K. Tamura, J. Dudley, M. Nei, and S. Kumar, "MEGA4: Molecular Evolutionary Genetics Analysis (MEGA) software version 4.0," *Molecular Biology and Evolution*, vol. 24, no. 8, pp. 1596–1599, 2007.

[29] H. R. Ashbee and E. G. V. Evans, "Immunology of diseases associated with *Malassezia* species," *Clinical Microbiology Reviews*, vol. 15, no. 1, pp. 21–57, 2002.

[30] C. M. Gemmer, Y. M. DeAngelis, B. Theelen, T. Boekhout, and T. L. Dawson, "Fast, noninvasive method for molecular detection and differentiation of *Malassezia* yeast species on human skin and application of the method to dandruff microbiology," *Journal of Clinical Microbiology*, vol. 40, no. 9, pp. 3350–3357, 2002.

[31] S. N. Sinha and M. Biswas, "Evaluation of antibacterial activity of some lichen from Ravangla, Sikkim, India," *International Journal of Pharma and Bio Sciences*, vol. 2, no. 4, pp. 23–28, 2011.

[32] M. C. B. Martins, M. J. G. de Lima, F. P. Silva, E. Azevedo-Ximenes, N. H. da Silva, and E. C. Pereira, "Cladia aggregata (lichen) from Brazilian northeast: chemical characterization and antimicrobial activity," *Brazilian Archives of Biology and Technology*, vol. 53, no. 1, pp. 115–122, 2010.

[33] S. K. Shahi, A. C. Shukla, D. K. Upreti, and A. Dikshit, "Use of lichens as antifungal drugs against superficial fungal infections," *Journal of Medicinal and Aromatic Plant Sciences*, vol. 22, and vol. 23, no. 1A, no. 4A, pp. 169–172, 2000.

[34] S. K. Shahi, A. C. Shukla, A. Dikshit, and D. K. Uperti, "Broad spectrum antifungal properties of the lichen *Heterodermia leucomela*," *Lichenologist*, vol. 33, no. 2, pp. 177–179, 2001.

[35] A. Dikshit, "Antifungal activity of some macrolichens," in *Proceedings of the International Conference on Global Environment and Diversification of Plants through Geological Time*, Abstract, p. 53, Allahabad, India, 1991.

[36] S. K. Shahi, M. Patra, A. Dikshit, and D. K. Upreti, "Parmelia cirrhatum: a potential source of broad spectrum natural antifungal," *Phytotherapy Research*, vol. 17, no. 4, pp. 399–400, 2003.

[37] R. Randhir, Y. Lin, and K. Shetty, "Stimulation of phenolics, antioxidant and antimicrobial activities in dark germinated mung bean sprouts in response to peptide and phytochemical elicitors," *Process Biochemistry*, vol. 39, no. 5, pp. 637–646, 2004.

[38] D. A. Vattem, Y.-T. Lin, R. G. Labbe, and K. Shetty, "Phenolic antioxidant mobilization in cranberry pomace by solid-state bioprocessing using food grade fungus *Lentinus edodes* and effect on antimicrobial activity against select food borne pathogens," *Innovative Food Science and Emerging Technologies*, vol. 5, no. 1, pp. 81–91, 2004.

[39] K. Müller, "Pharmaceutically relevant metabolites from lichens," *Applied Microbiology and Biotechnology*, vol. 56, no. 1-2, pp. 9–16, 2001.

[40] A. Dikshit, A. K. Tiwari, R. K. Mishra et al., "Botanicals for the management of dandruff," *Medicinal Plants*, vol. 4, no. 2, pp. 55–64, 2012.

10

Tramadol Pretreatment Enhances Ketamine-Induced Antidepressant Effects and Increases Mammalian Target of Rapamycin in Rat Hippocampus and Prefrontal Cortex

Chun Yang,[1] Wen-Yuan Li,[2] Hai-Yin Yu,[3] Zhi-Qin Gao,[3] Xiang-Liu Liu,[1] Zhi-Qiang Zhou,[1] and Jian-Jun Yang[1]

[1] *Department of Anesthesiology, School of Medicine, Jinling Hospital, Nanjing University, No. 305 East Zhongshan Road, Jiangsu Nanjing 210002, China*
[2] *Department of Anesthesiology, Affiliated Drum-Tower Hospital of Medical College of Nanjing University, No. 321 Zhongshan Road, Jiangsu Nanjing 210008, China*
[3] *The PLA 102nd Hospital and Mental Health Center of Military, No. 55 North Heping Road, Jiangsu Changzhou 213000, China*

Correspondence should be addressed to Jian-Jun Yang, yjyangjj@126.com

Academic Editor: Daniel T. Monaghan

Several lines of evidence have demonstrated that acute administration of ketamine elicits fast-acting antidepressant effects. Moreover, tramadol also has potential antidepressant effects. The aim of this study was to investigate the effects of pretreatment with tramadol on ketamine-induced antidepressant activity and was to determine the expression of mammalian target of rapamycin (mTOR) in rat hippocampus and prefrontal cortex. Rats were intraperitoneally administrated with ketamine at the dose of 10 mg/kg or saline 1 h before the second episode of the forced swimming test (FST). Tramadol or saline was intraperitoneally pretreated 30 min before the former administration of ketamine or saline. The locomotor activity and the immobility time of FST were both measured. After that, rats were sacrificed to determine the expression of mTOR in hippocampus and prefrontal cortex. Tramadol at the dose of 5 mg/kg administrated alone did not elicit the antidepressant effects. More importantly, pretreatment with tramadol enhanced the ketamine-induced antidepressant effects and upregulated the expression of mTOR in rat hippocampus and prefrontal cortex. Pretreatment with tramadol enhances the ketamine-induced antidepressant effects, which is associated with the increased expression of mTOR in rat hippocampus and prefrontal cortex.

1. Introduction

Mounting studies have demonstrated that ketamine, a widely used anesthetic agent, has antidepressant effects in animal models or patients [1–4]. Compared with conventional antidepressant agents, ketamine exerts fast-acting antidepressant effects within 1-2 h after administration. Moreover, ketamine also has therapeutic effects for patients with treatment-resistant depression [1, 5–9].

Mammalian target of rapamycin (mTOR) is a serine/threonine kinase that modulates the initiation of protein translation, which controls new protein synthesis as required for synaptogenesis [10]. Mounting studies have shown that mTOR plays a critical role in the process of ketamine-exerting antidepressant effects [10, 11]. A recent study has indicated that ketamine's antidepressant effects are associated with the upregulation of mTOR in prefrontal cortex [12], which is confirmed by a subsequent case report with an increase of mTOR in the peripheral blood in a depressed patient [13]. Moreover, Jernigan et al. [14] have detected decreased mTOR expression in depressed patients' brain in the postmortem study. These findings indicate that mTOR acts as a crticical role in the pathogenesis of depression.

On the other hand, tramadol is a widely used analgesic agent, which exerts therapeutic effects via activation of opioid receptors and elevating the plasma levels of serotonin and norepinephrine [15]. As we know, the most prescribed conventional antidepressant agents produce their efficacy also through increasing the monoamine levels, which share the identical mechanisms as tramadol. From this point of view, we thus suggested that tramadol also has potential to exert antidepressant effects.

However, there is no information available at present regarding the effects of pretreatment with tramadol on the ketamine-induced antidepressant activity. Therefore, this study aimed to evaluate the effects of tramadol pretreatment on ketamine-induced antidepressant activity and to determine the expression of mTOR in rat hippocampus and prefrontal cortex.

2. Materials and Methods

2.1. Animals. Eighty-six male Wistar rats weighing 180–220 g were purchased from Shanghai Animal Center, Shanghai, China. The rats were housed 5 per cage with food and water available *ad libitum* and were maintained on a 12 h light/dark cycle (lights on at 7:00 am). Animals were involved in this experiment in accordance with the Guide for Care and Use of Laboratory Animals of National Institutes of Health.

2.2. Drugs and Treatment. Ketamine was obtained from Gutian Pharmaceutical Company (Fujian, China). Tramadol was purchased from Grunenthal GmbH (Germany). One day before drug pretreatment, rats were involved in the FST for 15 min as pretest session. At the day of drug pretreatment, rats were intraperitoneally injected with tramadol at the dose of 5 mg/kg or saline, respectively. Thirty minutes later, rats were intraperitoneally injected with ketamine at the dose of 10 mg/kg or saline 1 h before the second episode of the FST, respectively. Another 30 min later, FST was conducted for 5 min as test session, and the immobility time was recorded. All the interventions were administrated in the same volume of 1 mL.

2.3. Open-Field Tests. Locomotor activity of rats was evaluated by using open-field tests, which were performed during light phase of the light-dark cycle. The open-field consisted of an arena of 100 × 100 cm square floor surrounded by 30 cm high wall. The floor of the arena was divided into 25 equal squares. Thirty minutes later after the drug or saline intervention, rats were placed in the center of the square, and the numbers of crossings and rearings were subsequently recorded [16].

2.4. Forced Swimming Test (FST). The FST included two separate exposures to a cylindrical tank with water in which rats cannot touch the bottom of the tank. The volume of the tank was 60 cm tall, 30 cm in diameter, and was filled with water in a depth of 40 cm. All the procedures were conducted between 9:00–15:00. Rats were placed in the water for 15 min without any administration. Twenty-four hours later, rats were treated as the first episode lasting 5 min, and the immobility time of rats was recorded. Rats were intraperitoneally administrated with intervents in the same volume at 30 min before the second episode of the FST. Each rat was judged to be immobile when it ceased struggling and remained floating motionless in the water, making only those movements necessary to keep its head above water. Immobility time was recorded by the same observer. Water in the tank was changed after the test of every rat.

2.5. Western Blotting. Immediately after the FST, the rats were sacrificed by decapitation, and the hippocampus and prefrontal cortex were rapidly dissected out on an ice-cold plate, frozen, and stored at −80°C until used. Samples of homogenates (15 μg of protein) were subjected to SDS-PAGE under reducing conditions. Proteins were transferred onto PDVF membranes, and the stripped blots were kept blocking solution for 1 hr and incubated with the antiphospho mTOR Ser 2448 (1 : 2000, Cell Signaling) directed against total levels of the mTOR (1 : 2000, Cell Signaling) for loading control. Densitometric analysis of immunoreactivity for each protein was conducted using Image J software.

2.6. Statistical Analysis. Statistical analysis was performed by Statistical Product for the Social Sciences (SPSS version 17.0). Data are expressed as mean ± standard deviation (SD). Comparisons were made by one-way analysis of variance (ANOVA) and post hoc comparisons were performed by the least significant difference tests. Differences were considered to be significant at $P < 0.05$.

3. Results

Different doses of tramadol were intraperitoneally injected to investigate its antidepressant effects. Rats showed a significant decrease in the immobility time during the FST after the administration of tramadol at the dose of 10 mg/kg (Figure 1, $P < 0.05$). However, tramadol at the doses of 2.5 and 5 mg/kg both did not elicit any changes of the immobility time as compared with saline-treated rats (Figure 1, $P > 0.05$).

Before the FST, open-field test was required to test whether locomotor activities were affected in the experimental rats. Compared with saline-treated rats, treatment with ketamine at the dose of 10 mg/kg did not induce any significant changes of crossings and rearings of rats in the open-field test (Figure 2(a), $P > 0.05$). Moreover, tramadol pretreatment also did not change the crossings and rearings of ketamine-treated rats as compared with saline (Figure 2(b), $P > 0.05$).

Ketamine-treated rats showed a significant decrease in immobility time during the FST as compared with saline (Figure 3, $P < 0.05$), and pretreatment with tramadol at the dose of 5 mg/kg further decreased immobility time of rats in the FST as compared with ketamine-treated alone (Figure 3, $P < 0.05$).

Compared with saline-treated rats, the administration of ketamine at the dose of 10 mg/kg significantly increased the levels of mTOR in rat hippocampus (Figure 4, $P < 0.05$), and pretreatment with tramadol at the dose of 5 mg/kg increased the levels of mTOR as compared with ketamine-treated rats (Figure 4, $P < 0.05$).

Compared with saline-treated rats, the administration of ketamine at the dose of 10 mg/kg significantly increased

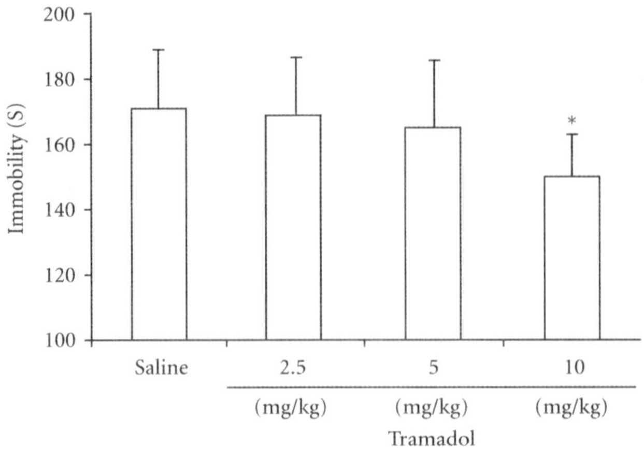

FIGURE 1: Immobility time of rats ($n = 10$) during the FST after intraperitoneal injection of tramadol at different doses. Tramadol administered at the dose of 10 mg/kg significantly decreased the immobility time as compared to saline ($^*P < 0.05$), while tramadol administered at the doses of 2.5 and 5 mg/kg both did not affect the immobility time ($P > 0.05$).

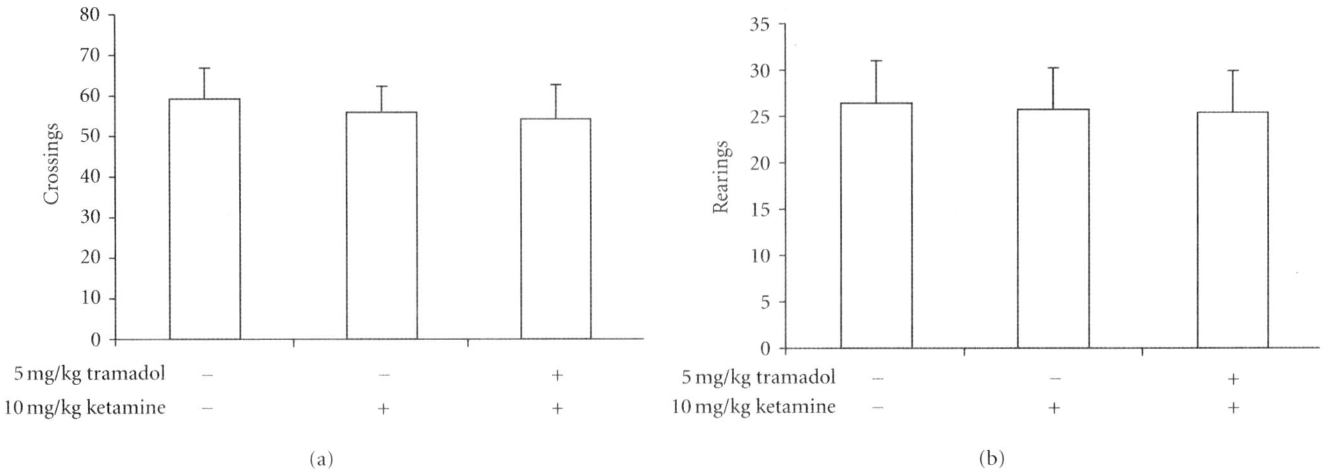

FIGURE 2: (a) The scores of crossings of rats ($n = 10$) during open-field tests. Ketamine administered at the dose of 10 mg/kg did not affect the scores of crossings, and pretreatment with 5 mg/kg tramadol did not affect any changes of scores of crossings ($P > 0.05$). (b) The scores of rearings of rats ($n = 10$) during open-field tests. Ketamine administered at the dose of 10 mg/kg did not affect the scores of rearings, and pretreatment with 5 mg/kg tramadol did not affect any changes of scores of rearings ($P > 0.05$).

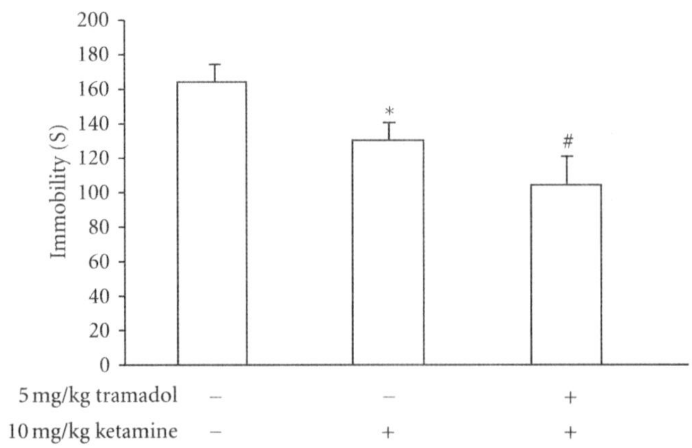

FIGURE 3: The immobility time of rats ($n = 10$) during the FST after intraperitoneal injection of ketamine and pretreatment with tramadol. Ketamine administered at the dose of 10 mg/kg significantly decreased the immobility time as compared with control ($^*P < 0.05$), and pretreatment with 5 mg/kg tramadol significantly decreased the immobility time as compared with ketamine administration ($^\#P < 0.05$).

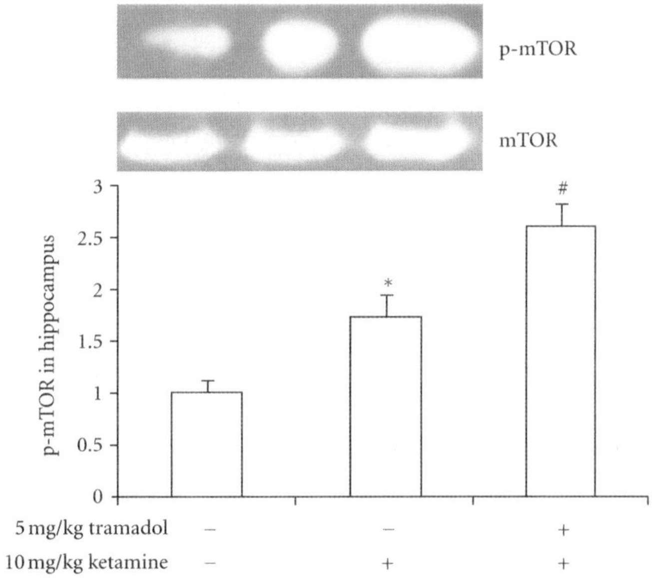

Figure 4: The expression of p-mTOR in rat hippocampus ($n = 3$). Ketamine administered at the 10 mg/kg significantly increased the expression of p-mTOR in rat hippocampus as compared with control ($^{*}P < 0.05$), and tramadol pretreated at the dose of 5 mg/kg significantly increased the expression of p-mTOR as compared with ketamine administered alone ($^{\#}P < 0.05$).

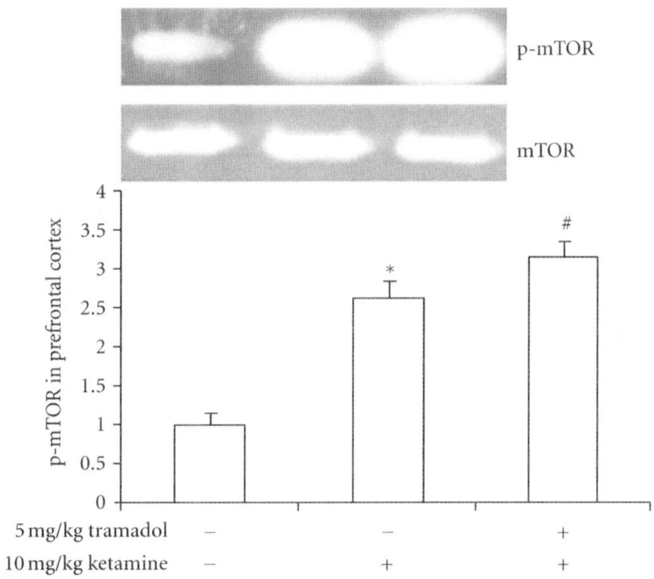

Figure 5: The expression of p-mTOR in rat prefrontal cortex ($n = 3$). Ketamine administered at the 10 mg/kg significantly increased the expression of p-mTOR in rat prefrontal cortex as compared with control ($^{*}P < 0.05$), and tramadol pretreated at the dose of 5 mg/kg significantly increased the expression of p-mTOR as compared with ketamine administered alone ($^{\#}P < 0.05$).

the levels of mTOR in rat prefrontal cortex (Figure 5, $P < 0.05$), and pretreatment with tramadol at the dose of 5 mg/kg increased the levels of mTOR in rat prefrontal cortex as compared with ketamine-treated rats (Figure 5, $P < 0.05$).

4. Discussion

The FST is a widely used behavioral test in rodents, which is sensitive and selective for clinically effective antidepressant agents [17]. In this study, the results showed that ketamine significantly decreased the immobility time of rats during the FST, suggesting that ketamine has exact antidepressant effects. More importantly, this study demonstrated that tramadol administrated alone at the dose of 10 mg/kg could elicit significant decrease in immobility time of rats during the FST, and our findings also showed that tramadol under the dose of 10 mg/kg did not induce a significant change of immobility time. Therefore, we administrated tramadol at the dose of 5 mg/kg in this study to avoid its potential antidepressant effects. Interestingly, although administration of tramadol at the dose of 5 mg/kg could not elicit any antidepressant effects, pretreatment with it could enhance ketamine-indued antidepressant effects. However, the exact mechanisms of pretreatment with tramadol-enhancing ketamine-induced antidepressant effects are unclear.

A previous study shows that ketamine suppresses the serotonin transporter and norepinephrine transporter in cultured human embryonic kidney 293 cells [18]. Moreover, Reeves and Burke [19] demonstrated that the increase of serotonin and norepinephrine neurotransmitter is the core mechanism of tramadol exerting its efficacy. Thus ketamine and tramadol may have synergistic effects to elevate the serotonin and norepinephrine levels in central nervous system, which then lead to the enhanced antidepressant effects.

Wang et al. [20] have shown that propofol, an anesthetic agent, administered alone does not elicit antidepressant effects, but may enhance ketamine-induced antidepressant effects. Réus et al. [21] have observed that the coadministration of ketamine and imipramine produces the enhanced antidepressant effects, and the authors attribute the underlying mechanisms of enhanced ketamine-induced antidepressant effects to the increased expression of glutamate-α-amino -3-hydroxy-5-methyl-4-isoxazolepropionic acid receptor-1 in rat hippocampus, cyclic adenosine monophosphate response element-binding and brain-derived neurotrophic factor protein levels, and protein kinase C and protein kinase A phosphorylation in rat brain, respectively. Interestingly, our study showed that pretreatment with tramadol-enhancing ketamine-induced antidepressant effects was associated with the increased expression of mTOR in rat hippocampus and prefrontal cortex.

As above mentioned, ketamine's antidepressant effects are mainly due to the upregulation of mTOR in rat prefrontal cortex, and the activation of mTOR can stimulate the synaptogenesis [12]. The induction of mTOR signaling occurs within 30 min after ketamine administration [10]. Collectively, these findings suggest that ketamine's antidepressant effects are associated with mTOR-dependent synaptogenesis in rat prefrontal cortex. Our findings exhibited an enhanced expression of mTOR in rat hippocampus and prefrontal cortex after pretreatment with tramadol. Until now, no data has shown that tramadol has effects on the expression of mTOR or synaptogenesis. So we supposed that tramadol has effects on stimulation of synaptogenesis via activating mTOR, which may contribute to the underlying mechanism of tramadol-enhancing ketamine-induced antidepressant effects.

In Conclusion, Ketamine exerts exactly antidepressant effects in rats during the FST, and tramadol pretreatment enhances its antidepressant effects. The relevant mechanisms are potentially ascribed to the activation of mTOR in rat hippocampus and prefrontal cortex. However, we did not evaluate whether tramadol-pretreatment-enhancing ketamine-induced antidepressant effects are related to synaptogenesis in rat hippocampus, and further studies are needed to understand the exact relevant mechanisms.

Acknowledgments

This work was supported by grants from the National Natural Science Foundation of China (Grant no. 30872424).

References

[1] N. Diazgranados, L. Ibrahim, N. E. Brutsche et al., "A randomized add-on trial of an N-methyl-D-aspartate antagonist in treatment-resistant bipolar depression," *Archives of General Psychiatry*, vol. 67, no. 8, pp. 793–802, 2010.

[2] R. Machado-Vieira, G. Salvadore, N. DiazGranados, and C. A. Zarate Jr, "Ketamine and the next generation of antidepressants with a rapid onset of action," *Pharmacology and Therapeutics*, vol. 123, no. 2, pp. 143–150, 2009.

[3] P. Skolnick, P. Popik, and R. Trullas, "Glutamate-based antidepressants: 20 years on," *Trends in Pharmacological Sciences*, vol. 30, no. 11, pp. 563–569, 2009.

[4] C. A. Zarate Jr, J. B. Singh, P. J. Carlson et al., "A randomized trial of an N-methyl-D-aspartate antagonist in treatment-resistant major depression," *Archives of General Psychiatry*, vol. 63, no. 8, pp. 856–864, 2006.

[5] M. aan het Rot, K. A. Collins, J. W. Murrough et al., "Safety and efficacy of repeated-dose intravenous ketamine for treatment-resistant depression," *Biological Psychiatry*, vol. 67, no. 2, pp. 139–145, 2010.

[6] N. DiazGranados, L. A. Ibrahim, N. E. Brutsche et al., "Rapid resolution of suicidal ideation after a single infusion of an N-methyl-D-aspartate antagonist in patients with treatment-resistant major depressive disorder," *Journal of Clinical Psychiatry*, vol. 71, no. 12, pp. 1605–1611, 2010.

[7] M. Liebrenz, A. Borgeat, R. Leisinger, and R. Stohler, "Intravenous ketamine therapy in a patient with a treatment-resistant major depression," *Swiss Medical Weekly*, vol. 137, no. 15-16, pp. 234–236, 2007.

[8] C. Zarate Jr, R. MacHado-Vieira, I. Henter, L. Ibrahim, N. Diazgranados, and G. Salvadore, "Glutamatergic modulators: the future of treating mood disorders," *Harvard Review of Psychiatry*, vol. 18, no. 5, pp. 293–303, 2010.

[9] R. B. Price, M. K. Nock, D. S. Charney, and S. J. Mathew, "Effects of intravenous ketamine on explicit and implicit measures of suicidality in Treatment-Resistant Depression," *Biological Psychiatry*, vol. 66, no. 5, pp. 522–526, 2009.

[10] R. S. Duman, N. Li, R. -J. Liu, V. Duric, and G. Aghajanian, "Signaling pathways underlying the rapid antidepressant actions of ketamine," *Neuropharmacology*, vol. 62, no. 1, pp. 35–41, 2012.

[11] K. Hashimoto, "Role of the mTOR signaling pathway in the rapid antidepressant action of ketamine," *Expert Review of Neurotherapeutics*, vol. 11, no. 1, pp. 33–36, 2011.

[12] N. Li, B. Lee, R. J. Liu et al., "mTOR-dependent synapse formation underlies the rapid antidepressant effects of NMDA antagonists," *Science*, vol. 329, no. 5994, pp. 959–964, 2010.

[13] M. C. Denk, C. Rewerts, F. Holsboer, A. Erhardt-Lehmann, and C. W. Turck, "Monitoring ketamine treatment response in a depressed patient via peripheral mammalian target of rapamycin activation," *American Journal of Psychiatry*, vol. 168, no. 7, pp. 751–752, 2011.

[14] C. S. Jernigan, D. B. Goswami, M. C. Austin et al., "The mTOR signaling pathway in the prefrontal cortex is compromised in major depressive disorder," *Progress in Neuro-Psychopharmacology and Biological Psychiatry*, vol. 35, no. 7, pp. 1774–1779, 2011.

[15] J. Barber, "Examining the Use of Tramadol Hydrochloride as an Antidepressant," *Experimental and Clinical Psychopharmacology*, vol. 19, no. 2, pp. 123–130, 2011.

[16] M. N. M. de Lima, D. C. Laranja, F. Caldana et al., "Selegiline protects against recognition memory impairment induced by neonatal iron treatment," *Experimental Neurology*, vol. 196, no. 1, pp. 177–183, 2005.

[17] M. J. Detke, J. Johnson, and I. Lucki, "Acute and chronic antidepressant drug treatment in the rat forced swimming test model of depression," *Experimental and Clinical Psychopharmacology*, vol. 5, no. 2, pp. 107–112, 1997.

[18] M. Nishimura, K. Sato, T. Okada et al., "Ketamine inhibits monoamine transporters expressed in human embryonic kidney 293 cells," *Anesthesiology*, vol. 88, no. 3, pp. 768–774, 1998.

[19] R. R. Reeves and R. S. Burke, "Tramadol: basic pharmacology and emerging concepts," *Drugs of Today*, vol. 44, no. 11, pp. 827–836, 2008.

[20] X. Wang, Y. Yang, X. Zhou et al., "Propofol pretreatment increases antidepressant-like effects induced by acute administration of ketamine in rats receiving forced swimming test," *Psychiatry Research*, vol. 185, no. 1-2, pp. 248–253, 2011.

[21] G. Z. Réus, R. B. Stringari, K. F. Ribeiro et al., "Ketamine plus imipramine treatment induces antidepressant-like behavior and increases CREB and BDNF protein levels and PKA and PKC phosphorylation in rat brain," *Behavioural Brain Research*, vol. 221, no. 1, pp. 166–171, 2011.

11

Amikacin Population Pharmacokinetics in Critically Ill Kuwaiti Patients

Kamal M. Matar,[1] Yousef Al-lanqawi,[2] Kefaya Abdul-Malek,[3] and Roger Jelliffe[4]

[1] *Department of Pharmacology & Therapeutics, Faculty of Pharmacy, Kuwait University, P.O. Box 24923, Kuwait City 13110, Kuwait*
[2] *Department of Pharmacy, Al-Amiri Hospital, Ministry of Health, P.O. Box 491, Kuwait City 32005, Kuwait*
[3] *Intensive Care Unit, Al-Amiri Hospital, Ministry of Health, P.O. Box 491, Kuwait City 32005, Kuwait*
[4] *Laboratory of Applied Pharmacokinetics, School of Medicine, University of Southern California, Los Angeles, CA 90033, USA*

Correspondence should be addressed to Kamal M. Matar; kamal@hsc.edu.kw

Academic Editor: Abdelwahab Omri

Amikacin pharmacokinetic data in Kuwaiti (Arab) intensive care unit (ICU) patients are lacking. Fairly sparse serum amikacin peak and trough concentrations data were obtained from adult Kuwaiti ICU patients. The data were analysed using a nonparametric adaptive grid (NPAG) maximum likelihood algorithm. The estimations of the developed model were assessed using mean error (ME) as a measure of bias and mean squared error (MSE) as a measure of precision. A total of 331 serum amikacin concentrations were obtained from 56 patients. The mean (±SD) model parameter values found were $V_c = 0.2302 \pm 0.0866$ L/kg, $k_{\text{slope}} = 0.004045 \pm 0.00705$ min per unit of creatinine clearance, $k_{12} = 2.2121 \pm 5.506\ \text{h}^{-1}$, and $k_{21} = 1.431 \pm 2.796\ \text{h}^{-1}$. The serum concentration data were estimated with little bias (ME = −0.88) and good precision (MSE = 13.08). The present study suggests that amikacin pharmacokinetics in adult Kuwaiti ICU patients are generally rather similar to those found in other patients. This population model would provide useful guidance in developing initial amikacin dosage regimens for such patients, especially using multiple model (MM) dosage design, followed by appropriate Bayesian adaptive control, to optimize amikacin dosage regimens for each individual patient.

1. Introduction

Amikacin is an aminoglycoside antibiotic that is most effective against Gram-negative bacteria. Its optimal dosing is highly variable and depends on the site and severity of infection, the susceptibility of the organism, and the body weight and renal function of the patient.

Like other aminoglycosides, amikacin has a very narrow therapeutic index, and the concentrations needed for optimal efficacy are close to those having a risk of toxicity. Amikacin is a concentration-dependent drug, with the rate of killing of microorganisms being proportional to the drug concentrations achieved in serum, especially peak concentrations [1]. However, abnormally high plasma or serum trough concentrations soon after commencing therapy is often associated with toxicity [1].

With multiple daily dosing of amikacin, the specific desired peak concentration for life-threatening Gram-negative sepsis usually ranges between 30 and 50 μg/mL, while the corresponding specific desired trough amikacin concentration ranges between 5 and 10 μg/mL.

Although aminoglycosides are extensively used, the accurate determination of their optimal dosage is complicated by marked intra-and interindividual variability in its pharmacokinetic behavior in patients with normal or abnormal renal function [2]. Management of intensive care unit (ICU) patients often requires general support of failing organs including specific treatment and administration of multiple drugs. All these situations may alter the pharmacokinetics of many drugs such as amikacin in critically ill patients. Large interindividual variations in the pharmacokinetics of amikacin in ICU patients have been described [3, 4]. Thus, amikacin is a drug for which therapeutic drug monitoring (TDM) has a well-established role. Individualized optimal dosage regimens should be designed and implemented as early as possible in therapy to yield maximal efficacy. It has been reported that severe sepsis modifies amikacin kinetics by increasing its apparent volume of distribution of the

TABLE 1: Demographic and biological characteristics of the patients included in the population model.

Parameter	Mean (range)
Gender (male : female)	32 : 24
Age (years)	57.4 (19–90)
Weight (kg)	72.6 (50–110)
Height (cm)	166.2 (148–182)
Serum creatinine (mg/dL)	1.50 (0.60–6.26)
Creatinine clearance (mL/min)	75.06 (7.81–177.10)
Total no. of peak concentrations collected	85
Total no. of trough concentrations collected	246

central compartment and decreasing its elimination rate, probably as a consequence of leaky capillaries and organ failure [5–7].

Population pharmacokinetic techniques are widely used to characterize the interindividual variability of pharmacokinetic parameter values among patients. The objective of the present study was to analyze a representative population of critically ill Kuwaiti patients receiving amikacin therapy using the nonparametric adaptive grid (NPAG) program, in the MM-USCPACK collection [8, 9]. This software has been incorporated into the Pmetrics software, which is now embedded in R.

2. Materials and Methods

2.1. Study Approval. All data for this study were obtained retrospectively during routine clinical care of ICU Kuwaiti patients. The study was approved by both Health Sciences Center (HSC) Ethics Committee (HSC, Kuwait University, Kuwait) and the Ministry of Health Ethics Committee (Ministry of Health, Kuwait). Informed consent was not needed since the blood samples were collected for routine care and therapeutic drug monitoring (TDM) of their amikacin therapy.

2.2. Patient Characteristics. From December 2008 to October 2010, fifty six Kuwaiti patients received amikacin therapy in the ICU of Al-Amiri Hospital in Kuwait and were included in this study. No additional blood samples were taken other than those requested for routine TDM of amikacin. The most frequent clinical conditions in these patients were septicemia (23 patients), pneumonia (6 patients), and severe trauma (27 patients). The patients' demographic data and characteristics are presented in Table 1.

2.3. Drug Administration. All patients received an initial standard Kuwaiti amikacin dosage regimen of 500 mg every 12 h. All doses were administered intravenously over 5 min, the standard practice in Kuwait. Exact dosing times were recorded.

2.4. Blood Sampling. Blood samples were withdrawn daily from the patients for determination of amikacin in serum. The trough level was taken within 30 min before a dose was administered, whereas the peak level was taken 1 h after the 5 min i.v. infusion was started. Exact blood sampling times were recorded. Blood samples were immediately centrifuged, and serum samples were collected and stored at −80°C pending analysis.

2.5. Drug Analysis. Serum amikacin samples as well as serum creatinine were measured by Kobas Integra 400 (Roche Diagnostics, Basel, Switzerland). Calibration standards of amikacin in serum were at concentrations of 0, 2.5, 5, 10, 20, and 40 μg/mL. Quality control samples at concentrations of 5.31, 14.8, and 26.9 μg/mL were assayed each time patient samples were assayed. The tests were performed according to the manufacturer's protocol [11]. The intra-run and interrun coefficients of variation for amikacin assay were less than 5% and 10%, respectively.

2.6. Assay Error. The standard deviation (SD) of the assay over its working range was determined using 5 replicates of each serum amikacin concentrations of 0, 2.5, 5, 10, 20, and 40 μg/mL. The relationship between serum amikacin concentrations and the assay SD was described by a polynomial equation using the MM-USCPACK software as follows:

$$\mathrm{SD} = A_0 C^0 + A_1 C^1 + A_2 C^2, \tag{1}$$

where A_0, A_1, A_2, are various coefficients and C^0, C^1, C^2 are the concentrations raised to the zero power, first power, and the second power, respectively. The coefficients of this polynomial equation were used to give proper weighting of each measured concentration by the reciprocal of the assay variance (SD^2) at each measured concentration, in performing the population analysis using the NPAG software.

2.7. Data Analysis. In the present study, the NPAG method of population pharmacokinetic analysis was selected for performing the population pharmacokinetic modeling for the following specific reasons. In contrast to parametric approaches such as NONMEM, for example, there is no need to make any constraining assumptions about the shape of the model parameter distributions such as normal and log normal. In addition, nonparametric (NP) models permit multiple model (MM) dosage design, which is always maximally precise [12], while dosage regimens developed using only single-point parameter values such as means or medians from parametric population modeling methods cannot do this, as they do not use the entire model parameter distributions and therefore cannot evaluate and maximize the expected precision with which the dosage regimen hits a clinically selected target goal. Moreover, NPAG software calculates the likelihood function exactly and thus possesses statistical consistency in contrast to parametric approaches, many of which (but certainly not all) use only approximate methods; first order (FO), first-order conditional estimation (FOCE), for example, to calculate the likelihood. They, therefore, do not have statistical consistency. This most desirable property of statistical consistency means that the more subjects one studies in the population, the closer the estimated parameter distributions approach the true ones. This means that the more subjects studied, the closer the predicted parameter value approaches the true value [9, 12].

Individual patient data including serum amikacin concentrations, age, weight, height, gender, serum creatinine, and dosage history were entered in the MM-USCPACK PC program. The software used the entire dosing history, amikacin peak and trough levels, and the estimated creatinine clearances [8]. The model pharmacokinetic parameter distributions for the population were computed by the NPAG nonparametric maximum likelihood method [9]. The model used was a two-compartment open model with elimination from the central compartment. The fitted parameters were the apparent volume of distribution of the central compartment (V_c, L/kg), the transfer rate constants (k_{12} and k_{21}) from the central to peripheral and from the peripheral back to central compartments, respectively, (in h^{-1}), k_{slope}, the renal component of K_{el}, the elimination rate constant, (in h^{-1} per unit of creatinine clearance), where

$$K_{el} = k_{nr} + k_{slope} * CL_{cr}. \quad (2)$$

In this analysis, the nonrenal elimination rate constant (k_{nr}) was fixed to zero, assuming no nonrenal elimination of amikacin. Creatinine clearance was estimated from serum creatinine concentrations using the MM-USCPACK software [8].

The population analysis began with a uniform prior distribution spread over 40009 grid points of equal probability between stated initial ranges for each parameter. It then proceeded iteratively to maximize the likelihood of the entire model parameter distributions given the observed serum amikacin concentrations. The program stopped when 2 successive estimations of the log likelihood differed by less than 0.001%. This was the criterion that the likelihood function had reached a maximum. The program also estimated mean, median, and standard deviations of each pharmacokinetic parameter, as well as the covariance matrix of the model parameters.

In addition, the nonparametric Bayesian posterior joint density was computed for each individual patient. In the nonparametric approach, this is done by computing the Bayesian posterior probability of each population model support point given the individual patient data. In this way, each patient's Bayesian posterior joint probability density is determined.

2.8. Evaluation of the Parameter Estimates. The performance of the parameter estimates was evaluated by comparing the estimated serum amikacin concentrations with the patient's measured data. The bias (weighted mean error, ME) and precision (bias-corrected weighted mean squared error, MSE) were assessed according to Sheiner and Beal [13]. The bias and precision were evaluated separately for peak and trough serum amikacin concentrations.

3. Results

A total of 331 serum amikacin samples comprising 85 peak levels and 246 trough levels were analyzed (Table 1).

TABLE 2: Population pharmacokinetic parameters of amikacin in 56 ICU patients.

Parameter	Mean	Median	S.D.	C.V., %
k_s (h^{-1} per unit of CLcr)	0.004045	0.002576	0.007054	174.389
k_{12} (h^{-1})	2.21207	0.584539	5.5061	248.912
k_{21} (h^{-1})	1.43121	0.23237	2.7957	195.338
V_c (L/kg)	0.23012	0.218929	0.08658	37.6236

The mean peak concentration was 22.32 μg/mL (95% CI; 19.7–24.9 μg/mL) and the mean trough concentration was 4.26 μg/mL (95% CI; 3.88–4.64 μg/mL). With the conventional amikacin dosage regimen, it was found that only 14% of the peak levels were within the therapeutic range of 30 to 50 μg/mL, and only 24% of the trough levels were within the therapeutic range of 5 to 10 μg/mL. This strongly suggests the advantage of population modeling and dosage individualization using tools such as NPAG and the MM-USCPACK software to maximize the precision of achievement of target serum amikacin concentrations.

3.1. Assay Error. The polynomial equation describing amikacin assay standard deviation (SD) was found to be

$$SD = 0.2451 + 0.0950 * C. \quad (3)$$

The C^2 term was set to zero.

The coefficients of this equation were then entered into the MM-USCPACK software and used for weighting the data as described earlier, using the NPAG software.

3.2. Population Model Results. Using the NPAG software, convergence was reached on cycle 669. The final log likelihood was −777.4437, and the number of active grid points decreased from an initial value of 40009 down to 27. The parameter values were essentially stable before the convergence criterion was reached. The marginal density plots of the pharmacokinetic parameters k_{slope} and V_c are displayed in Figures 1(a) and 1(b). The pharmacokinetic parameter summaries estimated from the final population model are presented in Table 2. As shown in Figures 1(a) and 1(b), there may be two possible subpopulations of adult and elderly patients or subpopulations of patients with renally impaired and normal function. As shown in Figure 1(a), for instance, two subpopulations appear to be present, a principal one with k_s values ranging from almost zero to 0.005 h^{-1} per unit of creatinine clearance and another small one with values ranging from about 0.033 to 0.039 h^{-1} per unit of creatinine clearance. Moreover, it is possible that two subpopulations may also be present in the volume of distribution of the central compartment (V_c). In this regard, the first subpopulation is centered at about 0.2 L/kg and another one centered at about 0.36 L/kg, a value seen somewhat more often in Caucasian ICU patients (Figure 1(b)).

The performance of the NPAG population and individualized Bayesian estimates are shown in the plots of the observed versus estimated serum amikacin concentrations (Figures 2 and 3). The scatter plots of estimated versus

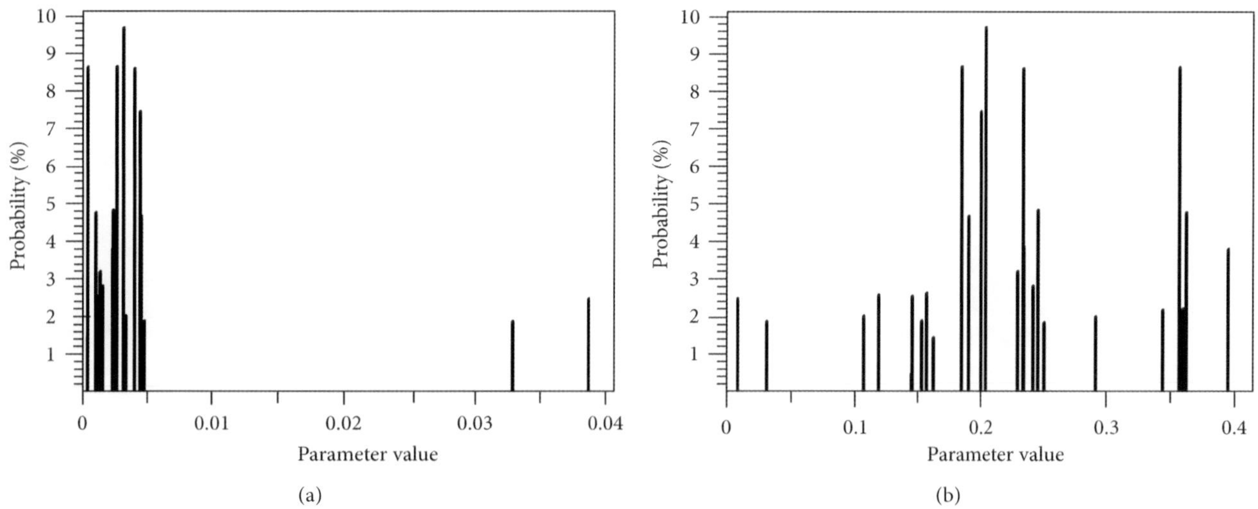

FIGURE 1: Marginal density plot of the parameters k_s (h^{-1} per unit of creatinine clearance); renal component of elimination rate constant (a) and V_c (L/kg); apparent volume of distribution of the central compartment (b) generated by NPAG program for adult ICU patients ($n = 56$) who received amikacin.

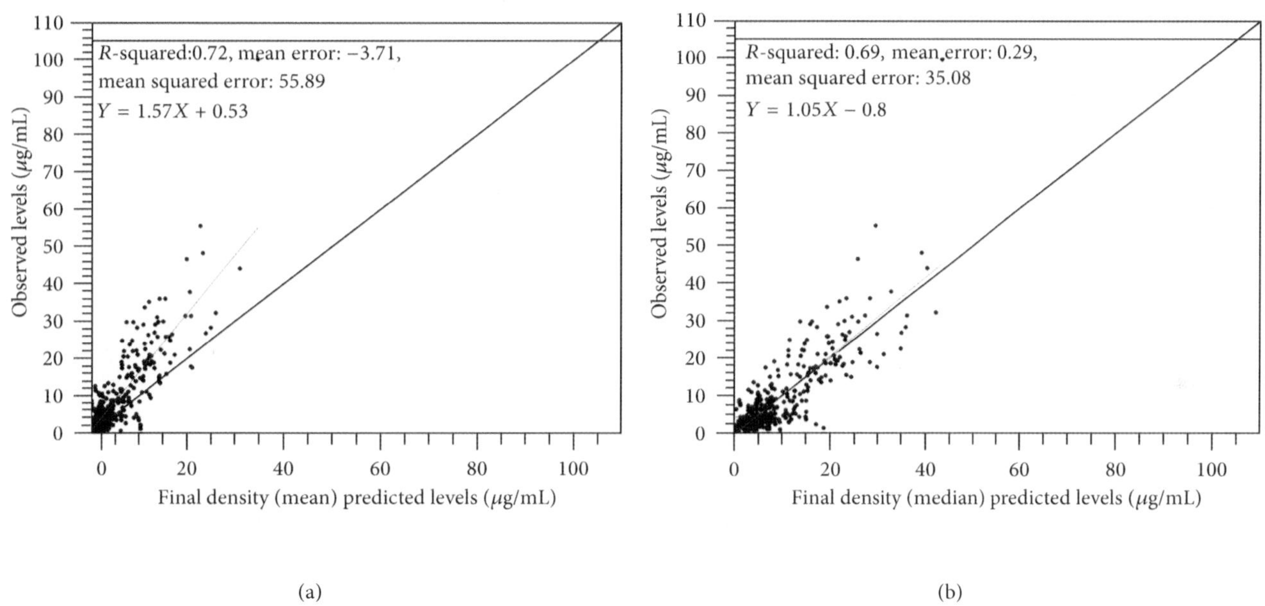

FIGURE 2: Scatter plot of predicted (x-axis) versus measured (y-axis) serum amikacin concentrations (μg/mL) based on means (a) and medians (b) of population parameter distributions. Pooled data from all patients ($n = 56$).

observed serum amikacin concentrations using the mean (Figure 2(a)) and median (Figure 2(b)) population model parameter values have been demonstrated. The relationship between the mean predicted and measured serum amikacin concentrations was found to be the following: measured conc = 1.57 ∗ predicted conc + 0.53; $r^2 = 0.72$; ME = −3.71; MSE = 55.89 (Figure 2(a)), whereas the relationship between the median predicted and measured serum amikacin concentrations was found to be the following: measured conc = 1.05 ∗ predicted conc − 0.8; $r^2 = 0.69$; ME = 0.29, MSE = 35.08 (Figure 2(b)). Similarly, the scatter plots based on the means (Figure 3(a)) and medians (Figure 3(b)) of each individual patient's Bayesian posterior parameter distributions have been presented. In this regard, the relationship between the mean predicted and measured serum amikacin concentrations was found to be the following: measured conc = 1.00 ∗ predicted conc + 0.89; $r^2 = 0.89$; ME = −0.88; MSE = 13.08 (Figure 3(a)), whereas the relationship between the median predicted and measured serum amikacin concentrations was found to be the following: measured conc = 0.93 ∗ predicted conc + 0.3; $r^2 = 0.85$; ME = 0.34; MSE = 17.30 (Figure 3(b)). The estimates based on the individual

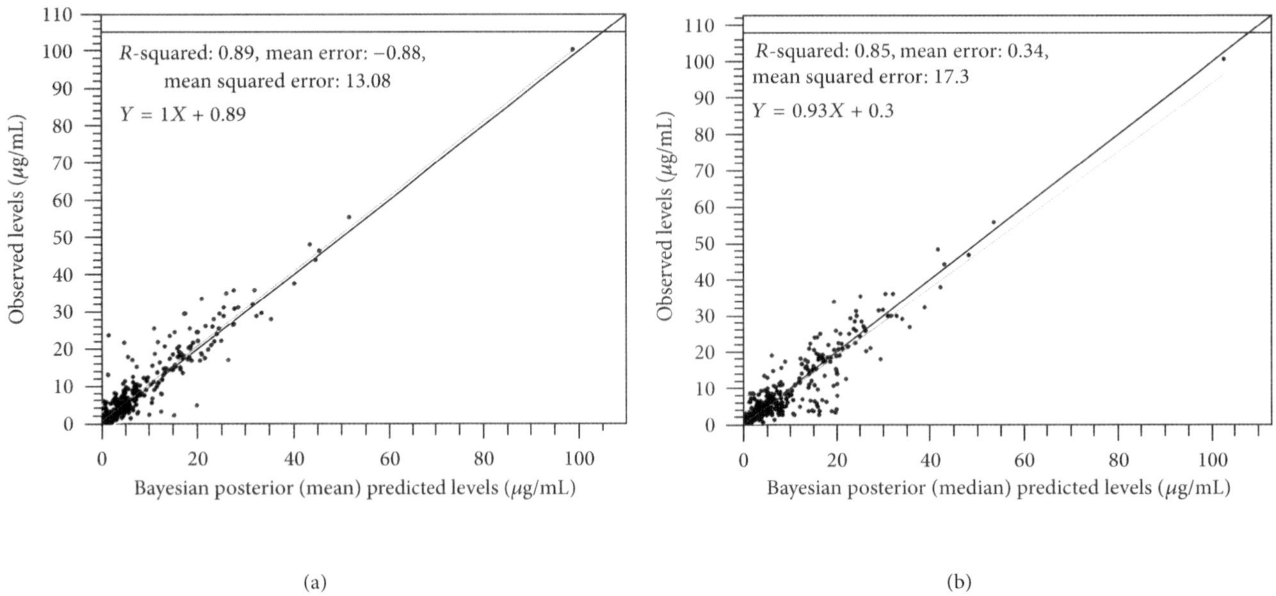

FIGURE 3: Scatter plot of predicted (x-axis) versus measured (y-axis) serum amikacin concentrations (μg/mL) based on means (a) and medians (b) of each individual patient's Bayesian posterior parameter distributions. Pooled data from all patients ($n = 56$).

TABLE 3: Assessment of absolute predictive performance of NPAG in amikacin population model. Figures in parenthesis are 95% confidence intervals.

Level	N	ME	MSE
T	246	0.24 (−0.03–0.51)	4.67 (2.93–6.42)
P	85	2.10 (1.18–3.01)	22.16 (13.46–30.87)

N: sample size; ME: weighted mean error; MSE: bias-corrected weighted mean squared error; T: trough; P: peak.

patient's Bayesian posterior parameter distributions were much better than those based on the population distributions. This illustrates the utility of Bayesian individualization of each patient's model based on his/her individual data using TDM.

Separating peaks from troughs, the mean (±SD) observed and predicted (based on individual patient's mean Bayesian posterior parameter values) serum amikacin trough concentrations were 4.38 ± 3.26 μg/mL and 4.14 ± 3.16 μg/mL, respectively; whereas those for the peak concentrations were 23.36 ± 12.32 μg/mL and 21.27 ± 12.42 μg/mL, respectively. The mean error (ME) was lowest for amikacin trough levels and highest for peak levels (based on individual patient's mean Bayesian posterior parameter values), just as the assay error was less for the troughs and more for the peaks as described by the assay SD polynomial. The precision, mean squared error (MSE), of the mean serum amikacin concentration predictions (based on individual patient's mean Bayesian posterior parameter values) ranged from 4.67 μg/mL (95% CI; 2.93–6.42) for trough levels to 22.16 μg/mL (95% CI; 13.46–30.87) for peak levels, Table 3.

Bland-Altman plots of the mean serum amikacin trough and peak concentrations (based on individual patient's mean Bayesian posterior parameter values) are displayed in Figures 4(a) and 4(b), respectively, and are consistent with the relationship between the more precisely measured troughs and the less precisely measured peaks. As shown, 94% of trough residual levels and 93% of peak residual levels were in the range of the mean (±2SD) overall difference between estimated and measured serum concentrations.

A three-dimensional plot of V_c versus k_s using NPAG software demonstrated the potential presence of two clusters of subpopulations (Figure 5). Moreover, a correlation exists between V_c and k_s ($r^2 = 0.44$).

4. Discussion

Amikacin pharmacokinetic parameter distributions have substantial interindividual variation among the patients treated with the drug. This interindividual variability is especially great in ICU patients [14], presumably owing to various physiological changes in ICU patients. The findings of the present study demonstrate that the V_c is not significantly increased in ICU patients, as its mean value of 0.23 L/kg (Table 2) is similar to that of normal patients and in agreement with previous studies [15]. However, except for our subgroup with the higher V_c, our results contrast with those of other investigators who reported increased values of V_d in ICU patients [16–18]. Nevertheless, the narrow therapeutic range and great interindividual variability of amikacin in all patients emphasize the need for therapeutic drug monitoring of its peak and trough levels for optimized dosing as well as optimal efficacy and prevention of serious side effects.

In this analysis, however, several possible subpopulations of patients were found, though there was no other information to identify why this should be so. The ability to detect such unsuspected subpopulations is a distinct strength of the nonparametric approach and is one of the

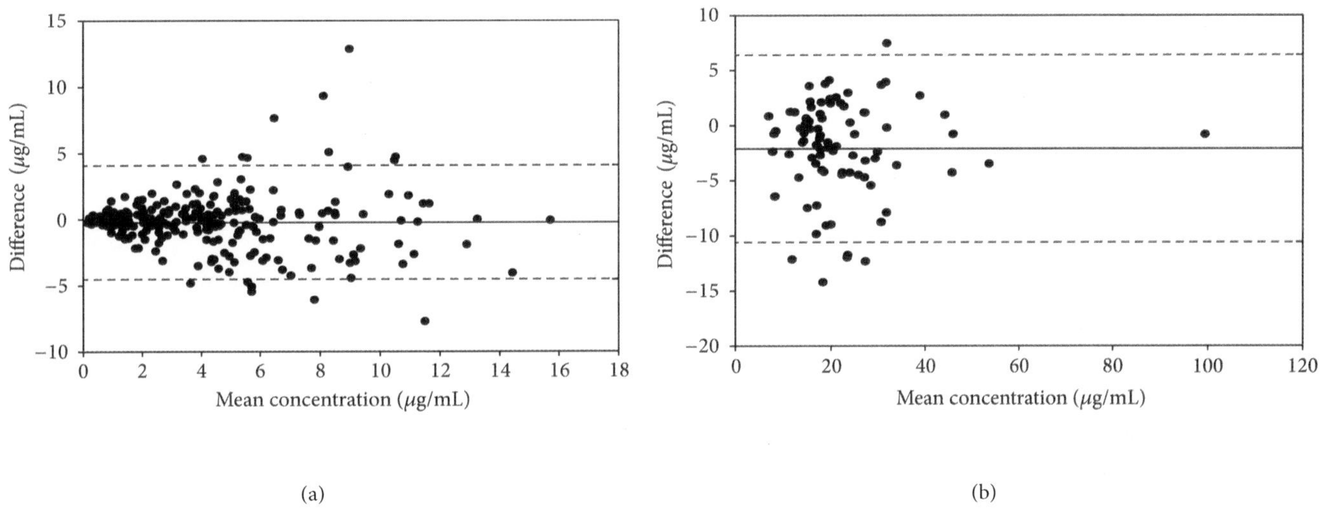

FIGURE 4: Bland-Altman plot of the mean serum amikacin (x-axis) trough concentrations (a) and peak concentrations (b) versus difference (y-axis) between predicted and observed amikacin concentrations. The solid line represents the mean difference; the dashed lines represent the limits of agreement (mean difference ±2 SD difference).

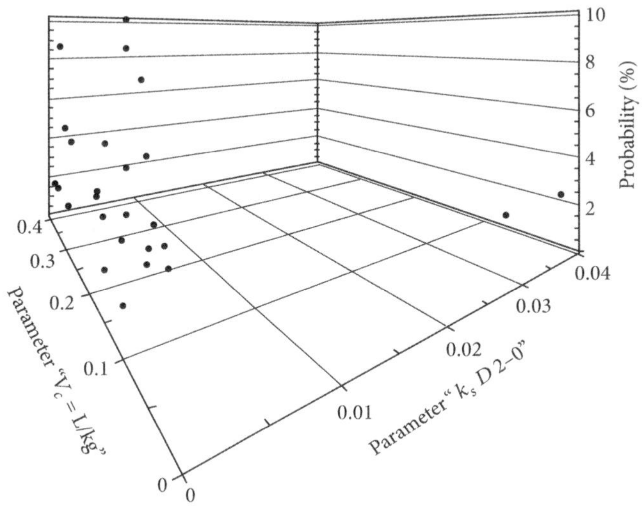

FIGURE 5: Three-dimensional plot of apparent volume of distribution of the central compartment (V_c; L/kg) versus renal component of elimination rate constant (k_s; h^{-1} per unit of creatinine clearance) for Kuwaiti ICU patients (n = 56) using NPAG program.

reasons why this method of analysis was selected for use here. These subpopulations might well have been missed by population analyses using parametric approaches, which only compute means and covariances of the assumed distributions of the model parameter values [9]. The Bayesian posterior parameter values would have had to be analyzed, and the population analysis would then have to be specifically set up to detect such anticipated multimodal distributions. In addition, the problem of subpopulations within a larger population is most important from the point of view of developing maximally precise dosage regimens for patients. When a patient belongs to a larger population in which the parameter distributions are not Gaussian, as found here, the use of parametric models based on only single-point parameter estimates has no way to evaluate and optimize the expected precision with which a dosage regimen will hit a target. This is a distinct limitation of what is known as separation principle control [19]. This principle states that whenever one seeks to control a system, first by getting single-point estimates of the model parameter values (rather than estimating the entire parameter distributions) and then using these single point estimates to control the system, the control is done suboptimally. This is because there is no method of estimating the degree of failure of the regimen to hit the target. It is simply assumed that the regimen is designed to hit the target exactly, and everyone of course knows that this will not be the case. In contrast, nonparametric population models, having multiple discrete support points which describe the entire model parameter distributions without having to make any assumptions about their shape, can easily compute the expected weighted squared error with which any dosage regimen fails to hit a desired target and can then find the regimen which specifically minimizes that error. This is Multiple Model (MM) dosage design [9, 12] and it is well known in the aerospace community for flight control and spacecraft guidance applications.

In the present RightDose clinical software, MM dosage design proceeds as follows: just as the process of weighted nonlinear least squares begins with an initial set of parameter estimates, so does MM dosage design begin with an initial estimate of the dosage regimen to be developed. This candidate regimen is given to each population model support point. Each point, having its own set of model parameter values, predicts future serum concentrations resulting from that regimen, with the probability estimated for each point in either the original population model or the Bayesian posterior joint density of an individual patient. At the time the desired target is to be achieved, one can compare each

Table 4: Comparative mean population amikacin pharmacokinetic parameters for Kuwaitis (Arabs) and other ethnic groups.

Parameter	Hispanic*	Asian*	Caucasians*	Arabs**
k_s (h^{-1} per unit of CLcr)	0.00404	0.00424	0.00394	0.00405
V_c (L/kg)	0.248	0.264	0.26	0.23

*Jhee et al., 1994 [10].
**Present study.

prediction, weighted by its own probability with the target goal, and the weighted squared error of the failure of that candidate regimen to hit the target is calculated. Then, just as in least squares, the dosage regimen is iteratively optimized until the regimen hitting the target with the minimum expected weighted squared error is found. This is MM dosage design. The combination of nonparametric population modeling and MM dosage design lends great strength to these applications. It can be seen that in addition to covariates, the MM dose regimen itself becomes a most important tool to minimize the variability of patient response when hitting a desired target goal. MM dosage design is unique to nonparametric models having their multiple support points. Such maximal precision can never be computed, and this process can never be done if only parametric models are used. In general, amikacin pharmacokinetic behavior in Kuwaiti ICU patients compares reasonably well with previously reported findings [10]. Table 4 presents the comparative mean population amikacin pharmacokinetic parameters of Kuwaiti patients in contrast to other ethnic groups including Hispanic, Asian, and Caucasian subjects. The results suggest that the Kuwaiti population is a part of a larger population comprising Hispanic, Asian, and Caucasian subjects.

In conclusion, a population pharmacokinetic model for amikacin was developed from 56 adult Kuwaiti ICU patients using the NPAG program. The present study demonstrates lack of significant differences in amikacin pharmacokinetic behavior in Kuwaiti patients in comparison with Asian, Hispanic, or Caucasian patients. The present study suggests that amikacin pharmacokinetics in adult Kuwaiti ICU patients are generally rather similar to those found in other patients. The distributions of the present population pharmacokinetic parameters can be utilized as population priors for developing initial amikacin dosage regimens in Kuwaiti patients, using the MM-USCPACK Rightdose PC software (http://www.lapk.org/). The findings of the present study will help clinicians to establish optimized amikacin dosing regimens for each individual Kuwaiti ICU patient, using MM Bayesian adaptive control. Further study is warranted to evaluate the clinical utility of these findings in Kuwaiti ICU patients.

Conflict of Interests

The authors declare that they have no conflicts of interests in this work.

Acknowledgments

The authors acknowledge Kuwait University Research Sector for funding the present research project (Grant no. PT02/07). The NPAG software was supported by NIH Grants (GM068968 and EB005803).

References

[1] C. Kummana and K. Yuen, "Parenteral aminoglycoside therapy. Selection, administrationandmonitoring," *Drugs*, vol. 47, pp. 902–913, 1994.

[2] S. M. Erdman, K. A. Rodvold, and R. D. Pryka, "An updated comparison of drug dosing methods. Part III: aminoglycoside antibiotics," *Clinical Pharmacokinetics*, vol. 20, no. 5, pp. 374–388, 1991.

[3] M. J. Beckhouse, I. M. Whyte, P. L. Byth, J. C. Napier, and A. J. Smith, "Altered aminoglycoside pharmacokinetics in the critically ill," *Anaesthesia and Intensive Care*, vol. 16, no. 4, pp. 418–422, 1988.

[4] M. D. M. F. De Gatta, S. R. Moreno, M. V. Calvo, R. Ardanuy, A. Domínguez-Gil, and J. M. Lanao, "Evaluation of population pharmacokinetic models for amikacin dosage individualization in critically ill patients," *Journal of Pharmacy and Pharmacology*, vol. 61, no. 6, pp. 759–766, 2009.

[5] J. A. Roberts and J. Lipman, "Antibacterial dosing in intensive care: pharmacokinetics, degree of disease and pharmacodynamics of sepsis," *Clinical Pharmacokinetics*, vol. 45, no. 8, pp. 756–773, 2006.

[6] F. Pea, P. Viale, and M. Furlanut, "Antimicrobial therapy in critically ill patients: a review of pathophysiological conditions responsible for altered disposition and pharmacokinetic variability," *Clinical Pharmacokinetics*, vol. 44, no. 10, pp. 1009–1034, 2005.

[7] R. Mehrotra, R. De Gaudio, and M. Palazzo, "Antibiotic pharmacokinetic and pharmacodynamic considerations in critical illness," *Intensive Care Medicine*, vol. 30, no. 12, pp. 2145–2156, 2004.

[8] R. Jelliffe, "Estimation of creatinine clearance in patients with unstable renal function, withoutaurinespecimen," *American Journal of Nephrology*, vol. 22, pp. 320–324, 2002.

[9] A. Bustad, D. Terziivanov, R. Leary, R. Port, A. Schumitzky, and R. Jelliffe, "Parametric and nonparametric population methods: their comparative performance in analysing a clinical dataset and two Monte Carlo simulation studies," *Clinical Pharmacokinetics*, vol. 45, no. 4, pp. 365–383, 2006.

[10] S. S. Jhee, J. P. Burm, and M. A. Gill, "Comparison of aminoglycoside pharmacokinetics in Asian, Hispanic, and Caucasian patients by using population pharmacokinetic methods," *Antimicrobial Agents and Chemotherapy*, vol. 38, no. 9, pp. 2073–2077, 1994.

[11] I. Domke, P. Cremer, and M. Huchtemann, "Therapeutic drug monitoring on COBAS INTEGRA 400—evaluation results," *Clinical Laboratory*, vol. 46, no. 9-10, pp. 509–515, 2000.

[12] R. W. Jelliffe, A. Schumitzky, D. Bayard et al., "Model-based, goal-oriented, individualised drug therapy. Linkage of population modelling, new "Multiple Model" dosage design, Bayesian feedback and individualised target goals," *Clinical Pharmacokinetics*, vol. 34, no. 1, pp. 57–77, 1998.

[13] L. B. Sheiner and S. L. Beal, "Some suggestions for measuring predictive performance," *Journal of Pharmacokinetics and Biopharmaceutics*, vol. 9, no. 4, pp. 503–512, 1981.

[14] D. E. Zaske, R. G. Strate, and P. R. Kohls, "Amikacin pharmacokinetics: wide interpatient variation in 98 patients," *Journal of Clinical Pharmacology*, vol. 31, no. 2, pp. 158–163, 1991.

[15] T. Gauthier, B. Lacarelle, F. Marre, P. H. Villard, J. Catalin, and A. Durand, "Predictive performance of two software packages (USC*PACK PC and Abbott PKS system) for the individualization of amikacin dosage in intensive care unit patients," *International Journal of Bio-Medical Computing*, vol. 36, no. 1-2, pp. 131–134, 1994.

[16] G. Lugo and G. Castañeda-Hernândez, "Amikacin Bayesian forecasting in critically ill patients with sepsis and cirrhosis," *Ther Drug Monit*, vol. 19, pp. 271–276, 1997.

[17] J. Debord, C. Pessis, J. C. Voultoury et al., "Population pharmacokinetics of amikacin in intensive care unit patients studied by NPEM algorithm," *Fundamental and Clinical Pharmacology*, vol. 9, no. 1, pp. 57–61, 1995.

[18] J. Debord, J. Voultoury, G. Lachâtre, C. Gay, J. Favereau, and R. Gay, "Population pharmacokinetic paramters for Bayesian monitoring of amikacintherapy in intensive care unit patients," *European Journal of Clinical Pharmacology*, vol. 43, pp. 435–436, 1992.

[19] D. Bertsekas, *Dynamic Programming: Deterministic and Stochastic Models*, Prentice-Hall, Englewood Cliffs, NJ, USA, 1987.

12

Plasma and Ocular Prednisolone Disposition after Oral Treatment in Cats

María J. Del Sole,[1,2] Paula Schaiquevich,[3] Marcelo A. Aba,[4] Carlos E. Lanusse,[2] and Laura Moreno[2]

[1] *Hospital de Pequeños Animales, CIVETAN-CONICET, Facultad de Ciencias Veterinarias (UNCPBA), Campus Universitario, Paraje Arroyo Seco s/n, 7000 Tandil, Buenos Aires, Argentina*
[2] *Laboratorio de Farmacología, CIVETAN-CONICET, Facultad de Ciencias Veterinarias (UNCPBA), 7000 Tandil, Argentina*
[3] *Unidad de Farmacocinética Clínica, CONICET, Hospital de Pediatría JP Garrahan, 1245 Buenos Aires, Argentina*
[4] *Laboratorio de Endocrinología, CIVETAN-CONICET, Facultad de Ciencias Veterinarias (UNCPBA), 7000 Tandil, Argentina*

Correspondence should be addressed to María J. Del Sole; mjdelsole@gmail.com

Academic Editor: Robert J. Lee

Objective. To evaluate the plasma and aqueous humor disposition of prednisolone after oral administration in cats. *Methods.* Six cats were administered with a single oral dose of prednisolone (10 mg). Blood and aqueous humor samples were serially collected after drug administration. Prednisolone concentrations in plasma and aqueous humor were measured at 0.25, 0.5, 1.0, 1.5, 2.0, 3.0, 4.0, and 5.0 h after administration by a high-performance liquid chromatographic analytical method developed and validated for this purpose. *Results.* Mean ± standard error (SE) of maximum plasma prednisolone concentration (300.8 ± 67.3 ng/mL) was reached at 1 h after administration. Prednisolone was distributed to the aqueous humor reaching a mean peak concentration of 100.9 ± 25.5 ng/mL at 1.25 h after administration. The mean ± SE systemic and aqueous humor exposure (AUC) was 553.3 ± 120.0 ng∗h/mL and 378.8 ± 64.9 ng∗h/mL, respectively. A high $AUC_{\text{aqueous humor}}/AUC_{\text{plasma}}$ ratio was observed (0.68 ± 0.13). The mean half-life time of elimination in plasma and aqueous humor was 0.87 ± 0.16 h and 2.25 ± 0.44 h, respectively. *Clinical Significance.* The observed high ratio between aqueous humor and plasma prednisolone concentrations indicates that extensive penetration of prednisolone to the anterior segment of the eye may occur. This is the first step that contributes to the optimization of the pharmacological therapeutics for the clinical treatment of uveitis.

1. Introduction

Uveitis is a frequent ophthalmic disorder in domestic cats commonly associated with perforating or blunt traumas, systemic diseases, neoplasia, intraocular surgery, and lens-induced uveitis [1]. Currently, the treatment of feline uveitis of any etiology is based on topical and/or systemic corticosteroid or anti-inflammatory nonsteroidal agents [1, 2]. Despite the fact that the use of potent anti-inflammatory drugs carries the risk of side effects, corticosteroids remain the mainstay of the prevention and treatment of many painful and potentially blinding ocular diseases in different species [3]. Prednisolone is a synthetic adrenocortical steroid used primarily due to its anti-inflammatory activity in several diseases [4]. In addition, due to the potential antiangiogenic, antiedematous, antiapoptotic, and antiproliferative effects of prednisolone, this steroid gained wide use in the treatment of both anterior and posterior ocular segment diseases [5].

Although topical administration of prednisolone is widely used in the treatment of anterior uveitis, oral administration is also used in traumatic, after intraocular surgery, and neoplastic uveitis [1]. However, there is limited information about ocular prednisolone disposition after its oral administration in small species including the cat.

Previous studies on plasma pharmacokinetics of prednisolone have been performed in humans, rats, rabbits, cows, sheep, horses, dogs, and cats [6–13], but there are no reports about ocular disposition of the corticoid after oral administration in any of those species. In order to characterize the pharmacokinetics of prednisolone in different biological matrices, an analytical technique needs to be developed to obtain precise and accurate results. Different techniques were previously reported in the literature to estimate steroids concentrations in biological samples [14–20]. However, the methodologies to measure prednisolone in aqueous humor are limited, and there are no previous reports about a specific high-performance liquid chromatographic (HPLC) analytical method to quantify prednisolone in plasma and/or aqueous humor of cats.

Thus, the main goal of the current work was to evaluate the systemic kinetic behaviour of prednisolone and its distribution to aqueous humor after oral administration to cats. The work included the development and validation of an analytical HPLC methodology to quantify prednisolone in cat plasma and aqueous humor.

2. Materials and Methods

2.1. Animals. Six intact young European short-hair male cats with an average ± standard deviation (SD) weight of 4.2 ± 0.5 kg, obtained from the research colony of Facultad de Ciencias Veterinarias (UNCPBA), were used in the present study. Animals were housed individually in a temperature- and light-controlled environment (fluorescent lights were automatically turned on and off every 12 h) and fed with a balanced diet and water *ad libitum*. They were acclimated to human contact for 4 to 6 weeks prior to the study. Previous to their inclusion in the study it was assured that the animals were in healthy physical and ocular condition, throughout physical and ocular examination. Ocular examination included Schirmer tear test measurements (Schirmer tear test strips, Schering-Plough Animal Health Corp., Union, New Jersey, USA), fluorescein staining (Love Sudamericana Laboratory, Argentina), applanation tonometry (Tono-Pen XL, Mentor, Norwell, MA, USA), slit lamp biomicroscopy (HLS 150, Heine Optotechnik, Herrsching, Germany), direct (Heine Beta 200, Heine Optotechnik, Herrsching, Germany) and indirect (20-D lens, Ocular Instruments, Bellevue, Wash; Heine Omega 150, Heine Optotechnik, Herrsching, Germany) ophthalmoscopies. During the sampling period and the following 24 h, the animals were evaluated for aqueous flare and others signs of uveitis by slit lamp biomicroscopy. The cats did not receive any medications containing prednisone or prednisolone prior to the study (including topical preparations). All animal procedures were conducted in strict accordance with the Association for Research in Vision and Ophthalmology Statement for the Use of Animals in Ophthalmic and Vision Research and Animal Welfare Policy (Act 087/02, Facultad de Ciencias Veterinarias, UNCPBA, http://www.vet.unicen.edu.ar).

2.2. Experimental Administration and Sample Collection. Immediately after oral administration of 10 mg of prednisolone (Prednisolona Syntex, Syntex S.A., Argentina), cats were anesthetized using I.M. ketamine (7 mg/kg)-xylazine (1 mg/kg) and maintained with I.V. ketamine (3.5 mg/kg)-xylazine (0.1 mg/kg) administered 5 minutes previous to each sample extraction. Blood samples (2 mL) were taken through preplaced cephalic antebrachial intravenous catheters before and at 0.25, 0.5, 1.0, 1.5, 2.0, 3.0, 4.0, and 5.0 h after prednisolone administration. Blood samples were centrifuged at 2000 ×g for 15 min, and the separated plasma was transferred to plastic tubes. Aqueous humor samples were obtained alternating between each eye by paracentesis of the anterior chamber at the same blood sampling times. Aqueous humor samples (450 μL) were collected slowly using a disposable 1 mL syringe with a 25 gauge needle, with the minimal vacuum needed to obtain the samples, as previously described [21]. Both plasma and aqueous humor samples were stored at −20°C until HPLC analysis.

2.3. Sample Preparation. All plasma and aqueous humor samples were vortexed, and aliquots of 300 μL of plasma or 450 μL of aqueous humor were placed into glass tubes. Plasma and aqueous humor samples were spiked with 40 μL and 45 μL of the internal standard (dexamethasone 1 μg/mL), respectively. Prednisolone was extracted by the addition of 1 mL of ethyl acetate under a high speed vortexing shaker over 10 min. After centrifugation at 2500 ×g for 10 min (4°C) to allow phase separation, the clear supernatant was transferred to a 5 mL glass tube. This volume was evaporated (45°C) to dryness in a vacuum concentrator and then reconstituted with 300 μL of mobile phase.

2.4. HPLC Analysis. Experimental and fortified plasma and aqueous humor samples were analysed for prednisolone by HPLC. After extraction, 100 μL aliquots were injected in a Shimadzu Chromatography system (Shimadzu Corporation, Kyoto, Japan). The equipment was composed of two LC-10AS solvent pumps, an automatic sample injector (SIL-10A) with a 100 μL loop, an ultraviolet visible spectrophotometer detector (UV) (SPD-10A), a column oven (Eppendorf TC-45, Eppendorf, Madison, WI, USA) set at 30°C, and a CBM-10A data integrator. Data and chromatograms were collected and analysed using the Class LC10 software (SPD-10A, Shimadzu Corporation, Kyoto, Japan). A C18 reversed-phase column (Kromasil, Eka Chemicals AB, NY, USA) of 250 mm × 4.6 mm with 5 μm particle size was used for separation. Elution from the stationary phase was carried out at a flow rate of 1.2 mL/min using acetonitrile and water (36 : 64) in isocratic mode as mobile phase during 11 min. The detector was set at 254 nm. A complete validation of the analytical procedures for the extraction and quantification of prednisolone in plasma and aqueous humor was performed before starting the analysis of the biological samples. Recovery of prednisolone was estimated by the comparison of the peak areas from spiked plasma and aqueous humor samples with the areas resulting from direct injections of standards in mobile phase. Precision (intra- and inter-assay) was determined by analyzing replicates of each matrix sample enriched with prednisolone standard to achieve 50, 100 and 200 ng/mL for plasma and 10, 50 and 100 ng/mL for aqueous humor. The intraday and interday precision and accuracy of the method were evaluated by coefficient of variation (CV) and relative error (RE; RE = 100 × [(predicted concentration − nominal concentration)/nominal concentration]).

The theoretical limit of quantification (LOQ) for prednisolone in plasma and aqueous humor were determined comparing the signal of zero samples of the different biological matrices fortified with the internal standard and measurement of the baseline noise at the retention time of prednisolone. The mean baseline noise plus six standard deviations was defined as the theoretical LOQ. The robustness was evaluated on the retention time (t_R), recovery and repeatability of the method (% CV) by deliberate variations of the column temperature (30 and 35°C), flow rate (1 and 1.2 mL/min), and brand columns (Kromasil, Eka Chemicals AB, NY, USA and Phenomenex, CA, USA).

2.5. Pharmacokinetic Analysis. The pharmacokinetic analysis of prednisolone after oral administration to cats was carried out using the program PK Solution (Summit Research Services, Ashland, USA). Pharmacokinetic analysis of the experimental data was performed by a noncompartmental analysis. The following equation [22] was used to describe the biexponential concentration versus time curves for prednisolone in plasma and aqueous humor for each cat after the oral administration: $C_p = Be^{-\beta t} - Ae^{-at}$, where C_p = concentration (ng/mL) in plasma or aqueous humor at time t after administration, A is concentration at time zero extrapolated from the absorption phase (ng/mL), B is concentration at time zero extrapolated from the elimination phase (ng/mL), e is base of the natural logarithm, β is terminal slope (h^{-1}), and a is the slope obtained by feathering which represents the first order absorption rate constant (k_{abs}) (h^{-1}). No lag time was observed for plasma or aqueous humor pharmacokinetics. The maximum concentration (C_{max}) was obtained from the observed data. The area under the concentration (AUC) versus time curves was calculated by the trapezoidal rule [23]. The absorption ($T_{1/2abs}$) and the elimination ($T_{1/2el}$) half-lives were calculated as $\ln 2/k_{abs}$ and $\ln 2/\beta$, respectively. Statistical moment theory was applied to calculate the mean residence time (MRT) in plasma and aqueous humor as follows [23]: MRT = AUMC/AUC, where AUC was defined previously and AUMC is the area under the curve for the first moment, obtained by the product of time and the plasma or aqueous humor drug concentrations versus time from zero to infinity [24].

2.6. Statistical Data Analysis. The pharmacokinetic parameters are reported as mean ± SE and the concentration data as mean ± SD. Student's t-test was used to compare parameters. A value of $P < 0.05$ was considered statistically significant.

3. Results

Prednisolone plasma and aqueous humor concentrations after oral administration of 10 mg of prednisolone to cats were quantified using the analytical assay developed in the present work. The calibration curves for prednisolone were linear in the range of 25–500 and 5–200 ng/mL (r^2 > 0.993 and 0.999) for plasma and aqueous humor, respectively. The linear regression was further supported by a homogeneous distribution of residuals and homoscedasticity of the variance.

Table 1: HPLC analytical validation.

Chromatographic parameter	Plasma	Aqueous humor
Absolute recovery range (%)	72–78	89–93
Intraday precision (%CV)	3.2–5.5	3.3–4
Interday precision (%CV)	4.2–7.6	2.3–11.1
Interday accuracy (%RE)	5.1–13.1	7.0–17.2
LOD (ng/mL)	4.3	1.3
LOQ (ng/mL)	25	5
Precision LOQ (%CV)	12.4	5.8
Stability (%CV)	3.8–4.5	0.9–4.6

CV: coefficient of variation; LOD: limit of detection; LOQ: limit of quantification; RE (relative error) = 100 × [(predicted concentration − nominal concentration)/nominal concentration].

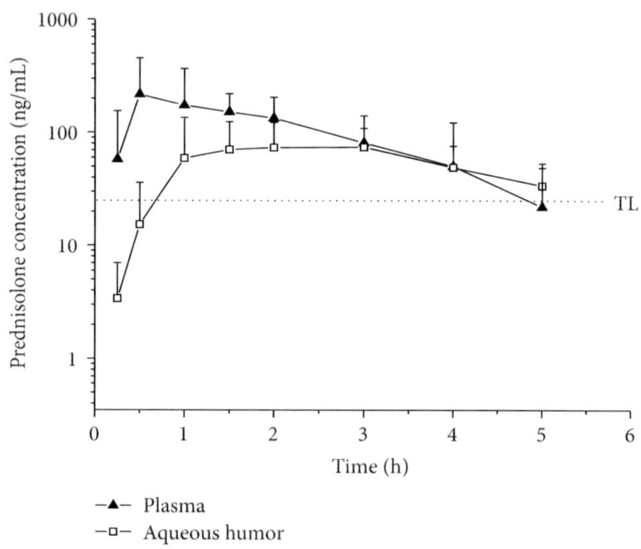

Figure 1: Mean ± SD prednisolone plasma and aqueous humor concentration profiles versus time obtained after its oral administration (10 mg) to cats. TL: therapeutic level concentration is reported as sufficient to suppress inflammation and minimise side effects in humans (25 ng mL^{-1}).

The theoretical LOQ of the method was 25 and 5 ng/mL for plasma and aqueous humor, respectively. The method exhibited a high degree of intraday and interday precision and accuracy as demonstrated by low CV and RE. The values of the main parameters determined in the validation methodology are shown in Table 1. Deliberate variation of the method conditions had no significant effect on assay data or on chromatographic performance, indicating the robustness of method and its suitability for routine use and transference to other laboratories.

Prednisolone concentrations were detected in both plasma and aqueous humor in all sampling periods after oral administration of 10 mg per cats. Mean plasma and aqueous humor concentration profiles versus time are shown in Figure 1. Prednisolone was detectable in plasma from 0.25 up to 5 h after administration. The mean ± SD plasma concentration at the first sampling time was 58.0±96.8 ng/mL

TABLE 2: Plasma and aqueous humor pharmacokinetic parameters for prednisolone after a single oral administration (10 mg) to cats.

Pharmacokinetic parameter	Plasma		Aqueous humor	
	Mean	SE	Mean	SE
$T_{1/2abs}$ (h)	0.37	0.07	0.55	0.09
C_{max} (ng/mL)	300.8	67.3	100.9	25.5
T_{max} (h)	1	0.25	2.25	0.31
MRT (h)	2.24	0.42	4.39	0.64
$T_{1/2el}$ (h)	0.87	0.16	2.25	0.44
AUC (ng·h/mL)	553.3	120.0	378.8	64.9

$T_{1/2abs}$: absorption half-life; C_{max}: maximum concentration; T_{max}: time to maximum concentration; MRT: mean residence time; $T_{1/2el}$: elimination half-life; SE: standard error; AUC: area under the concentration—time curve.

and reached a mean ± SE maximum (C_{max}) level of 300.8 ± 67.3 ng/mL at 1 ± 0.25 h (T_{max}, ±SE). In addition, the lowest mean ± SD plasma concentration of 22.0 ± 26.6 ng/mL was observed after 5 hours of drug administration. In aqueous humor, the concentration measured at 0.25 h after administration was lower than the LOQ, and the mean C_{max} was 100.9 ± 25.5 ng/mL at 1.25 ± 0.30 h (T_{max}). Prednisolone concentration was higher in plasma than in aqueous humor up to 2 hours after drug administration, and thereafter both concentrations were similar as shown in Figure 1. At the last sampling time (5 h), the concentration in aqueous humor was higher than that observed in plasma. Plasma and aqueous humor calculated pharmacokinetic parameters are summarized in Table 2. The prednisolone absorption process to the systemic circulation was fast with a mean absorption half-life ($T_{1/2abs}$, ±SE) of 0.37 ± 0.07 h. The mean half-life time of elimination ($T_{1/2el}$) in plasma was 0.87 ± 0.16 h, and meanwhile the prednisolone $T_{1/2el}$ in the aqueous humor was longer (2.25 ± 0.44 h). Prednisolone plasma and aqueous humor exposure, represented by the AUC ± SE, was 553.3 ± 120.0 ng∗h/mL and 378.8 ± 64.9 ng∗h/mL, respectively. The mean ± SE $AUC_{aqueous\ humor}/AUC_{plasma}$ ratio was 0.68 ± 0.13.

4. Discussion

In the present study, we developed an analytical assay for quantification of prednisolone in aqueous humor and plasma and characterized prednisolone pharmacokinetics in plasma and aqueous humor after oral administration to cats. This is the first study to evaluate the disposition of prednisolone in aqueous humor after oral administration.

After systemic administration, once absorbed, drug molecules are distributed throughout the body in the circulating blood, and they must diffuse into the target tissues to exert the pharmacological effect. The concentration attained at the desired target tissue depends on the delivery process of the drug to the tissues and the ability of the drug to penetrate capillary endothelium and diffuse across cell membranes [25], where factors such as lipophilicity and the binding of the drug to plasma proteins and other tissue components play a critical role [26]. Therefore, the tissue distribution process varies widely for different drug molecules and has to be studied in each case [27].

After oral prednisolone administration to cats, we observed that plasma and aqueous humor concentrations were quantifiable at 0.25 h, demonstrating that both prednisolone absorption and aqueous humor distribution processes were fast. In addition, it has been previously reported that a prednisolone concentration of 25 ng/mL has to be attained in human aqueous humor in order to suppress inflammation [28]. Currently, there is no information about the aqueous humor level that needs to be attained to obtain an anti-inflammatory response in cats. Apart from this limitation, if we considered the level reported in humans, we could expect that the prednisolone aqueous humor concentrations attained in the present work should be pharmacologically active for at least 5 hours after the oral administration of 10 mg of prednisolone in cats (Figure 1).

In the current work, the maximal concentration of prednisolone (C_{max}) in plasma was attained at 1 h and reached a mean ± SE value of 300.8 ± 67.3 ng/mL, and the mean prednisolone plasma exposure, represented by the AUC, was 553.3 ng∗h/mL. While higher systemic exposure of prednisolone was previously reported in cats [13], the rate of drug absorption and elimination was comparable to our present results. A feasible explanation for the different results could be attributed to differences in animal weight and, thus, in volume of distribution. Besides, plasma C_{max} values that were obtained after 10 mg oral prednisolone in rats (863 ng/mL) were higher than the values observed in the present experiment in cats. This is probably due to the lower volume of distribution of the rat [7].

In the present study, we reported plasma half-life time of elimination of 0.66 h, comparable to previous reports in cats [13]. On the contrary, longer $T_{1/2el}$ values (around 3 h) were reported after oral prednisolone in humans [6, 29]. When corrected for dose and considering the volume of distribution, the systemic exposure in human (AUC) is higher than that in cats probably because the 3-fold difference in $T_{1/2el}$ between species. The lower plasma C_{max} and AUC and the shorter prednisolone $T_{1/2el}$ in cats with respect to humans may be associated with a higher metabolism and/or elimination rate or a less protein-bound prednisolone (transcortin) in this species. With important interspecies variations, prednisolone protein binding may affect pharmacokinetic parameters such as drug concentration, volume of distribution, and elimination rate which could explain the differences in distribution process and volume between cats and humans [30].

The aqueous humor drug exposure to prednisolone was lower than that calculated for plasma (AUC = 553.3 ± 120 ng∗h/mL) leading to an $AUC_{aqueous\ humor}/AUC_{plasma}$ ratio of 0.68 ± 0.13, indicating an extensive prednisolone distribution into the aqueous humor after systemic administration to cats. Interestingly, aqueous humor $T_{1/2el}$ and mean residence time were much longer than those observed in plasma ($P < 0.01$), indicating a longer residence in the eye.

According to the results previously reported for dexamethasone, another corticosteroid widely used for uveitis treatment, after a single oral dose of 7.5 mg the drug penetrates into the posterior segment in humans and the ratio mean $C_{max\ vitreous}/C_{max\ plasma}$ was approximately equal to 0.084. Assuming that this ratio is comparable between dexamethasone and prednisolone and similar between humans and cats, based on the plasma C_{max} obtained in the present study (300.8 ± 67.3 ng/mL), the vitreous levels should be about 25 ng/mL. Hence, we suggest that a therapeutic drug level would be attained in the vitreous of our animal model after 10 mg of prednisolone [31]. If we considered this ratio, we can suppose that the vitreous humor level after oral administration of prednisolone should be lower than that in aqueous humor. Thus, assuming that the rate constant of drug transfer from the plasma to the vitreous is comparable between humans and cats, and that the therapeutic level in cats is similar to that in humans (25 ng/mL) [28], then based on the plasma C_{max} obtained in the present study (300.8 ± 67.3 ng/mL) we could hypothesize that a therapeutic drug level would be attained in the vitreous of our animal model after 10 mg of prednisolone. However, the interval of time during which prednisolone vitreous concentrations are higher than 25 ng/mL has to be determined.

Anaesthesia for short periods was necessary to obtain the aqueous humor samples. For this purpose, similar to previous works, the animals were administered at each sampling time with ketamine and xylazine, since no interaction between prednisolone and these anaesthetic drugs has been observed [32, 33]. As described previously, under our experimental conditions, a single paracentesis does not induce ocular inflammation in cats [21]. Although four repetitive paracenteses were performed in this study, with a minimal interval of 45 minutes and a maximal of 120 minutes between samples, we did not observe any clinical signs of blood ocular barriers (BOB) breakdown during the sampling period or during the next 24 h, when the cats were examined before reposition to the research colony. It could be possible that the prednisolone directly reduced PGE synthesis and increased vascular stability avoiding BOB breakdown [34]. However, subclinical BOB breakdown could have occurred during sampling in the present experiment, and this could have increased slightly the aqueous humor drug levels. To avoid this situation, a microdialysis sampling technique is being developed to be used in future studies of prednisolone disposition in the eye.

Although the low content of aqueous humor proteins could result in a greater fraction of free prednisolone with respect to the plasma content, the BOB subclinical breakdown may lead to increased transcortin levels over time compensating the physiologic low levels of proteins.

In conclusion, the simple, precise, and accurate method developed and validated to quantify prednisolone in plasma and aqueous humor allowed us to obtain novel pharmacology-based information on the distribution of prednisolone in cats. This is a useful first step to evaluate the potential of prednisolone as an anti-inflammatory systemic drug for use in feline anterior uveitis. The pharmacokinetic characterization of prednisolone in plasma and aqueous humor after oral administration to cats indicates that the drug penetrates into the anterior chamber of the eye. Follow-up studies to characterize the pattern of distribution in the vitreous humor and to determine the anti-inflammatory levels of prednisolone are required to further evaluate the potential of this drug as an anti-inflammatory drug in the treatment of uveitis.

Conflict of Interests

The authors confirm that there is no known conflict of interests associated with this publication and that there has been no significant financial support for this work that could have influenced its outcome. They also confirm that they do not have a direct financial relation with any commercial identity mentioned in their paper that might lead to a conflict of interests for any of the authors. They further confirm that any aspect of the work covered in this study that has involved experimental animals has been conducted with the ethical approval of all relevant bodies.

Acknowledgments

This work was partially supported by Consejo Nacional de Investigaciones Científicas y Técnicas (CONICET) and Agencia Nacional de Promoción Científica y Técnica (ANPCyT), both from Argentina.

References

[1] J. Stiles and W. M. Townsend, "Feline ophthalmology," in *Veterinary Ophthalmology*, K. N. Gelatt, Ed., pp. 1117–1127, Blackwell, Ames, Iowa, USA, 4th edition, 2007.

[2] W. M. Townsend, "Canine and feline uveitis," *Veterinary Clinics of North America—Small Animal Practice*, vol. 38, no. 2, pp. 323–346, 2008.

[3] B. J. Holmberg and D. J. Maggs, "The use of corticosteroids to treat ocular inflammation," *Veterinary Clinics of North America—Small Animal Practice*, vol. 34, no. 3, pp. 693–705, 2004.

[4] F. L. S. Tse and P. G. Welling, "Prednisolone bioavailability in the dog," *Journal of Pharmaceutical Sciences*, vol. 66, no. 12, pp. 1751–1754, 1977.

[5] M. A. Cunningham, J. L. Edelman, and S. Kaushal, "Intravitreal steroids for macular edema: the past, the present, and the future," *Survey of Ophthalmology*, vol. 53, no. 2, pp. 139–149, 2008.

[6] K.-H. Lee, "Bioavailability of oral prednisolone," *Seoul Journal of Medicine*, vol. 32, no. 3, pp. 131–137, 1991.

[7] A. Isowaki, A. Ohtori, Y. Matsuo, and K. Tojo, "Drug delivery to the eye with a transdermal therapeutic system," *Biological and Pharmaceutical Bulletin*, vol. 26, no. 1, pp. 69–72, 2003.

[8] J. D. Unadkat and M. Rowland, "Pharmacokinetics of prednisone and prednisolone at steady state in the rabbit," *Drug Metabolism and Disposition*, vol. 13, no. 4, pp. 503–509, 1985.

[9] P. L. Toutain, G. D. Koritz, and M. Alvinerie, "Prednisolone succinate and prednisolone acetate in cattle: pharmacokinetics and action on the adrenal gland," *American Journal of Veterinary Research*, vol. 46, no. 3, pp. 719–725, 1985.

[10] M. Alvinerie, G. Houin, and P. L. Toutain, "Prednisolone binding to plasma proteins in domestic species," *Journal of Pharmaceutical Sciences*, vol. 77, no. 11, pp. 937–938, 1988.

[11] P. L. Toutain, R. A. Brandon, and H. De Pomyers, "Dexamethasone and prednisolone in the horse: pharmacokinetics and

action on the adrenal gland," *American Journal of Veterinary Research*, vol. 45, no. 9, pp. 1750–1756, 1984.

[12] B. M. Frey, F. J. Frey, and N. H. G. Holford, "Prednisolone pharmacodynamics assessed by inhibition of the mixed lymphocyte reaction," *Transplantation*, vol. 33, no. 6, pp. 578–584, 1982.

[13] C. A. Graham-Mize and E. J. Rosser, "Bioavailability and activity of prednisone and prednisolone in the feline patient," *Veterinary Dermatology*, vol. 15, pp. 9–10, 2004.

[14] J. H. Andersen, L. G. Hansen, and M. Pedersen, "Optimization of solid phase extraction clean up and validation of quantitative determination of corticosteroids in urine by liquid chromatography-tandem mass spectrometry," *Analytica Chimica Acta*, vol. 617, no. 1-2, pp. 216–224, 2008.

[15] F. K. Główka, M. Karaźniewicz, and E. Lipnicka, "RP-HPLC method with fluorescence detection for determination of small quantities of triamcinolone in plasma in presence of endogenous steroids after derivatization with 9-anthroyl nitrile; pharmacokinetic studies," *Journal of Chromatography B*, vol. 839, no. 1-2, pp. 54–61, 2006.

[16] J. M. Lemus Gallego and J. Pérez Arroyo, "Determination of prednisolone and the most important associated compounds in ocular and cutaneous pharmaceutical preparations by micellar electrokinetic capillary chromatography," *Journal of Chromatography B*, vol. 784, no. 1, pp. 39–47, 2003.

[17] S. Noé, J. Böhler, E. Keller, and A. W. Frahm, "Determination of prednisolone in serum: method development using solid-phase extraction and micellar electrokinetic chromatography," *Journal of Pharmaceutical and Biomedical Analysis*, vol. 18, no. 3, pp. 471–476, 1998.

[18] H. Shibasaki, H. Nakayama, T. Furuta et al., "Simultaneous determination of prednisolone, prednisone, cortisol, and cortisone in plasma by GC-MS: estimating unbound prednisolone concentration in patients with nephrotic syndrome during oral prednisolone therapy," *Journal of Chromatography B*, vol. 870, no. 2, pp. 164–169, 2008.

[19] N. Shibata, T. Hayakawa, K. Takada, N. Hoshino, T. Minouchi, and A. Yamaji, "Simultaneous determination of glucocorticoids in plasma or urine by high-performance liquid chromatography with precolumn fluorimetric derivatization by 9-anthroyl nitrile," *Journal of Chromatography B*, vol. 706, no. 2, pp. 191–199, 1998.

[20] S. Tunn, G. Pappert, P. Willnow, and M. Krieg, "Multicentre evaluation of an enzyme-immunoassay for cortisol determination," *Journal of Clinical Chemistry and Clinical Biochemistry*, vol. 28, no. 12, pp. 929–935, 1990.

[21] M. J. Del Sole, P. H. Sande, A. E. Felipe et al., "Characterization of uveitis induced by use of a single intravitreal injection of bacterial lipopolysaccharide in cats," *American Journal of Veterinary Research*, vol. 69, no. 11, pp. 1487–1495, 2008.

[22] R. Notari, *Biopharmaceutics and Clinical Pharmacokinetics*, Marcel Dekker, New York, NY, USA, 1987.

[23] D. Perrier and M. Mayersohn, "Noncompartmental determination of the steady-state volume of distribution for any mode of administration," *Journal of Pharmaceutical Sciences*, vol. 71, no. 3, pp. 372–373, 1982.

[24] M. Gibaldi and D. Perrier, *Pharmacokinetics*, Marcel Dekker, New York, NY, USA, 1982.

[25] J. D. Baggot, *Principles of Drug Disposition: The Basis of Veterinary Clinical Pharmacology*, Saunders, Philadelphia, Pa, USA, 1977.

[26] J. T. DiPiro, W. J. Spruill, R. A. Blouin et al., *Concepts in Clinical Pharmacokinetics*, American Society of Health Systems Pharmacists, Bethesda, Md, USA, 2005.

[27] H. G. Eichler and M. Müller, "Drug distribution. The forgotten relative in clinical pharmacokinetics," *Clinical Pharmacokinetics*, vol. 34, pp. 95–99, 1998.

[28] C. N. J. McGhee, D. G. Watson, J. M. Midgley, M. J. Noble, G. N. Dutton, and A. I. Fern, "Penetration of synthetic corticosteroids into human aqueous humour," *Eye*, vol. 4, no. 3, pp. 526–530, 1990.

[29] K.-Y. Chien, T.-T. Chen, J. Hsu et al., "Sub-maximal exercise alters the prednisolone absorption pattern," *Journal of Pharmacy and Pharmaceutical Sciences*, vol. 13, no. 1, pp. 58–66, 2010.

[30] L. Shargel and A. Yu, *Applied Biopharmaceutics & Pharmacokinetics*, McGraw-Hill, New York, NY, USA, 2002.

[31] O. Weijtens, R. C. Schoemaker, A. F. Cohen et al., "Dexamethasone concentration in vitreous and serum after oral administration," *American Journal of Ophthalmology*, vol. 125, no. 5, pp. 673–679, 1998.

[32] K. Hippalgaonkar, R. Srirangam, B. Avula, I. A. Khan, and S. Majumdar, "Interaction between topically and systemically coadministered P-glycoprotein substrates/inhibitors: effect on vitreal kinetics," *Drug Metabolism and Disposition*, vol. 38, no. 10, pp. 1790–1797, 2010.

[33] W. J. Tranquilli, J. C. Thurmon, and G. J. Benson, "Lumb and Jones' veterinary anesthesia," in *Lumb and Jones*, W. J. Tranquilli, J. C. Thurmon, and G. J. Benson, Eds., Williams and Wilkins, Baltimor, Md, USA, 3rd edition, 1998.

[34] M. Goppelt-Struebe, D. Wolter, and K. Resch, "Glucocorticoids inhibit prostaglandin synthesis not only at the level of phospholipase A2 but also at the level of cyclo-oxygenase/PGE isomerase," *British Journal of Pharmacology*, vol. 98, no. 4, pp. 1287–1295, 1989.

13

Involvement of Nrf2-Mediated Upregulation of Heme Oxygenase-1 in Mollugin-Induced Growth Inhibition and Apoptosis in Human Oral Cancer Cells

Young-Man Lee,[1] Q-Schick Auh,[2] Deok-Won Lee,[3] Jun-Yeol Kim,[1] Ha-Jin Jung,[1] Seung-Ho Lee,[4] and Eun-Cheol Kim[1]

[1] *Department of Maxillofacial Tissue Regeneration and Research Center for Tooth & Periodontal Regeneration, School of Dentistry, Kyung Hee University, 1 Heogi-dong, Dongdaemun-gu, Seoul 130-701, Republic of Korea*
[2] *Department of Oral Medicine, School of Dentistry, Kyung Hee University, Heogi-dong, Dongdaemun-gu, Seoul 130-701, Republic of Korea*
[3] *Department of Oral and Maxillofacial Surgery, School of Dentistry, Kyung Hee University, Heogi-dong, Dongdaemun-gu, Seoul 130-701, Republic of Korea*
[4] *College of Pharmacy, College of Pharmacy, Yeungnam University, Gyeongsan 712-749, Republic of Korea*

Correspondence should be addressed to Eun-Cheol Kim; eckim@khu.ac.kr

Academic Editor: George Perry

Although previous studies have shown that mollugin, a bioactive phytochemical isolated from *Rubia cordifolia* L. (Rubiaceae), exhibits antitumor effects, its biological activity in oral cancer has not been reported. We thus investigated the effects and putative mechanism of apoptosis induced by mollugin in human oral squamous cell carcinoma cells (OSCCs). Results show that mollugin induces cell death in a dose-dependent manner in primary and metastatic OSCCs. Mollugin-induced cell death involved apoptosis, characterized by the appearance of nuclear shrinkage, flow cytometric analysis of sub-G_1 phase arrest, and annexin V-FITC and propidium iodide staining. Western blot analysis and RT-PCR revealed that mollugin suppressed activation of NF-κB and NF-κB-dependent gene products involved in antiapoptosis (Bcl-2 and Bcl-xl), invasion (MMP-9 and ICAM-1), and angiogenesis (FGF-2 and VEGF). Furthermore, mollugin induced the activation of p38, ERK, and JNK and the expression of heme oxygenase-1 (HO-1) and nuclear factor E2–related factor 2 (Nrf2). Mollugin-induced growth inhibition and apoptosis of HO-1 were reversed by an HO-1 inhibitor and Nrf2 siRNA. Collectively, this is the first report to demonstrate the effectiveness of mollugin as a candidate for a chemotherapeutic agent in OSCCs via the upregulation of the HO-1 and Nrf2 pathways and the downregulation of NF-κB.

1. Introduction

Oral squamous cell carcinoma (OSCC) represents the fifth most common cancer worldwide and is a significant cause of cancer morbidity and mortality. Each year, approximately 300,000 new cases are diagnosed with only a 50% survival rate over 5 years. Common treatments, including surgery, radiation therapy, and chemotherapy, have very low success rates [1]. Two of the most frequently used chemotherapeutic drugs, 5-fluorouracil and cisplatin, cause side effects such as bone marrow suppression, gastrointestinal toxicity, and renal damage, which remain problems that need to be resolved [2]. To overcome such side effects and limitations, the direction of present research into novel antitumor agents has turned to natural products, especially plants used in traditional medicine [3]. Previously, we demonstrated that highly purified sulfur [4] and herbal medicines, such as *Caesalpinia sappan* [5], *Coptidis rhizoma* [6], and verticinone [7], exerted antitumor effects on oral cancer cells *in vitro*. Moreover, we showed that a single compound isolated from *Caesalpinia sappan* heartwood, isoliquiritigenin 2′-methyl ether (ILME), had antioral cancer effects involving mitogen-activated protein kinases (MAPKs) and the nuclear factor-κB (NF-κB) pathway [8]. In addition, we reported that a flavonoid extracted from *Caesalpinia sappan*, sappanchalcone, suppressed oral cancer cell growth and induced apoptosis through activation of p53-dependent mitochondrial MAPK and NF-κB signaling [9].

The roots of *Rubia cordifolia* L. have been widely used as a traditional herbal medicine in Korea to treat cough, bladder and kidney stones, joint inflammation, uterine hemorrhage, and uteritis [10]. In addition, this plant has been used in traditional Chinese medicine for the treatment of arthritis, dysmenorrheal, hematorrhea, hemostasis, and psoriasis [11, 12]. Among the bioactive components from *Rubia cordifolia*, mollugin ($C_{17}H_{16}O_4$; methyl 2,2-dimethyl-6-hydroxy-*2H*-naphtho[1,2-*b*]pyran-5-carboxylate) has been reported to have antitumor and anti-inflammatory activities, and neuroprotective and apoptotic effects [13–16]. A recent study demonstrated that mollugin induced apoptosis through endoplasmic reticulum stress-mediated activation of c-Jun N-terminal kinase (JNK) and the mitochondria-dependent caspase cascade, regulated by Bcl-xL in human Jurkat T cells [14]. Moreover, mollugin inhibited proliferation and induced apoptosis by suppressing fatty acid synthase in HER2-overexpressing human breast and ovarian cancer cells [17].

Heme oxygenase-1 (HO-1) is an inducible cytoprotective enzyme that catalyzes the initial rate-limiting reaction in heme catabolism. Previously, we reported that the HO-1 pathway plays a key role in the adaptation of cells to stressful conditions and the recovery of dental pulp cells and periodontal ligament cells from injury [18–20]. Despite its cytoprotective properties, recent evidence suggests a role for HO-1 in promoting cancer [21]. HO-1 is overexpressed in various types of cancer and is further induced by radiation and chemotherapy [22, 23]. Regarding the mechanisms of HO-1 induction, several studies have suggested the involvement of MAPK and NF-κB pathways, as well as nuclear factor erythroid 2-related factor 2 (Nrf2) [18, 24]. However, the precise cellular mechanisms of mollugin on OSCCs are not completely understood.

The aim of this study was to investigate the chemotherapeutic effect of mollugin on human primary and metastatic OSCCs *in vitro*. In addition, we further explored whether the effect of mollugin is related to Nrf2 activation and HO-1 expression.

2. Materials and Methods

2.1. Reagents. Mollugin was isolated from root of heartwood of *Rubia cordifolia* L. as described previously [13]. Antibody against NF-κB p65, IκB, Nrf2, Bcl-xL, Bcl-2, p53, p21, or phosphorylated isoforms of IκB and horseradish peroxidase-conjugated secondary antibodies were purchased from Santa Cruz Biotechnology (Delaware Avenue, CA). ERK, JNK, p38 or phosphorylation of ERK, JNK, and p38 were purchased from Cell signaling, Inc. (Beverly, MA). Dulbecco's modified Eagle's medium (DMEM), fetal bovine serum (FBS), and other tissue culture reagents were purchased from Gibco BRL (Grand Island, NY). All other chemicals were obtained from Sigma (St. Louis, MO), unless indicated otherwise.

2.2. Cell Culture. The cell line HNSCC4 (HN4), from a primary OSCCs, and cell line HNSCC12 (HN12), from a metastatic carcinoma of the OSCCs [25], were derived in the laboratory of Dr. John F. Ensley (Wayne State University). Cells were cultured in DMEM supplemented with 10% FBS, 100 U/mL penicillin, and 100 μg/mL streptomycin in a humidified atmosphere of 5% CO_2 at 37°C. Cells were dissociated with 0.25% trypsin just before transferring for experiments and counted using a hemocytometer.

Human keratinocyte cell line HaCaT (nontransformed human cell line) were incubated in DMEM supplemented with 10% FBS, 1 mM sodium pyruvate, 50 μg/mL streptomycin, and 50 μg/mL penicillin at 37°C in 5% CO_2. Human gingival fibroblasts (HGFs) cell line by transfection with the E6/E7 open reading frames of HPV type 16 was cultured according to the following protocol, as reported by our study [26]. Briefly, HGFs were cultured in DMEM supplemented with 10% FBS, 100 U/mL penicillin, and 100 μg/mL streptomycin in a humidified atmosphere of 5% CO_2 at 37°C.

2.3. Antiproliferative Assay. Cell viability was determined by 3-(4,5-Dimethylthiazol-2-yl)-2,5-diphenyltetrazolium bromide (MTT) assay. Briefly, cells were seeded in flat-bottomed 96-well plates, at 1×10^5 cell/well 24 h prior to treatment. The cells were treated for various lengths of time with the agents indicated. Then 25 μL of 5 mg/mL MTT was added to each well. After 4 h incubation at 37°C, 100 μL of lysing buffer was added. The buffer consisted of 20% w/v of sodium dodecyl sulfate in 0.1% of HCl solution. The plates were incubated for a further analysis on an ELISA reader at 570 nm. The same experiment was repeated in three separate cultures, and the data were presented as the means ± SD of five observations.

2.4. Flow Cytometry

2.4.1. Propidium Iodide (PI) Staining. Cells were seeded at 5×10^5cells/well in six-well plates. After 24 h, cells were treated with mollugin the 3 days. After treatment, cells were harvested and pelleted by centrifugation (400 ×g, 4°C, 5 min). The cells were fixed with cold 75% ethanol for 24 h and then stained with PI solution, consisting of 45 mg/mL PI, 10 mg/mL RNase A, and 0.1% Triton X-100. After incubation in the dark at 4°C for 1 h, fluorescence-activated cells were sorted using the FACScan flow cytometer, and the data were analyzed using Cellfit Analysis Software.

2.5. Fluorescein-Isothiocyanate-(FITC-) Annexin V and Propidium Iodide (PI) Double Staining. Cells (5×10^5) were seeded in 6-well plates, incubated for 24 h, and then treated with or without mollugin, and the incubation was continued for 3 days. After treatment, the cell pellet was prepared in a FACStar tube containing annexin V-FITC solution and incubated in 5% CO_2 at 37°C. The PI solution (without NP 40) was then added, and the ratio of PI-positive and annexin V-positive cells was measured using the flow cytometer.

2.6. Morphological Analysis of Apoptosis by Staining with 4′,6-Diamino-2-Phenylindole Dihydrochloride (DAPI). To confirm that the nuclei underwent morphological changes, the cells were cultured in 60 mm dishes overnight and then washed twice in DMEM. The cells were then treated with mollugin and fixed in 4% paraformaldehyde, after which they were incubated in 1 μg/mL DAPI solution for 30 min in the dark. The cells were then examined using a fluorescence microscope (Zeiss, Oberköchen, Germany).

2.7. Western Blot Analysis. Western blot analysis was performed by lysing cells in 20 mM Tris-HCl buffer (pH 7.4) containing protease inhibitor mixture (0.1 mM phenylmethanesulfonyl fluoride, 5 mg/mL aprotinin, 5 mg/mL pepstatin A, and 1 mg/mL chymostatin). Protein concentration was determined using the Lowry protein assay kit (P5626; Sigma). An equal amount of protein for each sample was resolved using 7% or 12% sodium dodecyl sulfate-polyacrylamide gel electrophoresis (SDS-PAGE) and then electrophoretically transferred onto a Hybond-enhanced chemiluminescence (ECL) nitrocellulose membrane (Bio-Rad, Hercules, CA). The membrane was blocked with 5% skim milk and sequentially incubated with primary antibody (Santa Cruz Biotechnology) and horseradish peroxidase-conjugated secondary antibody followed by ECL detection (Amersham Pharmacia Biotech, Piscataway, NJ).

2.8. Isolation of RNA and RT-PCR. Total RNA was isolated using the TRIzol reagent (Invitrogen, Carlsbad, CA, USA) according to the manufacturer's instructions. It was then reverse-transcribed using AccuPower RT premix (Bioneer, Daejeon, Korea). The PCR amplification of the resulting cDNA samples was performed using a GeneAmp PCR System 2400 thermal cycler (PerkinElmer, Wellesley, MA, USA). The primers information is summarized in Table 1. The following PCR conditions were used: 34 cycles of denaturation at 95°C for 30 s, primer annealing at 60°C for 30 s, and extension at 72°C for 30 s. The PCR products were resolved on 1-2% agarose gels and stained with ethidium bromide.

2.9. HO-1 and Nrf2 siRNA Transfection. The target sequence for human HO-1 siRNA was 5′-AACUUUCAGAAGGGCCAGGUGTT-3′ (forward) and 5′-CACCUGGCCCUUCUGAAAGUUTT-3′ (reverse). Transfection of Nrf2 siRNA was performed using the target sequence 5′-AAGAGUAUGAGCUGGAAAAACTT-3′ (forward) and 5′-GUUUUUCCAGCUCAUACUCUUTT-3′ (reverse). Cells were transfected with siRNA using Lipofectamine RNAiMAX (Invitrogen) according to the manufacture's instruction. Silencer Negative Control siRNA (Invitrogen) was introduced into cells by the same method. Following transfection, cells were cultured in six-well plates at 37°C until required.

2.10. Statistical Analysis. Data are expressed as the mean ± standard deviation. Statistical comparisons of the results were made using analysis of variance (ANOVA). Significant differences ($P < 0.05$) between the means of control and sulfur-treated cells were analyzed using Dunnett's test.

TABLE 1: Reverse transcriptase-polymerase chain reaction primers.

Gene	Sequence 5′-3′	Size
MMP-9	Forward: GTTGGGGAGGGCTGTCCGTGA Reverse: CGTGGCGCTATCCAGCTCACC	911 bp
ICAM-1	Forward: CGCCCGATTGCTTTAGCTTG Reverse: CGACTCACCTGGGAACAGAG	320 bp
VEGF	Forward: TCAAGGTTGGCGGAAGTGAGG Reverse: CCCTTGCATCAGTAGGCTTCA	443 bp
FGF2	Forward: GCCTCATTTCCATTTCGTGG Reverse: CGGGGGTACTGGTTTACAG	224 bp
β-actin	Forward: CATGGATGATGATATCGCCGC Reverse: ACATGATCTGGGTCATCTTCT	319 bp

3. Results

3.1. Effect of Mollugin on HN4 and HN12 Cell Viability. To investigate the effect of mollugin on the proliferation of human OSCCs, the MTT assay was used. As shown in Figure 1, mollugin inhibited cellular proliferation in a dose- and time-dependent manner. Moreover, mollugin displayed higher cytotoxicity in primary OSCC HN4 cells compared with metastatic OSCC HN12 cells, although the overall trend of the effects of mollugin on HN4 and HN12 cells was similar. Furthermore, we tested whether mollugin has any toxic effect on nonneoplastic human skin keratinocytes (HaCaT) and gingival fibroblasts (GF). Interestingly, we did not find significant cytotoxicity or cell death by mollugin on HaCaT and GF (Figures 1(c) and 1(d)).

3.2. Effect of Mollugin on HN4 and HN12 Cell Apoptosis. To determine whether the cause of cell death was apoptosis, HN4 and HN12 cells were exposed to 40 μM mollugin for 3 days. This concentration was used because it reproducibly induced 50% growth inhibition in HN4 and HN12 cells cultured for 3 days. Cell nuclei were stained with 4′,6-diamidino-2-phenylindole (DAPI), a fluorescent DNA-binding dye (Figure 2(a)). DAPI staining showed that the control nuclei were large and round without condensation or fragmentation, whereas most of the nuclei of mollugin-treated cells were condensed and fragmented, as is typical during apoptosis. The onset of apoptotic cell death by mollugin was confirmed by flow cytometry of HN4 and HN12 cells (Figure 2(b)). Without treatment, only 3.88% HN4 and 2.80% HN12 cells were in the sub-G_1 region; however, mollugin treatment increased the proportions of cells in the sub-G_1 region to 20.26% and 31.46%, respectively. To determine whether the growth inhibitory effect of mollugin is associated with cell death, annexin V-propidium iodide (PI) double staining of HN4 and HN12 cells and flow cytometry was performed (Figure 2(c)). Treatment of cells with mollugin for 3 days increased the number of annexin V^+/PI^+ stained cells. These results demonstrate that the inhibition of cell growth by mollugin was caused by the induction of apoptosis.

3.3. Effect of Mollugin on NF-κB Activation and Expression of NF-κB-Regulated Genes. Since NF-κB transcription factors

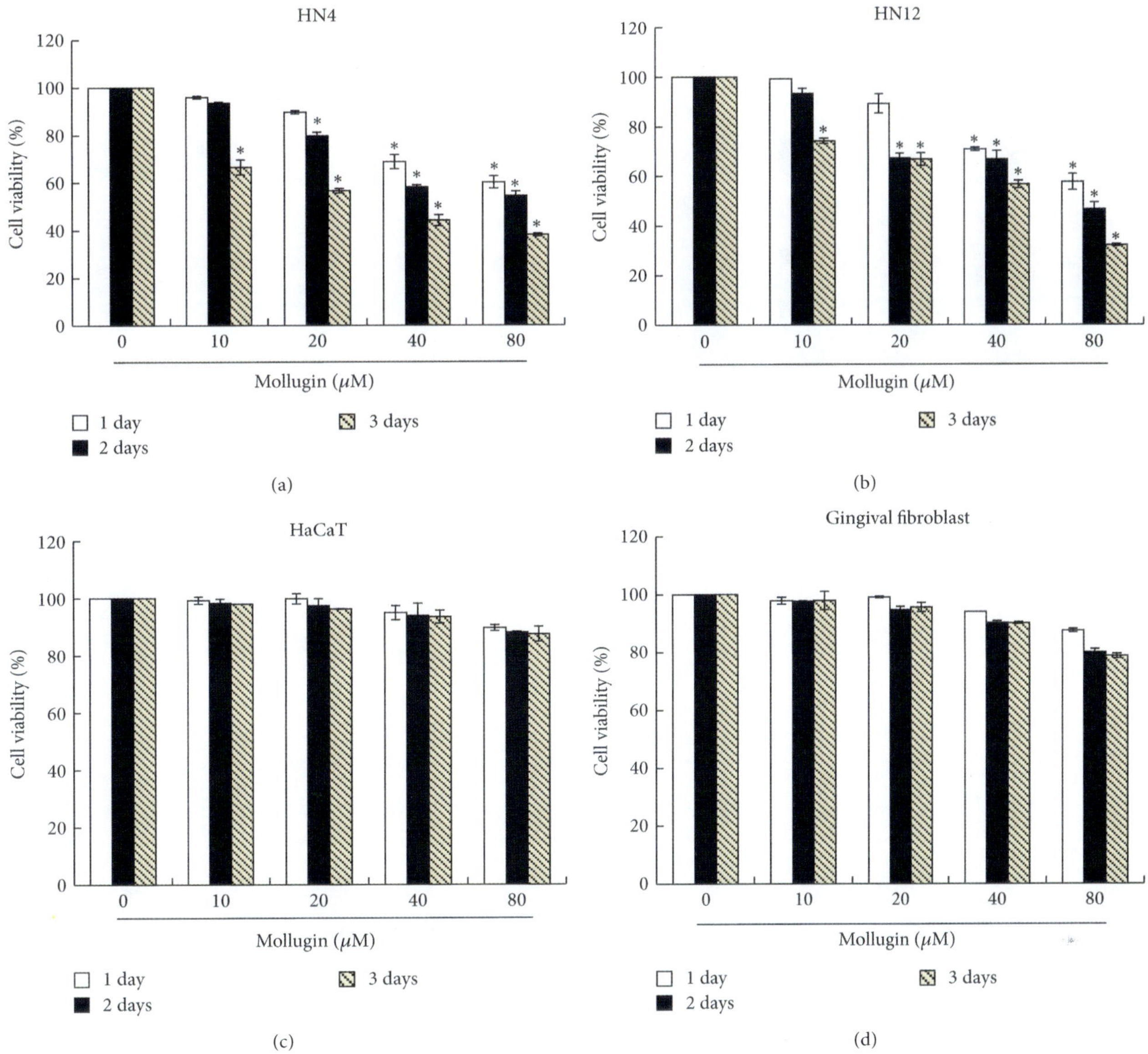

FIGURE 1: Effects of mollugin on cell viability in primary (HN4, (a)), metastatic oral cancer cells (HN12, (b)), skin keratinocytes (HaCaT, (c)), and gingival fibroblasts (d) as measured by MTT assay. *Statistically significant difference as compared to control, $P < 0.05$. The same experiment was repeated in three separate cultures, and the data were presented as the means ± SD of five observations.

and their upstream activating molecules are attractive targets for cancer therapeutics, we evaluated the effect of mollugin on NF-κB activation by measuring the phosphorylation and degradation of IκBα and NF-κB p65. As shown in Figure 3(a), treatment of HN4 and HN12 cells with mollugin decreased the steady-state levels of phosphorylated IκBα and nuclear NF-κB p65.

To clarify the molecular mechanism by which mollugin induces apoptosis in primary and metastatic OSCCs, we determined the levels of NF-κB-regulated gene products involved in apoptosis and antiapoptosis (Figure 3(b)). Mollugin treatment upregulated p53 and p21 expression in both HN4 and HN12 cells in a dose-dependent manner. In contrast, the expression of antiapoptotic Bcl-2 and Bcl-xl proteins was dose-dependently reduced by mollugin treatment in HN4 and HN12 cells. Next, we investigated whether mollugin could modulate levels of NF-κB-regulated gene products involved in invasion (ICAM-1 and MMP-9) and angiogenesis (VEGF and FGF-2) of OSCCs. The results show that mollugin downregulated the expression of NF-κB-regulated gene products, including MMP-9, ICAM-1, VEGF, and FGF-2 mRNA in a dose-dependent manner (Figure 3(c)).

3.4. Effect of Mollugin on MAPK and Nrf2 Activation. To clarify the mechanism underlying the apoptosis, we assessed the effect of mollugin on Nrf2 and NF-κB upstream pathways. Treatment with mollugin (40 μM) increased levels of phosphorylated (activated) ERK, p38, and JNK; the phosphorylated proteins were easily detectable by Western blot after 30

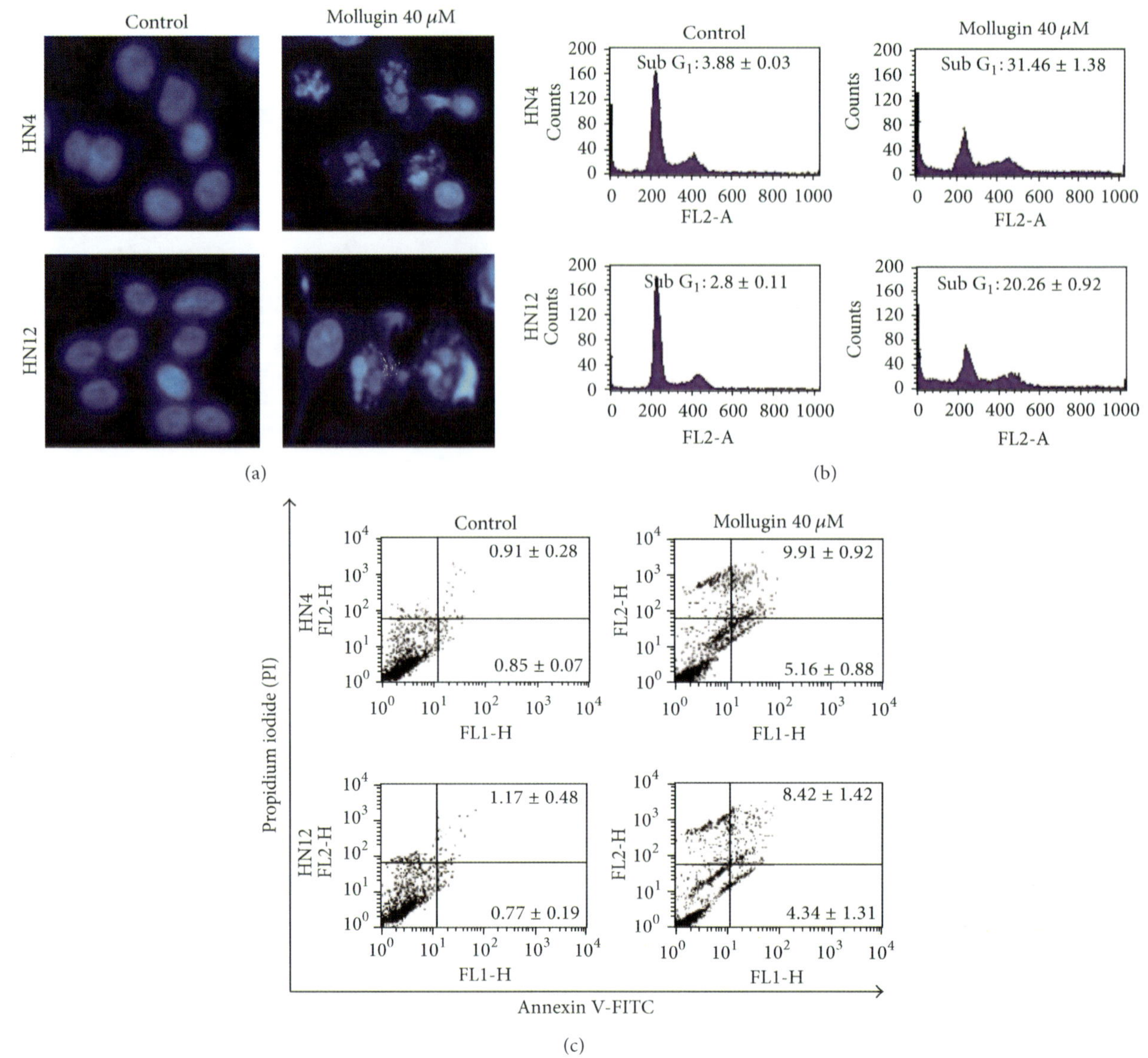

FIGURE 2: Confirmation of mollugin-induced apoptosis by DAPI staining (a), cell cycle analysis (b), and annexin V-PI staining (c) in OSCCs. Cells were incubated with 40 μM mollugin for 3 days. Data are presented as mean ± SD from triplicate determinations (b, c). Results are representative from three independent experiments (a)–(c).

or 60 min. In contrast, mollugin did not affect total p38, ERK, or JNK levels (Figure 4(a)).

Since the stress response element/Nrf2 transcription factor pathway is important for HO-1 expression [23], we next determined whether Nrf2 signaling is involved in mollugin-induced HO-1 expression and apoptosis. Initially, Nrf2 activation was assessed by the accumulation of Nrf2 in the nucleus. Treatment with mollugin resulted in an accumulation of Nrf2 in the nucleus in primary and metastatic OSCCs (Figure 4(b)).

To determine whether mollugin induces expression of antioxidant genes, HO-1 expression in oral cancer cells and the change in the pattern of HO-1 expression were evaluated. HO-1 protein expression in primary and metastatic OSCCs increased following mollugin treatment in a time-dependent manner (Figure 4(c)).

To confirm the involvement of MAPK pathways in the mollugin-driven activation of NF-κB and Nrf2, inhibitors of ERK (PD98059), JNK (SP6100126), and p38 (SB203580) MAPK signaling were used. Mollugin-induced NF-κB, Nrf2, and HO-1 expression was effectively inhibited by PD98059, SP600126, and SB203580 (Figure 4(d)), suggesting that p38, ERK1/2, and JNK play important roles in activating NF-κB, Nrf2, and HO-1 in HN4 and HN12 cells.

3.5. Involvement of the HO-1 Pathway in Mollugin-Induced Apoptosis. To examine the cytotoxic potential of tin protoporphyrin (SnPP), an HO-1 inhibitor, its effect on viability was initially measured by the MTT assay (Figure 5(a)). Although, 10 or 20 μM SnPP had no cytotoxicity effect for 3 h, we found that SnPP exhibited slight cytotoxicity on HN4 and

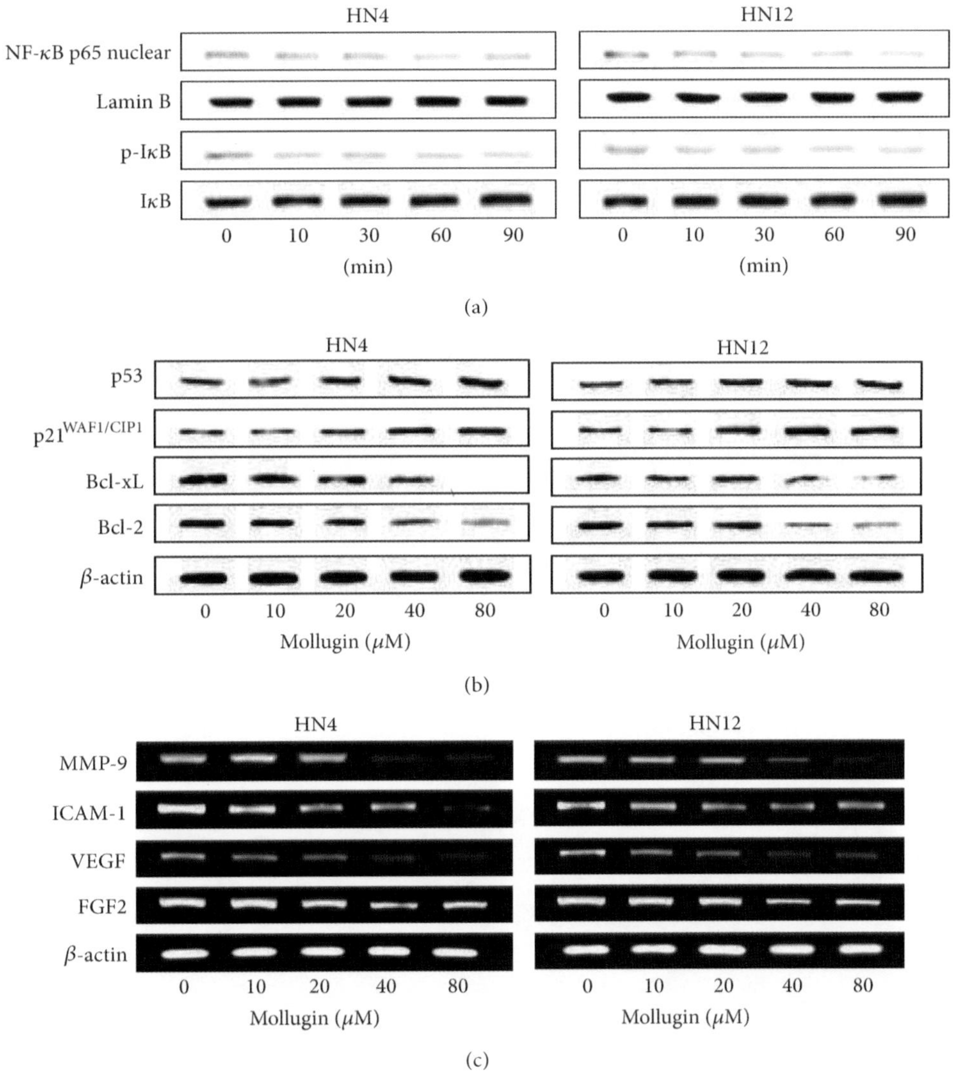

FIGURE 3: Effects of mollugin on activation of NF-κB (a), and expression of NF-κB-regulated gene products involved in apoptosis and antiapoptosis (b), metastasis, and angiogenesis (c) in OSCCs. Cells were treated with 40 μM mollugin for indicated times (a) or 3 days (b, c). The figure is representative of 3 independent experiments.

HN12 cells at 16 h. Based on these findings, we chose to use SnPP for 3 h.

To determine whether the induction of HO-1 plays a role in mollugin-induced growth inhibition and apoptosis in OSCCs, cells were treated with SnPP, an HO-1 inhibitor, for 3 h before incubation with mollugin for 3 days. MTT assays showed that mollugin-induced cytotoxicity and apoptosis in HN4 and HN12 cells were dose-dependently reversed by pretreatment with SnPP (Figures 5(a) and 5(b)). In addition, SnPP treatment abolished the induction of p53 and $p21^{WAF1/CIP1}$ expression by mollugin, but reversed the expression of Bcl-2 and Bcl-xl (Figure 5(c)).

Additionally, we used a siRNA-expressing plasmid to induce HO-1 gene silencing. HN4 and HN12 cells were transfected with an HO-1-targeting siRNA expression vector (Figure 6). The siRNA approach resulted in high silencing efficacies for HO-1, which was confirmed by Western blot analysis (Figure 6(c)). Silencing of HO-1 significantly attenuated mollugin-induced cytotoxicity (Figure 6(a)) and apoptosis (Figure 6(b)). Moreover HO-1 RNA blocked mollugin-induced Nrf2, p53, and p21 upregulation as well as Bcl-2 and Bcl-xl downregulation (Figure 6(c)).

3.6. Involvement of the Nrf2 Pathway in Mollugin-Induced HO-1 Induction and Apoptosis. To investigate whether mollugin-induced apoptosis and HO-1 expression were mediated by Nrf2 activation, a specific small interfering RNA (siRNA) against Nrf2 was used. As shown in Figure 7(c), transfection with Nrf2 siRNA for 5 h in HN4 and HN12 cells blocked mollugin-induced HO-1 and Nrf2 expression. However, Nrf2 siRNA did not affect the mollugin-induced p65 expression. Transfection with Nrf2 siRNA inhibited mollugin-induced cytotoxicity and apoptosis in HN4 and HN12 cells (Figures 7(a) and 7(b)). Moreover, transfection with Nrf2 siRNA in HN4 and HN12 cells reduced mollugin-induced apoptosis proteins (p53 and p21), but reversed antiapoptosis proteins (Bcl-2 and Bcl-xl) (Figure 7(c)).

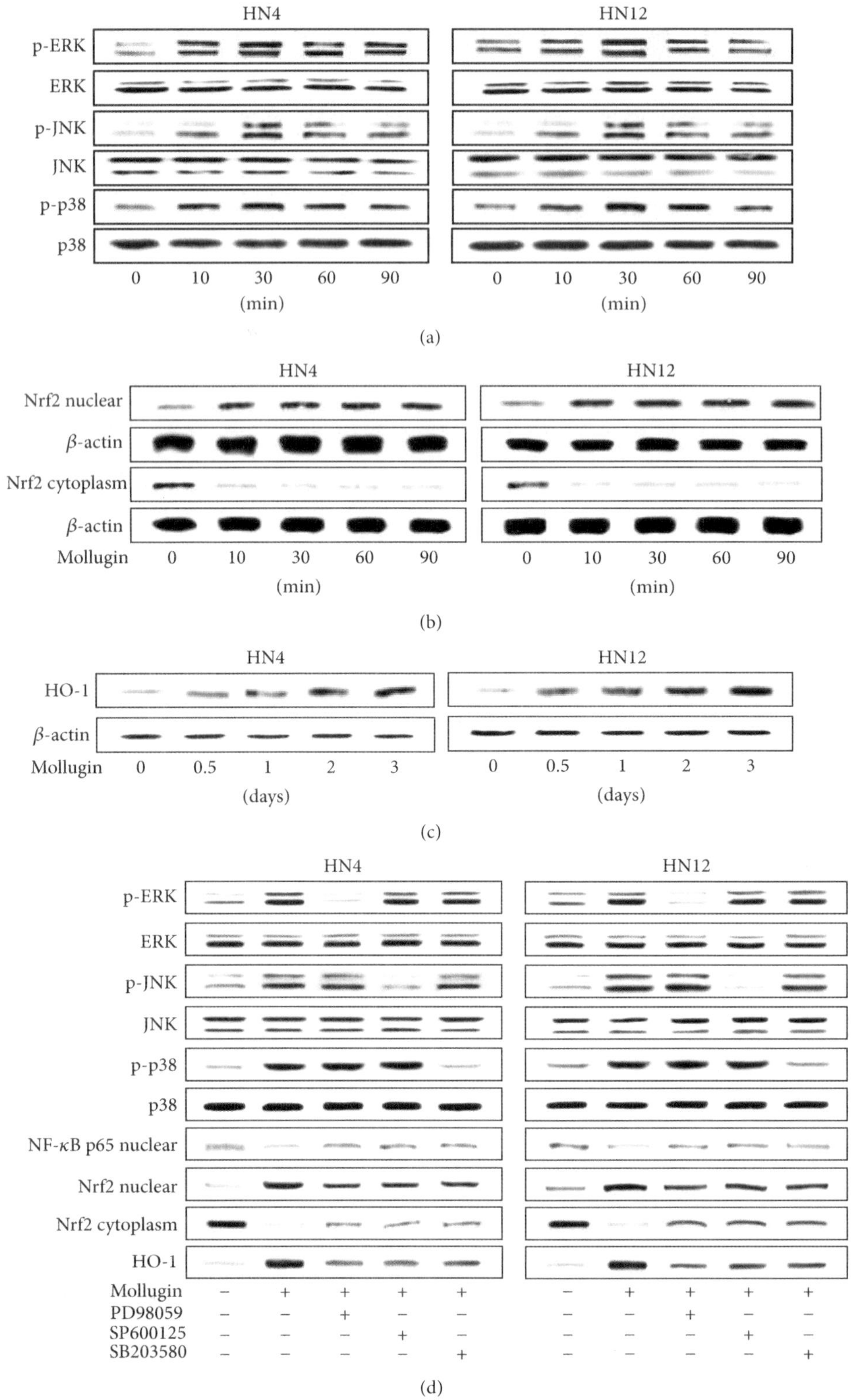

FIGURE 4: Effect of mollugin on phosphorylation of MAPK (a), activation of Nrf2 (b), and expression of HO-1 (c) in OSCCs. Effects of MAP kinase inhibitors on mollugin-induced activation of NF-κB, Nrf2, and HO-1 (d). Cells were treated with 40 μM mollugin for indicated times (a)–(c). Cells were pretreated with the p38 inhibitor SB203580 (20 μM/L), the ERK inhibitor PD98059 (20 μM/L), or the JNK inhibitor SP600125 (20 μM/L) for 1 hour and treated with 40 μM mollugin for 30 min (MAPK, Nrf2, and NF-κB) or 3 days (HO-1). The results are representative of three independent experiments.

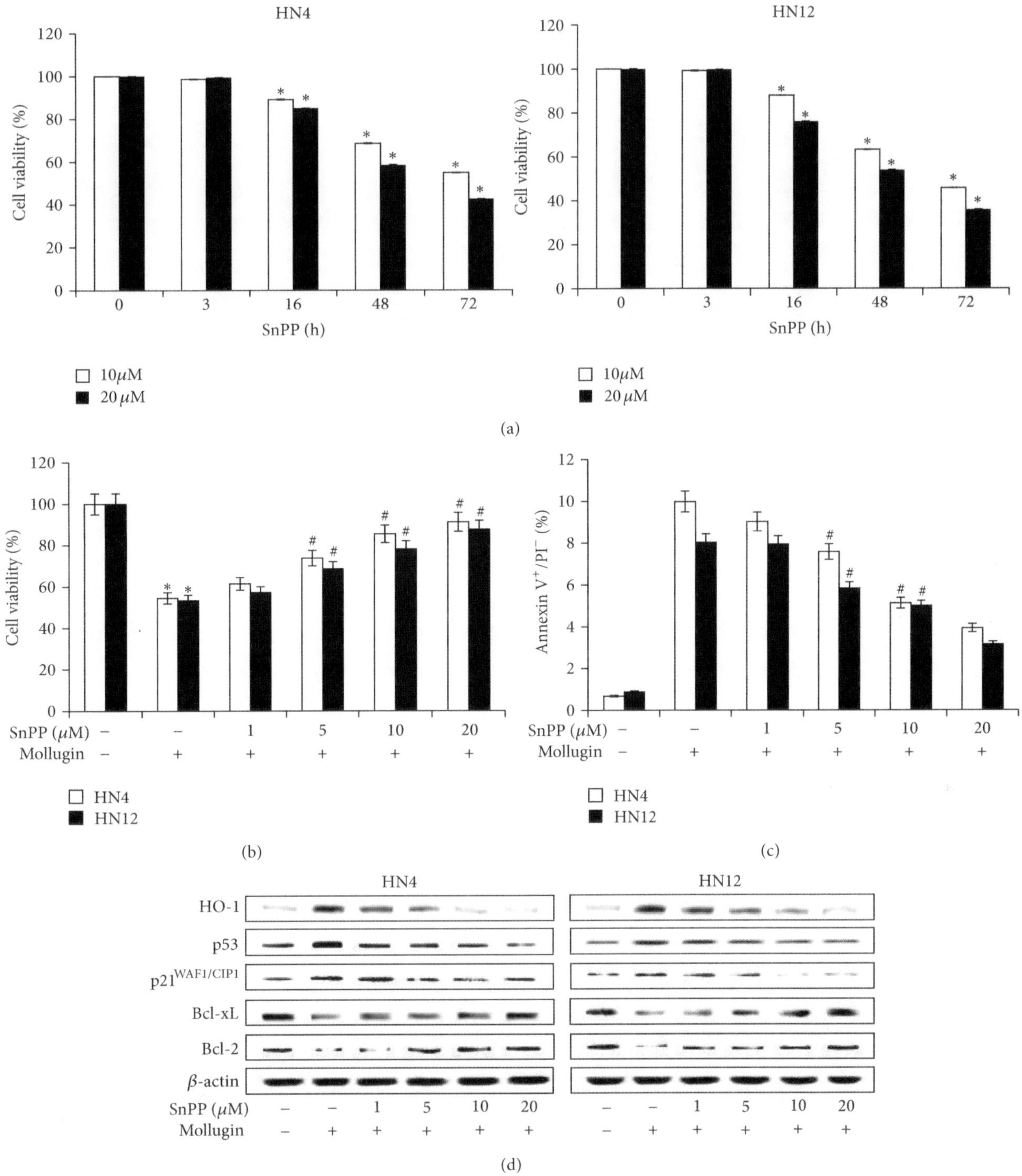

Figure 5: Effects of HO-1 inhibitor (SnPP) on cytotoxicity (a), mollugin-induced growth inhibition (b), apoptosis (c), and apoptosis-related proteins expression (d) in OSCCs. Cells were pretreated with SnPP for 3 h and treated for 3 days with mollugin (b)–(d). Cell viability was examined by MTT assay (a), and apoptosis was examined by flow cytometry (b), respectively. The same experiment was repeated in three separate cultures, and the data were presented as the means ± SD of five observations (a, b). Data are presented as mean values from triplicate determinations (c). Western data show one representative result of three independent experiments (d). *Statistically significant difference as compared to control, $P < 0.05$. #Statistically significant difference as compared to mollugin, $P < 0.05$.

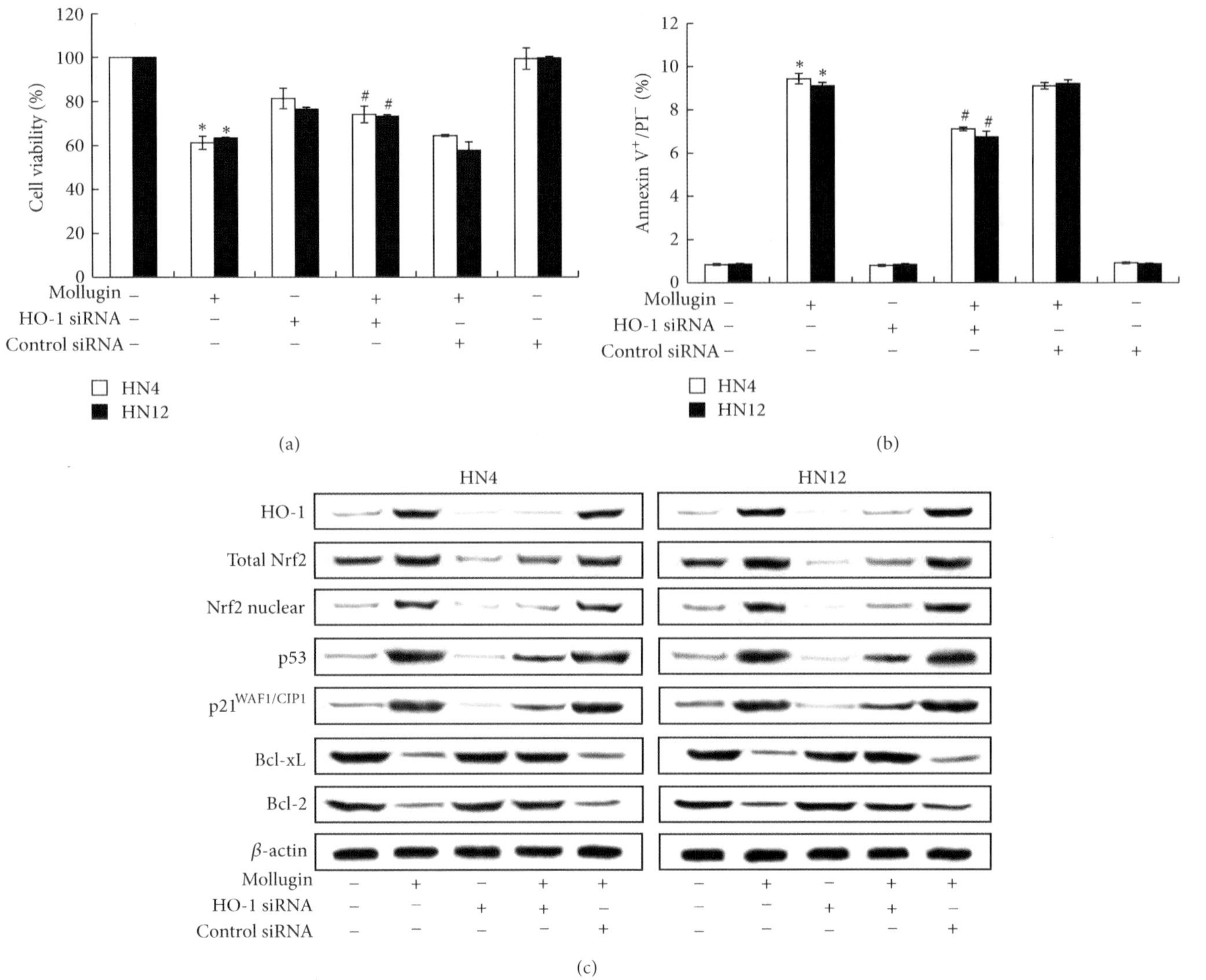

Figure 6: Effects of HO-1 siRNA on mollugin-induced growth inhibition (a), apoptosis (b), and apoptosis-related proteins expression (c) in OSCCs. Cells were pretreated with HO siRNA (30 nM) for 5 h and treated for 3 days with mollugin (a)–(c). Cell viability was examined by MTT assay (a), and apoptosis was examined by flow cytometry (b), respectively. The same experiment was repeated in three separate cultures, and the data were presented as the means ± SD of five observations (a). Data are presented as mean values from triplicate determinations (b). Western data show one representative result of three independent experiments (c). *Statistically significant difference as compared to control, $P < 0.05$. #Statistically significant difference as compared to mollugin, $P < 0.05$.

4. Discussion

This study is to our knowledge the first to demonstrate that mollugin directly induces growth inhibition and apoptosis in primary and metastatic OSCCs and to address the molecular basis of this effect.

With regard to antitumor activity, mollugin has been shown to exert cytotoxic effects on human colon cancer (Col2) cells (IC_{50} = 12.3 μM; [11]), human liver carcinoma (HepG2) cells (IC_{50} value = 60.2 μM; [10]), and basal HER2-expressing human breast cancer cells (IC_{50} value = 58 μM; [17]). In the present study, we found that mollugin (10–80 μM) resulted in significant growth inhibition, with an average IC_{50} value of 46.3 μM in metastatic OSCCs (HN12) and 43.9 μM in primary OSCCs (HN4) after 3 days. These antiproliferative properties of mollugin are consistent with previous reports in human acute leukemia Jurkat T cells [14] and HER2-overexpressing breast and ovarian cancer cell lines [17]. Moreover, we demonstrated that mollugin induced OSCC cell death by triggering apoptosis due to the presence of several apoptotic characteristics, including sub-G_1 phase accumulation, increase in annexin$^+$/PI$^+$ cells, and DNA fragmentation.

NF-κB signaling is a ubiquitous pathway in cell proliferation, survival, and apoptosis. Normally, NF-κB proteins are inhibited by binding to IκB proteins in the cytoplasm. Stress factors cause degradation of IκB proteins through the ubiquitin-proteosomal pathway, and NF-κB is released

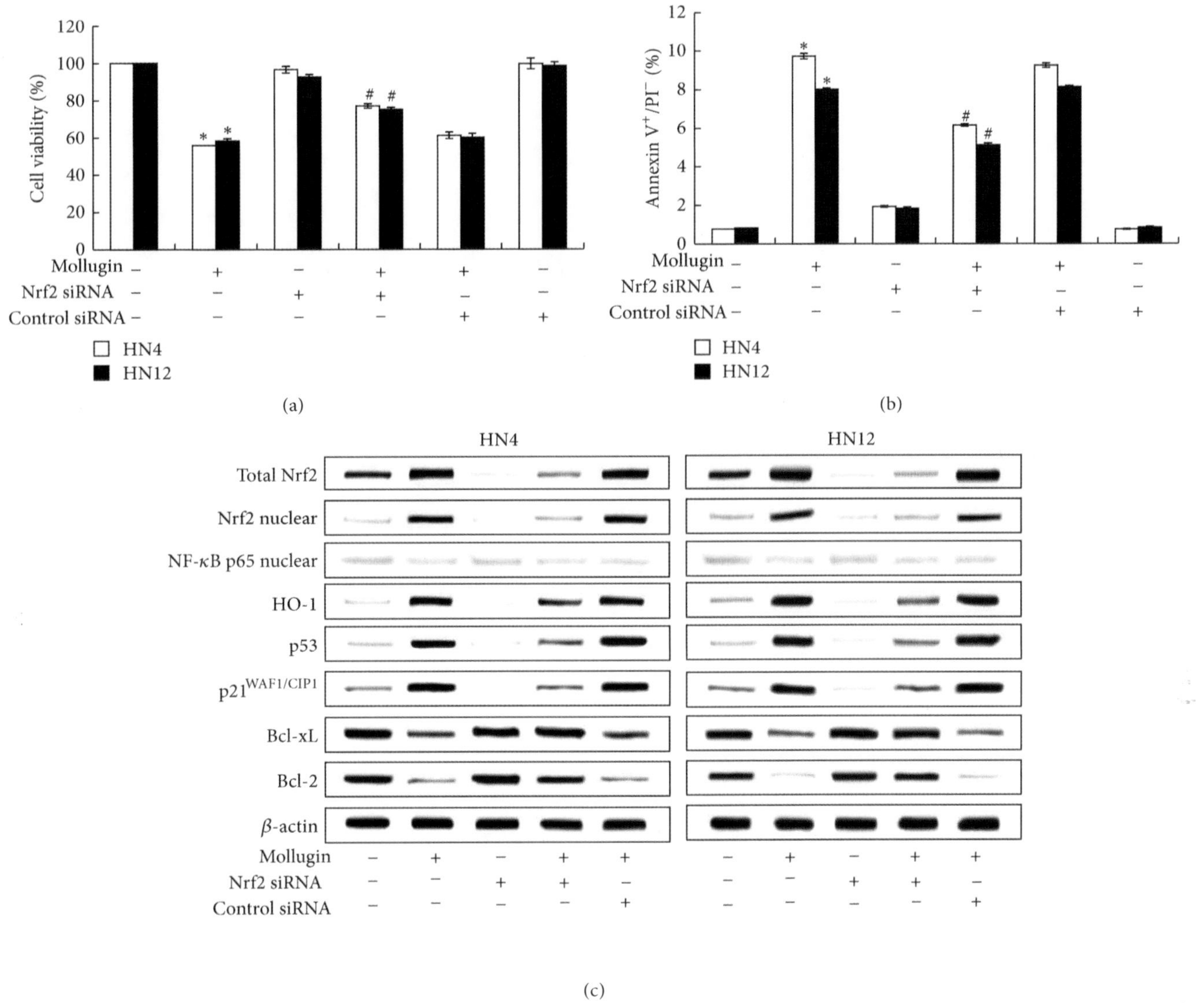

Figure 7: Effect of Nrf2 siRNA on mollugin-induced growth inhibition (a), apoptosis (b), and apoptosis-related proteins expression (c). Cells were treated with 40 μM mollugin for indicated times (a). Cells were pretreated with Nrf2 siRNA (250 nM) for 5 h and treated for 3 days with mollugin 40 μm (a)–(c). *Statistically significant difference as compared to control, $P < 0.05$. #Statistically significant difference as compared to mollugin, $P < 0.05$. Data are representative of 3 independent experiments.

to bind to the DNA of promoter regions of specific genes that increases their transcription rate [27, 28]. To explore the mechanism underlying mollugin-induced apoptosis in OSCCs, we examined NF-κB activation. In agreement with previous findings that mollugin suppressed NF-κB activation in HER2-overexpressing SK-BR-3 breast cancer cells [17], our results indicate that mollugin significantly inhibited NF-κB activation by reducing the level of phospho-IκBα, leading to blockage of the IκBα pathway in NF-κB activation in OSCCs. In addition, it was reported that mollugin significantly suppressed TNF-α-induced NF-κB transcriptional activation in HT-29 human colonic epithelial cells [13].

Genes involved in the proliferation, apoptosis, antiapoptosis, angiogenesis, and metastasis of cancer are regulated by NF-κB [29]. Constitutive activation of NF-κB negatively regulates the proapoptotic functions of p53 by inducing the expression of an array of antiapoptotic genes, including Bcl-2 and Bcl-xL [30]. In our study, treatment with mollugin induced the downregulation of antiapoptotic Bcl-2 and Bcl-xL levels as well as the upregulation of apoptotic p53 and p21 levels in OSCCs. Another hallmark of OSCC behavior is their propensity for local invasion and metastasis. MMP-9 is frequently overexpressed in OSCCs and is dependent upon NF-κB for expression [31]. Adhesion molecules such as ICAM-1 are regulated by NF-κB and are essential for the adhesion of tumor cells to endothelial cells and thus mediate tumor cell metastasis [32]. Angiogenesis is important for tumor growth and progression. The development of angiogenesis is stimulated by cytokines and growth factors, and the expression of these cytokines and growth factors is

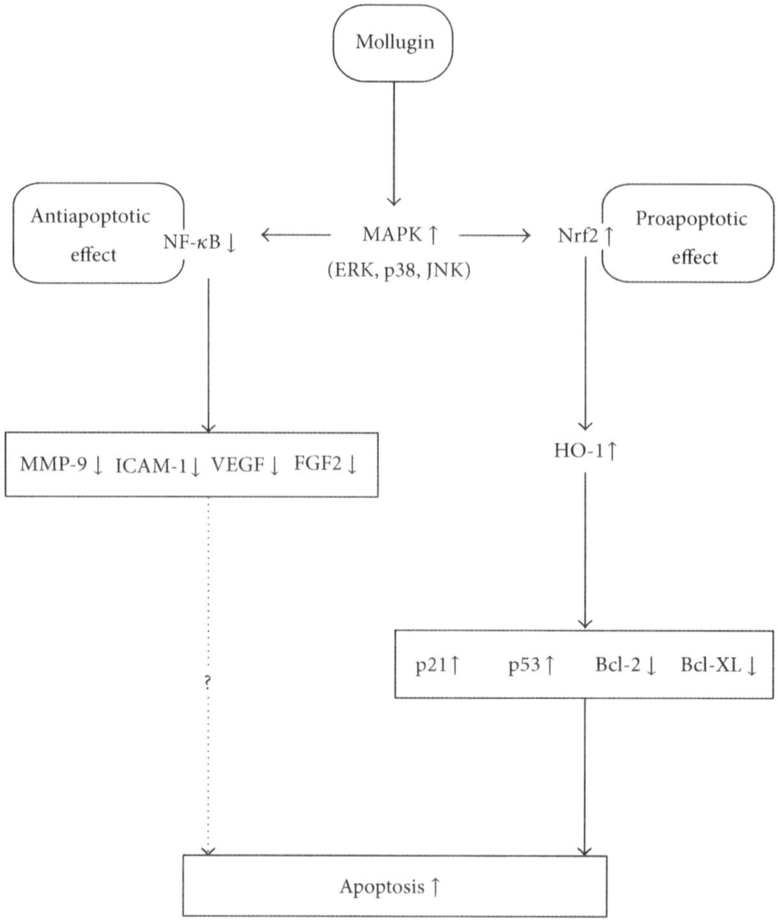

FIGURE 8: Schematic diagram illustrating the Nrf2 pathway and other signaling pathways triggered by exposure to mollugin in in OSCCs. Mollugin treatment leads to the activation of the cellular stress-dependent signaling pathways mediated by MAPK activation (ERK, JNK, and p38) and subsequent transcription factor activation (NF-κB and Nrf2). Ultimately, these transcription factors result in altered gene expression to produce cytoprotective gene HO-1, allowing lead to apoptosis.

correlated with the pathological neovascularization circumstances. Among these angiogenic factors, VEGF and FGF-2 are important angiogenic factors and essential for cancers [33]. In this study, we found that mollugin inhibited the expression of NF-κB-regulated gene products involved in invasion (MMP-9 and ICAM-1) and angiogenesis (FGF-2 and VEGF). Thus, our results demonstrate that mollugin inhibits NF-κB, leading to suppression of proliferation, invasion, and angiogenesis in OSCCs.

The MAPKs are proline-directed Ser/Thr protein kinases that regulate many cellular processes, including cell proliferation and death. JNK and p38 are activated by cellular stress and are associated with apoptosis [34]. The involvement of ERK in the induction of apoptosis by quercetin, resveratrol, and taxol has been reported [35, 36]. In the present study, phosphorylation of p38, ERK, and JNK was detected in mollugin-treated OSCCs, which is consistent with our previous reports that sappanchalcone may exert its effect on OSCCs through p38, ERK, and JNK activation [9]. Therefore, NF-κB regulation downstream of the MAPK (ERK1/2, p38, and JNK) pathways may be involved in mollugin-induced apoptosis in OSCCs. However, mollugin activated p38 MAPK in hippocampal and microglial cells [15] and ERK in HER2-overexpressing breast cancer cells [17]. Therefore, MAPK can be differentially activated, and its involvement in apoptosis is highly context and model dependent.

The role of HO-1 in tumor development is still not understood completely. Some recent reports demonstrate discordant or even completely contrasting results. Nevertheless, accumulating evidence indicates that HO-1 is expressed or overexpressed in a wide variety of human tumors and plays a critical role in the progression of neoplastic diseases [37]. For example, it has been shown that increased expression of HO-1 is associated with a higher rate of proliferation of various tumor cells [37, 38], although opposite effects have been observed in breast cancer cells [39]. Furthermore, the increased basal level of HO-1 expression in tumor cells can be further elevated by chemotherapeutics or phytochemicals, such as curcumin, carnosol, and ILME [8, 22, 23]. Our results show that mollugin upregulated HO-1 expression in a time- and dose-dependent manner (data not shown), consistent with results in hippocampal and microglial cells [15]. We found that growth inhibition and apoptosis of OSCCs by mollugin was reversed in the presence of an HO-1 inhibitor. In addition, mollugin induced downregulation of antiapoptotic Bcl-2 and Bcl-xL levels, while upregulation of apoptotic p53 and p21 levels was reversed by SnPP in a dose-dependent manner. These results suggest that the growth inhibition and apoptosis-inducing effect of mollugin is mediated via HO-1 expression.

Regarding HO-1, Nrf-2 is a relatively well-known transcription factor [40]. In response to diverse HO-1 inducers, Nrf2 translocates from the cytosol to the nucleus where it binds to the antioxidant response element in the promoter region of the HO-1 gene [41]. In our study, mollugin also induced the translocation of Nrf-2 into the nucleus, as evidenced by Western blot. Furthermore, the results of this study demonstrate a correlation between apoptotic gene upregulation and the suppression of antiapoptotic genes of OSCCs to undergo mollugin-induced growth inhibition and apoptosis when Nrf-2 is knocked down. Based on these observations, it is reasonable to conclude that Nrf2 activation mediates mollugin-induced growth inhibition and apoptosis in OSCCs.

Redox-sensitive transcription factor (NF-κB, AP-1, and Nrf2) pathways are known to be important molecular targets in chemoprevention. Activation of Nrf2 and NF-κB involves regulation of protein kinases, which may induce their nuclear translocation [42]. It was previously shown that mollugin induced apoptosis via JNK in human Jurkat T cells [14]. In this regard, specific protein kinase inhibitors of PI3 K and ERK repressed Nrf2 phosphorylation and nuclear translocation of Nrf2 and NF-κB in HepG2 cells, as previously reported in different cell types [43, 44]. The present results also suggest that the MAPK pathway plays a role in the mollugin-induced nuclear translocation of Nrf2 and NF-κB in HN4 and HN12 cells. A variety of anticarcinogenic phytochemicals suppress NF-κB signalling and activate the Nrf2-ARE pathway [45], suggesting that the suppression of NF-κB signalling and the activation of the Nrf2-ARE pathway may crosstalk with each other. Indeed, inhibition of NF-κB activation by phospholipid hydroperoxide glutathione peroxidase and 15-lipoxygenase is concomitant to upregulation of HO-1, probably via Nrf2 activation [46]. Thus, the findings support that the participation of NF-κB p65 in the negative regulation of Nrf2-ARE signalling, providing a new insight into a possible role of NF-κB in suppressing the expression of anti-inflammatory or antitumour genes [47]. Our results suggest that MAPK singnaling event mediates the link between NF-κB and Nrf2. Although the NF-κB pathway was inhibited by mollugin exposure, Nrf2 siRNA did not seem to participate in the translocation of NF-κB, suggesting that NF-κB and Nrf2 pathways might act in parallel in our *in vitro* model. A summary of our results is shown in Figure 8.

Colectivelly, our results demonstrate for the first time that mollugin inhibits cell growth and induces apoptosis in OSCCs through the NF-κB/MAPK/Nrf2/HO-1 signaling pathway. Therefore, mollugin may have potential as a chemotherapeutic agent for OSCCs. The activities of mollugin against multiple antitumor targets should be studied intensively for further clinical application either as a natural agent alone or in combination with other commonly used chemotherapeutics. Further investigation of mollugin in animal models of OSCCS will contribute to additional understanding of its *in vivo* activity toward malignant cells and its potential toxicity toward normal tissues.

Authors' Contribution

Y.-M. Lee and Q.-S. Auh contributed equally to this work as 1st author.

Acknowledgments

This work was supported by the National Research Foundation of Korea (NRF) Grant funded by the Korean Government (MEST) (no. 2012R1A5A2051384).

References

[1] H. Schliephake, "Prognostic relevance of molecular markers of oral cancer—a review," *International Journal of Oral and Maxillofacial Surgery*, vol. 32, no. 3, pp. 233–245, 2003.

[2] E. Yamachika, T. Habte, and D. Oda, "Artemisinin: an alternative treatment for oral squamous cell carcinoma," *Anticancer Research*, vol. 24, no. 4, pp. 2153–2160, 2004.

[3] J. McCann, "Texas center studies research alternative treatments," *Journal of the National Cancer Institute*, vol. 89, no. 20, pp. 1485–1486, 1997.

[4] J. Lee, H. J. Lee, J. D. Park et al., "Anti-cancer activity of highly purified sulfur in immortalized and malignant human oral keratinocytes," *Toxicology in Vitro*, vol. 22, no. 1, pp. 87–95, 2008.

[5] E. C. Kim, Y. S. Hwang, H. J. Lee et al., "Caesalpinia sappan induces cell death by increasing the expression of p53 and $p21^{WAF1/CIP1}$ in head and neck cancer cells," *The American Journal of Chinese Medicine*, vol. 33, no. 3, pp. 405–414, 2005.

[6] H. J. Lee, D. H. Son, S. K. Lee et al., "Extract of Coptidis rhizoma induces cytochrome-c dependent apoptosis in immortalized and malignant human oral keratinocytes," *Phytotherapy Research*, vol. 20, no. 9, pp. 773–779, 2006.

[7] Y. G. Yun, B. H. Jeon, J. H. Lee et al., "Verticinone induces cell cycle arrest and apoptosis in immortalized and malignant human oral keratinocytes," *Phytotherapy Research*, vol. 22, no. 3, pp. 416–423, 2008.

[8] Y. M. Lee, G. S. Jeong, H. D. Lim, R. B. An, Y. C. Kim, and E. C. Kim, "Isoliquiritigenin 2′-methyl ether induces growth inhibition and apoptosis in oral cancer cells via heme oxygenase-1," *Toxicology in Vitro*, vol. 24, no. 3, pp. 776–782, 2010.

[9] Y. M. Lee, Y. C. Kim, E. C. Kim et al., "Mechanism of sappanchalcone-induced growth inhibition and apoptosis in human oral cancer cells," *Toxicology in Vitro*, vol. 25, no. 8, pp. 1782–1788, 2011.

[10] J. K. Son, S. J. Jung, M. H. M. H. Woo et al., "Anticancer constituents from the roots of *Rubia cordifolia* L.," *Chemical Pharmacology Bulletin*, vol. 56, no. 2, pp. 213–216, 2008.

[11] L. C. Chang, D. Chavez, J. J. Gills, H. H. S. Fong, J. M. Pezzuto, and A. D. Kinghorn, "Rubiasins A-C, new anthracene derivatives from the roots and stems of *Rubia cordifolia*," *Tetrahedron Letters*, vol. 41, no. 37, pp. 7157–7162, 2000.

[12] W. P. Tse, C. H. K. Cheng, C. T. Che, M. Zhao, and Z. X. Lin, "Induction of apoptosis underlies the Radix Rubiae-mediated anti-proliferative action on human epidermal keratinocytes: implications for psoriasis treatment," *International Journal of Molecular Medicine*, vol. 20, no. 5, pp. 663–672, 2007.

[13] K. J. Kim, J. S. Lee, M. K. Kwak et al., "Anti-inflammatory action of mollugin and its synthetic derivatives in HT-29 human colonic epithelial cells is mediated through inhibition of NF-κB activation," *European Journal of Pharmacology*, vol. 622, no. 1-3, pp. 52–57, 2009.

[14] S. M. Kim, H. S. Park, D. Y. Jun et al., "Mollugin induces apoptosis in human Jurkat T cells through endoplasmic reticulum stress-mediated activation of JNK and caspase-12 and subsequent activation of mitochondria-dependent caspase cascade regulated by Bcl-xL," *Toxicology and Applied Pharmacology*, vol. 241, no. 2, pp. 210–220, 2009.

[15] G. S. Jeong, D. S. Lee, D. C. Kim et al., "Neuroprotective and anti-inflammatory effects of mollugin via up-regulation of heme oxygenase-1 in mouse hippocampal and microglial cells," *European Journal of Pharmacology*, vol. 654, no. 3, pp. 226–234, 2011.

[16] D. Y. Jun, C. R. Han, M. S. Choi, M. A. Bae, M. H. Woo, and Y. H. Kim, "Effect of mollugin on apoptosis and adipogenesis of 3T3-L1 preadipocytes," *Phytotherapy Research*, vol. 25, no. 5, pp. 724–731, 2011.

[17] M. T. Do, Y. P. Hwang, H. G. Kim, M. Na, and H. G. Jeong, "Mollugin inhibits proliferation and induces apoptosis by suppressing fatty acid synthase in HER2-overexpressing cancer cells through modulation of a HER2/Akt/SREBP-1c signaling," *Journal of Cell Physiology*, vol. 228, no. 5, pp. 1087–1097, 2012.

[18] S. K. Lee, H. I. Choi, Y. S. Yang et al., "Nitric oxide modulates osteoblastic differentiation with heme oxygenase-1 via the mitogen activated protein kinase and nuclear factor-κB pathways in human periodontal ligament cells," *Biological and Pharmaceutical Bulletin*, vol. 32, no. 8, pp. 1328–1334, 2009.

[19] S. K. Lee, S. H. Pi, S. H. Kim et al., "Substance P regulates macrophage inflammatory protein 3α/chemokine C-C ligand 20 (CCL20) with heme oxygenase-1 in human periodontal ligament cells," *Clinical and Experimental Immunology*, vol. 150, no. 3, pp. 567–575, 2007.

[20] S. H. Pi, S. C. Kim, H. T. Kim, H. J. Lee, S. K. Lee, and E. C. Kim, "Defense mechanism of heme oxygenase-1 against cytotoxic and receptor activator of nuclear factor-κB ligand inducing effects of hydrogen peroxide in human periodontal ligament cells," *Journal of Periodontal Research*, vol. 42, no. 4, pp. 331–339, 2007.

[21] K. D. Poss and S. Tonegawa, "Reduced stress defense in heme oxygenase 1-deficient cells," *Proceedings of the National Academy of Sciences of the United States of America*, vol. 94, no. 20, pp. 10925–10930, 1997.

[22] E. Balogun, M. Hoque, P. Gong et al., "Curcumin activates the haem oxygenase-1 gene via regulation of Nrf2 and the antioxidant-responsive element," *Biochemical Journal*, vol. 371, no. 3, pp. 887–895, 2003.

[23] D. Martin, A. I. Rojo, M. Salinas et al., "Regulation of heme Oxygenase-1 expression through the phosphatidylinositol 3-kinase/akt pathway and the Nrf2 transcription factor in response to the antioxidant phytochemical carnosol," *The Journal of Biological Chemistry*, vol. 279, no. 10, pp. 8919–8929, 2004.

[24] A. A. Anwar, F. Y. L. Li, D. S. Leake, T. Ishii, G. E. Mann, and R. C. M. Siow, "Induction of heme oxygenase 1 by moderately oxidized low-density lipoproteins in human vascular smooth muscle cells: role of mitogen-activated protein kinases and Nrf2," *Free Radical Biology and Medicine*, vol. 39, no. 2, pp. 227–236, 2005.

[25] M. Cardinali, H. Pietraszkiewicz, J. F. Ensley, and K. C. Robbins, "Tyrosine phosphorylation as a marker for aberrantly regulated growth-promoting pathways in cell lines derived from head and neck malignancies," *International Journal of Cancer*, vol. 61, no. 1, pp. 98–103, 1995.

[26] S. H. Pi, S. K. Lee, Y. S. Hwang, M. G. Choi, S. K. Lee, and E. C. Kim, "Differential expression of periodontal ligament-specific markers and osteogenic differentiation in human papilloma virus 16-immortalized human gingival fibroblasts and periodontal ligament cells," *Journal of Periodontal Research*, vol. 42, no. 2, pp. 104–113, 2007.

[27] S. Ghosh and M. Karin, "Missing pieces in the NF-κB puzzle," *Cell*, vol. 109, pp. S81–S96, 2002.

[28] Y. Suh, F. Afaq, J. J. Johnson, and H. Mukhtar, "A plant flavonoid fisetin induces apoptosis in colon cancer cells by inhibition of COX2 and Wnt/EGFR/NF-κB-signaling pathways," *Carcinogenesis*, vol. 30, no. 2, pp. 300–307, 2009.

[29] B. B. Aggarwal, "Nuclear factor κB, the enemy within," *Cancer Cell*, vol. 6, no. 3, pp. 203–208, 2004.

[30] G. Sethi, B. Sung, and B. B. Aggarwal, "Nuclear factor-κB activation: from bench to bedside," *Experimental Biology and Medicine*, vol. 233, no. 1, pp. 21–31, 2008.

[31] M. Bond, R. P. Fabunmi, A. H. Baker, and A. C. Newby, "Synergistic upregulation of metalloproteinase-9 by growth factors and inflammatory cytokines: an absolute requirement for transcription factor NF-κB," *FEBS Letters*, vol. 435, no. 1, pp. 29–34, 1998.

[32] C. Lawson, M. Ainsworth, M. Yacoub, and M. Rose, "Ligation of ICAM-1 on endothelial cells leads to expression of VCAM-1 via a nuclear factor-κB-independent mechanism," *Journal of Immunology*, vol. 162, no. 5, pp. 2990–2996, 1999.

[33] R. S. Kerbel, "Tumor angiogenesis: past, present and the near future," *Carcinogenesis*, vol. 21, no. 3, pp. 505–515, 2000.

[34] D. Xiao, S. Choi, D. E. Johnson et al., "Diallyl trisulfide-induced apoptosis in human prostate cancer cells involves c-Jun N-terminal kinase and extracellular-signal regulated kinase-mediated phosphorylation of Bcl-2," *Oncogene*, vol. 23, no. 33, pp. 5594–5606, 2004.

[35] Q. B. She, A. M. Bode, W. Y. Ma, N. Y. Chen, and Z. Dong, "Resveratrol-induced activation of p53 and apoptosis is mediated by extracellular-signal-regulated protein kinases and p38 kinase," *Cancer Research*, vol. 61, no. 4, pp. 1604–1610, 2001.

[36] A. Brozovic, G. Fritz, M. Christmann et al., "Long-term activation of SAPK/JNK, p38 kinase and fas-L expression by cisplatin is attenuated in human carcinoma cells that acquired drug resistance," *International Journal of Cancer*, vol. 112, no. 6, pp. 974–985, 2004.

[37] A. Jozkowicz, H. Was, and J. Dulak, "Heme oxygenase-1 in tumors: is it a false friend?" *Antioxidants and Redox Signaling*, vol. 9, no. 12, pp. 2099–2117, 2007.

[38] P. O. Berberat, Z. Dambrauskas, A. Gulbinas et al., "Inhibition of heme oxygenase-1 increases responsiveness of pancreatic cancer cells to anticancer treatment," *Clinical Cancer Research*, vol. 11, no. 10, pp. 3790–3798, 2005.

[39] M. Hill, V. Pereira, C. Chauveau et al., "Heme oxygenase-1 inhibits rat and human breast cancer cell proliferation: mutual cross inhibition with indoleamine 2,3-dioxygenase," *FASEB Journal*, vol. 19, no. 14, pp. 1957–1968, 2005.

[40] J. Alam and J. L. Cook, "Transcriptional regulation of the heme oxygenase-1 gene via the stress response element pathway," *Current Pharmaceutical Design*, vol. 9, no. 30, pp. 2499–2511, 2003.

[41] T. Ishii, K. Itoh, S. Takahashi et al., "Transcription factor Nrf2 coordinately regulates a group of oxidative stress-inducible genes in macrophages," *The Journal of Biological Chemistry*, vol. 275, no. 21, pp. 16023–16029, 2000.

[42] J. Pi, Y. Bai, J. M. Reece et al., "Molecular mechanism of human Nrf2 activation and degradation: role of sequential phosphorylation by protein kinase CK2," *Free Radical Biology and Medicine*, vol. 42, no. 12, pp. 1797–1806, 2007.

[43] T. Nguyen, P. J. Sherratt, H. C. Huang, C. S. Yang, and C. B. Pickett, "Increased protein stability as a mechanism that enhances Nrf2-mediated transcriptional activation of the antioxidant response element: degradation of Nrf2 by the 26 S proteasome," *The Journal of Biological Chemistry*, vol. 278, no. 7, pp. 4536–4541, 2003.

[44] G. Sethi, B. Sung, B. B. Aggarwal et al., "Nuclear factor-κB activation: from bench to bedside," *Experimental Biology and Medicine*, vol. 6, no. 5, pp. 515–524, 2006.

[45] J. H. Lim, H. S. Park, J. K. Choi, I. S. Lee, and J. C. Hyun, "Isoorientin induces Nrf2 pathway-driven antioxidant response through phosphatidylinositol 3-kinase signaling," *Archives of Pharmacal Research*, vol. 30, no. 12, pp. 1590–1598, 2007.

[46] W. Li, T. O. Khor, C. Xu et al., "Activation of Nrf2-antioxidant signaling attenuates NFκB-inflammatory response and elicits apoptosis," *Biochemical Pharmacology*, vol. 76, no. 11, pp. 1485–1489, 2008.

[47] A. Banning and R. Brigelius-Flohé, "NF-κB, Nrf2, and HO-1 interplay in redox-regulated VCAM-1 expression," *Antioxidants and Redox Signaling*, vol. 7, no. 7-8, pp. 889–899, 2005.

14

Antitumor Activity of Artemisinin and Its Derivatives: From a Well-Known Antimalarial Agent to a Potential Anticancer Drug

Maria P. Crespo-Ortiz[1] and Ming Q. Wei[2]

[1] *Department of Biomedical Science, Faculty of Basic and Health Science, Santiago de Cali University, Pampalinda Campus, Cali, Colombia*
[2] *Division of Molecular and Gene Therapies, Griffith Health Institute and School of Medical Science, Griffith University, Gold Coast Campus, Southport, QLD 4222, Australia*

Correspondence should be addressed to Maria P. Crespo-Ortiz, mdpcrespo@gmail.com

Academic Editor: Masa-Aki Shibata

Improvement of quality of life and survival of cancer patients will be greatly enhanced by the development of highly effective drugs to selectively kill malignant cells. Artemisinin and its analogs are naturally occurring antimalarials which have shown potent anticancer activity. In primary cancer cultures and cell lines, their antitumor actions were by inhibiting cancer proliferation, metastasis, and angiogenesis. In xenograft models, exposure to artemisinins substantially reduces tumor volume and progression. However, the rationale for the use of artemisinins in anticancer therapy must be addressed by a greater understanding of the underlying mechanisms involved in their cytotoxic effects. The primary targets for artemisinin and the chemical base for its preferential effects on heterologous tumor cells need yet to be elucidated. The aim of this paper is to provide an overview of the recent advances and new development of this class of drugs as potential anticancer agents.

1. Introduction

Cancer remains as a life-threatening disease and a leading cause of death as its control has been difficult. Although, a range of conventional therapies based on chemotherapy, surgery, and radiotherapy are available, these approaches are in many cases of limited efficacy [1]. Moreover, current anticancer regimens are frequently associated with significant levels of toxicity and the emergence of drug resistance. One major challenge to relieve cancer burden is to develop highly effective drugs with specificity on cancers but little or no side effects on normal mammalian cells.

Many research projects have been focused on developing new chemotherapies either by exploring the anticancer ability of novel compounds or by assessing drugs conventionally used in other clinical diseases. Natural products have been found to be a relevant source of novel and potent bioactive compounds with minimal side effects *in vivo*. Plant derivatives have been known to be effective against a range of diseases with broad antimicrobial activity, and some have also exhibited significant antitumor activity. One of the promising compounds is artemisinin, a naturally occurring antimalarial with anticancer properties [2]. Artemisinin and its derivatives, which are commonly used in malaria therapy, have also potent anticancer activity in the nano- to-micromolar range in sensitive and drug- or radiation-resistant cell lines [3–5]. Importantly, artemisinin is one of the very few drugs that have been widely used as antimalarials but has no significant side effects [6] or clinical resistance, although tolerance has been reported [7]. Recently, growing amount of research has focused on the mechanisms underlying the action and response to artemisinin-like drugs.

In this review, we will revisit some of the key issues in the development of artemisinin and its analogs as anticancer agents to better understand the mechanisms of their antitumor effects from the insights of new gained knowledge. By considering the benefits, limitations, and current and future development of artemisinins, we can then identify emerging questions and address future research needs in this promising field of cancer drug discovery.

2. Artemisinin and Its Derivatives

Artemisinin is a sesquiterpene lactone with a 1,2,4-tiroxane ring system (Figure 1). This endoperoxide compound is extracted from the Chinese herb *qinghaosu* (*Artemisia annua* or annual wormwood) which was used for treating fevers for over two millennia [8]. Despite its efficacy, the prototype drug, artemisinin, has pharmacokinetic limitations. Naturally, artemisinin has low solubility in water or oil, poor bioavailability, and a short half-life *in vivo* (~2.5 h) [9, 10]. To overcome some of these problems, three generations of artemisinin-like endoperoxides including semisynthetic derivatives and fully synthetic compounds have been developed. So far, two generations of semisynthetic derivatives of artemisinin such as artesunate, arteeter, artemether, and artemisone have been effectively used as antimalarials with good clinical efficacy and tolerability (Figure 1).

Semisynthetic artemisinins are obtained from dihydroartemisinin (DHA), the main active metabolite of artemisinin [11, 12]. The first generation of semisynthetic artemisinins includes arteeter and artemether, the lipophilic artemisinins, whereas artesunate is the water soluble derivative [11, 12]. Artemisone, a second-generation artemisinin, has shown improved pharmacokinetic properties including longer half-life and lower toxicity [13]. So far, artesunate is the derivative that is commonly used in the antimalarial combination therapy.

Fully synthetic artemisinin derivatives have also been designed by preserving the peroxide moiety which confers potent drug activity. These compounds are easily synthesized from simple starting materials, thus being currently under intense development [14–17].

3. Antitumor Mechanism of Action of Artemisinin

In the malaria parasite, the endoperoxide moiety of artemisinin has been shown to be pharmacologically important and responsible of the antimalarial activity [18, 19]. The endoperoxide bond is thought to be activated by reduced heme (FPFeII) or ferrous iron (FeII) [20], leading to cytotoxic carbon-centered radicals which are highly potent alkylating agents [21]. Radicals may target essential parasite macromolecules causing parasite's death. However, the precise mechanism of action and primary target of artemisinin remain under study. In *Plasmodium*, it has been postulated that artemisinin may target organelles such as the mitochondrion, endoplasmic reticulum, and the digestive vacuole (reviewed in [22]). Some postulated molecular targets include heme alkylation, protein alkylation, Ca^{2+} ATPase (SERCA) inhibition, membrane damage, and loss of mitochondrial potential (reviewed in [22]). Despite the continuous debate on artemisinin activation and specific targets, supporting evidence points that heme or ferrous iron is required for potent activity [23]. This observation has been substantiated in other systems. In *Schistosomas*, artemether has an exquisite action against the tegument; this activity is also enhanced by iron [24].

Interestingly, the potent anticancer action of artemisinin can also be attributed to the endoperoxide bond (red square in Figure 2) and shares the same parasitical chemical base. Lack of the endoperoxide moiety does not completely abrogate anticancer activity [25] but significantly reduces cytotoxicity to only fiftieth compared to those compounds with the trioxane ring [26–28]. Residual anticancer activity may be associated with an alternative peroxide-independent mechanism [26]. In a general consensus, iron and heme or heme-bound proteins have been involved in the bioreductive activation of artemisinin [29–31]. In most of the systems, preloading of cancer cells with iron or iron-saturated holotransferrin (diferric transferrin) triggers artemisinin cytotoxicity [32–35] with an increase in artemisinin activity up to 100-fold in some cell lines [36]. Moreover, artemisinins tagged to iron-carrying compounds exhibit greater activity compared with that of artemisinin alone [37–39]. Recently, it was shown that chemical modulation using succinylacetone, a heme synthesis inhibitor, decreases DHA cytotoxicity in HL-60 (human promyelocytic leukemia cells) [35]. This was consistent with previous studies showing that induction of heme oxidase followed by downregulation of the heme synthesis genes may also inhibit cytotoxicity of novel artemisinin dimers in the same cancer line [40]. Similarly, treatment with desferroxamine (DFO), an iron chelator, renders compounds inactive [41]. Iron and heme metabolism may have a relevant role in the selective antitumor activity of artemisinin. Continued proliferation and growth of malignant cells require higher iron metabolism to achieve processes of cell survival [35]. Therefore, cancer cells exhibit an increase in transferrin receptors (TfR) which are responsible for the iron uptake and regulation of intracellular concentrations. Levels of expression of TfR in cancer cells may vary depending on the cell line. However, they differ substantially from normal cells leading to a high selectivity index of artemisinin and its derivatives. Efferth et al. reported that leukemia (CCRF-CEM) and astrocytoma (U373) cells express TfR in 95% and 43% of the cell population, whereas normal monocytes only account for approximately 1% [42, 43]. Blocking the TfR by pretreatment with specific monoclonal antibodies abrogates artemisinin activity [43].

It has been hypothesized that iron-activated artemisinin induces damage by release of highly alkylating carbon-centered radicals and radical oxygen species (ROS) (Figure 2) [28, 35]. Radicals may play a role in the cell alterations reported in artemisinin-treated cancer cells such as enhanced apoptosis, arrest of growth, inhibition of angiogenesis, and DNA damage (Figure 2). Several studies have also associated artemisinin toxicity with impaired cytokinesis, enhanced levels of oxidative stress, inhibition of tumor invasion, migration, and metastasis (reviewed in [44]). ROS generation may contribute with the selective action of artemisinin on cancer cells. Tumor cells have enhanced vulnerability to ROS damage as they exhibit lower expression of antioxidant enzymes such as superoxide dismutase, catalase, and gluthatione peroxidase compared to that of normal cells [45, 46]. Hence, increasing oxidative stress is a common anticancer

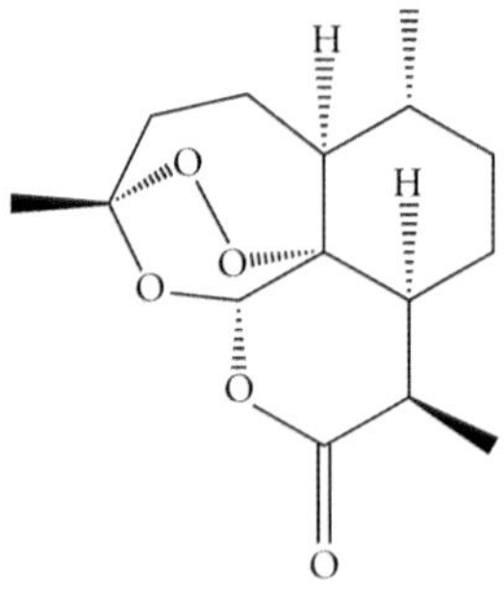

(1)

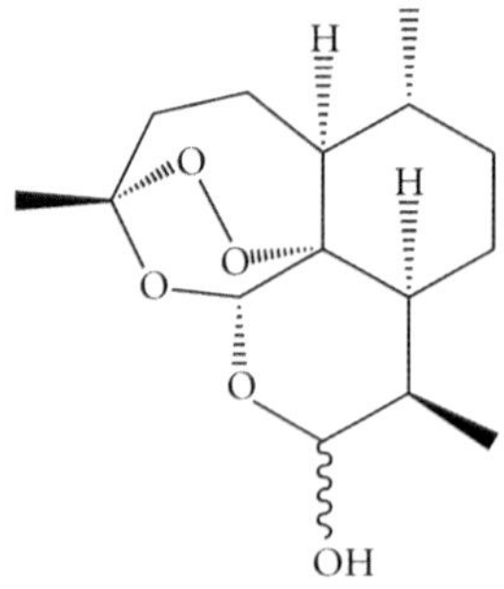

(2)

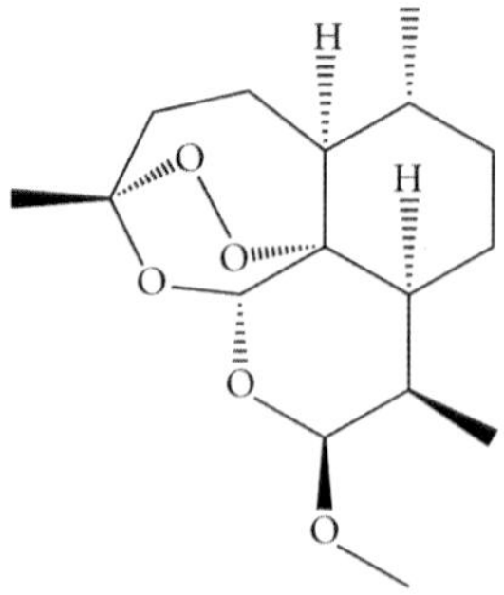

(3)

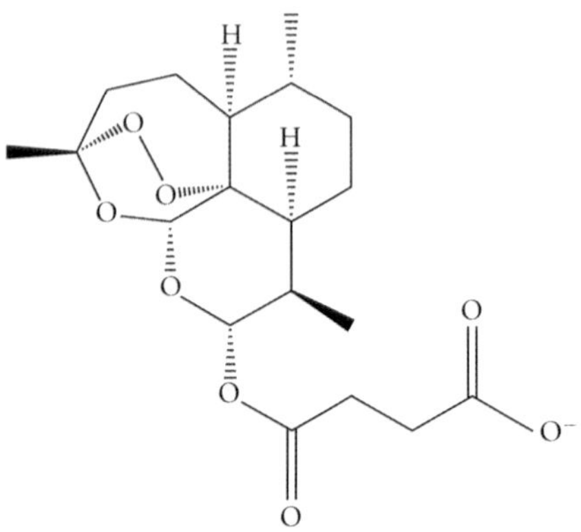

(4)

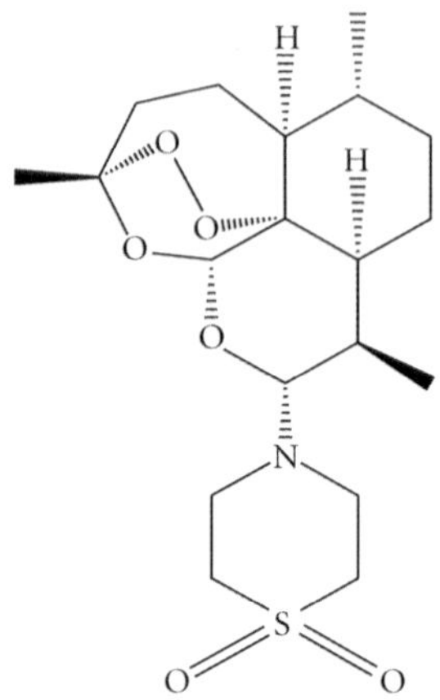

(5)

Figure 1: Chemical structure of artemisinin antimalarials (artemisinins) with anticancer activity. Artemisinin (1), dihydroartemisinin (DHA) (2), artemether (3), artesunate (4), and artemisone (5).

mechanism of antitumor agents [47]. In addition, the selectivity of artemisinin may be boosted by preferential targeting of cancer biomarkers or overexpressed cancer genes and proteins which are not detectable in normal differentiated tissues [48].

3.1. Generation of ROS as a Primary Effector of Cytotoxicity. As in *Plasmodium*, the artemisinin molecular targets in cancer cells are debatable. Although artemisinin-induced alterations in some tumor cells are consistent, it is not clear if this toxicity resides in defined molecular targets. Drug concentrations required to have an effect on cancer cells are often higher than those inducing toxicity in malaria parasites. Artemisinin, DHA, artesunate, and artemether exhibit 48 h IC_{50}s (fifty percent inhibitory concentration) up to 15 nM in malaria parasites [49, 50], whereas their anticancer activity is cell-line dependent and IC_{50}s fluctuate between 0.5 and $\geq 200\,\mu$M [5]. The exquisite sensitivity of malaria parasites to artemisinin points to the presence of specific parasitic targets. By contrast, in cancer cells, the artemisinin effect seems to be rather mediated by more general mechanisms through generation of ROS. However, it has been suggested that ROS-mediated damage may be triggered by an initiating event in the vicinity of artemisinin activation [35]. Microscopy analyses in artesunate-treated cells have shown early oncosis-like morphological changes at subcellular structures in which ROS generation may be triggered [51].

Microarray analyses found that the action of artemisinin seems to be modulated by the expression of oxidative stress enzymes including catalase, thioredoxin reductase, superoxide dismutase and the glutathione S-transferase family [5, 52]. Artemisinin-sensitive cells have downregulated oxidation enzymes whereas overexpression of these molecules renders cancer cells less sensitive [5]. Direct evidence in the HL-60 cell line has revealed that early and rapid generation (1 h) of ROS has been associated with apoptosis induction and artemisinin-induced damage. Furthermore, IC_{50} has been directly correlated with ROS levels [52]. Conversely, the action of artemisinin in several experimental systems has been reverted in presence of the antioxidant agents, N-acetyl cysteine, and 1,2-dihydroxybenzene-3,5-disulfonic acid (TIRON, an iron scavenger), which resulted in a delay in cell death [40, 52, 53]. A recent study has demonstrated that generation of ROS in artesunate-treated HeLa cells (16 h) occurring before cytotoxicity is being detected (48 h) [35], suggesting that this may be the starting event in artemisinin-induced damage. The electron transfer chain (ETC) in the mitochondrion has been proposed to play a role in the generation of ROS, however substantial cytotoxicity is still detected in HeLa cells devoid of ETC indicating that other sources of ROS may be available in the cells [35]. Indeed, emerging evidence has postulated that oxidative stress in breast cancer cells is initially generated in the lysosome as consequence of iron-activated artesunate in a process

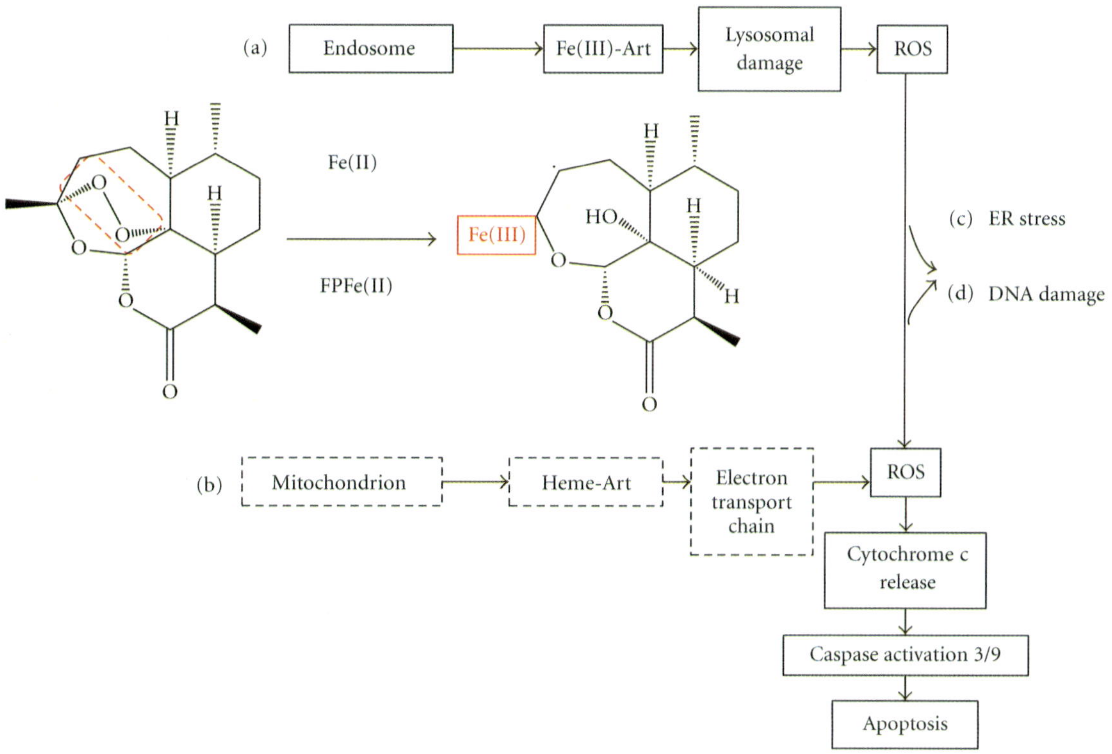

FIGURE 2: Postulated anticancer mechanisms of action of artemisinins. (a) It has been postulated that bioactivation of artemisinin occurs in the endosome after pH-induced release of iron from internalized transferrin. Iron activated-artemisinin generates carbon-centered radicals which may mediate lysosomal disruption and generation of ROS resulting in mitochondrial damage, activation of caspases, and cell death. (b) Alternatively, it has been suggested that only specific activation of artemisinin by heme or heme-bound protein generates cytotoxic-carbon-centered radicals. In the mitochondrion, these adducts interfere with the electron transfer chain (ETC) by interacting with heme or heme-bound proteins leading to generation of ROS and apoptosis. (c) ROS harboring may induce ER stress and (d) genotoxicity.

similar to that suggested in malaria parasites [31]. Thus, activation of the mitochondrial intrinsic apoptotic pathway is a downstream event leading to cell death [31] (Figure 2). In this model, artemisinins may be negatively controlling heme synthesis and further increase cytotoxicity [31].

Despite the growing evidence of ROS-mediated damage in many cell systems [31, 33, 35, 54], cell damage has been also independently associated with oxidative stress [35]. Particularly, novel artemisinin dimers seem to exert antitumor action with little or no ROS generation, however the underlying mechanism of cytotoxicity is still under study [26]. It also remains unclear if artemisinins-induced necrosis may be a ROS-independent mechanism of cell death [35].

The antineoplastic toxicity of artemisinins appears to be also modulated by calcium metabolism [40, 55–57], endoplasmic reticulum (ER) stress [33, 40], and the expression of the translationally controlled tumor protein, TCTP, a binding calcium protein which has been also postulated as a parasite target [5]. Although the expression of the TCTP gen, *tctp,* was initially correlated with cancer cell response to artemisinins, a functional role for TCTP in the artemisinin action has yet to be found [58].

As for malaria parasites, the role of sarcoendoplasmic Ca^{2+} ATPase (SERCA) as artemisinin target in cancer cells has also been explored [40]. Previous evidence has revealed that treatment with $10\,\mu$M artemisinin increases calcium concentrations as a result of SERCA inhibition [59]. However, studies on the mechanism of action of two artemisinin dimers have shown that potent ROS-mediated induced ER-stress after treatment was independent of SERCA inhibition [40]. Interestingly, the behavior of a highly active artemisinin dimer and thapsigargin, a well-known SERCA inhibitor, seems to be similar but mediated by different molecular events [40]. In fact, thapsigargin lacks the endoperoxide moiety and only generates discrete ROS levels. Nevertheless the ER appears to be a relevant site for artemisinin action as in HepG2 cells a fluorescent derivative has been shown to preferentially accumulate in this cell compartment [60].

Artemisinins have shown pleiotropic effects through different experimental systems. It is also possible that the underlying mechanisms mediating artemisinins cytotoxicity may vary upon specific hallmarks or shifting characteristics in cancer cell lines (Table 1). This will be only possible to elucidate if the molecular events involved in countering malignant cell proliferation are investigated in different cell lines under similar conditions.

4. Artemisinins as Anticancer Drugs

4.1. Antitumor Effects of Artemisinin and Its Derivatives. Significant antitumor activity of artemisinin and licensed semisynthetic artemisinin derivatives has been documented

TABLE 1: Factors that may influence artemisinins response in cancer cells.

System	Factor/characteristic
Cancer cell	Proliferating activity
	Expression of transferrin receptors
	Accumulation levels of iron
	Levels of gene expression (i.e., proapoptotic and antiapoptotic genes)
	Shifting hallmarks
	Overexpression of potential molecular targets in some tumors
	Cellular dependence on redox balance
	Expression of antioxidant enzymes
	Expression of estrogen receptors in breast cancer cells
Artemisinin compound	Dose and time of exposure
	Chemical structure: number of trioxane rings, for example, dimeric compounds can be up to >1000 fold-more potent than monomeric artemisinins [61]
	In dimeric endoperoxides: nature and stereochemistry of the linker
	In novel compounds, electrophilic substitutions in the ring or those conferring lipophilicity. Boat/chair conformation

in vitro and in animal models. Considerable research has been focused on the most active compounds, namely, DHA and artesunate. One study that tested 55 cell lines from the Developmental Therapeutics Program of the National Cancer Institute (NCI) showed that artesunate displays inhibitory activity against leukemia, colon, melanoma, breast, ovarian, prostate, central nervous system (CNS), and renal cancer cells [5]. Dihydroartemisinin has also remarkable antineoplastic activity against pancreatic, leukemic, osteosarcoma, and lung cancer cells [62]. Moreover, artemisone has shown better activity than artemisinin and considerable synergistic interactions with other anticancer agents [63].

Artemisinin has been found to act either directly by inducing DNA damage (genotoxicity) or indirectly by interfering with a range of signaling pathways involved in several hallmarks of malignancy. However, direct DNA damage is only described in specific systems, while indirect effects are more commonly refereed in the literature. In pancreatic cells (Panc-1), artesunate caused DNA fragmentation and membrane damage. Interestingly, low doses of artesunate were associated with oncosis-like cell death, whereas higher concentrations induce apoptosis [51]. Extend and type of damage seem to depend on the phenotype and the origin of cell line, and it may also vary in a time- and dose-dependent manner (Table 1). Notably, higher sensitivity to artesunate was observed in rapidly growing cell lines when compared with slow growing cancer cells [5].

Alternatively, DHA, artesunate, and artemether are likely to modulate genes and proteins coordinating growth signals, apoptosis, proliferation capacity, angiogenesis and tissue invasion, and metastasis. A complex network of interactions through different pathways may enhance the anticancer effect of these endoperoxide drugs leading to cancer control and cell death (Table 2).

4.1.1. Artemisinins Counter Cancer Proliferative Capacity. In normal cells, cyclin-dependent kinases (CDK) are the proteins translating signals in order to push cell through the cell cycle. Normal growth relies on the ability to translate signals in order to replicate and divide in an effective manner [64]. Uncontrolled proliferation in cancer cells is the result of mutations inducing amplification of growth signals, deregulation of checkpoints, and loss of sensitivity to growth inhibitors [65]. Abnormal cell growth is also triggered by deregulation of programmed cell death or apoptosis [65]. Artemisinin and its semisynthetic derivatives are able to effectively induce cell growth arrest in cancer lines either by disrupting the cell cycle kinetics or by interfering with proliferation-interacting pathways. Dihydroartemisinin and artesunate are very potent growth inhibitors with multiple studies pointing to DHA as the most potent anticancer artemisinin-like compound (DHA > artesunate > arteeter > artemether) [5, 66]. Recently, artemisone has shown impressive antitumor efficacy in 7 cells lines including melanoma and breast cancer cells [63]. Artemisinin compounds have been shown to exert cytostatic and cytotoxic action on cancer cells [63, 67]. Artemisinin-induced growth arrest has been reported at all cell cycle phases; however, arrest at G_0/G_1 to S transition seems to be more commonly affected [5] (Table 2). Arrest at all cell cycle phases at the same time has been interpreted as a cytostatic effect [63]. Disruption of the cell cycle at G_2/M was observed after DHA treatment in osteosacorma, pancreas, leukemia [68] and ovarian cancer cells [69] (Table 2). Similarly, artesunate interferes with G_2 in osteosarcoma, ovarian, and other different cancer lines (Table 2). The underlying mechanisms of artemisinins-induced growth arrest include alterations in the expression and activity of regulatory enzymes of the cell cycle, such as CDK2-4 and -6 and D type cyclins (G_1-to-S-phase transition) or CDK1, and A-type cyclin (G_2/M) [70–72]. The antiproliferative action of artemisinin induces downregulation of CDK transcription, inhibition of CDK promoters or increase of p21, p27, and CDK inhibitor [72] (Table 2). Inhibition of proliferation may be also attributed to downregulation of interacting proteins targeting multiple pathways [72]. It has

TABLE 2: Antitumor effects of artemisinins.

Cmpd	Cancer/cell line	Effect	Event/mechanism	Refs
DHA/ART	Osteosarcoma	Growth arrest	G_2/M, decreased survivin	[73]
	4 cell lines with different p53 status	Apoptosis	Increased Bax, activation of caspase 3,8,9 Decreased Bc12, Cdc25B, cyclin B1, NF-κB	[44]
DHA	Hepatoma (different cell lines)	Growth arrest	G_1, decreased cyclin D, E, CDK2-4, E2F1 Increased Cip 1/p21, Kip 1/p27	[67]
		Apoptosis	Increased Bax/Bcl2 ratio, activation of caspase 3 Increased poly ADP-ribose polymerase Decreased MDM2	
DHA/ART	Neuroblastoma	Growth arrest	G_1	[52]
		Apoptosis	Activation of caspase 3	
DHA	Pancreas (BxPC3 RFP)	Growth arrest	G_1, decreased cyclin D1, increased p21	[74]
		Apoptosis	Increased Bax, decreased Bcl2	[74, 75]
		Angiogenesis	Decreased VEGF	[75, 76]
			Decreased NF-κB DNA binding	[74, 76]
			IL-8, COX2, MMP9	[76]
DHA	Human promyelocytic	Growth arrest	G_1	[33, 34]
	Leukemia (HL-60)	Apoptosis	ER stress, degradation of c-MYC	[33]
	Colorectal cancer (HT116)		Increased GRP78	[34]
			DNA damage	[33]
DHA	Lung cancer (SPCA1)	Apoptosis	Decreased survivin	[56]
	(PC-14)		Increased calcium levels, increased p38 MAPK	[57]
	(ASTC-a-l)		Increased oxidation, activation caspase 3,9,8 Bax translocation	[54]
DHA/ARS	Human ovarian cancer (cell panel, A2780, OVCAR-3)	Growth arrest	G_2	[69]
		Apoptosis	Increased Bax-Bad, decreased Bclx-Bcl2	[69, 77]
			Activation caspase 3/9 pathway	[69, 77]
DHA	Lymphatic endothelial cells	Apoptosis	Increased Bax, decreased Bcl2 Decreased VEGFR-3/FL-4	[78]
DHA	Melanoma (A375, G361, LOX)	Apoptosis	Increased oxidative stress, increased NOXA Activation caspase 3	[79]
DHA	Jurkat T Lymphoma	Apoptosis	DNA damage Increased oxidation, increased NOXA Increased Bak, activation of caspase 9	[80]
DHA	Fibrosarcoma (HT 1080)	Migration/invasion	Decreased NF-κB, AP-1 Decreased activation of MMP2, MMP9 Decreased PKC α/Raf/ERK and JNK	[81]
DHA	Glioma cells (C6)	Apoptosis	Decreased HIF 1α, VEGF	[41]
DHA	Chronic myeloid leukemia (K562 cells)	Growth arrest	G_2, decreased PCNA, cyclin B1, D1, E1	[82]
			CDK2-4, E2F1, DNA-PK, DNA-topo1, JNK VEGF	[68]
ART		Angiogenesis	Decreased VECF	[82]
DHA	Lewis lung carcinoma	Angiogenesis	Decreased VEGF-C, IL-1 β-induced p38 MAPK activation	[83]
			Decreased VEGF receptor KDR/flk-1	[84]
DHA/ART	Cervix carcinoma (HeLa) Human papillomavirus immortalized/transformed cells	Apoptosis	Activation of caspase 9	[85]
ART	Leukemia, melanoma, non-small cell lung cancer, colon, renal, ovarian, prostate, CNS; prostate, breast cancer (NIC cell panel)	Growth arrest	G_0/G_1, decreased CDK2, CDC25A G_2/M, decreased cyclin B1	[5]

Table 2: Continued.

Cmpd	Cancer/cell line	Effect	Event/mechanism	Refs
ART	Endometrial carcinoma (HEC-1B)	Growth arrest	G_0/G_1	[86]
		Apoptosis	Activation of caspase 3, decreased COX-2	
		Angiogenesis	Increased E-cadherin	
ART	Pancreatic cancer (BxPC3, MiaPaCa-2)	Apoptosis	Activation of caspases 3, 7 Inhibition of topoisomerase II a	[87]
ART	Non-small cell lung cancer (SPC-A1)	Metastasis	Decreased MMP2, transactivation of AP-1	[56, 88]
			NF-κB	
			uPA promoter	[88]
			MMP7	[56]
ART	Colorectal (CLY, HT29, Lovo)	Metastasis	Increased E cadherin Decreased Wnt-signalling pathway	[89]
ART	Mouse myeloma cell line SP2/0	Growth arrest	G_0/G_1	[90]
		Apoptosis	Decreased NF-κB p65, increased IκBα	
ARS	Hepatocellular cancer cells (HepG2, SMMC-7721)	Metastasis	Increased TIMP2, Cdc42, E cadherin	[91]
			Decreased MMP2	
	Nasopharyngeal cancer lines (CNE-1 and CNE-2)	Growth arrest	G_1	[92]
	Melanoma (A375P, A375M)	Growth arrest	—	[93]
		Migration	Decreased MMP2, $\alpha v\beta 3$ integrin	
ATM	Colorectal (HCT116, SW480)	Growth arrest	G_1, S, G_2, decreased CDK1	[63]
			All phases	
	Breast (MCF-7)		G_1, decreased CDK4, cyclin D1	

Abbreviations: Cmpd: compound; DHA: Dihydroartemisinin; ART: artesunate, ARS: artemisinin, ATM: artemisone.

been shown that DHA treatment in pancreatic cells (BxPC3, AsPC-1) inhibits viability by decreasing levels of proliferating cell nuclear antigen (PCNA) and cyclin D with parallel increase in p21 [74]. Another study in the same system shows that DHA counters NF-κB factor activation leading to inhibition of its targets in the proliferation (c-myc, cyclin D) and apoptotic pathways (Bcl2, Bcl-xl) [94]. Downregulation of survivin, a protein modulating apoptosis and G_2/M cell cycle progression [95], was observed after treatment with DHA in lung cancer cells (SPC-A1) [94]. A similar effect was described by Qiang et al. in artesunate- treated osteosarcoma cells [44]. In prostate cancer, DHA induces cell cycle arrest by disrupting the interaction of Sp1 (specificity protein 1) and the CDK4 promoter [96]. Dissociation of the Sp1-CDK4 complex promotes caspase activation and cell death. In addition one work has identified artesunate as a topoisomerase II, an inhibitor which inhibits growth by interaction with multiple pathways [87]. Overall, artemisinins seem to be interfering with several pathways that are common to different cancer entities.

4.1.2. Proapoptotic Effect of Artemisinins. Apoptosis is a widely studied mechanism in antitumor therapy as its manipulation is an effective strategy for cancer control. This cellular process is mediated by a balance between the Bcl2 family genes, the proapoptotic Bax, and the antiapoptotic Bcl2 and their effects on the mitochondria [97, 98]. An increase in the Bax/Bcl2 ratio induces the release of cytochrome c followed by sequential activation of caspases and culminating with cell death [98].

Apoptosis is a common and rapid artemisinin-induced effect observed in many cancer and cell lines. Treatment with 200 μM DHA in leukemia cells induced apoptosis after 1 hour of exposure [32]. Artemisinin sensitivity has been correlated to the level of expression of antiapoptotic (Bcl2) and proapoptotic genes (Bax) in a cancer cell line [61, 97, 99] (Table 1). In general, the apoptotic effects of artemisinin have been attributed to activation of the intrinsic pathway. Hence, mitochondrial membrane damage is thought to have a pivotal role in the cascade of cell death events. Many studies have revealed that artemisinin-like compounds induce apoptosis by modulating the Bax/Bcl2 ratio [33, 44, 54, 63, 75, 77, 78, 86, 99]. Consistent with these observations, DHA and artesunate, in a panel of osteosarcoma cells, caused cytochrome c release, Bax overexpression, increase in Bax/Bcl2 ratio [44, 73], and activation of caspases 3 and 9. DHA also activates caspase 8 and decreases the levels of CDC25B, cyclin B1, and NF-κB [73]. In the same system, artesunate exposure depletes survivin which has also been involved in the apoptotic DHA response in lung cancer cells [56]. Similar events have been described in hepatoma cancer lines treated with DHA, particularly in this system DHA and the prototype drug artemisinin seem to have similar potency [67]. A microarray analysis has correlated the expression levels of c-MYC with enhanced DHA-induced apoptosis. Leukemia (HL-60) and colon cancer cells (HCT116) expressing high levels of c-MYC are significantly more sensitive to the DHA proapoptotic action. Moreover, knockdown of *c-myc* in HCT116 depleted DHA-associated cell death [33]. Downregulation of *c-myc* may also correlate with induced G_1 arrest in this cell line [33]. Studies in metastatic melanoma (A375, G361 cell line) and Jurkat T lymphoma cells have associated the elevated apoptotic action of DHA with upregulation of NOXA (a proapoptotic protein), caspase 3 activation, and oxidative stress [79, 80]. In lung cells, the apoptotic effect of DHA occurs with increasing calcium concentration and activation of p38 [56, 57].

In some studies alterations on molecules acting on the extrinsic apoptotic pathway have also been described [54]. DHA seems to increase the transcription of the cell death receptor 5 (DR5) promoter and induces DR5 in different prostate cancer lines. In fact, a combination treatment with TRAIL, a DR5 ligand, strongly enhances DHA proapoptotic action by up to 35% on this system [100].

Artemisinins usually promote apoptosis rather than necrosis in most of the systems, however in some cases both apoptosis and necrosis have been reported. Induction of apoptosis is a major benefit of artemisinins' antitumor action as it prevents the collateral effects of inflammation and cell damage caused by necrosis. Artemisinin-induced necrosis has been associated with low levels of ATP and defective apoptotic mechanisms in some cell lines [35].

4.1.3. Artemisinins and Metastasis/Invasion Inhibition. The ability of malignant cells to invade has been associated with high mortality and morbidity in cancer patients. The spread of cancer cells to other organs is a process in which malignant cells readily invade through the extracellular matrix, reach and survive in the bloodstream, and finally seed at distant organs [101]. To achieve invasion, the cancer cell requires the loss of expression or function of E-cadherin, a calcium-binding transmembrane molecule involved in cell-cell adhesion. A range of genes encoding extracellular matrix processing proteases, motility factors, and adhesion proteins are also acting at different steps in the metastatic process [101]. Recently, PAI-1 and TIMP-1 known as endogenous protease inhibitors have also been shown to be involved in cancer metastasis [102]. An invaluable benefit of artemisinin is its relevant antimigratory activity in highly aggressive and invasive cancer entities [56, 59, 88, 91]. Antimetastatic activity of artemisinins has been correlated with modified expression of the matrix metalloproteinases (MMP) gene family and their effects on $\alpha v\beta 3$ integrins [93]. In hepatoma cells (HepG2 and SMMC 7721), treatment with 12.5 μM artemisinin depleted migration linked to a decrease in MMP2 with concomitant increase in TIMP-2. Inhibition of metastasis is achieved as artemisinin increases cell-cell adhesion by enhancing E-cadherin activity and Cdc42 activation [91]. In addition, it has been found that some cancer cells may have specific proteins cointeracting at different pathways. For example, in non-small cell lung cancer [56] and fibrosarcoma, DHA treatment induced low levels of MMP2, MMP7, or MMP9 driven by AP-1 and NF-κB transactivation or inactivation [81]. Previous studies have shown that MMP2 is regulated by Sp-1 transcription factor activity [103], moreover DHA-induced disruption of Sp-1 molecular interactions has been postulated as a crucial event for DHA regulation effects on different pathways [72]. Other investigations have found that in mouse lung Lewis cancer, lymphoid node metastasis and lymphangiogenesis were retarded by artemisinin-mediated inhibition of vascular endothelial growth factor C (VGF-C) [83].

4.1.4. Artemisinins and Angiogenesis Inhibition. As malignant tissues grow, metastases and solid tumors require extra blood supply for thriving and survival. Thus, cancer cells induce neovascularisation by regulating proteins and pathways involved in the generation and restructure of new vasculature [101]. Angiogenesis process leads to enhanced proliferation of endothelial cells through induction of vascular endothelial growth factor (VEGF), fibroblast growth factor (FGF), its receptors, and cytokines [101]. This event occurs via multiple mechanisms including hypoxia-driven activation of expression of HIF-1α and the aryl hydrocarbon receptor nuclear translocator (ARNT) [104]. Angiogenesis control is mediated by angiostatin, endostatin, thrombospondin, TIMPs, PAI-1, and others [101]. Due to their role in tumor survival, the proangiogenic factors and the molecules involved in their regulatory networks are relevant drug targets. A microarray-based study revealed that artemisinins, artesunate and other derivatives inhibit neovascularisation by modulating gene expression of angiogenic factors [105]. Artemisinins responses seem to be mediated by downregulation of growth factors (VEGF, FGF) [82, 106], HIF-1α [107], new vessel mediator angiogenin (ANG), the cysteine-rich angiogenic inducer (CYR61), some metalloproteinases (MMP9, MMP11, and BMP1), and collagens [105]. In parallel, artemisinins- induced upregulation of angiogenesis inhibitors was observed [105]. These findings have been supported by experimental investigation in different systems, unveiling other molecular interactions. Exposure of human umbilical vein endothelial cells to 50 μM DHA prevents angiogenesis by depleting the levels of the VEGF flt-1 and KDR/flk-1-receptors. Similar effects were reproduced in lymphatic endothelial cells and Lewis lung carcinoma [78, 84]. In pancreatic cells (BxPc-3) and BalB/c nude mice, DHA induced inhibition of NF-κB DNA binding and downregulation of its angiogenic-related targets such as VEGF, IL-8, COX2, and MMP9 [76]. Reduced levels of NF-κB have been previously associated with proliferation and metastasis inhibition [33, 81, 90, 94] suggesting that NF-κB regulation may be a key role in the multimodal action of DHA in this system. NF-κB is a crucial factor regulating multiple processes and it has a key role in the anticancer drug response. It is activated by DNA damage and it is a mediator of apoptosis resistance in response to drug pressure.

Other anticancer properties have also been attributed to artemisinins. Artesunate has shown its ability to revert cellular transitions allowing re-differentiation of tissues by negative control of Wnt-signaling pathway [89]. Notably, artesunate has been found to be more effective in less differentiated cell lines [89].

4.2. Antitumor Action of Artemisinins in Resistant Cancer Cells. One major obstacle for a successful anticancer therapy is the development of resistance over time. Many aggressive tumors become refractory to anticancer therapy with hardly any chemotherapeutic alternatives. A leading cause of drug resistance is the drug efflux generated by overexpression of membrane protein pumps, which results in ineffective low drug concentrations [108]. Anticancer activity of artemisinins has shown to be unaffected in otherwise resistant and multiresistant cancer cells. One study using the 55 NCI cell lines and microarray analysis revealed that genes related with resistance to the established anticancer drugs such as *MDR1 (Pgp), MRP1,* and *BCRP* showed no impact on the activity of artemisinins [5]. This was substantiated when no effects on the artesunate growth inhibition profile were observed in multidrug resistance HL-60 cell lines overexpressing *MRP-1* and *BCRP*-overexpressing cells, suggesting that antitumor activity of artemisinin is preserved when resistance to other agents is present [5]. Artemisinins are effective in a broad range of resistant cancer lines including doxorubicin, metrotexate, and hydroxyurea-resistant lines with no cross-resistance [5]. Further investigation has shown that artesunate proapoptotic effect is not affected in a doxorubicin-resistant leukemia cell line; instead artesunate potentiates doxorubicin apoptotic effects [4]. In another study, anticancer potency of artesunate is preserved in chemoresistant and chemosensitive neuroblastoma cell lines and primary neuroblastoma cultures [52]. In this system, sensitivity to artesunate was not affected in vincristin, doxorubicin, cisplastin, topotecan, mephalan, and ectoposide-adapted cells with IC_{50}s ranging from 1.4–2.7 μM similar to that of the parent sensitive cell line [52]. Only one cell line showed low sensitivity to artesunate which was related to low ROS formation and increased expression of gluthatione cysteine ligase (GCL) [52]. Depletion of glutathione mediated by a GCL inhibitor improved artesunate sensitivity in this cell line [52]. P-glycoprotein (Pgp) or p53 attenuation did not affect sensitivity to artesunate [52]. DHA has shown the lowest IC_{50} in some cell lines such as cholangiocarcinoma (CL-6) and hepatocarcinoma (Hep G2) compared to other anticancer agents; moreover, upregulation of *MDR1, MRP1-2,* or *MRP3* shows no effect on potency [109]. Lack of cross resistance between anticancer agents and artemisinins might be based on different mechanisms of drug action and/or resistance. Most of the conventional anticancer agents are nucleoside analogs, whereas artemisinins action is thought to be mediated by a ROS-dependent mechanism. Furthermore, in erythromyelogenous leukemia and human small cell lung cancer, artemisinins show no significant inhibition towards Pgp or MRP1 [4], thus in principle overexpression of protein pump may not affect artemisinin's potency. In another system however, artemisinin (the prototype drug) increases doxorubicin resistance by upregulating *mdrp* through a mechanism that will be discussed later.

4.3. Interactions of Artemisinins and Standard Anticancer Chemotherapy: Artemisinin Combination Therapy (ACT) for Cancer? Existing anticancer therapies predominantly target cancer proliferation either with chemotherapeutic agents, ionizing radiation or direct toxicity on growth factor signaling pathways. In a combination therapy for cancer, the antineoplastic action of artemisinin may contribute to an independent antitumor activity with no additional side effects. The benefits of combining artemisinins with other anticancer agents have been investigated showing that multifactorial action of artemisinin in different pathways may improve overall activity (synergism).

It has been reported that resistant cancer cell lines become sensitive by adding artemisinin to the conventional treatment (chemosensitization). Interestingly, DHA and artesunate have exhibited the strongest chemosensitizing/synergistic effects [4, 110], whereas the prototype drug artemisinin shows only additive and antagonistic interactions (Table 3). DHA significantly improves the anticancer effect of gemcitabine, an anticancer drug used in pancreatic cancer which develops resistance over time. *In vitro* and *in vivo* analysis in pancreatic cells demonstrated a DHA-induced increase in growth inhibition and apoptosis by 4- and 2-fold, respectively, compared with those obtained with gemcitabine alone [94]. A dual action of DHA in potentiating gemcitabine activity and possibly counteracting resistance has been attributed to DHA inhibition of gemcitabine- induced NF-κB activation and subsequent action on its targets [94]. A similar effect has been shown in hepatoma cancer cell lines irrespective of their p53 status [67]. DHA synergistically enhances tumor growth inhibition by 45% when in combination with gemcitabine, whereas artemisinin, the prototype, only induces additive effects [94].

Consistent with this observation, a greater antitumor activity was observed when DHA was used in a combination with cyclosphosphamide in murine Lewis lung carcinoma cell line or in combination with cisplatin in non-small cell lung cancer A549 in mice [84]. In rat C6 glioma cells, addition of 1 μM DHA increased by 177% the cytotoxic effect of temozolomide, a DNA-alkylating agent used in the treatment of brain cancer. Further investigation found that DHA promotes apoptotic and necrotic activity of temozolomide through ROS generation [107]. Recently, an enhancement of artesunate anticancer activity has been observed in different combination regimens. A striking synergy was achieved in combinations of artesunate and the immunomodulator drug, lenalidomide [111].

However, the benefits of an artemisinin combination therapy need to be carefully dissected. Therapeutic effects are influenced by the mode of action of the drugs and multiple interactions in particular systems and schedules. Recently, Graveth et al. showed that gemcitabine has only additive effects when combining gemcitabine and artemisone in colon and breast cancer cells [63]. In cancer colon cells (HT-29), it has been suggested that artemisinin may impair doxorubicin activity possibly by countering the doxorubicin effect on NF-κB inhibition [59]. The same authors have reported artemisinin-induced resistance in the same system through a different mechanism. Thus, it has been postulated that artemisinin exposure inhibits SERCA with subsequent accumulation of calcium. As a result, Pgp is upregulated and leads to generation of doxorubicin resistance cells [59]. By contrast, pretreatment with a calcium chelator reverted the cells to a sensitive phenotype [59]. Notably, DHA and artesunate have not been evaluated in this system; it remains to be elucidated whether the most potent chemosensitizers have similar effects on this cell line. So far, artesunate or DHA

Table 3: Drug interactions of artemisinins.

Drug combination	Cancer/cell line	Effect	Refs
DHA + Temozolomide	Rat C6 glioma cells	Increased apoptosis, ROS Induced necrosis	[107]
DHA + Cyclophosphamide	Lewis lung carcinoma	Increased apoptosis, decreased VEGF receptor KDR/flk-1 Apoptosis	[84]
DHA + Cisplatin	Human non-small cell lung cancer (A549)	Decreased metastasis	[84]
DHA + Gemcitabine	Pancreas (Panc-1)	Inhibition of proliferation, decreased cyclin D1 Increased apoptosis, increased Bax/Bcl2 ratio, activation of caspase 3	[94]
	Hepatoma (cell panel)	Increased growth inhibition by 45%	[67]
DHA + Butyric acid	Human lymphoblastoid leukemia (Molt-4)	Synergistic. Depletion of cancer cells	[110]
DHA + Radiation	Glioma cells U373MG	Increased cytotoxicity Inhibition of radiation-induced GST	[53]
DHA + Carboplatin	Ovarian cancer cells (A2780, OVCAR-3)	Increased growth inhibition through death receptor and mitochondrial mediated pathways	[77]
DHA + TRAIL	Prostate cancer (DU145, PC-3, LNCaP)	Increased apoptosis extrinsic and intrinsic pathways	[100]
ART/DHA + Doxorubicin + Pirarubicin	Leukemia (K562/adr) Small cell lung cancer (GLC4/adr)	Synergistic	[4]
ART + Lenalidomide	Lung (A549) and breast (MCF-7)	Decreased IC50 by 48%	[111]
ART + Oxiplatin	Colon (HT 1116)	Additive. Sensitising effect	[111]
ART + Gemcitabine	Breast (MCF-7)	Additive	
	Lung (A549)	Additive	
ATM + Oxiplatin ATM + Thalidomide ATM + Gemcitabine	Colon (HCTl16, SW480) Breast (MCF-7)	All additive	[63]
ARS + Hyperbaric oxygen (HBO_2)	Molt-4 human leukemia	22% decrease in growth	[112]
ARS + Doxorubicin	Colon cancer(HT29)	Predicted as antagonic, mediated by activation of NF-κB/overexpression of Pgp	[59]
ARS + Oxiplatin	Colon (HCTl16, SW480)	Antagonism	[63]
ARS + Thalidomide		Additive	
ARS + Gemcitabine	Breast (MCF-7)	Antagonism	

Abbreviations: HBO_2: hyperbaric oxygen.

in combination with doxorubicin and pirarubicin showed chemosensitizing effect in leukemia and human-small-cell cancer-resistant cell lines, but no further increase of sensitivity was observed in the sensitive parent cell lines [4]. The chemosensitising effect was independent of Pgp inhibition [4]. Overall, this evidence suggests that DHA and artesunate have remarkable ability to potentiate antitumor agents and to counter tumor resistance.

Artemisinins also improve ionizing-based therapies. In glioma cells U373MG, DHA treatment inhibits the radiation-induced expression of GST with concomitant ROS generation. A combination treatment with DHA has been shown to be more effective than radiation or DHA alone [53]. The adjuvant effect of artemisinin in other cancer treatments including hyperbaric oxygen has also been reported [112].

4.4. Artemisinin Resistance. A salient feature of artemisinin is that artemisinin resistance *in vitro* or in the field has yet to be confirmed after 30 years of use as an antimalarial. Clinically, tolerance has been reported in patients with therapeutic failure. However, *in vitro* tolerant strains are usually unstable and only develop after several years of continuous drug exposure [113]. The multimodal action of artemisinins at different cancer pathways might also predict a delay of induced resistance in malignant cells. Indeed, only few cell lines have shown intrinsic low sensitivity or no response to artemisinin or its derivatives. For example, artemisinin (the prototype drug) seems to be less active in breast cancer cells (MCF-7) and gastric cancer (MKN) [93]. Some studies in breast cancer cells have suggested that artemisinin response may be mediated by estrogen receptors (ERα and ERβ) which are involved in cell proliferation (reviewed in [72]). Interestingly, it has been documented that in breast cancer cells, disruption of iron metabolism may enhance potency of doxorubicin and cisplatin [114]. The low response to artemisinin has been also associated with overexpression of BMI-1 in highly metastatic nasopharyngeal cancer cell lines (CNE-1, CNE-2) [92]. A recent study found some levels of cross resistance to artesunate and DHA in a unique cisplatin chemo-resistant cell line. This effect was partially reverted by L-buthionine-S,R-sulfoximine, an inhibitor of the antioxidant GLC [52].

However, *in vitro* resistance has already been developed under experimental conditions. Microarray and experimental studies using knockouts and transfected cells indicate that upregulation of the tumor suppressor $p16^{INK4A}$ and the antioxidant protein, catalase, may confer resistance to artesunate independent of the p53 status [115]. Recently, concerns have arisen after Baechmeier et al. showed that a 24 h preincubation with 20 μM artesunate induces resistance in highly metastatic breast cancer cells. Pretreated MDA-MB-231 metastatic cells were completely refractory to further artesunate treatment, whereas a similar treatment in MDA-MB-468, a non-metastatic cell line, renders less sensitive cells. Further investigation on the mechanism of artesunate-acquired resistance indicates that upregulated transcription of NF-κB, AP-1, and NMP-1 overcome artesunate apoptotic and antimetastatic action and allows tumor progression [116]. It is not clear, however, whether artesunate-induced resistance and loss of sensitivity are preserved after long-term cell subculturing. It also remains to elucidate if other semisynthetic endoperoxides may induce a similar effect or whether a combinational therapy may delay or revert the effect on cell lines bearing this phenotype.

4.5. Artemisinins Toxicity. Dose-dependent toxicity is a major drawback that hampers anticancer therapy. This problem may be overcome by enhancing anticancer activity and thus reducing toxic drug concentrations. DHA is the most active and neurotoxic artemisinin derivative [117]. Neurotoxicity has been reported in animal studies in a dose- and time-dependent manner ($\geq$7 days) [118–120]. The toxicity of artemisinin-like compounds has been associated with long-term availability, whereas short-term peak concentrations are not toxic [121]. Thus, rapid elimination of artemisinin in oral formulations is safer than slow-release or oil-based intramuscular formulations [6, 121]. Remarkably, although artemisinins derivatives have been widely used as antimalarials, their toxicity in humans have been shown to be negligible. In cancer therapy, artemisinin may have multiple benefits as it can be used in combination with no additional side effects, but also it enhances potency and reduces doses of more toxic anticancer partners. Clinical doses used in malaria treatment after administration of 2 mg/kg in patients rise plasma concentrations of 2640 ± 1800 μg/mL (approximately 6.9 ± 4.7 mM) which can be considered up to 3 orders of magnitude higher than those artemisinin concentrations with antitumor activity [5]. It becomes relevant to closely monitor the safety of long-term artemisinin-based therapies as severe side effects may be highly unusual but significant. So far, artemisinin treatments for as long as 12 months have been reported with no relevant side effects [30, 122, 123]. However, an extremely rare case of toxic brainstem encephalopathy was described in a patient after a 2-week herbal/artemisinin combination (400 mg) regimen for breast cancer [124]. Brainstem neurotoxicity has been reported in animal studies and associated with long-term (>28 days) and high-dose treatments [118]. Recently, a fatal case of overdosing in a child who was taking antimalarial treatment was reported [125].

4.6. Artemisinins in Clinical Trials. Antitumor activity of artemisinin has also been documented in human trials [126] and individual clinical cases [30, 122]. Artemether and artesunate have been used in cancer therapy with good tolerability and lack of significant side effects.

Artesunate was successfully used in the treatment of laryngeal squamous cell carcinoma and substantially reduced the size of the tumor (by 70%) after two months of treatment [122]. Furthermore, artesunate increased survival and substantial metastasis reduction when used in combination with standard chemotherapy in patients with malignant skin cancer [30]. Another report describes a beneficial improvement in a patient with pituitary macroadenoma who was treated with artemether for 12 months [123]. Artemether has longer half-life and easily crosses the blood-brain barrier which is crucial for brain tumor treatment.

Similarly, a clinical trial in 120 patients with advanced non-small cell lung cancer has shown that artesunate in combination with a chemotherapy regimen of vinorelbine and cisplatin elevated 1-year survival rate by 13% with a significant improvement in disease control and time to progression [126]. No additional artesunate-related side effects were reported [126]. In Germany, a trial in patients with advanced breast cancer is currently ongoing. Tolerability to a combination therapy of 4-week artesunate will be assessed in this trial. Another trial in UK in colorectal adenocarcinoma to evaluate anticancer action and tolerability of artesunate was completed last year, but the results have not been published.

5. Anticancer Action of Novel Artemisinins Derivatives

5.1. Novel Semisynthetic Derivatives with Antitumor Action. Imperative need of highly effective compounds with enhanced pharmacological properties has led to the design of novel endoperoxide compounds with selective toxicity toward cancer cells. Considerable progress has been made in the design of novel compounds with enhanced potency at the nanomolar range, increased selectivity, and low toxicity *in vitro*. It has been reported that triazolyl substituted artemisinins-induced significant growth inhibitory effect [127]. Independent of stereo- or region-chemistry, strong inhibition was influenced by the functional group attached to the triazole ring. Substituted compounds with a penthyl benzene group showed the highest antiproliferative activity ranging from 0.07 to 0.39 μM 72 h IC_{50} in 6 cancer lines [127]. Recently, Feng et al. synthesized a series of dihydroartemisinin derivatives via an aza-Michael addition reaction with high selectivity index and

IC_{50} in the nanomolar range against HeLa cells (0.37 μM) [128]. In a series of deoxoartemisinins and carboxypropyldeoxoartemisinins, antitumor effect was associated with boat/chair conformations and drug-receptor interactions [129].

Different from their antiparasitic activity, it has been found that dimeric and trimeric artemisinin derivatives display much higher antitumor activity than their monomeric counterparts. In the last decade, an increase in the number of outputs in artemisinin dimeric compounds with anticancer activity has been observed. These compounds have shown IC_{50} ranging from 0.014 to 6 μM [130, 131]. Potent anticancer toxicity has been correlated with the nature of the linker [132] and with lipophilicity or electrophilic substitutions [66]. Posner et al. developed a series of artemisinin-trioxane derivate dimers from which two phosphate esters displayed nanomolar growth inhibitory values in the NCI 60 human cell line screen. Further investigation *in vitro* showed that in HL-60 cells, these compounds are more potent than doxorubicin, whereas their strongly anti-parasitic monomeric counterparts showed no anticancer activity. As suggested by the authors, two trioxane units in addition to the nature of the linker may be relevant in conferring potent anticancer activity [132]. Homodimers of artesunic acid have also nanomolar inhibitory values when tested in chemo-resistant and sensitive leukemia cells. Notably, the artesunic dimer seems to be 6-fold more potent in the multiresistant Pgp overexpressing cells (CEM/ADR500) than in its sensitive counterparts. Anticancer activity was attributed to apoptosis induction, arrest of cell cycle at G_0/G_1, and ROS generation [131]. In prostate cancer cells (LNCaP, TRAMP CIA, and C2H), two C10 non-acetal trioxane dimers displayed a 3-fold increase in potency compared to doxorubicin (17-18 nM versus 45.3 nM resp.). The dimers induced arrest at G_0/G_1 mediated by decreasing cyclin D1, cyclin E, CDK2, and an increase in p21 and p27. They also show proapoptotic action through upregulation in Bax expression [130].

In many studies, there has been an emphasis on the nature and stereochemistry of the dimer linker which may influence anticancer activity. However, it has also been shown that the linker by its own is inactive. Morrisey et al. have described that an artemisinin dimer exhibits up to 30-fold more activity than artemisinin in prostate cancer lines [61]. This dimer selectively exerted highly antigrowth potential and apoptosis in C4-2 (a cell line derived from LNCaP) and LNCaP cells compared to artemisinin [61]. An enhanced anticancer activity seems to be given by the stereoisomery of the linker [130]. In another study, C12 non-acetal dimers and one trimer of deoxoartemisinin showed similar potency to that of the conventional anticancer drugs against many cell lines. The linker with one amide or one sulfur-centered 2 ethylene groups was essential for potent anticancer activity [133]. Diastomeric-cholic-acid-derived 1,2,4,5-tetraoxanes were also tested and found to have high anticancer activity against human melanoma (Fem X), and cervix cancer (HeLa) [134] cis stereoisomers were twofold more active. The authors further suggested that an amide terminus in the linker confers increased anticancer activity.

Interestingly, Beckman et al. showed that the stereochemistry of the ether linkage of the dimers, of dihydroartemisinin (diDHA), and dihydrodeoxyartemisinin (the respective endoperoxide lacking dimer) was as important for antitumor activity as the endoperoxide moiety. Dimers were tested against 60 cells from 9 different cancers showing that although in general the diDHA was more active than dihydrodeoxyartemisinin toward anticancer growth, asymmetrical dimers of either diDHA or dihydrodeoxyartemisinin were similarly toxic [26]. The mechanism underlying the antiproliferative action of the artemisinin-derived dimers needs further study.

Recently, a series of potent artemisinin-like derivatives of easy synthesis and anticancer activity has been identified. These endoperoxides exhibit high chemical stability and greater cytotoxicity than artesunate. These compounds also exhibit relevant antiangiogenic properties as judged by studies in a zebrafish model [135].

5.2. Fully Synthetic Artemisinins. It is important to recall that some limitations of artemisinins such as short half-life (between 1 and 5 hours [136, 137]), limited affordability, and solubility need to be further addressed. Although semisynthetic compounds have partially overcome these issues, they still rely on the availability of natural precursors. In malaria, some trioxolanes and ozonides with remarkable improved pharmacokinetics are under clinical development [138]. Recently, it has been found that synthetic trioxolanes with enhanced pharmacokinetic properties may exhibit a similar toxicity than artesunate in *Schistosomas* [139]. Given that artemisinins may be potentially used as anticancer drugs and possibly in other parasitic and viral infections, the development of novel compounds with enhanced pharmacokinetic properties and targeted anticancer actions is also paramount. Although novel semisynthetic artemisinins have shown substantial antineoplastic activity, there is still limited information regarding the cytotoxicity of fully synthetic endoperoxides. A series of tetraoxacyclohexanes have been shown to potentially exhibit anticancer properties. A triol substituted compound has displayed prominent antitumor action *in vivo* toward melanoma (LOX IMVI) and ovarian (IGROV1) cancer in nanomolar concentrations (LC_{50} 60 nM) [140]. Other authors have synthesized compounds with dual action (antimalarial/anticancer effect). These deoxycholic-acid-(DCA-)—and cholic acid (CA)—derived mixed tetraoxanes are cytotoxic at very low concentrations and particularly potent against melanoma cancer (LOX IMVI, LC_{50} up to 69 nM) [141].

6. Future Development of Artemisinins as Anticancer Drugs

Artemisinins have been recommended and widely used as antimalarials for several years [142]. This drug class has shown many biological activities, in particular, strong anticancer growth activity. Supporting evidence indicates that artemisinin-like compounds may be a therapeutic alternative in highly metastatic and aggressive cancers [44] with no long-term effective therapy [44, 61] and commonly developing drug resistance [94]. Furthermore, antimalarial endoperoxides may act synergistically with other anticancer drugs with no additional side effects [143].

6.1. What Do We Need to Know? The ability of artemisinins to kill cancer cells through multiple and heterogeneous molecular events has been well documented. However, some questions about the molecular base of artemisinin-induced cell death need further study. Growing research has been focusing on determination of the mechanism of bioactivation and molecular events underlying the artemisinin effects. However, how the antitumor activity is exerted following artemisinin activation is still not well understood. So far, the precise molecular events involved in how, when, and where ROS production is initially triggered in cancer cells remain to be defined. In addition, the relevance of any ROS- independent mechanism should be also addressed; these might not be obvious but possibly important for artemisinin cytotoxicity in some cancer cells. Some other aspects such as the direct DNA damage induced by artemisinin-like compounds and the role of p53 status in genotoxicity need to be further analysed.

One relevant aim in anticancer therapy is cotargeting multiple pathways minimizing shifting cell hallmarks and side effects. Whereas it remains important to characterize the anticancer effects of existing and novel artemisinins derivatives, research also needs to be focused on unveiling the mechanisms of cytotoxicity by identifying their relation to a particular cancer biomarkers and molecules. Artemisinins seems to regulate key players participating in multiple pathways such as NF-κB, survivin, NOXA, HIF-1α, and BMI-1. These molecules and others are to be revealed, which in turn may be involved in drug response, drug interactions, mechanisms of resistance, and collateral effects in normal cells. A better understanding of common mechanisms under similar conditions in different cell systems will greatly aid the development of targeted artemisinin derivatives. This will improve artemisinins cytotoxicity by lowering IC_{50}, emerging of resistance, drug associated toxicity, and potentiating drug interactions.

It is important to connect the molecular interactions and the regulatory effects of artemisinin on the cancer hallmarks and particularly in those tumors with poor prognosis. Some cancer cell biomarkers may be potentially useful to predict success on an artemisinin-based treatment in specific systems. Furthermore, novel endoperoxide compounds and combinational therapies can be addressed to target or cotarget markers of carcinoma progression and prevent invasiveness and metastatic properties in highly recurrent and aggressive tumors or advanced stage cancers.

Although the benefits of artemisinins in the clinical setting have been already assessed, specific interactions with established chemotherapy need to be further dissected in different cancer cells and their phenotypes. This will be crucial to implement clinical trials and treatment of individual cases. In this regard, long-term therapy with artemisinins also requires close monitoring. It is important to note that the prototype drug, artemisinin, seems to modulate responses leading to antagonistic interactions with other anticancer drugs. However, whereas it may be useful to have the prototype drug as a control *in vitro*, its pharmacokinetic properties may differ from the semisynthetic artemisinins. Therefore, artemisinin antagonistic reactions and resistance must be cautiously validated using different semisynthetic derivatives. DHA, artesunate, and artemether are the endoperoxides currently licensed for therapeutic use. So far, artemether has been shown to share similar anticancer properties than DHA and artesunate [144].

Cancer research drives a permanent discovery of new genes and interactions. The study of how artemisinin drives tumor control may become even more complex as immunological hallmarks are also involved in the generation of tumors. Immunological hallmarks in cancer cells include the ability to induce chronic inflammatory response, evasion of tumor recognition, and ability to induce tolerance [145]. Whether artemisinin may participate in the mechanisms involved in these events has yet to be determined.

Overall, the real potential and benefits of the artemisinin drug class remain yet to be uncovered. The imminent possibility of artemisinins being included in the arsenal of anti cancer drugs has opened the door for challenging research in this area, one that seems to fulfill many expectations.

Abbreviations

ADP-ribose polymerase:	Adenosine diphosphate ribose polymerase
AP-1:	Activator protein 1
BAK:	Proapoptotic member of the BCL2 protein family
BAX:	BCL2-associated protein
BCL2:	B-cell lymphoma 2
BCRP:	Breast cancer resistant protein gen
BCLX:	Bcl-2-like protein 1
CDC25B:	Dual specific phosphatase involved in the activation of cyclin-dependent kinases
CDK:	Cyclin-dependent kinase
Cip 1/p21:	Cyclin-dependent kinase inhibitor 1
CDC25A:	Dual specific phosphatase involved in the activation of cyclin-dependent kinases
COX2:	Cyclooxygenase 2
Cdc42:	GTPase of the Rho family
c-MYC:	Transcription factor
DNA-PK:	DNA-dependent protein kinase
DNA topo 1:	DNA topoisomerase 1
E2F1:	Transcription factor
ER:	Endoplasmic reticulum
GST:	Glutathione S-transferase
GRP78:	78 kDa glucose-regulated protein
HIF 1α:	Hypoxia-inducible factor 1 alpha
$\alpha v\beta 3$ integrin:	Transmembrane heterodimeric protein expressed on sprouting endothelial cells
IκBα:	Inhibitor of NF-κB
IL-1β:	Interleukin 1 beta

IL8:	Interleukin 8
JNK:	Jun N-terminal kinase
Kip1/p27:	Cyclin-dependent kinase inhibitor 1B
KDR:	Kinase insert domain protein receptor
MMP:	Matrix metalloproteinase
MRP1:	Multidrug resistance-associated protein gene
MDM2:	Murine doble minute oncogene protein
NK-κB:	Nuclear factor of kappa light polypeptide gene enhancer in B cells
NOXA:	Proapoptotic protein, a member of the BH3-only Bcl-2 protein family
p38-MAPK:	Mitogen-activated protein kinase
PAI-1:	Plasminogen activator inhibitor 1
PCNA:	Proliferating cell nuclear antigen
PKCa:	Serine/threonine kinase
ROS:	Radical oxygen species
Raf/ERK:	Signaling pathway
uPA:	Urokinase plasminogen
TIMP2:	Tissue inhibitor of metalloproteinases
TRAIL:	The tumor necrosis factor-related apoptosis-inducing ligand
VEGF:	Vascular endothelial growth factor
VEGFR-3/FL-4:	Vascular endothelial growth factor receptor
Wnt:	Wingless-type signaling pathway.

References

[1] W. L. W. Hsiao and L. Liu, "The role of traditional Chinese herbal medicines in cancer therapy from TCM theory to mechanistic insights," *Planta Medica*, vol. 76, no. 11, pp. 1118–1131, 2010.

[2] T. Efferth, H. Dunstan, A. Sauerbrey, H. Miyachi, and C. R. Chitambar, "The anti-malarial artesunate is also active against cancer," *International Journal of Oncology*, vol. 18, no. 4, pp. 767–773, 2001.

[3] H. J. Woerdenbag, T. A. Moskal, N. Pras et al., "Cytotoxicity of artemisinin-related endoperoxides to Ehrlich ascites tumor cells," *Journal of Natural Products*, vol. 56, no. 6, pp. 849–856, 1993.

[4] P. Reungpatthanaphong and S. Mankhetkorn, "Modulation of multidrug resistance by artemisinin, artesunate and dihydroartemisinin in K562/adr and GLC4/adr resistant cell lines," *Biological and Pharmaceutical Bulletin*, vol. 25, no. 12, pp. 1555–1561, 2002.

[5] T. Efferth, A. Saverbrey, A. Olbrich et al., "Molecular modes of action of artesunate in tumour cell lines," *Molecular Pharmacology* , vol. 64, no. 2, pp. 382–394, 2003.

[6] T. Gordi and E. I. Lepist, "Artemisinin derivatives: toxic for laboratory animals, safe for humans?" *Toxicology Letters*, vol. 147, no. 2, pp. 99–107, 2004.

[7] A. M. Dondorp, F. Nosten, P. Yi et al., "Artemisinin resistance in *Plasmodium falciparum* malaria," *New England Journal of Medicine*, vol. 361, no. 5, pp. 455–467, 2009.

[8] Qinghaosu Antimalaria Coordinating Research Group, "Antimalaria studies on Qinghaosu," *Chinese Medical Journal*, vol. 92, no. 12, pp. 811–816, 1979.

[9] M. Ashton, N. D. Sy, N. van Huong et al., "Artemisinin kinetics and dynamics during oral and rectal treatment of uncomplicated malaria," *Clinical Pharmacology and Therapeutics*, vol. 63, no. 4, pp. 482–493, 1998.

[10] Q. Li, P. J. Weina, and W. K. Milhous, "Pharmacokinetic and pharmacodynamic profiles of rapid-acting artemisinins in the antimalarial therapy," *Current Drug Therapy*, vol. 2, no. 3, pp. 210–223, 2007.

[11] R. K. Haynes, H. W. Chan, M. K. Cheung et al., "C-10 ester and ether derivatives of dihydroartemisinin - 10-α artesunate, preparation of authentic 10-β artesunate, and of other ester and ether derivatives bearing potential aromatic intercalating groups at C-10," *European Journal of Organic Chemistry*, vol. 2002, no. 1, pp. 113–132, 2002.

[12] D. L. Klayman, "Qinghaosu (artemisinin): an antimalarial drug from China," *Science*, vol. 228, no. 4703, pp. 1049–1055, 1985.

[13] R. K. Haynes, "From artemisinin to new artemisinin antimalarials: biosynthesis, extraction, old and new derivatives, stereochemistry and medicinal chemistry requirements," *Current Topics in Medicinal Chemistry*, vol. 6, no. 5, pp. 509–537, 2006.

[14] D. J. Creek, W. N. Charman, F. C. K. Chiu et al., "Relationship between antimalarial activity and heme alkylation for spiro- and dispiro-1,2,4-trioxolane antimalarials," *Antimicrobial Agents and Chemotherapy*, vol. 52, no. 4, pp. 1291–1296, 2008.

[15] C. W. Jefford, "New developments in synthetic peroxidic drugs as artemisinin mimics," *Drug Discovery Today*, vol. 12, no. 11-12, pp. 487–495, 2007.

[16] A. P. Ramirez, A. M. Thomas, and K. A. Woerpel, "Preparation of bicyclic 1,2,4-trioxanes from γ,δ-unsaturated ketones," *Organic Letters*, vol. 11, no. 3, pp. 507–510, 2009.

[17] D. K. Taylor, T. D. Avery, B. W. Greatrex et al., "Novel endoperoxide antimalarials: synthesis, heme binding, and antimalarial activity," *Journal of Medicinal Chemistry*, vol. 47, no. 7, pp. 1833–1839, 2004.

[18] C. W. Jefford, J. Velarde, and G. Bernardinelli, "Synthesis of tricyclic arteannuin-like compounds," *Tetrahedron Letters*, vol. 30, no. 34, pp. 4485–4488, 1989.

[19] G. H. Posner, Chang Ho Oh, L. Gerena, and W. K. Milhous, "Extraordinarily potent antimalarial compounds: new, structurally simple, easily synthesized, tricyclic 1,2,4-trioxanes," *Journal of Medicinal Chemistry*, vol. 35, no. 13, pp. 2459–2467, 1992.

[20] S. R. Meshnick, A. Thomas, A. Ranz, C. M. Xu, and H. Z. Pan, "Artemisinin (qinghaosu): the role of intracellular hemin in its mechanism of antimalarial action," *Molecular and Biochemical Parasitology*, vol. 49, no. 2, pp. 181–189, 1991.

[21] P. L. Olliaro, R. K. Haynes, B. Meunier, and Y. Yuthavong, "Possible modes of action of the artemisinin-type compounds," *Trends in Parasitology*, vol. 17, no. 3, pp. 122–126, 2001.

[22] P. M. O'Neill, V. E. Barton, and S. A. Ward, "The molecular mechanism of action of artemisinin—the debate continues," *Molecules*, vol. 15, no. 3, pp. 1705–1721, 2010.

[23] N. Klonis, M. P. Crespo-Ortiz, I. Bottova et al., "Artemisinin activity against *Plasmodium falciparum* requires hemoglobin uptake and digestion," *Proceedings of the National Academy of Sciences of the United States of America*, vol. 108, no. 28, pp. 11405–11410, 2011.

[24] X. Shuhua, S. Binggui, J. Utzinger, J. Chollet, and M. Tanner, "Ultrastructural alterations in adult Schistosoma mansoni caused by artemether," *Memorias do Instituto Oswaldo Cruz*, vol. 97, no. 5, pp. 717–724, 2002.
[25] A. M. Galal, S. A. Ross, M. A. ElSohly et al., "Deoxyartemisinin derivatives from photooxygenation of anhydrodeoxydihydroartemisinin and their cytotoxic evaluation," *Journal of Natural Products*, vol. 65, no. 2, pp. 184–188, 2002.
[26] A. C. Beekman, P. K. Wierenga, H. J. Woerdenbag et al., "Artemisinin-derived sesquiterpene lactones as potential antitumour compounds: cytotoxic action against bone marrow and tumour cells," *Planta Medica*, vol. 64, no. 7, pp. 615–619, 1998.
[27] B. Meunier and A. Robert, "Heme as trigger and target for trioxane-containing antimalarial drugs," *Accounts of Chemical Research*, vol. 43, no. 11, pp. 1444–1451, 2010.
[28] A. E. Mercer, J. L. Maggs, X. M. Sun et al., "Evidence for the involvement of carbon-centered radicals in the induction of apoptotic cell death by artemisinin compounds," *Journal of Biological Chemistry*, vol. 282, no. 13, pp. 9372–9382, 2007.
[29] S. Zhang and G. S. Gerhard, "Heme mediates cytotoxicity from artemisinin and serves as a general anti-proliferation target," *PLoS ONE*, vol. 4, no. 10, Article ID e7472, 2009.
[30] T. G. Berger, D. Dieckmann, T. Efferth et al., "Artesunate in the treatment of metastatic uveal melanoma–first experiences," *Oncology Reports*, vol. 14, no. 6, pp. 1599–1603, 2005.
[31] A. Hamacher-Brady, H. A. Stein, S. Turschner et al., "Artesunate activates mitochondrial apoptosis in breast cancer cells via iron-catalyzed lysosomal reactive oxygen species production," *Journal of Biological Chemistry*, vol. 286, no. 8, pp. 6587–6601, 2011.
[32] N. P. Singh and H. C. Lai, "Artemisinin induces apoptosis in human cancer cells," *Anticancer Research*, vol. 24, no. 4, pp. 2277–2280, 2004.
[33] J. J. Lu, L. H. Meng, U. T. Shankavaram et al., "Dihydroartemisinin accelerates c-MYC oncoprotein degradation and induces apoptosis in c-MYC-overexpressing tumor cells," *Biochemical Pharmacology*, vol. 80, no. 1, pp. 22–30, 2010.
[34] J. J. Lu, S. M. Chen, X. W. Zhang, J. Ding, and L. H. Meng, "The anti-cancer activity of dihydroartemisinin is associated with induction of iron-dependent endoplasmic reticulum stress in colorectal carcinoma HCT116 cells," *Investigational New Drugs*, vol. 7, pp. 1–8, 2010.
[35] A. E. Mercer, I. M. Copple, J. L. Maggs, P. M. O'Neill, and B. K. Park, "The role of heme and the mitochondrion in the chemical and molecular mechanisms of mammalian cell death induced by the artemisinin antimalarials," *Journal of Biological Chemistry*, vol. 283, no. 2, pp. 987–996, 2011.
[36] H. Lai and N. P. Singh, "Selective cancer cell cytotoxicity from exposure to dihydroartemisinin and holotransferrin," *Cancer Letters*, vol. 91, no. 1, pp. 41–46, 1995.
[37] H. Lai, I. Nakase, E. Lacoste, N. P. Singh, and T. Sasaki, "Artemisinin-transferrin conjugate retards growth of breast tumors in the rat," *Anticancer Research*, vol. 29, no. 10, pp. 3807–3810, 2009.
[38] I. Nakase, H. Lai, N. P. Singh, and T. Sasaki, "Anticancer properties of artemisinin derivatives and their targeted delivery by transferrin conjugation," *International Journal of Pharmaceutics*, vol. 354, no. 1-2, pp. 28–33, 2007.
[39] H. Lai, T. Sasaki, and N. P. Singh, "Targeted treatment of cancer with artemisinin and artemisinin-tagged iron-carrying compounds," *Expert Opinion on Therapeutic Targets*, vol. 9, no. 5, pp. 995–1007, 2005.
[40] L. H. Stockwin, B. Han, S. X. Yu et al., "Artemisinin dimer anticancer activity correlates with heme-catalyzed reactive oxygen species generation and endoplasmic reticulum stress induction," *International Journal of Cancer*, vol. 125, no. 6, pp. 1266–1275, 2009.
[41] X. J. Huang, Z. Q. Ma, W. P. Zhang, Y. B. Lu, and E. Q. Wei, "Dihydroartemisinin exerts cytotoxic effects and inhibits hypoxia inducible factor-1α activation in C6 glioma cells," *Journal of Pharmacy and Pharmacology*, vol. 59, no. 6, pp. 849–856, 2007.
[42] J. C. Kwok and D. R. Richardson, "The iron metabolism of neoplastic cells: alterations that facilitate proliferation?" *Critical Reviews in Oncology/Hematology*, vol. 42, no. 1, pp. 65–78, 2002.
[43] T. Efferth, A. Benakis, M. R. Romero et al., "Enhancement of cytotoxicity of artemisinins toward cancer cells by ferrous iron," *Free Radical Biology and Medicine*, vol. 37, no. 7, pp. 998–1009, 2004.
[44] Q. Xu, Z. -X. Li, H. -Q. Peng et al., "Artesunate inhibits growth and induces apoptosis in human osteosarcoma HOS cell line *In vitro* and *In vivo*," *Biomedicine and Biotechnology*, vol. 12, no. 4, pp. 247–255, 2011.
[45] W. S. May and P. Cuatrecasas, "Transferrin receptor: its biological significance," *Journal of Membrane Biology*, vol. 88, no. 3, pp. 205–215, 1985.
[46] D. G. Bostwick, E. E. Alexander, R. Singh et al., "Antioxidant enzyme expression and reactive oxygen species damage in prostatic intraepithelial neoplasia and cancer," *Cancer*, vol. 89, no. 1, pp. 123–134, 2000.
[47] U. N. Das, "A radical approach to cancer," *Medical Science Monitor*, vol. 8, no. 4, pp. RA79–RA92, 2002.
[48] J. B. Hansen, N. Fisker, M. Westergaard et al., "SPC3042: a proapoptotic survivin inhibitor," *Molecular Cancer Therapeutics*, vol. 7, no. 9, pp. 2736–2745, 2008.
[49] M. D. P. Crespo, T. D. Avery, E. Hanssen et al., "Artemisinin and a series of novel endoperoxide antimalarials exert early effects on digestive vacuole morphology," *Antimicrobial Agents and Chemotherapy*, vol. 52, no. 1, pp. 98–109, 2008.
[50] I. D. Ferreira, D. Lopes, A. Martinelli, C. Ferreira, V. E. Do Rosário, and P. Cravo, "*In vitro* assessment of artesunate, artemether and amodiaquine susceptibility and molecular analysis of putative resistance-associated mutations of *Plasmodium falciparum* from São Tomé and Príncipe," *Tropical Medicine and International Health*, vol. 12, no. 3, pp. 353–362, 2007.
[51] J. H. Du, H. D. Zhang, Z. J. Ma, and K. M. Ji, "Artesunate induces oncosis-like cell death *In vitro* and has antitumor activity against pancreatic cancer xenografts *In vivo*," *Cancer Chemotherapy and Pharmacology*, vol. 65, no. 5, pp. 895–902, 2010.
[52] M. Michaelis, M. C. Kleinschmidt, S. Barth et al., "Anticancer effects of artesunate in a panel of chemoresistant neuroblastoma cell lines," *Biochemical Pharmacology*, vol. 79, no. 2, pp. 130–136, 2010.
[53] S. J. Kim, M. S. Kim, J. W. Lee et al., "Dihydroartemisinin enhances radiosensitivity of human glioma cells *In vitro*," *Journal of Cancer Research and Clinical Oncology.*, vol. 132, no. 2, pp. 129–135, 2006.
[54] Y. Y. Lu, T. S. Chen, X. P. Wang, and L. Li, "Single-cell analysis of dihydroartemisinin-induced apoptosis through reactive oxygen species-mediated caspase-8 activation and mitochondrial pathway in ASTC-a-1 cells using fluorescence imaging techniques," *Journal of Biomedical Optics*, vol. 15, no. 4, p. 046028, 2010.

[55] S. Noori, Z. M. Hassan, M. Taghikhani, B. Rezaei, and Z. Habibi, "Dihydroartemisinin can inhibit calmodulin, calmodulin-dependent phosphodiesterase activity and stimulate cellular immune responses," *International Immunopharmacology*, vol. 10, no. 2, pp. 213–217, 2010.

[56] D. Mu, W. Chen, B. Yu, C. Zhang, Y. Zhang, and H. Qi, "Calcium and survivin are involved in the induction of apoptosis by dihydroartemisinin in human lung cancer SPC-A-1 cells," *Methods and Findings in Experimental and Clinical Pharmacology*, vol. 29, no. 1, pp. 33–38, 2007.

[57] D. Mu, W. Zhang, D. Chu et al., "The role of calcium, P38 MAPK in dihydroartemisinin-induced apoptosis of lung cancer PC-14 cells," *Cancer Chemotherapy and Pharmacology*, vol. 61, no. 4, pp. 639–645, 2008.

[58] T. Efferth, "Willmar Schwabe Award 2006: antiplasmodial and antitumor activity of artemisinin from bench to bedside," *Planta Medica*, vol. 73, no. 4, pp. 299–309, 2007.

[59] C. Riganti, S. Doublier, D. Viarisio et al., "Artemisinin induces doxorubicin resistance in human colon cancer cells via calcium-dependent activation of HIF-1α and P-glycoprotein overexpression," *British Journal of Pharmacology*, vol. 156, no. 7, pp. 1054–1066, 2009.

[60] Y. Liu, C. N. Lok, B. C. B. Ko, T. Y. T. Shum, M. K. Wong, and C. M. Che, "Subcellular localization of a fluorescent artemisinin derivative to endoplasmic reticulum," *Organic Letters*, vol. 12, no. 7, pp. 1420–1423, 2010.

[61] C. Morrissey, B. Gallis, J. W. Solazzi et al., "Effect of artemisinin derivatives on apoptosis and cell cycle in prostate cancer cells," *Anti-Cancer Drugs*, vol. 21, no. 4, pp. 423–432, 2010.

[62] Y. Y. Lu, T. S. Chen, J. L. Qu, W. L. Pan, L. Sun, and X. B. Wei, "Dihydroartemisinin (DHA) induces caspase-3-dependent apoptosis in human lung adenocarcinoma ASTC-a-1 cells," *Journal of Biomedical Science*, vol. 16, no. 1, article 16, 2009.

[63] A. M. Gravett, W. M. Liu, S. Krishna et al., "*In vitro* study of the anti-cancer effects of artemisone alone or in combination with other chemotherapeutic agents," *Cancer Chemotherapy and Pharmacology*, pp. 569–577, 2010.

[64] E. R. McDonald 3rd. E.R. and W. S. El-Deiry, "Cell cycle control as a basis for cancer drug development (Review)," *International Journal of Oncology*, vol. 16, no. 5, pp. 871–886, 2000.

[65] B. Vogelstein and K. W. Kinzler, "Cancer genes and the pathways they control," *Nature Medicine*, vol. 10, no. 8, pp. 789–799, 2004.

[66] H. J. Woerdenbag, T. A. Moskal, N. Pras et al., "Cytotoxicity of artemisinin-related endoperoxides to Ehrlich ascites tumor cells," *Journal of Natural Products*, vol. 56, no. 6, pp. 849–856, 1993.

[67] J. Hou, D. Wang, R. Zhang, and H. Wang, "Experimental therapy of hepatoma with artemisinin and Its derivatives: *In vitro* and *In vivo* activity, chemosensitization, and mechanisms of action," *Clinical Cancer Research*, vol. 14, no. 17, pp. 5519–5530, 2008.

[68] L. Yao, H. Xie, Q.-Y. Jin, W.-L. Hu, and L.-J. Chen, "Analyzing anti-cancer action mechanisms of dihydroartemisinin using gene chip," *China Journal of Chinese Materia Medica*, vol. 33, no. 13, pp. 1583–1586, 2008.

[69] Y. Jiao, C. M. Ge, Q. H. Meng, J. P. Cao, J. Tong, and S. J. Fan, "Dihydroartemisinin is an inhibitor of ovarian cancer cell growth," *Acta Pharmacologica Sinica*, vol. 28, no. 7, pp. 1045–1056, 2007.

[70] M. Malumbres and M. Barbacid, "To cycle or not to cycle: a critical decision in cancer," *Nature Reviews Cancer*, vol. 1, no. 3, pp. 222–231, 2001.

[71] D. G. Johnson and C. L. Walker, "Cyclins and cell cycle checkpoints," *Annual Review of Pharmacology and Toxicology*, vol. 39, pp. 295–312, 1999.

[72] G. L. Firestone and S. N. Sundar, "Anticancer activities of artemisinin and its bioactive derivatives," *Expert Reviews in Molecular Medicine*, vol. 11, p. e32, 2009.

[73] Y. Ji, Y. C. Zhang, L. B. Pei, L. L. Shi, J. L. Yan, and X. H. Ma, "Anti-tumor effects of dihydroartemisinin on human osteosarcoma," *Molecular and Cellular Biochemistry*, vol. 351, no. 1-2, pp. 99–108, 2011.

[74] H. Chen, B. Sun, S. Pan, H. Jiang, and X. Sun, "Dihydroartemisinin inhibits growth of pancreatic cancer cells *In vitro* and *In vivo*," *Anti-Cancer Drugs*, vol. 20, no. 2, pp. 131–140, 2009.

[75] W. Aung, C. Sogawa, T. Furukawa, and T. Saga, "Anticancer effect of dihydroartemisinin (DHA) in a pancreatic tumor model evaluated by conventional methods and optical imaging," *Anticancer Research*, vol. 31, no. 5, pp. 1549–1558, 2011.

[76] S. -J. Wang, B. Sun, Z. -X. Cheng et al., "Dihydroartemisinin inhibits angiogenesis in pancreatic cancer by targeting the NF-κB pathway," *Cancer Chemotherapy and Pharmacology*. In press.

[77] T. Chen, M. Li, R. Zhang, and H. Wang, "Dihydroartemisinin induces apoptosis and sensitizes human ovarian cancer cells to carboplatin therapy," *Journal of Cellular and Molecular Medicine*, vol. 13, no. 7, pp. 1358–1370, 2009.

[78] J. Wang, Y. Guo, B. C. Zhang, Z. T. Chen, and J. F. Gao, "Induction of apoptosis and inhibition of cell migration and tube-like formation by dihydroartemisinin in murine lymphatic endothelial cells," *Pharmacology*, vol. 80, no. 4, pp. 207–218, 2007.

[79] C. M. Cabello, S. D. Lamore, W. B. Bair III et al., "The redox antimalarial dihydroartemisinin targets human metastatic melanoma cells but not primary melanocytes with induction of NOXA-dependent apoptosis," *Investigational New Drugs*. In press.

[80] R. Handrick, T. Ontikatze, K. D. Bauer et al., "Dihydroartemisinin induces apoptosis by a bak-dependent intrinsic pathway," *Molecular Cancer Therapeutics*, vol. 9, no. 9, pp. 2497–2510, 2010.

[81] Y. P. Hwang, H. J. Yun, H. G. Kim, E. H. Han, G. W. Lee, and H. G. Jeong, "Suppression of PMA-induced tumor cell invasion by dihydroartemisinin via inhibition of PKCα/Raf/MAPKs and NF-κB/AP-1-dependent mechanisms," *Biochemical Pharmacology*, vol. 79, no. 12, pp. 1714–1726, 2010.

[82] H. J. Zhou, W. Q. Wang, G. D. Wu, J. Lee, and A. Li, "Artesunate inhibits angiogenesis and downregulates vascular endothelial growth factor expression in chronic myeloid leukemia K562 cells," *Vascular Pharmacology*, vol. 47, no. 2-3, pp. 131–138, 2007.

[83] J. Wang, B. Zhang, Y. Guo et al., "Artemisinin inhibits tumor lymphangiogenesis by suppression of vascular endothelial growth factor C," *Pharmacology*, vol. 82, no. 2, pp. 148–155, 2008.

[84] H. J. Zhou, J. L. Zhang, A. Li, Z. Wang, and X. E. Lou, "Dihydroartemisinin improves the efficiency of chemotherapeutics in lung carcinomas *In vivo* and inhibits murine Lewis lung carcinoma cell line growth *In vitro*," *Cancer Chemotherapy and Pharmacology*, vol. 66, no. 1, pp. 21–29, 2010.

[85] G. L. Disbrow, A. C. Baege, K. A. Kierpiec et al., "Dihydroartemisinin is cytotoxic to papillomavirus-expressing epithelial cells *In vitro* and *In vivo*," *Cancer Research*, vol. 65, no. 23, pp. 10854–10861, 2005.
[86] W. Lijuan, "Effect of artesunate on human endometrial carcinoma," *Journal of Medical Colleges of PLA*, vol. 25, no. 3, pp. 143–151, 2010.
[87] M. Youns, T. Efferth, J. Reichling, K. Fellenberg, A. Bauer, and J. D. Hoheisel, "Gene expression profiling identifies novel key players involved in the cytotoxic effect of Artesunate on pancreatic cancer cells," *Biochemical Pharmacology*, vol. 78, no. 3, pp. 273–283, 2009.
[88] S. A. K. Rasheed, T. Efferth, I. A. Asangani, and H. Allgayer, "First evidence that the antimalarial drug artesunate inhibits invasion and *In vivo* metastasis in lung cancer by targeting essential extracellular proteases," *International Journal of Cancer*, vol. 127, no. 6, pp. 1475–1485, 2010.
[89] L. N. Li, H. D. Zhang, S. J. Yuan, D. X. Yang, L. Wang, and Z. X. Sun, "Differential sensitivity of colorectal cancer cell lines to artesunate is associated with expression of beta-catenin and E-cadherin," *European Journal of Pharmacology*, vol. 588, no. 1, pp. 1–8, 2008.
[90] S. Li, F. Xue, Z. Cheng et al., "Effect of artesunate on inhibiting proliferation and inducing apoptosis of SP2/0 myeloma cells through affecting NFκB p65," *International Journal of Hematology*, vol. 90, no. 4, pp. 513–521, 2009.
[91] T. Weifeng, S. Feng, L. Xiangji et al., "Artemisinin inhibits *In vitro* and *In vivo* invasion and metastasis of human hepatocellular carcinoma cells," *Phytomedicine*, vol. 18, no. 2-3, pp. 158–162, 2011.
[92] J. Wu, D. Hu, G. Yang et al., "Down-regulation of BMI-1 cooperates with artemisinin on growth inhibition of nasopharyngeal carcinoma cells," *Journal of Cellular Biochemistry*, vol. 112, no. 7, pp. 1938–1948, 2011.
[93] E. Buommino, A. Baroni, N. Canozo et al., "Artemisinin reduces human melanoma cell migration by down-regulating $\alpha v\beta 3$ integrin and reducing metalloproteinase 2 production," *Investigational New Drugs*, vol. 27, no. 5, pp. 412–418, 2008.
[94] S. J. Wang, Y. Gao, H. Chen et al., "Dihydroartemisinin inactivates NF-κB and potentiates the anti-tumor effect of gemcitabine on pancreatic cancer both *In vitro* and *In vivo*," *Cancer Letters*, vol. 293, no. 1, pp. 99–108, 2010.
[95] A. G. Uren, L. Wong, M. Pakusch et al., "Survivin and the inner centromere protein INCENP show similar cell-cycle localization and gene knockout phenotype," *Current Biology*, vol. 10, no. 21, pp. 1319–1328, 2000.
[96] J. A. Willoughby, S. N. Sundar, M. Cheung, A. S. Tin, J. Modiano, and G. L. Firestone, "Artemisinin blocks prostate cancer growth and cell cycle progression by disrupting Sp1 interactions with the cyclin-dependent kinase-4 (CDK4) promoter and inhibiting CDK4 gene expression," *Journal of Biological Chemistry*, vol. 284, no. 4, pp. 2203–2213, 2009.
[97] D. Karnak and L. Xu, "Chemosensitization of prostate cancer by modulating Bcl-2 family proteins," *Current Drug Targets*, vol. 11, no. 6, pp. 699–707, 2010.
[98] S. Elmore, "Apoptosis: a review of programmed cell death," *Toxicologic Pathology*, vol. 35, no. 4, pp. 495–516, 2007.
[99] T. Efferth, M. Glaisi, A. Merling, P. H. Krammer, and M. Li-Weber, "Artesunate induces ROS-mediated apoptosis in Doxorubicin-resistant T leukemia cells," *PLoS ONE*, vol. 2, no. 8, article e693, 2007.
[100] Q. He, J. Shi, X. L. Shen et al., "Dihydroartemisinin upregulates death receptor 5 expression and cooperates with TRAIL to induce apoptosis in human prostate cancer cells," *Cancer Biology and Therapy*, vol. 9, no. 10, pp. 817–823, 2010.
[101] P. S. Steeg, "Tumor metastasis: mechanistic insights and clinical challenges," *Nature Medicine*, vol. 12, no. 8, pp. 895–904, 2006.
[102] M. J. Duffy, P. M. McGowan, and W. M. Gallagher, "Cancer invasion and metastasis: changing views," *Journal of Pathology*, vol. 214, no. 3, pp. 283–293, 2008.
[103] W. C. Hung and H. C. Chang, "Indole-3-carbinol inhibits Sp1-induced matrix metalloproteinase-2 expression to attenuate migration and invasion of breast cancer cells," *Journal of Agricultural and Food Chemistry*, vol. 57, no. 1, pp. 76–82, 2009.
[104] E. Hur, H. H. Kim, S. M. Choi et al., "Reduction of hypoxia-induced transcription through the repression of hypoxia-inducible factor-1α/aryl hydrocarbon receptor nuclear translocator DNA binding by the 90-kDa heat-shock protein inhibitor radicicol," *Molecular Pharmacology*, vol. 62, no. 5, pp. 975–982, 2002.
[105] L. Anfosso, T. Efferth, A. Albini, and U. Pfeffer, "Microarray expression profiles of angiogenesis-related genes predict tumor cell response to artemisinins," *Pharmacogenomics Journal*, vol. 6, no. 4, pp. 269–278, 2006.
[106] H. H. Chen, H. J. Zhou, W. Q. Wang, and G. D. Wu, "Antimalarial dihydroartemisinin also inhibits angiogenesis," *Cancer Chemotherapy and Pharmacology*, vol. 53, no. 5, pp. 423–432, 2004.
[107] X. J. Huang, C. T. Li, W. P. Zhang, Y. B. Lu, S. H. Fang, and E. Q. Wei, "Dihydroartemisinin potentiates the cytotoxic effect of temozolomide in rat C6 glioma cells," *Pharmacology*, vol. 82, no. 1, pp. 1–9, 2008.
[108] R. O'Connor, "The pharmacology of cancer resistance," *Anticancer Research*, vol. 27, no. 3 A, pp. 1267–1272, 2007.
[109] W. Chaijaroenkul, V. Viyanant, W. Mahavorasirikul, and K. Na-Bangchang, "Cytotoxic activity of artemisinin derivatives against cholangiocarcinoma (CL-6) and hepatocarcinoma (Hep-G2) cell lines," *Asian Pacific Journal of Cancer Prevention*, vol. 12, no. 1, pp. 55–59, 2011.
[110] N. P. Singh and H. C. Lai, "Synergistic cytotoxicity of artemisinin and sodium butyrate on human cancer cells," *Anticancer Research*, vol. 25, no. 6 B, pp. 4325–4331, 2005.
[111] W. M. Liu, A. M. Gravett, and A. G. Dalgleish, "The antimalarial agent artesunate possesses anticancer properties that can be enhanced by combination strategies," *International Journal of Cancer*, vol. 128, no. 6, pp. 1471–1480, 2011.
[112] Y. Ohgami, C. A. Elstad, E. Chung, D. Y. Shirachi, R. M. Quock, and H. C. Lai, "Effect of hyperbaric oxygen on the anticancer effect of artemisinin on molt-4 human leukemia cells," *Anticancer Research*, vol. 30, no. 11, pp. 4467–4470, 2010.
[113] B. Witkowski, J. Lelièvre, M. J.L. Barragán et al., "Increased tolerance to artemisinin in *Plasmodium falciparum* is mediated by a quiescence mechanism," *Antimicrobial Agents and Chemotherapy*, vol. 54, no. 5, pp. 1872–1877, 2010.
[114] J. F. Head, F. Wang, and R. L. Elliott, "Antineoplastic drugs that interfere with iron metabolism in cancer cells," *Advances in Enzyme Regulation*, vol. 37, pp. 147–169, 1997.
[115] S. Sertel, T. Eichhorn, S. Sieber et al., "Factors determining sensitivity or resistance of tumor cell lines towards artesunate," *Chemico-Biological Interactions*, vol. 185, no. 1, pp. 42–52, 2010.

[116] B. Bachmeier, I. Fichtner, P. H. Killian, E. Kronski, U. Pfeffer, and T. Efferth, "Development of resistance towards artesunate in MDA-MB-231 human breast cancer cells," *PLoS ONE*, vol. 6, no. 5, article e20550, 2011.

[117] W. McLean and S. A. Ward, "*In vitro* neurotoxicity of artemisinin derivatives," *Médecine Tropicale*, vol. 58, no. 3, pp. 28–31, 1998.

[118] G. Schmuck, E. Roehrdanz, R. K. Haynes, and R. Kahl, "Neurotoxic mode of action of artemisinin," *Antimicrobial Agents and Chemotherapy*, vol. 46, no. 3, pp. 821–827, 2002.

[119] E. Kissinger, T. T. Hien, N. T. Hung et al., "Clinical and neurophysiological study of the effects of multiple doses of artemisinin on brain-stem function in vietnamese patients," *American Journal of Tropical Medicine and Hygiene*, vol. 63, no. 1-2, pp. 48–55, 2000.

[120] Y. Si, Q. Li, L. Xie et al., "Neurotoxicity and toxicokinetics of artelinic acid following repeated oral administration in rats," *International Journal of Toxicology*, vol. 26, no. 5, pp. 401–410, 2007.

[121] T. Efferth and B. Kaina, "Toxicity of the antimalarial artemisinin and its dervatives," *Critical Reviews in Toxicology*, vol. 40, no. 5, pp. 405–421, 2010.

[122] N. P. Singh and K. B. Verma, "Case report of a laryngeal squamous cell carcinoma treated with artesunate," *Archive of Oncology*, vol. 10, no. 4, pp. 279–280, 2002.

[123] N. P. Singh and V. K. Panwar, "Case report of a pituitary macroadenoma treated with artemether," *Integrative Cancer Therapies*, vol. 5, no. 4, pp. 391–394, 2006.

[124] L. A. Panossian, N. I. Garga, and D. Pelletier, "Toxic brainstem encephalopathy after artemisinin treatment for breast cancer," *Annals of Neurology*, vol. 58, no. 5, pp. 812–813, 2005.

[125] S. Campos, P. de la Cerda, and A. Rivera, "Fatal artesunate toxicity in a child," *Journal of Pediatric Infectious Diseases*, vol. 3, no. 1, pp. 69–75, 2008.

[126] Z. Y. Zhang, S. Q. Yu, L. Y. Miao et al., "Artesunate combined with vinorelbine plus cisplatin in treatment of advanced nonsmall cell lung cancer: a randomized controlled trial," *Journal of Chinese Integrative Medicine*, vol. 6, no. 2, pp. 134–138, 2008.

[127] S. Lee, "Synthesis of 10B-Substituited triazolyl artemisinins and their growth inhibitory activity against various cancer cells," *Bulletin of the Korean Chemical Society*, vol. 32, no. 2, pp. 737–740, 2011.

[128] F. S. Feng, E. M. Guantai, M. J. Nell, C. E. J. van Rensburg, H. Hoppe, and K. Chibale, "Antiplasmodial and antitumor activity of dDHA analogs derived via the aza-Michael addition reaction," *Bioorganic and Medicinal Chemistry Letters*, vol. 21, no. 10, pp. 2882–2886, 2000.

[129] C. H. Lee, H. Hong, J. Shin et al., "NMR studies on novel antitumor drug candidates, deoxoartemisinin and carboxypropyldeoxoartemisinin," *Biochemical and Biophysical Research Communications*, vol. 274, no. 2, pp. 359–369, 2000.

[130] A. A. Alagbala, A. J. McRiner, K. Borstnik et al., "Biological mechanisms of action of novel C-10 non-acetal trioxane dimers in prostate cancer cell lines," *Journal of Medicinal Chemistry*, vol. 49, no. 26, pp. 7836–7842, 2006.

[131] C. Horwedel, S. B. Tsogoeva, S. Wei, and T. Efferth, "Cytotoxicity of artesunic acid homo- and heterodimer molecules toward sensitive and multidrug-resistant CCRF-CEM leukemia cells," *Journal of Medicinal Chemistry*, vol. 53, no. 13, pp. 4842–4848, 2010.

[132] J. P. Jeyadevan, P. G. Bray, J. Chadwick et al., "Antimalarial and Antitumor Evaluation of Novel C-10 Non-Acetal Dimers of 10β-(2-Hydroxyethyl)deoxoartemisinin," *Journal of Medicinal Chemistry*, vol. 47, no. 5, pp. 1290–1298, 2004.

[133] M. Jung, S. Lee, J. Ham, K. Lee, H. Kim, and S. Kie Kim, "Antitumor activity of novel deoxoartemisinin monomers, dimers, and trimer," *Journal of Medicinal Chemistry*, vol. 46, no. 6, pp. 987–994, 2003.

[134] D. Opsenica, G. Pocsfalvi, Z. Juranic et al., "Cholic acid derivatives as 1,2,4,5-tetraoxane carriers: structure and antimalarial and antiproliferative activity," *Journal of Medicinal Chemistry*, vol. 43, no. 17, pp. 3274–3282, 2000.

[135] S. Soomro, T. Langenberg, A. Mahringer et al., "Design of novel artemisinin-like derivatives with cytotoxic and antiangiogenic properties," *Journal of Cellular and Molecular Medicine*, vol. 15, no. 5, pp. 1122–1135, 2011.

[136] P. J. de Vries and T. K. Dien, "Clinical pharmacology and therapeutic potential of artemisinin and its derivatives in the treatment of malaria," *Drugs*, vol. 52, no. 6, pp. 818–836, 1996.

[137] S. Krishna, A. C. Uhlemann, and R. K. Haynes, "Artemisinins: mechanisms of action and potential for resistance," *Drug Resistance Updates*, vol. 7, no. 4-5, pp. 233–244, 2004.

[138] S. A. Charman, S. Arbe-Barnes, I. C. Bathurst et al., "Synthetic ozonide drug candidate OZ439 offers new hope for a single-dose cure of uncomplicated malaria," *Proceedings of the National Academy of Sciences of the United States of America*, vol. 108, no. 11, pp. 4400–4405, 2011.

[139] S. -H. Xiao, J. Keiser, J. Chollet et al., "*In vitro* and *In vivo* activities of synthetic trioxolanes against major human schistosome species," *Antimicrobial Agents and Chemotherapy*, vol. 51, no. 4, pp. 1440–1445, 2007.

[140] I. Opsenica, D. Opsenica, K. S. Smith, W. K. Milhous, and B. A. Šolaja, "Chemical stability of the peroxide bond enables diversified synthesis of potent tetraoxane antimalarials," *Journal of Medicinal Chemistry*, vol. 51, no. 7, pp. 2261–2266, 2008.

[141] N. Terzić, D. Opsenica, D. Milić et al., "Deoxycholic acid-derived tetraoxane antimalarials and antiproliferatives," *Journal of Medicinal Chemistry*, vol. 50, no. 21, pp. 5118–5127, 2007.

[142] World Health Organization, *Guidelines for the Treatment of Malaria*, WHO press, Geneva, Switzerland, 2006.

[143] A. R. Yuen, G. Zou, A. T. Turrisi et al., "Reproductive functions in female patients treated with adjuvant and neoadjuvant chemotherapy for localized osteosarcoma of the extremity," *Cancer*, vol. 89, no. 9, pp. 1961–1965, 2000.

[144] Z. P. Wu, C. W. Gao, Y. G. Wu et al., "Inhibitive effect of artemether on tumor growth and angiogenesis in the rat C6 orthotopic brain gliomas model," *Integrative Cancer Therapies*, vol. 8, no. 1, pp. 88–92, 2009.

[145] F. Cavallo, C. de Giovanni, P. Nanni, G. Forni, and P. -L. Lollini, "2011: the immune hallmarks of cancer," *Cancer Immunology, Immunotherapy*, vol. 60, no. 3, pp. 319–326, 2011.

15

Therapeutic Approach in the Improvement of Endothelial Dysfunction: The Current State of the Art

Miroslav Radenković,[1] Marko Stojanović,[1] Tatjana Potpara,[2] and Milica Prostran[1]

[1] *Department of Pharmacology, Clinical Pharmacology and Toxicology, Medical Faculty, University of Belgrade, P.O. Box 38, 11129 Belgrade, Serbia*
[2] *Cardiology Clinic, Clinical Center of Serbia, Medical Faculty, University of Belgrade, 11000 Belgrade, Serbia*

Correspondence should be addressed to Miroslav Radenković; mradenkovic@med.bg.ac.rs

Academic Editor: Paul Higgins

The endothelium has a central role in the regulation of blood flow through continuous modulation of vascular tone. This is primarily accomplished by balanced release of endothelial relaxing and contractile factors. The healthy endothelial cells are essential for maintenance of vascular homeostasis involving antioxidant, anti-inflammatory, pro-fibrinolytic, anti-adhesive, or anticoagulant effects. Oppositely, endothelial dysfunction is primarily characterized by impaired regulation of vascular tone as a result of reduced endothelial nitric oxide (NO) synthase activity, lack of cofactors for NO synthesis, attenuated NO release, or increased NO degradation. So far, the pharmacological approach in improving/reversal of endothelial dysfunction was shown to be beneficial in clinical trials that have investigated actions of different cardiovascular drugs. The aim of this paper was to summarize some of the latest clinical findings related to therapeutic possibilities for improving endothelial dysfunction in different pathological conditions. In the majority of presented clinical investigations, the assessment of improvement or reversal of endothelial dysfunction was performed through the flow-mediated dilatation measurement, and in some of those endothelial progenitor cells' count was used for the same purpose. Still, given the fast and continuous development of this field, the evidence acquisition included the MEDLINE data base screening and the selection of articles published between 2010 and 2012.

1. Introduction

The endothelium has a central role in the regulation of blood pressure and flow through continuous modulation of vascular tone [1]. This is primarily accomplished by timely and balanced production and release of endothelial relaxing factors, namely, nitric oxide, prostacyclin, or endothelium-derived hyperpolarizing factor [2–4], as well as endothelium-derived contracting autacoids, such as endothelin-1, thromboxane A_2, angiotensin II, or superoxide anion. The response of different blood vessels to action of various relaxing and contractile vasoactive substances can be partly or entirely endothelium dependent, as well completely endothelium independent [5–8]. Endothelial cells are highly specialized to detect diverse physical, chemical, or mechanical stimuli, such as pulsatile changes in blood flow-induced shear stress, which is pivotal for physiological autoregulation of vascular tone. Apart from the key role in the regulation of vascular tone, healthy endothelial cells continuously adapt to local requirements and are essential for the maintenance of entire vascular homeostasis involving antioxidant, anti-inflammatory, profibrinolytic, and anticoagulant effects. Moreover, in physiological conditions leukocyte adhesion and migration, smooth muscle cell migration and proliferation, secretion of vasoconstrictive factors, and platelet aggregation and adhesion are negatively regulated by undamaged endothelium.

In contrast to previous facts, it is well established that hypertension, smoking, diabetes mellitus, hypercholesterolemia, obesity, or sedentary lifestyle represents major risk factors leading to endothelial dysfunction, atherosclerosis, and other cardiovascular clinical manifestations. Endothelial dysfunction is primarily characterized by impaired regulation of vascular tone as a result of reduced endothelial nitric oxide synthase activity, lack of cofactors for nitric oxide synthesis, attenuated nitric oxide release, or increased nitric oxide degradation. In addition, in this pathological process endothelial cells are directly affected by oxidative stress, increase of endogenous nitric oxide synthesis inhibitors, inflammation, increased adipocytokines, increased release of aldosterone, or depletion of tetrahydrobiopterin [9]. Finally, endothelial dysfunction is also characterized by increased production of endothelium-derived contracting factors, including angiotensin II, endothelins, superoxide anions, and cyclooxygenase-derived prostanoids [10]. In the early stages, endothelial function may be partly maintained by compensatory upregulation of prostacyclin and/or EDHF [11, 12]. Still, the balance between release of endothelial relaxing and contractile factors is shifted toward the vasoconstrictive autacoides. Hence, endothelial dysfunction is expressed in increased interactions with leukocytes, growth and proliferation of smooth muscle cells, prevailing vasoconstriction, impaired coagulation, vascular inflammation, thrombosis, and atherosclerosis [13]. Pharmacological approach in improving/reversal of endothelial dysfunction was shown to be beneficial in clinical trails that have investigated actions of angiotensin converting enzyme inhibitors, angiotensin receptor blockers, statins and other lipid lowering agents, calcium channel blockers, some β-receptor blockers, thiazolidinediones, erythropoietin, L-arginine, antioxidants, vitamins, tetrahydrobiopterin, or stimulators of endothelial progenitor cells [9, 14, 15].

The measurement of flow-mediated dilation represents a simple approach to examine vasodilator function in *in vivo* conditions. In particular, flow-mediated dilatation induced by reactive hyperemia has been known to be endothelium dependent, and this can be detected during reactive hyperemia by high-resolution ultrasound in superficial arteries noninvasively [16]. Although many different guidelines are present in the literature, one of the latest comprehensive methodological and physiological guidelines for the assessment of flow-mediated dilation in humans was presented by Thijssen et al. [17]. As outlined in this paper, flow-mediated dilation reflects endothelium-dependent and largely nitric oxide-mediated arterial function and has been used as a surrogate marker of vascular health. This technique has been used to compare groups of subjects and to evaluate the impact of interventions within individuals. Moreover, flow-mediated dilation has become broadly used in clinical studies, in part, because it strongly predicts cardiovascular events in asymptomatic subjects and in patients with established cardiovascular disease. This method is inexpensive, represents a repeatable measure of endothelial function, and can actually provide a fair chance for early assessment of possible cardiovascular outcomes. A blunted vasodilator response to flow-mediated dilation implies a decrease in nitric oxide bioavailability, which may be evoked by different risk factors and pathological conditions that are linked with alterations of signaling pathways in endothelial cells. Thus, improvement of flow-mediated dilation after specific therapeutic approach is translated to the improvement in clinical prognosis. Moreover, the use of flow-mediated dilatation early in drug development programmes provides the possibility to identify not only benefit, but also potential adverse effects on the vessel wall [18].

Endothelial progenitor cells, another powerful marker of endothelial function, are circulating cells with the ability to differentiate into mature endothelium and participate in neoangiogenesis. The circulating endothelial progenitor cells count is now considered to be a predictor of endothelial function and cardiovascular health. Thus, the measurement of endothelial progenitor cells may be a surrogate biologic marker for vascular function and cumulative cardiovascular risk, suggesting further that endothelial injury in the absence of sufficient circulating progenitor cells may unfavorably affect the progression of cardiovascular disease [19]. Furthermore, the assessment of flow-mediated brachial artery reactivity showed a notable relationship between the number of progenitor cells and endothelial function [19].

The aim of this paper was to review and summarize the latest clinical findings related to therapeutic possibilities for improving and restoring endothelial dysfunction in different pathological conditions. In the vast majority of presented clinical investigations the assessment of an improvement or complete reversal of endothelial dysfunction was performed through the flow-mediated dilatation measurement, and in some of those endothelial progenitor cells count was used for the same purpose. Still, given the fast and continuous development of this field, the evidence acquisition involved the MEDLINE data base screening and the selection of articles published between 2010 and 2012. The main findings connected to the improvement of endothelial dysfunction from the reviewed clinical studies were summarized in the Table 1.

2. Chronic Heart Failure

The production of nitric oxide has been established to be attenuated in chronic heart failure patients, most probably because of the reduced availability of endothelial nitric oxide synthase and nitric oxide inactivation induced by oxidative stress. Besides, there is an evident decrease of circulating endothelial progenitor cells required for the cellular restoration, too. On the other hand, various pharmacodynamic-unrelated (pleiotropic) actions of statins on patients with chronic heart failure are currently under investigation, given that statins are established to increase vascular nitric oxide production, reduce the production of reactive oxygen species, and promote vasculogenesis.

In randomized, placebo-controlled, and double-blind study reported by Erbs et al. [20], it was of interest to evaluate the pleiotropic effects of rosuvastatin on vascular and tissue regeneration, as well its impact on endothelial function and hemodynamics in chronic heart failure, as a result of ischemic heart disease or dilated cardiomyopathy. Forty-two age-, gender-, and cardiac medication-matched patients clinically stable for at least one month before enrollment were randomized to 12 weeks of oral rosuvastatin (40 mg/day) or placebo. The inclusion and exclusion criteria were in accordance with the clinical status of participants, as well as with the goal of the study, and were appropriately applied. In consideration to endothelial dysfunction, endothelium-dependent flow-mediated dilatation, vascular endothelial growth factor level, oxidized LDL, and the count of circulating progenitor cells were assessed at baseline and

TABLE 1: The main findings connected to the improvement of endothelial dysfunction from the reviewed clinical studies.

Pathological condition	Drug	Main effects	Corresponding reference
Chronic heart failure	Rosuvastatin	Oxidized LDL ↓ Lipid peroxidation ↓ Stem and progenitor cells ↑ FMD ↑	Erbs et al. [20]
Acute coronary syndrome	Perindopril	Apoptosis ↓ CD34+ mobilization ↑ VEGF ↑ TNF-α ↓ Bradykinin ↑	Cangiano et al. [21]
Cardiac syndrome X	Nebivolol	FMD ↔ High-sensitivity C-reactive protein ↓ von Willebrand factor ↓ Fibrinogen ↓	Kayaalti et al. [22]
Hypertensive left ventricular hypertrophy	Carvedilol	FMD ↑ Endothelin-1 ↓ Nitric oxide ↑	Xiaozhen et al. [23]
Coronary artery disease and impaired glucose tolerance	Pioglitazone	FMD ↑ TNF-α ↓ Triglycerides ↓ HMW adiponectin ↑	Rizza et al. [24]
Hypertension and impaired glucose tolerance	Telmisartan	FMD ↑ Insulin resistance ↓ Glucose tolerance ↑	Perl et al. [25]
Type 2 diabetes	Gliclazide	FMD ↑ Endothelial progenitor cells ↑	Chen et al. [26]
Obesity	Pitavastatin	FMD ↑ Triglycerides ↓	Nagashima and Endo [27]
Peripheral artery disease	Telmisartan	Maximum walking distance ↑ FMD ↑	Zankl et al. [28]
Behçet's disease	Atorvastatin Lisinopril	FMD ↑	Inanc et al. [29]
Polycystic ovary syndrome	Spironolactone	FMD ↑	Bajuk Studen et al. [30]
Subclinical hypothyroidism	L-thyroxin	FMD ↑ FT4 ↑ TSH ↓ Total cholesterol ↓	Alibaz Oner et al. [31]
Ankylosing spondylitis	Infliximab	FMD ↑ Serum nitrite ↓ Erythrocyte sedimentation rate ↓ C-reactive protein ↓	Syngle et al. [32]
Chronic hemodialysis	Simvastatin	FMD ↑ Oxidized LDL ↓ VCAM-1 ↓ 8-epi-PG F2 ↓ Nitric oxide bioavailability ↑	Kishimoto et al. [33]

FMD: flow-mediated dilatation; VEGF: vascular endothelial growth factor; TNF-α: tumor necrosis factor-α; TSH: thyroid-stimulating hormone; VCAM-1: vascular cell adhesion molecule 1.

after 12 weeks. Rosuvastatin exerted evident antioxidative action. This was substantiated by significant decrease of oxidized LDL levels and lipid peroxidation if compared to placebo group. This was accompanied with notable increase of circulating stem and progenitor cells in rosuvastatin group. Rosuvastatin treatment was also associated with increased plasma vascular endothelial growth factor level. Finally, in rosuvastatin group a significant improvement of flow-mediated dilatation was obtained in contrast to the baseline values in rosuvastatin-treated and the values obtained in placebo group. Although this study provided valuable results considering clinical improvement of chronic heart failure, taking into account only the part considering improvement of endothelial function it can be assumed that rosuvastatin via nonlipid-associated actions notably contributed to neovascularisation and to the enhancement of endothelial function in patients with chronic heart failure.

3. Acute Coronary Syndrome

In patients with coronary artery disease angiotensin-converting enzyme (ACE) inhibitors reduce cardiovascular mortality and myocardial infarction rate, most probably by producing beneficial action on functionally damaged endothelial cells and by reversing atherosclerotic process to some point. It is known that decrease in circulating endothelial progenitor cells (mostly characterized by the presence of specific assessment of surface markers, such as CD34 and vascular endothelial growth factor receptor-2) contributes to impaired angiogenesis as well as progression of atherosclerosis, and that patients at risk for coronary artery disease have decreased number of circulating endothelial progenitor cells with impaired activity [19]. On the other hand, vascular endothelial growth factor signaling activity and related angiogenesis plays a protective role in ischemic heart disease and myocardial infarction [34]. Moreover, pharmacotherapy by means of angiotensin II type 1 receptor antagonists or angiotensin-converting enzyme inhibitors has varying effects on progenitor cell levels and function [35].

In the study reported by Cangiano et al. [21] the effect of treatment on endothelial function with perindopril (ACE inhibitor) or valsartan (angiotensin II receptor blocker) at baseline and after 7, 15, and 30 days in patients with non-ST-segment elevation myocardial infarction, and also in normal sex- and age-matched healthy subject controls was investigated. Endothelial apoptosis was determined by cultivating serum samples *in vitro* with human umbilical vein endothelial cells (HUVECs), while endothelial renewal was assessed by necrosis-induced mobilization of CD34+ bone marrow cells. CD34+ cell mobilization is known to be linked with improved prognosis and reduced left ventricular remodeling in postmyocardial infarction patients. At the baseline, postmyocardial infarction patients had around 10 time higher rates of apoptosis if compared with the control group. In the perindopril group the observed parameter significantly declined after 30 days, but not in the group treated with valsartan. Similar results and trends were found for another serum indicator of apoptosis rate, namely, the Bax/Bcl-2 (proapoptotic/antiapoptotic) ratio. CD34+ mobilization was significantly increased in group treated with perindopril, whereas in the valsartan group CD34+ mobilization did not change notably. Positive findings in the perindopril group were associated with an increase in vascular endothelial growth factor, and a reduction in tumor necrosis factor-α and its soluble receptors, versus no change in the control. In this paper vascular endothelial growth factor values were strongly correlated with CD34+ cells, and tumor necrosis factor-α with the rate of apoptosis. Perindopril also reduced the proapoptotic charge of the serum by increasing the plasma concentration of bradykinin, while angiotensin II concentration was reduced. Thus, it can be suggested that perindopril, unlike valsartan, reduces the proapoptotic effect of serum on the endothelium and increases endothelial renewal in patients with acute coronary syndromes.

4. Cardiac Syndrome X

An important clinical entity termed cardiac syndrome X is usually described as angina pectoris with a normal coronary arteriogram [36]. Endothelial dysfunction and inflammation are known to be involved in pathophysiology of this syndrome primarily affecting coronary microvasculature. Treatment options would for example include angiotensin-converting enzyme inhibitors or nitrates. However, the effect of β-adrenoceptor antagonists in cardiac syndrome X is still under investigation. Nebivolol belongs to a group of cardioselective β-adrenoceptor antagonists having beneficial effects on endothelial function via stimulation of endothelial L-arginine/nitric oxide transduction pathway and augmentation of nitric oxide release [37], which is decreased in plasma of cardiac syndrome X patients.

The action of nebivolol in 38 patients diagnosed with cardiac syndrome X was evaluated in a prospective and randomized clinical trial [22]. The inclusion and the exclusion criteria were adequately defined and appropriately applied. The control group consisted of 18 patients, while the treatment group involved 20 patients receiving nebivolol hydrochloride (5 mg/day *per os*) within the four-week time frame. All ultrasonographic and biochemical analysis were done at baseline and four weeks later. All patients completed the study without any side effects during the followup. Thus, after the nebivolol therapy, there was a significant increase in both brachial artery baseline lumen diameter and lumen diameter after reactive hyperemia, yet without significant change in flow-mediated endothelium-dependent or endothelium-independent dilatation. On the other hand, the levels of serum inflammatory markers indirectly indicating the degree or severity of endothelial function, such as high-sensitivity C-reactive protein, von Willebrand factor, and fibrinogen were significantly decreased, thus leading to a suggestion that nebivolol therapy may have a beneficial effect on endothelial function in patients with cardiac syndrome X.

5. Hypertension and Left Ventricular Hypertrophy

Carvedilol belongs to a group of third-generation beta-blockers with nonselective β-adrenoceptor, selective $\alpha(1)$-adrenoceptor, and calcium channel blocking activity. This drug was shown to have other beneficial properties on vascular function; including anti-proliferative action on smooth muscle cells or scavenging of free-oxygen species in endothelial cells. In regard to the established association between left ventricular hypertrophy and the presence of endothelial dysfunction [15], possible beneficial action of carvedilol in this setting was not fully investigated.

In a single-centre, randomized, open, endpoint-blinded, and parallel-group clinical investigation conducted by Xiaozhen et al. [23], the primary goal was to compare the effects of carvedilol on coronary flow reserve in patients with hypertensive left ventricular hypertrophy. However, it was also of interest to investigate endothelium-dependent and endothelium-independent reactivity of the brachial artery through an ultrasound measuring of flow-mediated vasodilatation. In order to further evaluate changes in endothelial function, levels of plasma endothelin-1, nitric oxide, and several other metabolites were monitored and analyzed at baseline and after 6-month therapy. With regards to correctly designed inclusion and exclusion criteria, sixty-three female and male patients, with mean age of 61, were randomly assigned into two groups for treatment with carvedilol (10 mg twice daily) or metoprolol (50 mg). Because of several common beta-receptor blocker-associated side effects, at the end of 6-month therapy, 28 patients remained in the carvedilol group and 29 in the metoprolol group. Antihypertensive action of both drugs was comparable in the final statistical evaluation. Still, taking into account only results regarding the endothelial function, it was found that in carvedilol group endothelium function of the brachial artery was higher than after metoprolol regimen. Namely, in the carvedilol group, flow-mediated arterial dilation increased significantly by approximately 2.5%, as did glyceryl trinitrate-induced endothelium-independent dilatation by approximately 3.3%. Moreover, with the carvedilol treatment, plasma level of endothelin-1 was notably lower, while nitric oxide significantly higher if compared to the metoprolol group or baseline values in both investigated clusters, thus suggesting beneficial and protective effects of carvedilol on endothelial dysfunction in patients with hypertensive left ventricular hypertrophy. This is in accordance with known facts that endothelial dysfunction is usually characterized by decreased release of endothelial relaxing factors, such as nitric oxide, and on the other hand accompanied with increased plasma levels of different endogenous vasoconstrictor substances, such as endothelin-1.

6. Coronary Artery Disease and Impaired Glucose Tolerance

It has been established that glitazone-induced activation of PPARγ (peroxisome-proliferator activated receptor-gamma) is positively connected for example with an increase and decrease of adiponectin and TNF-alpha expression, respectively [38]. Pioglitazone belongs to a thiazolidinediones family of antidiabetic drugs having a PPARγ agonistic activity with beneficial effect on insulin sensitivity. PPARγ were first identified as a transcription factor integral to adipocyte differentiation, however, PPARγ are also present in endothelial and vascular smooth muscle cells and they are linked with increased nitric oxide bioavailability, as well with decreased proinflammatory/proatherogenic molecules, primarily through selective regulation of target genes expression [39].

In the study of Rizza et al. [24] the hypothesis that modulation of adipocyte function through PPARγ (peroxisome-proliferator activated receptor γ) activation may improve insulin sensitivity and adipose/endothelial function was tested. Fifty-four male and female patients with stable coronary artery disease and with a recent-onset impaired glucose tolerance status characterized mainly by insulin resistance but not compromised by glucose toxicity due to hyperglycemia were initially enrolled. In the further course twenty-five coronary artery disease age- and body-mass-index-matched patients with impaired glucose tolerance received either pioglitazone (30 mg/day) or placebo for 12 weeks. Ultrasound assessment of endothelium-dependent and endothelium-independent vasodilator brachial artery reactivity was performed at day one and after 12 weeks. Insulin sensitivity was assessed following the same time-frame. The baseline parameters did not change over the study course in the placebo group. On the other hand, flow-mediated dilatation was significantly improved by approximately 2% at the end of the treatment with pioglitazone. This was also the case with insulin sensitivity connected to significant decrease of tumor necrosis factor-alpha and triglycerides, and increase of high molecular weight adiponectin, as well. The additional analysis suggested that changes in high molecular weight adiponectin levels appeared to be an independent and significant predictor of increased flow-mediated dilatation after pioglitazone treatment. The significance of this result is also connected with the fact that in endothelial cells adiponectin enhances production of nitric oxide, suppresses production of reactive oxygen species, and protects cells from inflammation that results from exposure to high glucose levels or tumor necrosis factor [40].

7. Hypertension and Impaired Glucose Tolerance

Treatment-induced reversal of endothelial dysfunction has been confirmed to increase beneficial outcome in hypertensive patients. In consideration to angiotensin-receptor antagonists it has been suggested that telmisartan in serum concentrations obtained in clinical use possesses PPARγ (peroxisome-proliferator activated receptor γ) agonistic properties, which is typical for antidiabetic action of glitazones, and improves insulin resistance as well as vascular endothelial dysfunction. This would imply both vascular and metabolic effects of telmisartan, which would be in accordance with recent finding that PPARγ activation inhibited Ang II type 1 receptor expression and protected endothelial function for example by stimulation of endothelial nitric oxide production [41].

In the randomized, double-blind, prospective, and cross-over trial 24 hypertensive patients with impaired glucose tolerance were involved [25]. The patients were 40–75 years old with for at least three months stable parameters including body weight, smoking behavior, physical activity, concomitant medication, and nutritional habits. The exclusion criteria were appropriately defined too. Before an entry into the active period, antihypertensive treatment was switched to amlodipine. Patients were then randomised to telmisartan 80 mg or losartan 50 mg daily for 12 weeks (amlodipine was stopped) in a crossover fashion. At the baseline and after 12 weeks endothelial function testing was performed via ultrasound measuring of flow-mediated vasodilatation, and endothelium-independent, nitroglycerin-mediated vasodilatation, as well. Although both agents showed comparable antihypertensive clinical action, endothelial function improved significantly by telmisartan treatment, but not by losartan administration. Moreover, losartan treatment did not alter flow-mediated vasodilatation recordings if compared to the already low baseline values, indicating initial presence of endothelial dysfunction. The authors also reported that insulin resistance improved significantly after telmisartan only, as did glucose tolerance. This result was independent regarding the improvement of endothelial function. It was also underlined that the effect of telmisartan on insulin resistance and endothelial function is most pronounced in those patients with high insulin resistance and endothelial dysfunction at baseline.

8. Type 2 Diabetes

The prevention and appropriate treatment of type 2 diabetes are today's major issues, given the continuous increase of type 2 diabetes worldwide and consequent vascular complications. Hence, endothelial dysfunction provoked by underlying insulin resistance has been associated with reduced nitric oxide bioavailability, increased production of reactive oxygen species and also with alterations of reparative processes which mediate endothelial regeneration via endothelial progenitor cells [42]. Gliclazide belongs to a second generation of sulfonylurea antidiabetic drugs with additional antioxidant characteristics, most probably connected to free radical scavenging properties of its azabicyclo-octyl ring. This may be also linked with beneficial decrease of low-density lipoprotein oxidation and monocyte adhesion on endothelial cells evoked by diabetic pathological process.

Gliclazide action on possible improvement of flow-mediated dilatation and increase in number of circulating endothelial progenitor cells in type 2 diabetic patients was investigated by Chen et al. [26]. Apart from the inclusion and exclusion criteria, important confounding factors were taken into consideration during the recruitment process. Gliclazide was administered in male and female 33 newly diagnosed type 2 diabetes patients during 12 weeks in a daily dose of 30–90 mg, whereas control group consisted of 25 nondiabetic age- and gender-matched randomly selected subjects. Endothelial function was evaluated by flow-mediated vasodilatation recorded in brachial artery, which was accompanied with measurements of endothelium-independent dilatation induced by sublingual administration nitroglyceride. The number of circulating endothelial progenitor cells co-expressing three characteristic surface antigens ($CD45^{low}/CD34^{+}/VEGFR2^{+}$) and oxidative stress via malondialdehyde levels and superoxide dismutase activity was also determined. At baseline flow-mediated dilatation, the flow-mediated dilatation/nitroglyceride-mediated dilatation ratio, and the circulating endothelial progenitor cells count were significantly lower in the diabetic group. All quoted parameters were notably improved after 12-week-long gliclazide treatment, yet remained lower then in the control subjects. Still, the percentage increase in flow-mediated dilatation was positively correlated with the percentage increase of endothelial progenitor cells count in the diabetic group. Nitroglyceride-mediated dilatation was comparable in diabetic (before and after the treatment) and the control group. In diabetic patients gliclazide treatment reduced malondialdehyde levels compared to the baseline values. The obtained reduction still remained insufficient to match the values obtained in the control group. Similar trend was observed with the improvement of superoxide dismutase activity. The obtained results were indicative for the assumption that gliclazide could improve endothelial function in diabetes, which may be related to its antioxidative properties.

9. Obesity

Obesity has been shown to be one of the most important risk factors for the occurrence or the progression of metabolic syndrome and numerous cardiovascular diseases [43]. Moreover, postprandial hypertriglyceridemia and hyperglycemia are the contributing factors leading to acutely impaired endothelium-dependent vasodilatation and endothelial dysfunction as well. On the other hand, statins are known to improve endothelial function due to lipid-lowering or other pleiotropic actions, involving increased expression of endothelial nitric oxide synthase, negative action of intracellular oxidative stress, or attenuation of proinflammatory pathways [44]. Postprandial hyperlipemia is a phenomenon usually occurring if the dietary sources of fat went above physiological needs and is positively correlated with incidence of obesity, metabolic syndrome, or diabetes.

In a study including twenty-four obese and drug-naïve male subjects it was of interest to examine if pitavastatin, belonging to a statin group of drugs, can affect postprandial hypertriglyceridemia induced by oral fat loading test and improve endothelial function measured via flow-mediated dilatation methodological procedure [27]. The presence of metabolic syndrome was initially diagnosed in the half of enrolled subjects. During two weeks the participants (age range 29–68; body mass index $\geq 25\,kg/m^2$) with comparable baseline clinical characteristics received either 2 mg/day pitavastatin or placebo. Flow-mediated dilatation was measured before and after four hours of the oral fat load (74 mg of cholesterol per 100 g) in consideration to the fact that serum triglyceride and remnant-like particle cholesterol reach the peak within the same timeframe. Thus, in regard to postprandial response at baseline, after an oral fat load, a notable decrease in endothelium-dependent flow-mediated dilation was observed in all the participants, whereas endothelium-independent nitroglycerin-induced mediated dilation was unaffected. A marked increase of the serum triglyceride level was recorded in all subjects too. Secondly, in the fasting state the pitavastatin group of participants was shown to have an evident increase in the calculated percentages of flow-mediated dilatation and notable decrease in serum triglyceride level, while this was not the case in the placebo group. Finally, in postprandial state the pitavastatin group of subjects was determined to have the complete abolishment of initial decrease of postprandial flow-mediated dilatation at baseline and the further attenuation of the increase in postprandial serum triglyceride level, while oppositely in the placebo group the statistical significance was not observed.

The authors also reported that nominal change in postprandial serum triglyceride remained significantly correlated with nominal change in postprandial flow-mediated dilatation among the covariates, including nominal change in postprandial serum low-density lipoprotein cholesterol, triglyceride, and high-density lipoprotein cholesterol. Therefore, it was suggested that the prevention of postprandial endothelial dysfunction by pitavastatin could be at least partly caused by lowering of triglyceride-induced deteriorating actions on endothelial cells.

10. Peripheral Artery Disease

Peripheral artery disease is characterized by partial or complete obstruction of the arteries in the lower limbs. This pathological condition is known to be associated with endothelial dysfunction [45], a damaging vascular process that can be significantly linked with an increased inflammatory status, which also predicts future ischemic events, such as myocardial infarction and stroke [46]. Apart from increased risk for different cardiovascular events, peripheral artery disease is commonly accompanied with the high rate of the quality of life deterioration in affected patients. On the other hand, the preservation of quality of life is for the most part essential to encourage the patients for regular and adequately adjusted physical activity, which is in point of fact a basis of noninvasive treatment of peripheral artery disease—affected population. The angiotensin-converting-enzyme system plays an important role in the pathogenesis and progression of endothelial dysfunction, and ACE inhibitors were shown to be useful for reducing the risk of cardiovascular events in clinical and subclinical peripheral artery disease [47].

The aim of the recent single centre, single-blinded, randomized, and prospective study conducted by Zankl et al. [28] was to analyze the effects of telmisartan (AT_1-receptor blocker) on absolute walking distance and endothelial function in patients with peripheral artery disease. The authors hypothesized that telmisartan can improve endothelial function, which may further translate into longer maximum walking distance over a period of 12 months. Hence, thirty-six patients between 18 and 80 years of age with documented peripheral artery disease, at least stage Fontaine IIa, were assigned to a telmisartan or placebo group for 12 months, which included four visits (baseline visit, after four weeks, and finally after six and twelve months). Telmisartan was initially administered in a standard dose of 40 mg/day and up-titrated after four weeks to 80 mg/day, if clinically necessary. Absolute walking distance was measured at baseline visit and after six and 12 months by standard treadmill exercise test. In order to measure local endothelial release of nitric oxide, vascular ultrasound scans of the right brachial artery blood flow were recorded following standard flow-mediated vasodilatation protocol with ischemia and reactive hyperemia episodes. After 12 months, maximum walking distance increased by 26% (from 132 m at baseline to 191 m) in the telmisartan group, whereas in the placebo group it was comparable to baseline. At the same time flow-mediated vasodilatation was augmented by 40% (from 0.06 mm at baseline to 0.08 mm) in the telmisartan group, while it actually deteriorated in the placebo group (from 0.05 mm to 0.04 mm). Even though a questionnaire-estimated disease-related quality of life scores remained unchanged in the telmisartan group, placebo treatment was associated with a marked decline by 30%. In this pilot study there was a clear beneficial effect on brachial artery endothelial function in patients with peripheral artery disease subjected to treatment with telmisartan. The improvement of endothelial function was also shown to be translated into clinical advantages from which patients would benefit, that is to say walking capacity and the quality of life.

11. Behçet's Disease

Behçet's disease is rare multisystem disorder, which affects mostly young adults and it is described as a chronic immune-inflammatory vasculitis with perivascular infiltration affecting vessels of various sizes [48]. Vascular invasion by activated leucocytes and consequential production of free-oxygen species provides an excellent ground for the pathological activation and final dysfunction of endothelial cells. Although recurrent oral and genital ulcers and uveitis are the clinical trial of the disease, the vascular system involvement represents the main cause of mortality. The treatment of Behçet's disease is usually individualized and adjusted to the specific clinical findings in each patient, yet mostly symptomatic and empirical.

The effect of atorvastatin (HMG-CoA reductase inhibitor) and lisinopril (ACE inhibitor) on endothelium dysfunction was investigated in patients with Behçet's disease [29]. The undertaken investigation was designed as a prospective, randomized, double-blind, and placebo-controlled study enrolling 92 male and female patients diagnosed with Behçet's disease, and with ultrasonographically documented endothelial dysfunction as well. Patients clearly presenting pathological conditions or other risk factors known to contribute to occurrence and/or progress of endothelial dysfunction were initially excluded. Age, body mass index, systolic blood pressure, diastolic blood pressure, total cholesterol, HDL cholesterol, LDL cholesterol, fibrinogen, and erythrocyte sedimentation rate were comparable between the participants. Endothelial dysfunction was evaluated by brachial artery flow-mediated dilatation at baseline and after three months of atorvastatin (20 mg/day), lisinopril (10 mg/day), or placebo regimen. The obtained recordings were expressed as the percentage change in the brachial artery diameter from baseline to the subsequent reactive hyperemia. Thus, a notable improvement in endothelium-dependent flow-mediated dilatation by 7.8% was observed in atorvastatin group. This was also the case in patients with Behçet's disease initially assigned to lisinopril administration, where baseline results improved by 6.4%. Still, only partial enhancement of 0.8% was observed in placebo group. Apart from the previous findings, it was shown that reduced LDL level before and after three months was notably linked with an improvement of flow-mediated dilatation in atorvastatin group. In consideration to endothelium-independent vasodilatation provoked by sublingual nitroglycerine, there was a similar trend in improvement of dilatation in participants receiving lisinopril and atorvastatin. The obtained results were indicative for the assumption that atorvastatin and lisinopril improved endothelial functions in Behçet's disease patients, thus augmenting therapeutic possibilities for better treatment of this pathological condition.

12. Polycystic Ovary Syndrome

Polycystic ovary syndrome, representing a common endocrine disorder in women of reproductive age, has been established to have a positive correlation with increased risk of gestational diabetes, type 2 diabetes and other associated cardiovascular pathological conditions [49]. As a marker of pathological vascular damage, endothelial dysfunction was associated with polycystic ovary syndrome, as well. One of the possible reasons for endothelial dysfunction in this pathological condition could be related to androgens' proinflammatory and oxidative stress-related actions [50]. One of the accepted approaches for polycystic ovary syndrome treatment involves spironolactone, an androgen and mineralocorticoid receptor blocking drug, especially in patients with hirsutism or other androgen excess-associated clinical aberrations.

The assumption that treatment with spironolactone might reverse endothelial dysfunction in nonobese polycystic ovary syndrome patients was recently examined by Bajuk Studen et al. [30]. Thirty nonobese patients with polycystic ovary syndrome were compared with twenty healthy body mass index-matched women having a regular menstrual cycles and no clinical androgenism or biochemical hyperandrogenemia. All the inclusion and the exclusion criteria were appropriately defined and applied. Polycystic ovary syndrome patients were given spironolactone 100 mg daily in 21-day long intervals followed by a 7-day pause regardless of menstrual bleeding, for 6 months. In the hemodynamic examination an endothelium-dependent flow-mediated dilatation and endothelium-independent glyceryl trinitrate-induced dilatation of the brachial artery were studied. At baseline flow-mediated dilatation was significantly lower in polycystic ovary syndrome group comparing to healthy women (9.0 versus 10.2%, resp.). This was also the case with glyceryl trinitrate-induced dilatation (polycystic ovary syndrome (21.3%) versus control (26.6%)). After six months of spironolactone administration, all participants of the study were reevaluated and the flow-mediated dilatation was found to be notably improved in polycystic ovary syndrome group, while it remained unchanged in controls. Furthermore, the obtained percentages for flow-mediated dilatation after six months were comparable between treated and untreated women (8.3 versus 9.4%, resp.). Endothelium-independent glyceryl trinitrate-induced dilatation of the brachial artery remained unchanged. It was proposed that in this study, six months of spironolactone treatment reversed endothelial dysfunction in nonobese polycystic ovary syndrome patients primarily through its antiandrogenic effects and partly via aldosterone antagonism.

13. Subclinical Hypothyroidism

Subclinical hypothyroidism is medical condition, which involves normal serum free T4 (FT4) and free T3 (FT3) levels, while serum thyroid-stimulating hormone (TSH) levels are increased [51]. This endocrine pathological condition is considered to be one of the risk factors for atherosclerotic cardiovascular disease, and has been associated with dysfunction of endothelial cells, as well. The increase in cardiovascular risk, most clearly associated with hyper- and hypothyroidism, is due not only to alterations in lipid profile, but also to hemodynamic changes, endothelial dysfunction, coagulation disturbances, hormonal and metabolic changes, and changes in measurable factors such as homocysteine and C-reactive protein, which are known to increase risk for atherosclerotic disease [52]. Although it has been shown that thyroid hormone replacement therapy improves endothelial function in patients with hypothyroidism [53], the potential beneficial effects of L-thyroxin on damaged endothelium are still under investigation.

In the prospective study reported by Alibaz Oner et al. [31] it was of interest to evaluate endothelial functions and the effect of L-thyroxin therapy on endothelial functions in young adults without any cardiovascular disease concomitantly diagnosed with subclinical hypothyroidism. Twenty-seven patients with newly diagnosed subclinical hypothyroidism were prospectively enrolled. They were age- and sex-matched with twenty-two healthy subjects, representing a control group. The exclusion criteria were adequately applied. TSH, FT3, and FT4 levels were determined in all participants at baseline. Thus, TSH levels were significantly higher, while FT4 levels were notably lower in subclinical hypothyroidism group. Baseline brachial artery ultrasonographic parameters of endothelium-dependent flow-mediated dilatation where significantly lower in subjects with subclinical hypothyroidism compared to healthy controls, while endothelium-independent nitrate-induced dilatation remained comparable between examined groups. Oral L-thyroxin (L-T4) was administered at daily dose of 0.5 μg/kg and the patients were followed up and repeatedly tested in regard to thyroid function until euthyroidism was restored. Brachial ultrasonography was performed again 4–6 weeks after the restoration of euthyroidism with L-T4 therapy. Thus, baseline diameter of brachial artery, flow-mediated dilatation value, and nitrate-induced dilatation all significantly improved after the L-T4 treatment in subclinical hypothyroidism patients if compared to the baseline values. This was accompanied with significant increase of FT4 levels and decrease of TSH and total cholesterol levels. This investigation showed that L-T4 treatment in subclinical hypothyroidism patients was associated with significant improvement of endothelial dysfunction. Moreover, the improvement of nitrate-induced endothelium-independent dilatation suggests positive action of L-T4 on vascular smooth muscle cells too.

14. Ankylosing Spondylitis

Ankylosing spondylitis is defined as a chronic inflammatory rheumatic disease affecting sacroiliac joints and spine, which is associated with an increased cardiovascular risk, especially atherosclerosis and coronary artery disease. It is considered that the inflammatory component underlying ankylosing spondylitis pathological process contributes at least in one part to the overall cardiovascular risk and specifically to endothelial dysfunction, most probably as a consequence of increased proinflammatory cytokines levels, for example tumor necrosis factor alpha (TNF-α), which in turn negatively regulates endothelial function with resulting decrease of endogenous nitric oxide bioavailability [54]. Thus, as previously outlined, targeting of adhesion molecules, chemokines, and angiogenesis by administering nonspecific immunosuppressive drugs as well as monoclonal antibodies or small molecular compounds inhibiting the action of a single mediator may control inflammation and prevent tissue destruction [55].

The hypothesis that chronic inflammation in ankylosing spondylitis is associated with endothelial dysfunction despite treatment with conventional disease modifying antirheumatic drugs, which can be reversed with intravenous (i.v.) infusion of infliximab (anti-TNF-α agent) was tested in the prospective, uncontrolled, open-label, pilot study by Syngle et al. [32]. The study participants were twelve anti-TNF-naïve ankylosing spondylitis patients with high disease activity, lacking an adequate response to conventional disease modifying antirheumatic drugs. The inclusion criteria were well applied and only patients on stable dose of disease modifying antirheumatic drugs (diclofenac or indomethacin + sulfasalazine) for at least 6 months were included in the study. These patients were administered infliximab 5 mg/kg as a single i.v. infusion. The exclusion criteria were presented in detail and were in accordance with overall design and aim of the study. In consideration to the endothelial function, serum nitrite (nitric oxide surrogate metabolite marker) concentration and flow-mediated, as well as nitroglycerin-induced dilatation of brachial artery were evaluated at baseline and 12 weeks after single-dose treatment with infliximab. Thus, flow-mediated dilation was significantly improved by approximately 17% after 12 weeks, whereas endothelium-independent nitroglycerin-induced dilatation and baseline brachial artery diameter remained unchanged. Twelve weeks after single-dose treatment with infliximab serum nitrite concentration was notably decreased (approximately 4 μmol/L) if compare to the baseline. Infliximab also reduced markers of inflammatory disease activity (erythrocyte sedimentation rate and C-reactive protein levels). This all was indicative for the assumption that the protective effect of infliximab was preserved for at least 12 weeks after initial infusion. The authors suggested that in ankylosing spondylitis, endothelial dysfunction is a part of the disease process and infliximab improves both endothelial dysfunction and inflammatory disease activity, thus providing a promising approach to manage spondylitis and its atherosclerotic complications.

15. Chronic Hemodialysis

One of the principal origins of cardiovascular morbidity in patients undergoing hemodialysis is associated with the occurrence and the progression of atherosclerotic pathological process with ischemic heart disease and myocardial infarction as resulting consequences. The reasons for end-stage renal disease patients having signs of endothelial dysfunction are multifactorial, including increased oxidative stress, hyperhomocysteinemia, dyslipidemia, hyperglycemia, hypertension, or retention of L-arginine [56]. On the other hand, statins are confirmed to reduce risk of coronary events through decrease of plasma lipid levels and improving endothelial dysfunction via upregulation of endothelial nitric oxide and antioxidant activity, as well.

The effects of simvastatin on lipids, flow-mediated endothelium-dependent and nitroglycerin-induced endothelium-independent dilatation, and markers of oxidant stress and atherosclerosis were investigated in 37 patients on hemodialysis (lasting approximately 4 years) with or without mild hyperlipidemia, as well without lipid-lowering drugs for at least six weeks before the study beginning, and also without any acute coronary events for at least three months prior to the study [33]. The participants were age- and gender-matched and based on the plasma LDL levels they were enrolled into (a) 5 mg/day simvastatin group (n = 14), (b) 10 mg/day simvastatin group (n = 14), and (c) the control group without prescription (n = 9) for 16-week interval. All groups were matched in consideration to associated pathological conditions and regular use of medications that can affect endothelium-mediated physiological functions. Hence, the endothelium-dependent flow-mediated dilatation in simvastatin groups notably increased at week 1 and 16, while nitroglycerin-induced endothelium-independent dilatation remained unchanged over the study course. Markers associated with endothelial dysfunction, such as oxidized LDL, soluble vascular cell adhesion molecule 1, and 8-epi-prostaglandin F2, significantly decreased after 16 weeks in both statin groups, while on the other hand plasma nitrite/nitrate increased, thus indicating increased nitric oxide bioavailability. It was concluded that simvastatin improved the impaired endothelial function of dialysis patients by decreasing oxidized LDL, improving the lipid profile and, at least in part, enhancing nitric oxide bioavailability.

16. Conclusion

The knowledge about the risk factors, molecular mechanisms and related intracellular signaling pathways, and nonpharmacological and pharmacological treatment options regarding endothelial dysfunction is still accumulating. Although this paper covered some of the recent findings obtained with the clinical administration of primarily conventional drugs, such as statins, angiotensin-converting enzyme inhibitors, angiotensin receptor blockers, beta-adrenoceptor antagonists or oral antidiabetic drugs, quite a few articles were published involving the investigation of different dietary supplements, naturally-occurring compounds, food ingredients or related substances on endothelial function. Thus, over the last two years positive correlations considering the improvement of endothelial function in regard to flow-mediated dilation were confirmed, or newly established after enteral or parenteral use of polyphenols (resveratrol, hesperidin), folic acid, N^1-methylnicotinamide, antioxidant agents (vitamin C, E, α-lipoic acid, co-enzyme Q10), omega-3-polyunsaturated fatty acids, then after consumption of flavanol-rich cocoa, walnut-enriched *ad libitum* diet or flavonoid- and nitrates-rich food, as well after induction of tetrahydrobiopterin synthesis [57–68]. Taken together, clinical investigations aiming the improvement and/or complete reversal of endothelial dysfunction are constantly being undertaken, thus giving the additional input to adequate prevention, diagnosis, and nonpharmacological and pharmacological treatment of different cardiovascular diseases and pathological conditions associated with later cardiovascular pathology.

Conflict of Interests

The authors have no conflict of interests to declare.

Acknowledgment

This article was supported by the Ministry of Education and Science, Republic of Serbia, with Grant 175023.

References

[1] F. Ribeiro, A. J. Alves, M. Teixeira, V. Ribeiro, J. A. Duarte, and J. Oliveira, "Endothelial function and atherosclerosis: circulatory markers with clinical usefulness," *Revista Portuguesa de Cardiologia*, vol. 28, no. 10, pp. 1121–1151, 2009.

[2] R. G. Dias, C. E. Negrão, and M. H. Krieger, "Nitric oxide and the cardiovascular system: cell activation, vascular reactivity and genetic variant," *Arquivos Brasileiros de Cardiologia*, vol. 96, no. 1, pp. 68–75, 2011.

[3] R. J. Gryglewski, "Prostacyclin among prostanoids," *Pharmacological Reports*, vol. 60, no. 1, pp. 3–11, 2008.

[4] M. Radenković, "Endothelium-derived hyperpolarizing factor and pregnancy: possible contribution in regulation of vascular signaling mechanisms in normotensive and hypertensive settings," in *Pregnancy: Risk Factors, Management and Recovery*, T. Altamirano Frias and M. J. Cano, Eds., pp. 205–220, NOVA Publishers, New York, NY, USA, 2012.

[5] L. Grbović, M. Radenković, M. Prostran, and S. Pešić, "Characterization of adenosine action in isolated rat renal artery. Possible role of adenosine A(2A) receptors," *General Pharmacology*, vol. 35, no. 1, pp. 29–36, 2001.

[6] M. Radenković, M. Stojanović, R. Janković, M. Topalović, and M. Stojiljković, "Combined contribution of endothelial relaxing autacoides in the rat femoral artery response to CPCA: an adenosine A_2 receptor agonist," *The Scientific World Journal*, vol. 2012, Article ID 143818, 7 pages, 2012.

[7] M. Radenković, L. Grbović, N. Radunović, and P. Momčilov, "Pharmacological evaluation of bradykinin effect on human umbilical artery in normal, hypertensive and diabetic pregnancy," *Pharmacological Reports*, vol. 59, no. 1, pp. 64–73, 2007.

[8] M. Radenković, M. Stojanović, and M. Topalović, "Contribution of thromboxane A_2 in rat common carotid artery response to serotonin," *Scientia Pharmaceutica*, vol. 78, no. 3, pp. 435–443, 2010.

[9] Y. Hirata, D. Nagata, E. Suzuki, H. Nishimatsu, J. I. Suzuki, and R. Nagai, "Diagnosis and treatment of endothelial dysfunction in cardiovascular disease: a review," *International Heart Journal*, vol. 51, no. 1, pp. 1–6, 2010.

[10] D. Versari, E. Daghini, A. Virdis, L. Ghiadoni, and S. Taddei, "Endothelium-dependent contractions and endothelial dysfunction in human hypertension," *British Journal of Pharmacology*, vol. 157, no. 4, pp. 527–536, 2009.

[11] A. J. Flammer and T. F. Lüscher, "Three decades of endothelium research: from the detection of nitric oxide to the everyday implementation of endothelial function measurements in cardiovascular diseases," *Swiss Medical Weekly*, vol. 140, Article ID w13122, 2010.

[12] S. Taddei, D. Versari, A. Cipriano et al., "Identification of a cytochrome P450 2C9-derived endothelium-derived hyperpolarizing factor in essential hypertensive patients," *Journal of the American College of Cardiology*, vol. 48, no. 3, pp. 508–515, 2006.

[13] I. A. M. van den Oever, H. G. Raterman, M. T. Nurmohamed, and S. Simsek, "Endothelial dysfunction, inflammation, and apoptosis in diabetes mellitus," *Mediators of Inflammation*, vol. 2010, Article ID 792393, 15 pages, 2010.

[14] H. A. R. Hadi and J. Al Suwaidi, "Endothelial dysfunction in diabetes mellitus," *Journal of Vascular Health and Risk Management*, vol. 3, no. 6, pp. 853–876, 2007.

[15] D. Versari, E. Daghini, A. Virdis, L. Ghiadoni, and S. Taddei, "Endothelial dysfunction as a target for prevention of cardiovascular disease," *Diabetes Care*, vol. 32 , supplement 2, pp. S314–321, 2009.

[16] M. Hashimoto, Y. Miyamoto, Y. Matsuda, and H. Akita, "New methods to evaluate endothelial function: non-invasive method of evaluating endothelial function in humans," *Journal of Pharmacological Sciences*, vol. 93, no. 4, pp. 405–408, 2003.

[17] D. H. J. Thijssen, M. A. Black, K. E. Pyke et al., "Assessment of flow-mediated dilation in humans: a methodological and physiological guideline," *American Journal of Physiology*, vol. 300, no. 1, pp. H2–H12, 2011.

[18] M. Charakida, S. Masi, T. F. Lüscher, J. J. P. Kastelein, and J. E. Deanfield, "Assessment of atherosclerosis: the role of flow-mediated dilatation," *European Heart Journal*, vol. 31, no. 23, pp. 2854–2861, 2010.

[19] S. Devaraj and I. Jialal, "Dysfunctional endothelial progenitor cells in metabolic syndrome," *Experimental Diabetes Research*, vol. 2012, Article ID 585018, 5 pages, 2012.

[20] S. Erbs, E. B. Beck, A. Linke et al., "High-dose rosuvastatin in chronic heart failure promotes vasculogenesis, corrects endothelial function, and improves cardiac remodeling—results from a randomized, double-blind, and placebo-controlled study," *International Journal of Cardiology*, vol. 146, no. 1, pp. 56–63, 2011.

[21] E. Cangiano, J. Marchesini, G. Campo et al., "ACE inhibition modulates endothelial apoptosis and renewal via endothelial progenitor cells in patients with acute coronary syndromes," *American Journal of Cardiovascular Drugs*, vol. 11, no. 3, pp. 189–198, 2011.

[22] F. KayaaltI, N. Kalay, E. Basar et al., "Effects of nebivolol therapy on endothelial functions in cardiac syndrome X," *Heart and Vessels*, vol. 25, no. 2, pp. 92–96, 2010.

[23] H. Xiaozhen, Z. Yun, Z. Mei, and S. Yu, "Effect of carvedilol on coronary flow reserve in patients with hypertensive left-ventricular hypertrophy," *Blood Pressure*, vol. 19, no. 1, pp. 40–47, 2010.

[24] S. Rizza, M. Cardellini, O. Porzio et al., "Pioglitazone improves endothelial and adipose tissue dysfunction in pre-diabetic CAD subjects," *Atherosclerosis*, vol. 215, no. 1, pp. 180–183, 2011.

[25] S. Perl, I. Schmölzer, H. Sourij et al., "Telmisartan improves vascular function independently of metabolic and antihypertensive effects in hypertensive subjects with impaired glucose tolerance," *International Journal of Cardiology*, vol. 139, no. 3, pp. 289–296, 2010.

[26] L. L. Chen, F. Yu, T. S. Zeng, Y. F. Liao, Y. M. Li, and H. C. Ding, "Effects of gliclazide on endothelial function in patients with newly diagnosed type 2 diabetes," *European Journal of Pharmacology*, vol. 659, no. 2-3, pp. 296–301, 2011.

[27] H. Nagashima and M. Endo, "Pitavastatin prevents postprandial endothelial dysfunction via reduction of the serum triglyceride level in obese male subjects," *Heart and Vessels*, vol. 26, no. 4, pp. 428–434, 2011.

[28] A. R. Zankl, B. Ivandic, M. Andrassy et al., "Telmisartan improves absolute walking distance and endothelial function in patients with peripheral artery disease," *Clinical Research in Cardiology*, vol. 99, no. 12, pp. 787–794, 2010.

[29] M. T. Inanc, N. Kalay, T. Heyit et al., "Effects of atorvastatin and lisinopril on endothelial dysfunction in patients with Behçet's disease," *Echocardiography*, vol. 27, no. 8, pp. 997–1003, 2010.

[30] K. Bajuk Studen, M. Šebeštjen, M. Pfeifer, and J. Preželj, "Influence of spironolactone treatment on endothelial function in non-obese women with polycystic ovary syndrome," *European Journal of Endocrinology*, vol. 164, no. 3, pp. 389–395, 2011.

[31] F. Alibaz Oner, S. Yurdakul, E. Oner, A. Kubat Uzum, and M. Erguney, "Evaluation of the effect of l-thyroxin therapy on endothelial functions in patients with subclinical hypothyroidism," *Endocrine*, vol. 40, no. 2, pp. 280–284, 2011.

[32] A. Syngle, K. Vohra, A. Sharma, and L. Kaur, "Endothelial dysfunction in ankylosing spondylitis improves after tumor necrosis factor-α blockade," *Clinical Rheumatology*, vol. 29, no. 7, pp. 763–770, 2010.

[33] N. Kishimoto, T. Hayashi, I. Sakuma et al., "A hydroxymethylglutaryl coenzyme a reductase inhibitor improves endothelial function within 7-days in patients with chronic hemodialysis," *International Journal of Cardiology*, vol. 145, no. 1, pp. 21–26, 2010.

[34] D. Kajdaniuk, B. Marek, W. Foltyn, and B. Kos-Kudła, "Vascular endothelial growth factor (VEGF)—part 1: in physiology and pathophysiology," *Endokrynologia Polska*, vol. 62, no. 5, pp. 444–455, 2011.

[35] C. Qian, R. G. Schoemaker, W. H. van Gilst, and A. J. M. Roks, "The role of the renin-angiotensin-aldosterone system in cardiovascular progenitor cell function," *Clinical Science*, vol. 116, no. 4, pp. 301–314, 2009.

[36] I. A. C. Vermeltfoort, P. G. H. M. Raijmakers, I. I. Riphagen et al., "Definitions and incidence of cardiac syndrome X: review and analysis of clinical data," *Clinical Research in Cardiology*, vol. 99, no. 8, pp. 475–481, 2010.

[37] J. E. Toblli, F. DiGennaro, J. F. Giani, and F. P. Dominici, "Nebivolol: impact on cardiac and endothelial function and clinical utility," *Journal of Vascular Health and Risk Management*, vol. 8, no. 1, pp. 151–160, 2012.

[38] A. M. Sharma and B. Staels, "Review: peroxisome proliferator-activated receptor γ and adipose tissue—understanding obesity-related changes in regulation of lipid and glucose metabolism," *The Journal of Clinical Endocrinology and Metabolism*, vol. 92, no. 2, pp. 386–395, 2007.

[39] J. Plutzky, "The PPAR-RXR transcriptional complex in the vasculature: energy in the balance," *Circulation Research*, vol. 108, no. 8, pp. 1002–1016, 2011.

[40] B. J. Goldstein, R. G. Scalia, and X. L. Ma, "Protective vascular and myocardial effects of adiponectin," *Nature Clinical Practice Cardiovascular Medicine*, vol. 6, no. 1, pp. 27–35, 2009.

[41] A. Sugawara, A. Uruno, M. Kudo, K. Matsuda, C. W. Yang, and S. Ito, "PPARγ agonist beyond glucose lowering effect," *The Korean Journal of Internal Medicine*, vol. 26, no. 1, pp. 19–24, 2011.

[42] R. M. Cubbon, M. B. Kahn, and S. B. Wheatcroft, "Effects of insulin resistance on endothelial progenitor cells and vascular repair," *Clinical Science*, vol. 117, no. 5, pp. 173–190, 2009.

[43] J. A. Barbosa, A. B. Rodrigues, C. C. Mota, M. M. Barbosa, and A. C. Simões e Silva, "Cardiovascular dysfunction in obesity and new diagnostic imaging techniques: the role of noninvasive image methods," *Journal of Vascular Health and Risk Management*, vol. 7, no. 1, pp. 287–295, 2011.

[44] J. A. Lardizabal and P. C. Deedwania, "The anti-ischemic and anti-anginal properties of statins," *Current Atherosclerosis Reports*, vol. 13, no. 1, pp. 43–50, 2011.

[45] G. Brevetti, V. Schiano, and M. Chiariello, "Endothelial dysfunction: a key to the pathophysiology and natural history of peripheral arterial disease?" *Atherosclerosis*, vol. 197, no. 1, pp. 1–11, 2008.

[46] G. Brevetti, G. Giugliano, L. Brevetti, and W. R. Hiatt, "Inflammation in peripheral artery disease," *Circulation*, vol. 122, no. 18, pp. 1862–1875, 2010.

[47] G. Coppola, G. Romano, E. Corrado, R. M. Grisanti, and S. Novo, "Peripheral artery disease: potential role of ACE-inhibitor therapy," *Journal of Vascular Health and Risk Management*, vol. 4, no. 6, pp. 1179–1187, 2008.

[48] N. Ceylan, S. Bayraktaroglu, S. M. Erturk, R. Savas, and H. Alper, "Pulmonary and vascular manifestations of Behçet disease: imaging findings," *American Journal of Roentgenology*, vol. 194, no. 2, pp. W158–W164, 2010.

[49] S. Aust and J. Ott, "The impact of polycystic ovarian syndrome on gestational diabetes," in *Gestational Diabetes*, M. Radenković, Ed., pp. 183–200, InTech, Rijeka, Croatia, 2011.

[50] S. Samavat, P. Ahmadpoor, and F. Samadian, "Aldosterone, hypertension, and beyond," *Iranian Journal of Kidney Diseases*, vol. 5, no. 2, pp. 71–76, 2011.

[51] V. Fatourechi, "Subclinical hypothyroidism: an update for primary care physicians," *Mayo Clinic Proceedings*, vol. 84, no. 1, pp. 65–71, 2009.

[52] C. Neves, M. Alves, J. L. Medina, and J. L. Delgado, "Thyroid diseases, dyslipidemia and cardiovascular pathology," *Revista Portuguesa de Cardiologia*, vol. 27, no. 10, pp. 1211–1236, 2008.

[53] S. Taddei, N. Caraccio, A. Virdis et al., "Impaired endothelium-dependent vasodilatation in subclinical hypothyroidism: beneficial effect of levothyroxine therapy," *The Journal of Clinical Endocrinology and Metabolism*, vol. 88, no. 8, pp. 3731–3737, 2003.

[54] C. Zhang, "The role of inflammatory cytokines in endothelial dysfunction," *Basic Research in Cardiology*, vol. 103, no. 5, pp. 398–406, 2008.

[55] Z. Szekanecz and A. E. Koch, "Vascular involvement in rheumatic diseases: 'vascular rheumatology'," *Arthritis Research and Therapy*, vol. 10, no. 5, article 224, 2008.

[56] H. A. Hadi, C. S. Carr, and J. Al Suwaidi, "Endothelial dysfunction: cardiovascular risk factors, therapy, and outcome," *Journal of Vascular Health and Risk Management*, vol. 1, no. 3, pp. 183–198, 2005.

[57] R. H. Wong, P. R. Howe, J. D. Buckley, A. M. Coates, I. Kunz, and N. M. Berry, "Acute resveratrol supplementation improves flow-mediated dilatation in overweight/obese individuals with mildly elevated blood pressure," *Nutrition, Metabolism and Cardiovascular Diseases*, vol. 21, no. 11, pp. 851–856, 2011.

[58] K. Fujitaka, H. Otani, F. Jo et al., "Modified resveratrol Longevinex improves endothelial function in adults with metabolic syndrome receiving standard treatment," *Nutrition Research*, vol. 31, no. 11, pp. 842–847, 2011.

[59] S. Rizza, R. Muniyappa, M. Iantorno et al., "Citrus polyphenol hesperidin stimulates production of nitric oxide in endothelial cells while improving endothelial function and reducing inflammatory markers in patients with metabolic syndrome," *The Journal of Clinical Endocrinology and Metabolism*, vol. 96, no. 5, pp. E782–E792, 2011.

[60] Y. Ma, V. Y. Njike, J. Millet et al., "Effects of walnut consumption onendothelial function in type 2 diabetic subjects: a randomized controlled crossover trial," *Diabetes Care*, vol. 33, no. 2, pp. 227–232, 2010.

[61] Y. L. Dai, T. H. Luk, K. H. Yiu et al., "Reversal of mitochondrial dysfunction by coenzyme Q10 supplement improves endothelial function in patients with ischaemic left ventricular systolic dysfunction: a randomized controlled trial," *Atherosclerosis*, vol. 216, no. 2, pp. 395–401, 2011.

[62] D. Moertl, A. Hammer, S. Steiner, R. Hutuleac, K. Vonbank, and R. Berger, "Dose-dependent effects of omega-3-polyunsaturated fatty acids on systolic left ventricular function, endothelial function, and markers of inflammation in chronic heart failure of nonischemic origin: a double-blind, placebo-controlled, 3-arm study," *American Heart Journal*, vol. 161, no. 5, pp. 915.e1–915.e9, 2011.

[63] S. Westphal and C. Luley, "Flavanol-rich cocoa ameliorates lipemia-induced endothelial dysfunction," *Heart and Vessels*, vol. 26, no. 5, pp. 511–515, 2011.

[64] T. B. Domagala, A. Szeffler, L. W. Dobrucki et al., "Nitric oxide production and endothelium-dependent vasorelaxation ameliorated by N^1-methylnicotinamide in human blood vessels," *Hypertension*, vol. 59, no. 4, pp. 825–832, 2012.

[65] D. W. Wray, S. K. Nishiyama, R. A. Harris et al., "Acute reversal of endothelial dysfunction in the elderly after antioxidant consumption," *Hypertension*, vol. 59, no. 4, pp. 818–824, 2012.

[66] A. Z. Hoch, S. L. Lynch, J. W. Jurva, J. E. Schimke, and D. D. Gutterman, "Folic acid supplementation improves vascular function in amenorrheic runners," *Clinical Journal of Sport Medicine*, vol. 20, no. 3, pp. 205–210, 2010.

[67] C. P. Bondonno, X. Yang, K. D. Croft et al., "Flavonoid-rich apples and nitrate-rich spinach augment nitric oxide status and improve endothelial function in healthy men and women: a randomized controlled trial," *Free Radical Biology & Medicine*, vol. 52, no. 1, pp. 95–102, 2012.

[68] C. Antoniades, C. Cunnington, A. Antonopoulos et al., "Induction of vascular GTP-cyclohydrolase I and endogenous tetrahydrobiopterin synthesis protect against inflammation-induced endothelial dysfunction in human atherosclerosis," *Circulation*, vol. 124, no. 17, pp. 1860–1870, 2011.

16

The Indolic Diet-Derivative, 3,3′-Diindolylmethane, Induced Apoptosis in Human Colon Cancer Cells through Upregulation of NDRG1

A. Lerner,[1,2] M. Grafi-Cohen,[1,2] T. Napso,[3] N. Azzam,[4] and F. Fares[4,5]

[1] *Pediatric Gastroenterology and Nutrition Unit, Carmel Medical Center, Haifa 34362, Israel*
[2] *B. Rappaport School of Medicine, Technion-Israel Institute of Technology, Haifa 31096, Israel*
[3] *Department of Evolutionary and Environmental Biology, University of Haifa, Mount Carmel, Haifa 31905, Israel*
[4] *Department of Human Biology, University of Haifa, Mount Carmel, Haifa 31905, Israel*
[5] *Department of Molecular Genetics, Carmel Medical Center, Haifa 34362, Israel*

Correspondence should be addressed to F. Fares, ffares@sci.haifa.ac.il

Academic Editor: Masa-Aki Shibata

N-myc downstream regulated gene-1 participates in carcinogenesis, angiogenesis, metastases, and anticancer drug resistance. In the present study, we analyzed the expression pattern of N-myc downstream regulated gene-1 following treatment of human colonic cancer cell lines; HCT-116 (well differentiated with wild-type p53 gene) and Colo-320 (poorly differentiated with mutant p53 gene), with 3,3′-diindolylmethane, a well-established proapoptotic agent product derived from indole-3-carbinol. Treatment of Colo-320 and HCT-116 with 3,3′-diindolylmethane disclosed inhibition of cell viability in a dose-dependent manner, mediated through apoptosis induction. The increased expression of N-myc downstream regulated gene-1 was detected only in poorly differentiated colon cancer cells, Colo-320 cell line. Our results suggest that N-myc downstream regulated gene-1 expression is enhanced by 3,3′-diindolylmethane in poorly differentiated cells and followed by induction of apoptosis. 3,3′-diindolylmethane induced apoptosis may represent a new regulator of N-myc downstream regulated gene-1 in poorly differentiated colonic cancer cells.

1. Introduction

N-myc downstream regulated 1 gene (NDRG1) is a 43-kDa protein located mainly in the cytoplasm but occasionally translocates into the nucleus in a p53-dependent manner [1]. This protein interacts with many cell elements and consequently participates in various processes in the cells, such as differentiation, response to stress conditions, involvement in carcinogenesis, angiogenesis, and metastasis. NDRG1 is induced, among others, by stress conditions, inhibition of DNA methylation, and histone deacetylation [2–7]. Furthermore, NDRG1 is necessary for caspase-3 activation and is required for p53-dependent apoptosis in a cell type-specific manner [8]. Nevertheless, the precise function of NDRG1 and its regulation in cancer cells is far from being clear.

In colon cancer, NDRG1 protein levels appear to be decreased with the progression from normal colonic epithelium to carcinoma [9, 10]. Moreover, NDRG1 expression is associated with a more aggressive tumor phenotype and poor outcome in colorectal cancer [11].

NDRG1 mediates apoptosis in several tissues [8, 12, 13]. However, the regulation of NDRG1 during apoptosis state in cancer cells in general, and in colon cancer in particular, was not explored previously. The purpose of the current study was to investigate the NDRG1 expression pattern in human colon cancer cell lines which vary in their differentiation level and in their p53 status. For apoptosis induction, we used 3,3′-diindolylmethane (DIM), a well-established proapoptotic agent product derived from indole-3-carbinol (I3C). In a low environmental pH, I3C is converted into polymeric products, among which 3,3′-diindolylmethane (DIM) is the main one. Studies showed that DIM induced cell-cycle arrest in human prostate cancer through, the upregulation of cycline-dependent kinases [14] and apoptosis via mitochondrial pathway [15–21].

2. Materials and Methods

2.1. Cell Culture and Treatment. Two human colon cancer cell lines HCT-116 (well differentiated, p53 wild type) and Colo-320 (poorly differentiated, p53 mutant) were grown in a medium 10% fetal calf serum and 100 U/mL penicillin-streptomycin in the presence of DIM (10–100 μM). Cell viability (XTT) [22], cytotoxicity, and leakage of lactate dehydrogenase [23, 24] were tested 24, 48, and 72 hours after treatment.

DAPI staining for visualization of chromatin condensation [25] were conducted after treatment with 60 μM DIM for 72 hr [26].

2.2. RNA Isolation and Real-Time PCR. RNA from colon cancer cells was isolated using Tri-reagent (Tal-Ron). Total RNA (3 μg) was reverse-transcribed to cDNA. 1197 bp product of NDRG1 was amplified by real-time PCR (ABI Prism 7900) using probe and the following primers: 5′-AGGGACATGTCTCGGGAGATGCAGGAT-3′ and 5′-GGCCGCCTAGCAGGAGACCTCCATGG-3′. As a control gene, we amplified β-actin (838 bp) with 5′-ATCTGGCACCACACCTTCTACAATGAGCTGCG-3′ and 5′-CGTCATACTCCT GCTTGCTGATCCACATCTGC-3′.

Alkaline phosphatase activity assay [27] was conducted 4 and 8 h after treatment with 60 μM DIM.

2.3. Statistical Analysis. Data analyses were carried out using SPSS version 17. Experiments were repeated three times, each performed in triplicate, and the data are presented as means ± SD (Standard Deviation). Statistical analysis of the differences between controls and treated groups were performed using Student's t-test. $P < 0.05$ was considered significant.

3. Results

3.1. DIM Reduced Cell Viability by Apoptosis Induction. We observed that the two colon cancer cells treated with DIM (10–80 μM) for 72 hr had a significant inhibitory effect ($P < 0.001$) in a dose-dependent manner (Figure 1). The IC_{50} values were 52 μM for HCT-116 and 56 μM for Colo-320. Furthermore, no toxic effects were manifested for these concentrations, as it was determined with LDH enzyme activity (Data not shown).

Following the reduced viability, apoptosis was tested in cells treated with DIM (60 μM) for 72 hr (Figure 2(a)). Both cell lines showed DNA fragmentation, a main feature of apoptosis occurrence. In addition, cell treatment with 60 μM DIM for 48 h followed by DAPI staining (Figure 2(b)) showed apoptotic cells that exhibited typical apoptotic morphology, condensation, and fragmentation of the nucleus, in comparison to untreated cells.

3.2. Alteration in NDRG1 Expression in Colo 320. Basal expression of NDRG1 prior treatment showed low levels of mRNA and no expression of protein in Colo 320 cell lines; alternatively, high levels of both mRNA and protein were detected in HCT-116 cell line (Data not shown).

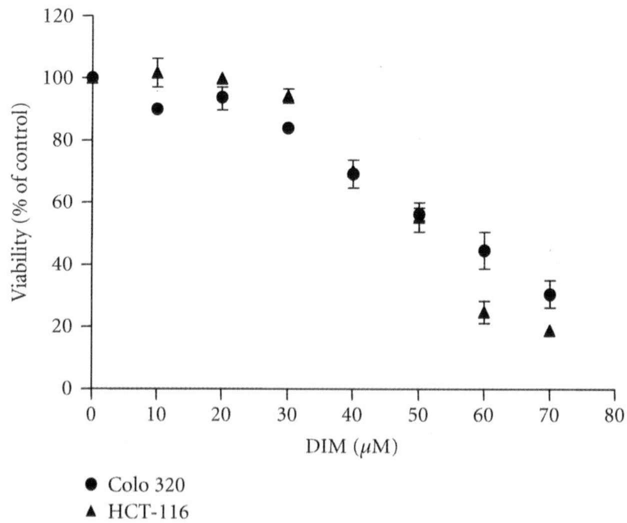

FIGURE 1: Effect of DIM on cell viability. Exponentially growing cells were incubated in the presence of 10 to 100 μM of DIM for 72 hours, and the viable cells were detected by XTT assay. The results are presented as percentage of control and expressed as means ± SD of three independent experiments.

Exposure of the Colo 320 to DIM for 24–72 hr resulted in a significant increase (9-fold for 24 h, 10-fold for 48 h, and 15-fold for 72 h following treatment) of the NDRG1 mRNA levels (Figure 3). However, exposure of HCT-116 to DIM resulted in uninfluenced expression of the NDRG1 mRNA compared to control cells.

3.3. Effect of DIM and NDRG1 Expression on Cell Differentiation. Alkaline phosphatase activity, a molecular marker of colon epithelial cells differentiation was used to determine whether the increase in NDRG1 expression is related to differentiation alteration in the cells. The results revealed that treated cells had a nonsignificant increase of alkaline phosphatase activity in Colo 320 cells and had no effect in HCT-116 cells (Figure 4).

4. Discussion

In the present study, we examined NDRG1 expression in human colon cancer cells during apoptosis induced upon DIM application. First, we showed that indol derivative found in crucifers (DIM) induced apoptosis in both human colon cancer cells HCT-116 and Colo 320. We have previously shown that DIM has a suppressive effect on the growth of breast cancer and prostate cell lines [15, 16, 20]. The IC_{50} values for DIM on growth inhibition of colon cancer cells (50–60 μM) were similar to those found for prostate and breast cancer cells (20–40 μM and 17–30 μM, resp.) [15, 28]. DIM affected the viability of the cancer cell in a time- and dose-dependent manner irrespective of their p53 phenotype. The effect was mediated by apoptosis as shown morphologically and by DNA fragmentation. Thus, colonic

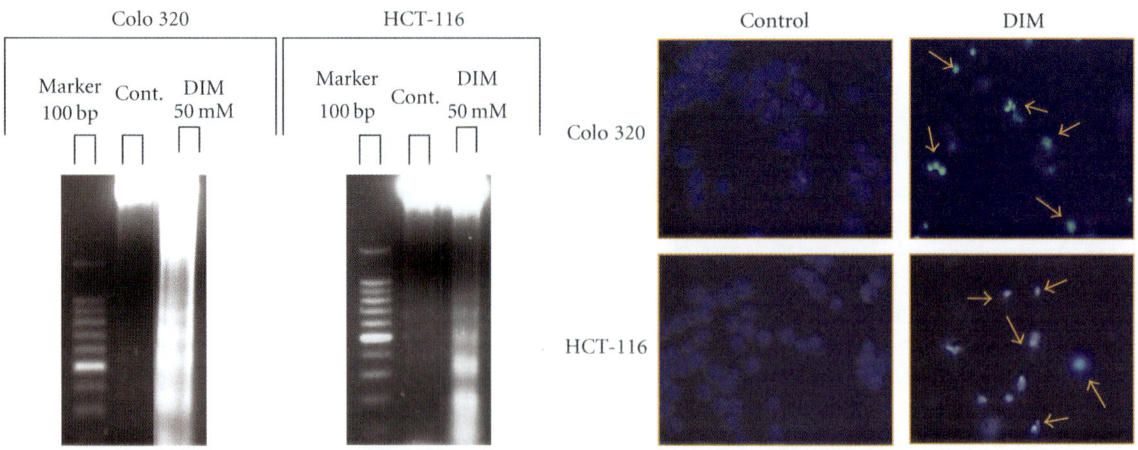

(a) (b)

Figure 2: Apoptosis formation by DIM in Colo 320 and HGT116 cell lines. Cells were treated with DIM 60 μM for 72 hours. DNA was extracted and separated on a 1.5% Agarose gel. The data shown were repeated three times (a). Morphologic changes, denoting apoptotic cells were shown by cell morphological changes. Cells were incubated in the presence of 60 μM DIM for 48 hours and stained with DAPI. Morphologic changes are shown by arrows (b). The data shown were repeated three times.

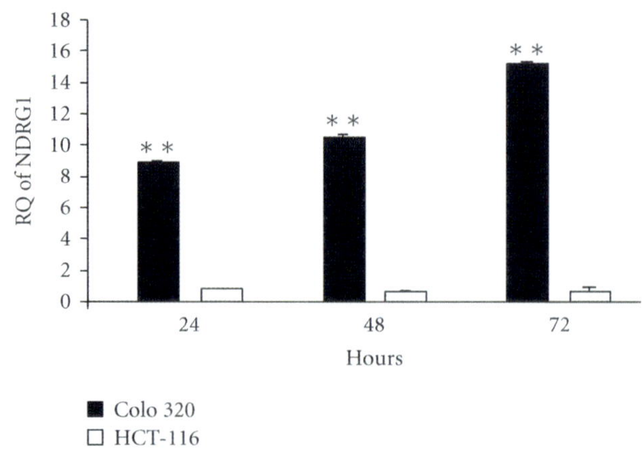

Figure 3: Expression of *NDRG1*. Cells treated with 60 μM DIM for 24, 48 and 72 h. The levels of mRNA were examined by real-time PCR and are represented as RQ (relative quantification) = 2^{-ddCt}. $^{*}P$ value <0.01, $^{**}P$ value <0.001.

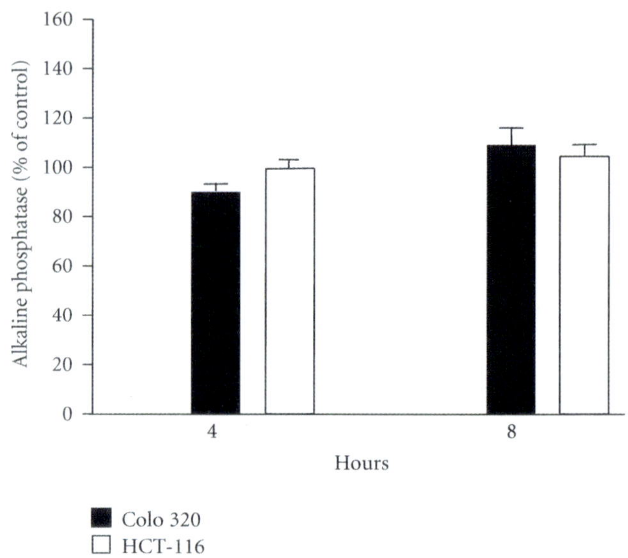

Figure 4: DIM treatment effect on alkaline phosphatase activity. Alkaline phosphatase activity (differentiation factor of colon cells) was detected after 4 and 8 hours of treatment. The results are presented as percentage of control and expressed as means ± SD of three independent experiments. $^{**}P$ value <0.001.

cell lines can be added to an increasing list of other organs' cell lines, namely, prostate and breast [16, 21, 29] that are affected by environmental factors which induce apoptosis.

The basal expression of NDRG1 reported here, high levels in well-differentiated cells (HCT-116) and low levels in poorly differentiated cells (Colo-320), was reported in colon [30], gastric cancer specimens [31], and in esophageal squamous cell carcinoma [32].

Quantization of NDRG1 expression showed that NDRG1 mRNA is increased 9–15-fold ($P < 0.001$) during treatment of the Colo-320 cells with DIM for 24–72 hr compared to control cells, indicating NDRG1 upregulation during apoptosis induced by DIM.

Up to now, it was known that NDRG1 expression is induced by DNA damage in a p53-dependent fashion, and it is necessary but not sufficient for p53-mediated caspase activation and apoptosis [8]. The present study shows for the first time that DIM increased NDRG1 expression in a p53 independent pathway followed by induction of apoptosis.

In conclusion, in this study, we provide evidence that the indole diet-derived DIM induce apoptosis in two human colon cancer cell lines, well- and poorly differentiated. However, induction of apoptosis by DIM is followed by increased NDRG1 expression only in a poorly differentiated and p53 mutant cells. On the other hand, DIM induced apoptosis in well-differentiated cells in a NDRG1-independent pathway. Our results may contribute to a better understanding of the molecular mechanisms by which DIM exerts its effects in colon cancer cells and tumors. It is suggested that NDRG1 is not only a differentiation factor but might impact the apoptotic process. In all the NDRG1 transfection studies, apoptotic effects should be taken in account. In fact, NDRG1 is on the list of metastatic-related/cancer suicide genes drug development in the battle against cancer [33, 34]. Further studies are needed in order to examine NDRG1 role in colon cancer genesis. Results from the present research may contribute to the development of new and efficient strategies for colon cancer therapy.

Conflict of Interests

The authors declare no potential conflict of interests with respect to the authorship and/or publication of this paper.

References

[1] S. K. Kurdistani, P. Arizti, C. L. Reimer, M. M. Sugrue, S. A. Aaronson, and S. W. Lee, "Inhibition of tumor cell growth by RTP/rit42 and its responsiveness to p53 and DNA damage," *Cancer Research*, vol. 58, no. 19, pp. 4439–4444, 1998.

[2] T. P. Ellen, Q. Ke, P. Zhang, and M. Costa, "NDRG1, a growth and cancer related gene: regulation of gene expression andfunction in normal and disease states," *Carcinogenesis*, vol. 29, no. 1, pp. 2–8, 2008.

[3] K. Kokame, H. Kato, and T. Miyata, "Homocysteine-respondent genes in vascular endothelial cells identified by differential display analysis: GRP78/BiP and novel genes," *Journal of Biological Chemistry*, vol. 271, no. 47, pp. 29659–29665, 1996.

[4] H. Park, M. A. Adams, P. Lachat, F. Bosman, S. C. Pang, and C. H. Graham, "Hypoxia induces the expression of a 43-kDa protein (PROXY-1) in normal and malignant cells," *Biochemical and Biophysical Research Communications*, vol. 276, no. 1, pp. 321–328, 2000.

[5] W. Ulrix, J. V. Swinnen, W. Heyns, and G. Verhoeven, "The differentiation-related gene 1, Drg1, is markedly upregulated by androgens in LNCaP prostatic adenocarcinoma cells," *FEBS Letters*, vol. 455, no. 1-2, pp. 23–26, 1999.

[6] D. Zhou, K. Salnikow, and M. Costa, "Cap43, a novel gene specifically induced by Ni2+ compounds," *Cancer Research*, vol. 58, no. 10, pp. 2182–2189, 1998.

[7] A. Kitowska and T. Pawełczyk, "N-myc downstream regulated 1 gene and its place in the cellular machinery," *Acta Biochimica Polonica*, vol. 57, no. 1, pp. 15–21, 2010.

[8] S. Stein, E. K. Thomas, B. Herzog et al., "NDRG1 is necessary for p53-dependent apoptosis," *Journal of Biological Chemistry*, vol. 279, no. 47, pp. 48930–48940, 2004.

[9] H. Cangul, "Hypoxia upregulates the expression of the NDRG1 gene leading to its overexpression in various human cancers," *BMC Genetics*, vol. 5, article 27, 2004.

[10] M. A. Shah, N. Kemeny, A. Hummer et al., "Drg1 expression in 131 colorectal liver metastases: correlation with clinical variables and patient outcomes," *Clinical Cancer Research*, vol. 11, no. 9, pp. 3296–3302, 2005.

[11] B. Strzelczyk, A. Szulc, R. Rzepko et al., "Identification of high-risk stage II colorectal tumors by combined analysis of the NDRG1 gene expression and the depth of tumor invasion," *Annals of Surgical Oncology*, vol. 16, no. 5, pp. 1287–1294, 2009.

[12] E. Angst, D. W. Dawson, D. Stroka et al., "N-myc downstream regulated gene-1 expression correlates with reduced pancreatic cancer growth and increased apoptosis in vitro and in vivo," *Surgery*, vol. 149, no. 5, pp. 614–624, 2011.

[13] X. Yan, M. S. Chua, H. Sun, and S. So, "N-Myc down-regulated gene 1 mediates proliferation, invasion, and apoptosis of hepatocellular carcinoma cells," *Cancer Letters*, vol. 262, no. 1, pp. 133–142, 2008.

[14] O. I. Vivar, C. L. Lin, G. L. Firestone, and L. F. Bjeldanes, "3,3′-Diindolylmethane induces a G1 arrest in human prostate cancer cells irrespective of androgen receptor and p53 status," *Biochemical Pharmacology*, vol. 78, no. 5, pp. 469–476, 2009.

[15] X. Ge, S. Yannai, G. Rennert, N. Gruener, and F. A. Fares, "3,3′-diindolylmethane induces apoptosis in human cancer cells," *Biochemical and Biophysical Research Communications*, vol. 228, no. 1, pp. 153–158, 1996.

[16] F. A. Fares, X. Ge, S. Yannai, and G. Rennert, "Dietary indole derivatives induce apoptosis in human breast cancer cells," *Advances in Experimental Medicine and Biology*, vol. 451, pp. 153–157, 1998.

[17] C. Bonnesen, I. M. Eggleston, and J. D. Hayes, "Dietary indoles and isothiocyanates that are generated from cruciferous vegetables can both stimulate apoptosis and confer protection against DNA damage in human colon cell lines," *Cancer Research*, vol. 61, no. 16, pp. 6120–6130, 2001.

[18] D. Z. Chen, M. Qi, K. J. Auborn, and T. H. Carter, "Indole-3-carbinol and diindolylmethane induce apoptosis of human cervical cancer cells and in murine HPV16-transgenic preneoplastic cervical epithelium," *Journal of Nutrition*, vol. 131, no. 12, pp. 3294–3302, 2001.

[19] S. R. Chinni, Y. Li, S. Upadhyay, P. K. Koppolu, and F. H. Sarkar, "Indole-3-carbinol (I3C) induced cell growth inhibition, G1 cell cycle arrest and apoptosis in prostate cancer cells," *Oncogene*, vol. 20, no. 23, pp. 2927–2936, 2001.

[20] M. Nachshon-Kedmi, S. Yannai, A. Haj, and F. A. Fares, "Indole-3-carbinol and 3,3′-diindolylmethane induce apoptosis in human prostate cancer cells," *Food and Chemical Toxicology*, vol. 41, no. 6, pp. 745–752, 2003.

[21] M. Nachshon-Kedmi, F. A. Fares, and S. Yannai, "Therapeutic activity of 3,3′-diindolylmethane on prostate cancer in an in vivo model," *Prostate*, vol. 61, no. 2, pp. 153–160, 2004.

[22] T. Mosmann, "Rapid colorimetric assay for cellular growth and survival: application to proliferation and cytotoxicity assays," *Journal of Immunological Methods*, vol. 65, no. 1-2, pp. 55–63, 1983.

[23] A. R. Goeptar, E. J. Groot, H. Scheerens, J. N. M. Commandeur, and N. P. E. Vermeulen, "Cytotoxicity of mitomycin C and Adriamycin in freshly isolated rat hepatocytes: the role of cytochrome P450," *Cancer Research*, vol. 54, no. 9, pp. 2411–2418, 1994.

[24] J. H. Moran and R. G. Schnellmann, "A rapid β-NADH-linked fluorescence assay for lactate dehydrogenase in cellular death," *Journal of Pharmacological and Toxicological Methods*, vol. 36, no. 1, pp. 41–44, 1996.

[25] P. M. O'Connor, K. Wassermann, M. Sarang, I. Magrath, V. A. Bohr, and K. W. Kohn, "Relationship between DNA cross-links, cell cycle, and apoptosis in Burkitt's lymphoma cell lines differing in sensitivity to nitrogen mustard," *Cancer Research*, vol. 51, no. 24, pp. 6550–6557, 1991.

[26] B. Almog, O. Fainaru, R. Gamzu et al., "Placental apoptosis in discordant twins," *Placenta*, vol. 23, no. 4, pp. 331–336, 2002.

[27] G. A. Turowski, Z. Rashid, F. Hong, J. A. Madri, and M. D. Basson, "Glutamine modulates phenotype and stimulates

proliferation in human colon cancer cell lines," *Cancer Research*, vol. 54, no. 22, pp. 5974–5980, 1994.

[28] M. Nachshon-Kedmi, S. Yannai, A. Haj, and F. A. Fares, "Indole-3-carbinol and 3,3′-diindolylmethane induce apoptosis in human prostate cancer cells," *Food and Chemical Toxicology*, vol. 41, no. 6, pp. 745–752, 2003.

[29] J. V. Higdon, B. Delage, D. E. Williams, and R. H. Dashwood, "Cruciferous vegetables and human cancer risk: epidemiologic evidence and mechanistic basis," *Pharmacological Research*, vol. 55, no. 3, pp. 224–236, 2007.

[30] N. Van Belzen, W. N. M. Dinjens, M. P. G. Diesveld et al., "A novel gene which is up-regulated during colon epithelial cell differentiation and down-regulated in colorectal neoplasms," *Laboratory Investigation*, vol. 77, no. 1, pp. 85–92, 1997.

[31] K. Jiang, Z. Shen, Y. Ye, X. Yang, and S. Wang, "A novel molecular marker for early detection and evaluating prognosis of gastric cancer: N-myc downstream regulated gene-1 (NDRG1)," *Scandinavian Journal of Gastroenterology*, vol. 45, no. 7-8, pp. 898–908, 2010.

[32] T. Ando, H. Ishiguro, M. Kimura et al., "Decreased expression of NDRG1 is correlated with tumor progression and poor prognosis in patients with esophageal squamous cell carcinoma," *Diseases of the Esophagus*, vol. 19, no. 6, pp. 454–458, 2006.

[33] M. Iiizumi, W. Liu, S. K. Pai, E. Furuta, and K. Watabe, "Drug development against metastasis-related genes and their pathways: a rationale for cancer therapy," *Biochimica et Biophysica Acta*, vol. 1786, no. 2, pp. 87–104, 2008.

[34] L. Teimoori-Toolabi, K. Azadmanesh, A. Amanzadeh, and S. Zeinali, "Selective suicide gene therapy of colon cancer exploiting the urokinase plasminogen activator receptor promoter," *BioDrugs*, vol. 24, no. 2, pp. 131–146, 2010.

17

Comparative Study of the Effect of Baicalin and Its Natural Analogs on Neurons with Oxygen and Glucose Deprivation Involving Innate Immune Reaction of TLR2/TNFα

Hui-Ying Li,[1] Jun Hu,[1] Shuang Zhao,[1] Zhi-Yi Yuan,[1] Hong-Jiao Wan,[2] Fan Lei,[1] Yi Ding,[3] Dong-Ming Xing,[1] and Li-Jun Du[1]

[1] *Protein Science Laboratory of the Ministry of Education, Laboratory of Pharmaceutical Sciences, School of Life Sciences and School of Medicine, Tsinghua University, Beijing 100084, China*
[2] *Jiangxi University of Traditional Chinese Medicine, Nanchang 330004, China*
[3] *Drug Discovery Facility, School of Life Sciences, Tsinghua University, Beijing 100084, China*

Correspondence should be addressed to Li-Jun Du, lijundu@mail.tsinghua.edu.cn

Academic Editor: Ikhlas A. Khan

This work is to study the baicalin and its three analogs, baicalin, wogonoside, and wogonin, on the protective effect of neuron from oxygen-glucose deprivation (OGD) and toll-like receptor 2 (TLR2) expression in OGD damage. The results showed that baicalin and its three analogs did protect neurons from OGD damage and downregulated protein level of TLR2. D-Glucopyranosiduronic acid on site 7 in the structure played a core of cytotoxicity of these flavonoid analogs. The methoxyl group on carbon 8 of the structure had the relation with TLR2 protein expression, as well as the anti-inflammation. In addition, we detected caspase3 and antioxidation capability, to investigate the effect of four analogs on cell apoptosis and total antioxidation competence in OGD model.

1. Introduction

Scutellariae radix, a Chinese medicine, has various pharmacological effects such as antibacterial, antivirus, anti-inflammation, antioxidation, and antistroke in clinic [1–4]. Its active ingredient is a kind of flavones, consisting of baicalin, baicalein, wogonin, and wogoniside briefly (Figure 1) [5]. It is reported that Scutellariae radix protects neurons from the injury of ischemia and reperfusion [6]. Baicalin, the major component of the flavones, was confirmed with the neuroprotection of the damage by ischemia and reperfusion and the action on central nerve system [7–10]. Recently, baicalein was studied with a promising effect of neuroaction on multiple sites [11–17]. However, no report presented the effect of baicalin and TLR2 expression on neurons. A few researches reported that wogonin and wogonoside acted on the neurons [18–20]. Baicalin and baicalein were studied as an antioxidant; in a few models baicalein was even stronger than baicalin in reducing several free redials [21]. Comparing them, baicalein and baicalin significantly attenuated the cellular injury induced by hydrogen peroxide, but wogonin and wogonoside acted more weakly [22]. It is suggested that there must be other mechanisms of wogonin and wogonoside on neuroprotection.

As the anti-inflammation of baicalin and baicalein was confirmed, the researches on the innate immune response were studied in cerebral ischemia reperfusion and presented the reason partly why the anti-inflammation of baicalin and baicalein was one of the major assays for the protection of brain from the ischemia reperfusion damage [23–27]. Several receptors were indicated as the key targets of ischemic reperfusion injury in the glia, such as toll like receptors (TLRs) and the NODs (nucleotide-binding oligomerisation domain) [28–30]. Our prior experiment showed baicalin attenuated the expression of NOD2 and TNFα in neurons with the ischemia and reperfusion damage *in vivo* and

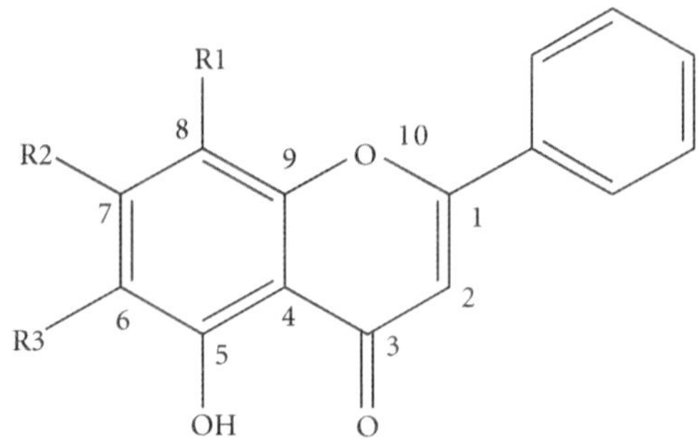

Compounds	R1	R2	R3
Baicalin	–H	–O–Glu	–OH
Baicalein	–H	–OH	–OH
Wogonoside	$–OCH_3$	–O–Glu	–H
Wogonin	$–OCH_3$	–OH	–H

Figure 1: Chemical structures of baicalin and its natural analogs, baicalein, wogonoside, and wogonin.

in vitro [31]. Wogonoside was reported with inhibition of lipopolysaccharide-induced angiogenesis via toll-like receptor 4 (TLR4) signal transduction [32]. However, TLR2 has not been investigated by baicalin and its natural analogs.

Based on the previously mentioned information, we investigated the regulation behavior of baicalin and its analogs through one kind of neuron cell PC12 in order to explore the possible targets of baicalin and its analogs in innate immune reactions during the oxygen and glucose deprivation (OGD) and the relations between the chemical structure and the effect among baicalin and its natural analogs. Since TLR2 is one of the initial receptors in innate immunity and the inflammatory activation, as well as TNFα, can be inhibited by baicalin in lung cells [33, 34], the protein expression of TLR2 and TNFα were tested to find out the role of baicalin and its analogs in this nerve injury models. Meanwhile, caspase3 is a well-known index of apoptosis, and several studies reported that a few flavones could induce apoptosis of inflammatory cells [35–37], so we detected the expression of caspase3 protein. Additionally, the effect of the four analogs on the total antioxidation capability of cells in OGD model was also detected in this paper, which further compared the whole competence of these flavones [38].

2. Materials and Methods

2.1. Chemicals and Materials. Baicalin (purity was 98%) was presented by Dr. Lujun Zhang, Laboratory of Pharmaceutical Sciences, Tsinghua University. Wogonoside (purity was 98%) was presented by Dr. Xiuwei Yang, School of Pharmaceutical Science, Peking university. Baicalein and wogonin, all with purity of 98% (batch number 111595-200604 and 111514-200403), were purchased from China National Institute for the Control of Pharmaceutical and Biological Products. Deionised water was used throughout the experiment. Other organic solvents and reagents were of analytical-reagent grade. PBS buffer with pH7.4 was prepared in our laboratory. PC12 cells were provided by the Cell Bank of the Institute of Fundamental Medicine, Chinese Academy of Medical Science (Beijing, China). Fetal bovine serum (FBS) and RPMI 1640 medium was purchased from GIBCO. Anti-TLR2/TNFα/caspase3/β-actin antibodies were purchased from Santa Cruz Company (USA). The secondary antibody was purchased from Zhongshan Company (Beijing, China). The Total antioxidation capability (T-AOC) detection kit was purchased from Nanjing Jiancheng Bioengineering Institute (Nanjing, China).

2.2. Cell Culture. PC12 cells were adjusted to about 1×10^6 cells/mL with 2 mL inoculate into each well of 6-well plates (Costar) in RPMI 1640 supplemented with 10% fetal bovine serum (FBS) and 5% horse serum and penicillin/streptomycin (100 U/mL each). Cells were cultured in a humidified incubator (5% CO_2) (Sanyo, Japan) at 37°C and allowed to attached for at least 48 h.

2.3. Cytotoxicity Assays In Vitro. The safe dosages of baicalin and its three analogs to the cells were evaluated by MTT (methylthiazol tetrazolium) assay *in vitro*. After 24 h of cells incubation in 96-well plates, baicalin and its analogs were added with the dosage from 10 mg/mL to 0.001 mg/mL. 24 h later of the compounds added, culture medium in 96-well plates were incubated with MTT (5 mg/mL, 200 μL per well) at 37°C for 4 h. Then the medium was carefully aspirated, and 200 μL dimethylsulfoxide (DMSO) per well was added to dissolve the blue formazan products. The values of absorbance at 490 nm were measured using a microplate reader (Model 550Bio-RadUSA). The results of the absorbance of the test wells were expressed as cell alive. The 50% cytotoxicity concentration (CC_{50}) was calculated [39].

2.4. Cells for Oxygen-Glucose Deprivation. For the oxygen-glucose deprivation (OGD) [40], we replaced the growth medium with glucose-free culture medium (2 mL per well) and put the plates into an incubator (YCP-30Q, Changsha, China) full of 95% N_2/5% CO_2 at 37°C for 120 min. Then cells were returned to the normal feeding medium and incubated under normal conditions at 37°C (Sanyo, Japan) for the specific time for later experiments. Control cell cultures not deprived of oxygen and glucose were incubated under normal conditions in the medium with glucose.

For protective effect of the compounds from OGD damage, the cell living assay was carried out as previously described. After 24 h of cells incubation in 96-well plates, baicalin and its analogs were added with the dosages from 10 mg/mL to 0.001 mg/mL. 24 h later from adding the compounds, culture medium in 96-well plates was incubated with MTT (5 mg/mL, 200 μL per well) at 37°C for 4 h. The medium was carefully aspirated, and 200 μL DMSO per well was added to dissolve the blue formazan products. The values of absorbance at 490 nm were measured using a microplate reader. The results of the absorbance of the test wells were expressed as cell alive. The 50% effective concentration (EC_{50}) was calculated [39]. Combined with cytotoxicity (CC_{50}) of the compounds, the safety indices (SIs) were calculated by EC_{50}/CC_{50} [41].

For TLR2/TNFα and caspase3 study, the minimum safety concentration of baicalin and its analogs was ordered as 10 μg/mL. These compounds (10 μg/mL) were added when culture medium was exchanged with glucose solution and cells were cultured in normal condition. The cells were picked up for protein experiment at the specific reperfusion time (0.5, 1, 3, 6 h) after baicalin and its analogs added. In control, medium was used as a vehicle and the cells were picked up at the reperfusion time of 6 h.

2.5. Preparation of Samples. Two groups without medicines were employed as control. One group of the cells was seeded in the medium with normal growth medium during all the experimental process without oxygen-glucose deprivation. The second group was seeded in the medium with process of oxygen-glucose deprivation as the model control. At each time point, the cell sample was prepared the same as previous description. The medium was drawn out from each well, and cells were washed three times with cold PBS (pH 7.4) and used with 100 μL RIPA to gather total protein for Western blotting.

2.6. Western Blot. Western blot assay for protein expression of β-actin, TLR2, TNFα, and Caspase3 was referenced in [42] with minimodification as follows: loaded samples into the gel (10%), was run until the marker (purchased from Fermentas Republic of Lithuania) and went to the end of the gel. The transfer should be semidry for 60 min at 12 volts and 280 mA. Then the membrane was blocked with 10% milk in PBST (1 $\times$ PBS + 0.1% Tween20) for 60 min shaking slowly at room temperature. The membrane was put in 1 mL PBST with antibody in a 1 : 1000 dilution, incubated for 60 min at room temperature on the shaker, and washed for 3 times using PBST after the primary antibody incubation. After that, the membrane was incubated for 60 min in PBST with the secondary antibody with the concentration 1 : 3000. The membrane was washed 3 times with PBST at last.

2.7. Total Antioxidation Capability Detection. The principle of this experiment was to detect the color change following the reduction of Fe^{3+} to Fe^{2+} by the reducing components in the samples. The reducing components might include the enzyme and nonenzymatic molecules such as lipid-soluble antioxidant vitamin E and water-soluble antioxidants vitamin C, bilirubin, and uric acid. Then the optical density was measured at 520 nm with a microplate reader [43]. The cell sample was prepared the same as previous description and picked at the specific reperfusion time (6 h) after baicalin and its analogs added. The medium was drawn out from each well, and the cells were washed three times with cold PBS (pH 7.4). These cells in the plate were resolved with PBS (1 mL/well) by repeated freezing and thawing. The supernatant was collected for T-AOC test after centrifuge 12 000 rpm/min.

2.8. Data Analysis. All values were expressed as mean $\pm$ S.D. Data were statistically analyzed by ANOVA. The Newman-Keuls comparisons were used to determine the source of significant differences where appropriate. P values below 0.05 were considered statistically significant. The software of CALC 2.0 (The China Association of Pharmacology) was employed for CC_{50} and EC_{50} calculation.

3. Results

3.1. Cell Growing Profile. The cells were seeded in the plates of the medium with 10% FBS for 48 h. They would not be used for the experiments till they grew well and attached to each other tightly in the flat of multiwell plates.

3.2. MTT Tests of Cytotoxicity. In order to examine the cytotoxicity and determine the safe dosages of baicalin and its analogs, MTT assay was conducted on PC12 cells *in vitro*. Based on the experiments, 10 μg/mL of baicalin and wogonoside was the highest in safety concentration on normal PC12 cells, and 1 μg/mL of baicalein and wogonin was the highest in safety concentration on normal PC12 cells (Figure 2).

In PC12 cells treated with oxygen-glucose deprivation, only less than 40% cells survived with comparison of normal control ($P < 0.05$). Compared with model control, the minimum effective concentration (MEC) of baicalin and wogonin was 10 μg/mL, while the MEC of both wogonoside and baicalein was the same at 1 μg/mL. The maximum effective concentration (MAXEC) of baicalin and woronin was the same at 1 mg/mL, implying the same safety of them. The MAXEC of wogonoside was 1 mg/mL, but the MAXEC of baicalein was only at 10 μg/mL. It was suggested that baicalein was more cytotoxic than that of wogonoside. All these compounds were not shown in the concentration-dependent manner distinctly (Figure 3).

The CC_{50} of baicalin (188.4 μg/mL or 0.422 mmol/L) showed large differences from other three compounds. Baicalein showed more cellular toxicity with CC_{50} 8.9 μg/mL (equal to 0.0329 mmol/L). Wogonin and wogonoside displayed toxicity similar to CC_{50} 10.6 μg/mL (equal to 0.0373 mmol/L) and 13.7 μg/mL (equal to 0.0298 mmol/L), respectively. However, baicalein was more effective of protection of the cells from OGD damage. The minimum effective dosage of baicalein was 1 μg/mL (equal to 0.0037 mmol/L). The EC_{50} of baicalin was 1.2 μg/mL (equal to 0.0027 mmol/L), and the EC_{50} of Wogonin and wogonoside was 4.3 μg/mL (equal to 0.0151 mmol/L) and 7.4 μg/mL (equal to 0.0161 mmol/L). Comparing between the toxicity and the effect, the safety indices of the four compounds were 156 (baicalin), 8.89 (baicalein), 2.47 (wogonin), and 1.85 (wogonoside), respectively (Table 1).

3.3. Effect on the Expressions of TLR2, TNFα, and Caspase3. Injured by OGD, the proteins of TLR2 and TNFα in the cells were expressed distinctly which means the OGD stimulated the innate immune reaction, causing inflammation. The caspase3 protein in OGD model was upregulated in

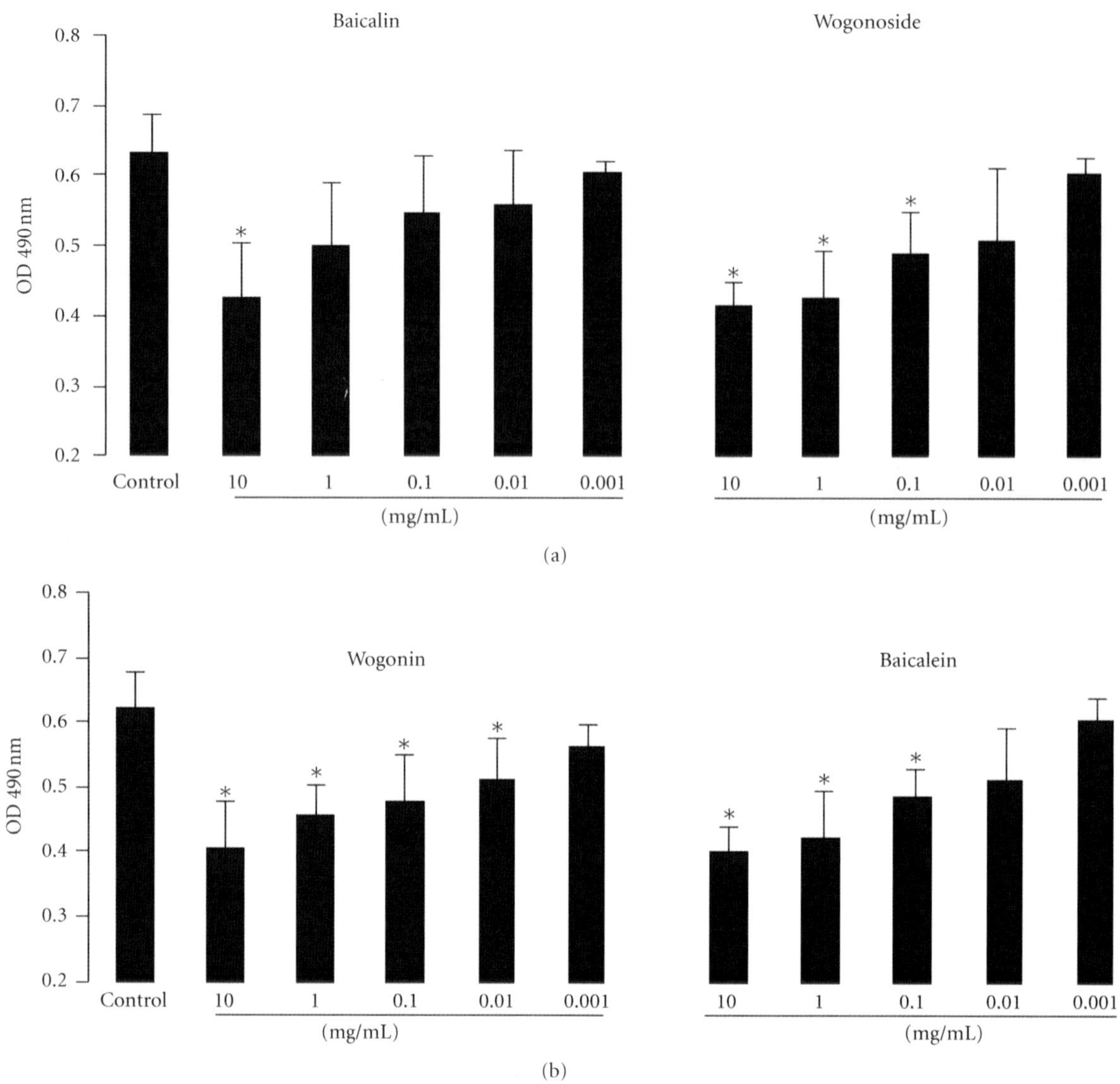

FIGURE 2: Cytotoxcity of baicalin, wogonoside, baicalein, and wogonin in normal PC12 cells (MTT assay). After 24 h of cells incubation in 96-well plates, the chemicals were added with the dosage from 10 mg/mL to 0.001 mg/mL. $^*P < 0.05$ versus normal control. Data were presented as mean ± S.D. from seven independent experiments.

TABLE 1: Values of CC_{50} and EC_{50} of baicalin, baicalein, wogonoside, and wogonin.

Compounds	CC_{50} μg/mL (mmol/L)	EC_{50} μg/mL (mmol/L)	SI
Baicalin	188.4 (0.422)	1.2 (0.0027)	156
Wogonoside	13.7 (0.0298)	7.4 (0.0161)	1.85
Baicalein	8.9 (0.0329)	1.0 (0.0037)	8.89
Wogonin	10.6 (0.0373)	4.3 (0.0151)	2.47

CC_{50} means the 50% cytotoxic concentration.
EC_{50} means the 50% effective concentration.
SI (the safety index) was calculated by CC_{50}/EC_{50}.

some degree, but there was no significant statistical value (Figure 4). Baicalin attenuated the protein expression of TLR2 and TNFα 3 hours after the administration. When baicalin took effect for 0.5 h, the expression of TLR2 showed statistical significance no matter when compared with the normal or comparing with the model ($P < 0.05$), and the TLR2 expression of 1 h increased (comparing with the normal, $P < 0.05$); however, its expression of 3 h or 6 h showed no obvious difference comparing with the normal (comparing with the model, $P < 0.05$). The expression of TNFα of 0.5 h was still higher than the control ($P < 0.05$), and its expressions of 1 h, 3 h, and 6 h were downregulated obviously, which showed significant difference from the model level ($P < 0.05$). Baicalin did not apparently affect the expression of protein caspase3, which was shown in Figure 4(a).

After the addition of wogonoside (10 μg/mL), TLR2 and TNFα were downregulated apparently. The expression of TLR2 was much lower than that of the model, even than the normal level ($P < 0.05$). Accordingly, the expression of

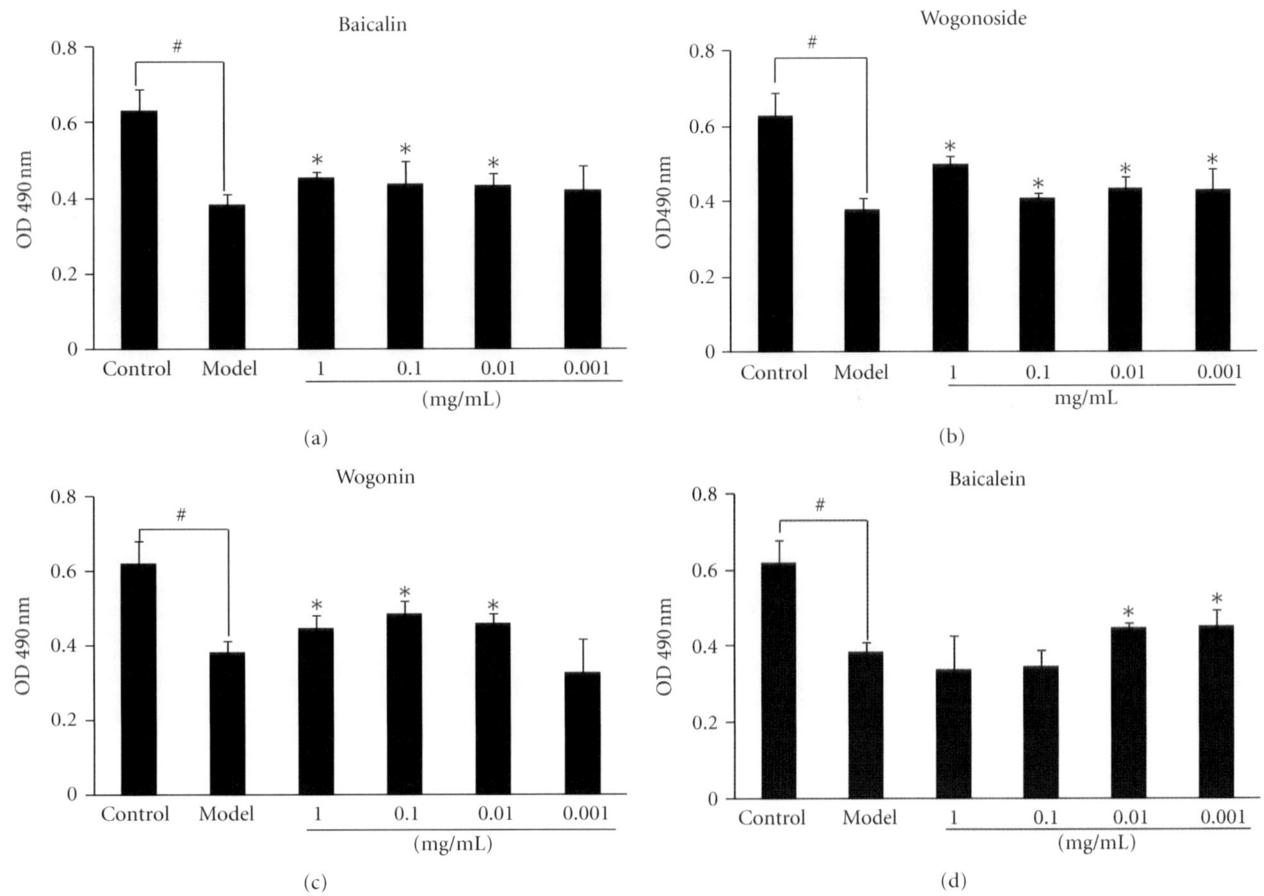

FIGURE 3: Protection of baicalin, wogonoside, baicalein, and wogonin in PC12 cell with oxygen-glucose deprivation (OGD) (MTT assay). After 24 h of cells incubation in 96-well plates and 2 h oxygen-glucose deprivation, the compounds were added with the dosage from 1 mg/mL to 0.001 mg/mL. $^{\#}P < 0.05$ versus normal control. $^{*}P < 0.05$ versus model. Data were presented as mean ± S.D. from seven independent experiments.

TNFα was inhibited by wogonoside apparently from 0.5 h after its administration till the timepoint of 6 h ($P < 0.05$). Wogonoside also did not show obvious effect on the expression of caspase3 (Figure 4(b)).

After baicalein administration, TLR2 was still upregulated significantly 0.5 h and 1 h after the addition of baicalein ($P < 0.05$), and it decreased down to the normal at 3 h and 6 h. Comparing with the model, TNFα was upregulated at 0.5 h and decreased gradually later. Like TLR2, it was expressed down to the normal at 3 h and 6 h (Figure 4(c)).

In wogonin group, the two factors decreased apparently. TLR2 decreased to the normal after 0.5 h of the addition of wogonin (comparing with the model, $P < 0.05$), and it stayed at a lower level during the experiment course. In the 0.5 h and 1 h time points, TNFα was expressed more than the normal ($P < 0.05$) but less than the model ($P < 0.05$), and at 3 h and 6 h, it came close to the normal level like TLR2 expression (Figure 4(d)).

Similar to baicalin and wogonoside groups, the expression of caspase3 showed no significant change in baicalein and wogonin groups (Figures 4(c) and 4(d)).

3.4. Assay of Total Antioxidation Competence (T-AOC). Utilizing the T-AOC kit, we found that the antioxidation competence of the normal cells was about 2.5 U/mg, and one of the cells treated by oxygen-glucose deprivation was far below 0.5 U/mg. In baicalin group, the detection value was 1.8 U/mL, showing a significant difference no matter comparing with the normal or comparing with the OGD model. In wogonoside, baicalein, and wogonin groups, the values were 1.6, 0.8, and 0.6 U/mg, respectively, which all showed a significant difference comparing with the normal or the model (Figure 5).

4. Discussions

Baicalin is a glycosylated compound derived from baicalein, and it has a functional group of D-glucopyranosiduronic acid on site 7 of baicalein (Figure 1), so that it will exhibit more biological function. The basic structure of baicalin consists of benzopyran with three hydroxyl groups at site 5, 6, and 7 and a phenyl group at the other side of the benzopyran (site 2). Baicalin also has an enol structure on the benzopyran ring to maintain the conjugation. The two differences between baicalin and wogonin lie in methoxyl group on carbon 8 of wogonin and hydroxyl group on carbon 6 of baicalein. The constitution of three hydroxyl groups in baicalin may account for more hydrophilic characters.

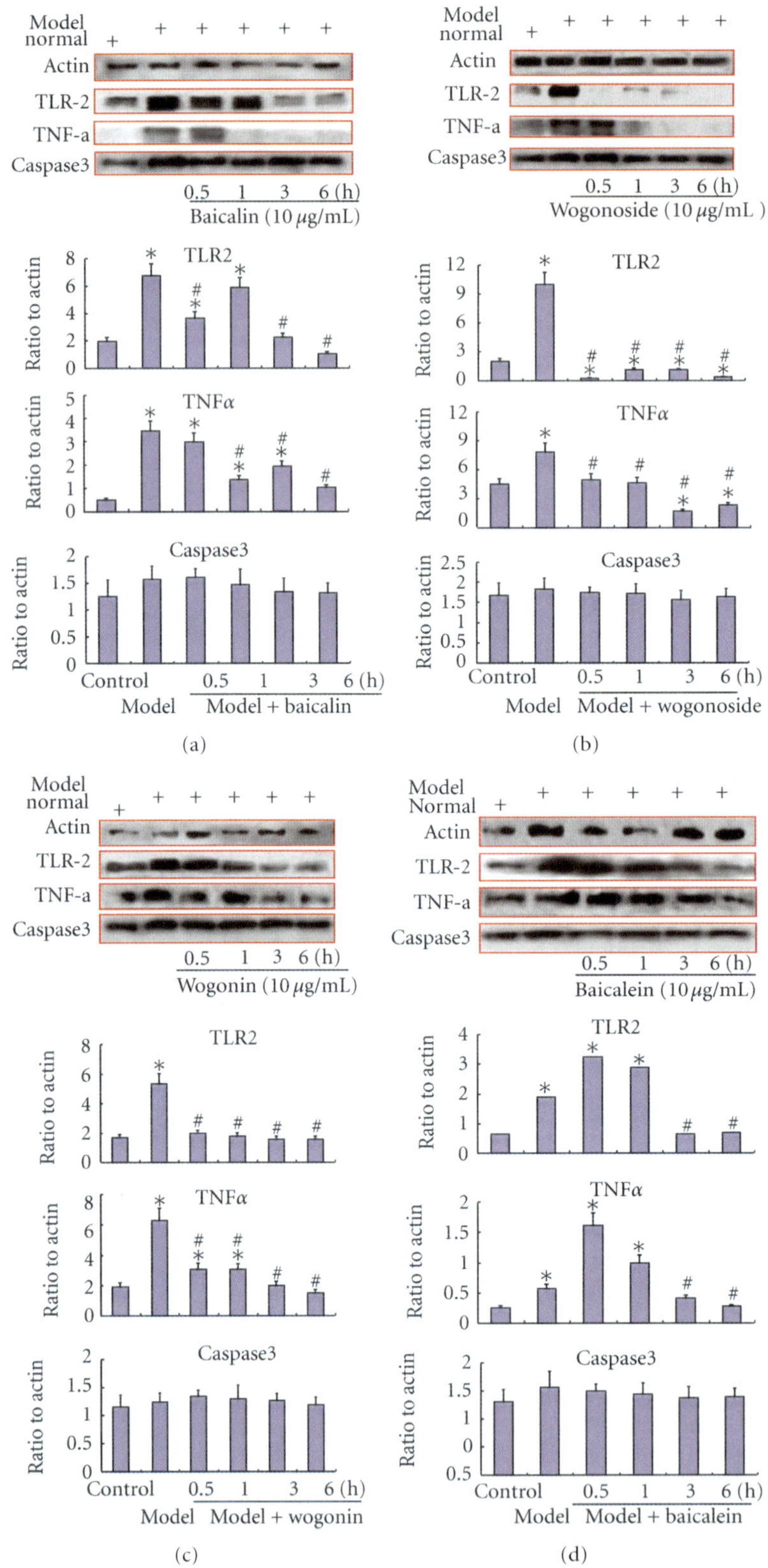

FIGURE 4: Effect of the four analogs on the protein expressions of TLR2, TNFα, and caspase3 in PC12 cells with oxygen-glucose deprivation (OGD). The protein level was measured by Western blot. Model means treatment with oxygen-glucose deprivation. 0.5, 1, 3, and 6 h mean the time of reperfusion process after OGD. (a) stands for baicalin effect; (b) stands for wogonoside effect; (c) stands for baicalein effect; (d) stands for wogonin effect. Baicalin, wogonoside, and wogonin were used in a concentrating of 10 μg/mL, and the baicalein was used in a concentrating of 1 μg/mL. $^{*}P < 0.05$ versus normal control. $^{\#}P < 0.05$ versus model group. Data were presented as mean ± SD from three independent experiments.

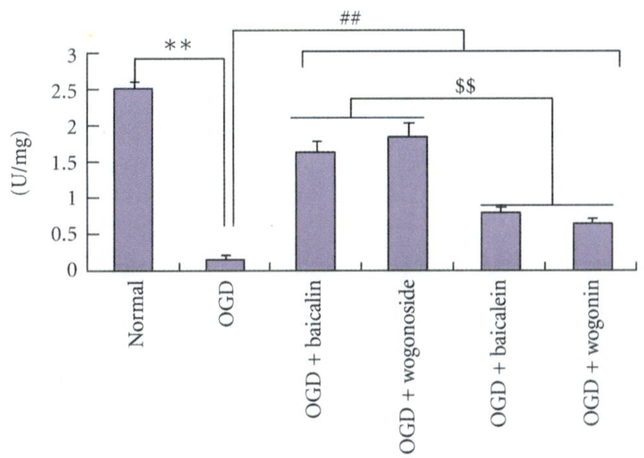

FIGURE 5: Effect of baicalin and its three analogs on the total antioxidation competence of the PC12 cells treated with oxygen-glucose deprivation. Model means treatment with oxygen-glucose deprivation. Baicalin, wogonoside, and wogonin were used in a concentrating of 10 μg/mL, the baicalein was used in a concentrating of 1 μg/mL. $^{**}P < 0.01$ versus normal control. $^{\#\#}P < 0.01$ versus model group. $^{\$\$}P < 0.01$ versus baicalin and wogonoside groups. Data were presented as mean ± S.D. from eight independent experiments.

Moreover, wogonoside is a glycosylated form of wogonin with D-glucopyranosiduronic acid on carbon 7. All four compounds share similar carbon skeleton with a benzopyran structure and also a hydroxyl group on carbon 5; baicalein and baicalin have hydroxyl groups on carbon 6, while wogonin and wogonoside does not have; baicalein and wogonin have hydroxyl groups on carbon 7, while wogonoside and baicalin are both glycosylated on the hydroxyl group at site 7; last, wogonin and wogonoside have methoxyl groups on carbon 8, but baicalein and baicalin does not have the functional groups [44, 45].

By the result of cytotoxicity and neuroprotection, D-glucopyranosiduronic acid on site 7 was important for reducing cytotoxicity, in which baicalin was less cytotoxic than baicalein and wogonoside was less cytotoxic than wogonin. Methoxyl group on carbon 8 and hydroxyl group on carbon 6 were the major factor influencing the neuroprotective effect, by which the EC_{50} of baicalin and baicalein was less than that of wogonoside and wogonin (Figure 1 and Table 1) after they were administered.

In this study, we found that TLR2 was highly expressed during the oxygen and glucose deprivation (OGD) damage in PC12 cells, which suggested that the receptor was activated in the damaged neurons (Figure 4). TLR2 had been identified as a key mediator of immune responses and inflammatory reactions, and it mediated proinflammatory responses through activating of TNFα [46–48]. The receptor was significantly up-regulated comparing with the normal level, indicating it joined neuron injury induced by OGD.

By the literature of research, TLR2 in the central nerve system (CNS) is realized as the direct source of the damaging signal and an important potential therapeutic target [49]. In our results, the expressions of TLR2 and TNFα decreased apparently a few hours after we added the compounds. In the same profile, the expressions of TLR2 and TNFα with wogonin and wogonoside were more inhibited than those with baicalin and baicalein. The inhibition of the expression started from 0.5 h after wogonin and wogonoside administration; however the inhibition of TLR2 and TNFα expression appeared later at 3 h after baicalin and baicalein administration. Therefore, wogonin and wogonoside were realized to have preference with TLR2. Combined with their chemical structures, all the results implied that methoxyl group on carbon 8 in the structure is the pharmacophore hypothesis of the effect of TLR2 inhibition, relating to inflammation inhibition.

Conditioning the oversuppression on TLR2 and TNFα by these analogs, we detected caspase3 to confirm whether there existed apoptosis with the addition of the analogs. Comparing with the normal, the expression of caspase3 protein in OGD model indeed increased in some degree, but showed no statistical difference. With the administration of the four analogs, the level caspase3 protein showed no obvious change, although it showed the tendency to decrease at 6 h time point and near to the normal control (comparing with the normal or the model, $P > 0.05$). The above results suggested the injured PC12 cells in OGD model had no apparent apoptosis, and the four analogs also could not induce apoptosis in the injured PC12 cells. According to the literature, baicalin attenuated global cerebral ischemia reperfusion injury in gerbils via antioxidative and antiapoptotic pathways [50], and baicalein and wogonin could both induce the apoptosis in human pancreatic cancer cells and HL-60 leukemia cells [51, 52]. Therefore, our results of apoptosis by these compounds need to be studied further.

Referring to the T-AOC detection, we found that the total antioxidation capability sequence was baicalin and wogonoside > baicalein and wogonin, indicating that a glycosylated form on site 2 of baicalin and wogonoside played a key role in overall antioxidation.

Taken together, baicalin and its three analogs presented comprehensively the protection of neuron cells from OGD damage and the inhibition of TLR2 expression and TNFα (the factor in the downstream), suggesting the possibility of these compounds used in stroke therapy by targeting TLR2, one of the major mechanisms of the cerebral damage. There is a structure-activity relationship among them with safety, efficacy, and specificity of drug targeting of TLR2. This is the first time to study baicalin and its natural analogs on molecular targets of TLR2 and TNFα, as well as T-AOC. All that will have benefit in elucidating and developing them for the new drugs.

Authors' Contribution

The first two authors contributed equally.

Acknowledgments

The author thank all members in their laboratory. The study was supported partly by the National Natural Science Foundation of China (30801523, 81073092), the National S&T Major Special Project for New Drug R&D

of China (2012ZX09103-201-041, 2012ZX09102-201-008, and 2011ZX09101-002-11), and Special Foundation for Laboratory of Tsinghua University (LF 20103579).

References

[1] L. L. Liu, L. K. Gong, H. Wang et al., "Baicalin inhibits macrophage activation by lipopolysaccharide and protects mice from endotoxin shock," *Biochemical Pharmacology*, vol. 75, no. 4, pp. 914–922, 2008.

[2] S. H. Jung, K. D. Kang, D. Ji et al., "The flavonoid baicalin counteracts ischemic and oxidative insults to retinal cells and lipid peroxidation to brain membranes," *Neurochemistry International*, vol. 53, no. 6–8, pp. 325–337, 2008.

[3] K. J. Woo, J. H. Lim, S. I. Suh et al., "Differential inhibitory effects of baicalein and baicalin on LPS-induced cyclooxygenase-2 expression through inhibition of C/EBPβ DNA-binding activity," *Immunobiology*, vol. 211, no. 5, pp. 359–368, 2006.

[4] Y. C. Chen, J. M. Chow, C. W. Lin, C. Y. Wu, and S. C. Shen, "Baicalein inhibition of oxidative-stress-induced apoptosis via modulation of ERKs activation and induction of HO-1 gene expression in rat glioma cells C6," *Toxicology and Applied Pharmacology*, vol. 216, no. 2, pp. 263–273, 2006.

[5] J. Zhu, Z. Wang, Q. Zhang, J. Niu, and F. Li, "A quantitative method for simultaneous assay of four flavones with one marker in Radix Scutellariae," *China Journal of Materia Medica*, vol. 34, no. 24, pp. 3229–3234, 2009.

[6] W. J. Xu and Q. L. Ding, "Pharmacological research of baicalin," *Jiangsu Pharmaceutical and Clinical Research*, vol. 14, no. 2, pp. 103–107, 2006.

[7] T. Tarragó, N. Kichik, B. Claasen, R. Prades, M. Teixidó, and E. Giralt, "Baicalin, a prodrug able to reach the CNS, is a prolyl oligopeptidase inhibitor," *Bioorganic and Medicinal Chemistry*, vol. 16, no. 15, pp. 7516–7524, 2008.

[8] X. Wang, L. Zhang, L. Hua, D. Xing, and L. Du, "Effect of flavonoids in Scutellariae Radix on depression-like behavior and brain rewards: possible in dopamine system," *Tsinghua Science and Technology*, vol. 15, no. 4, pp. 460–466, 2010.

[9] L. Chen, L. Zhang, X. Wang, H. Lin, and L. Du, "Determination of dopamine and its relativity of baicalin in rat nuclei after intravenous administration of flavonoids from Scutellariae radix," *Biomedical Chromatography*, vol. 21, no. 1, pp. 84–88, 2007.

[10] C. H. Ouyang and J. L. Wu, "Protective effect of baicalin on inflammatory injury following transient focal cerebral ischemia-reperfusion in rats," *Chinese Journal of Pharmacology and Toxicology*, vol. 20, no. 4, pp. 288–294, 2006.

[11] S. J. Park, D. H. Kim, J. M. Kim et al., "Mismatch between changes in baicalein-induced memory-related biochemical parameters and behavioral consequences in mouse," *Brain Research*, vol. 1355, pp. 141–150, 2010.

[12] X. Mu, G. He, Y. Cheng, X. Li, B. Xu, and G. Du, "Baicalein exerts neuroprotective effects in 6-hydroxydopamine-induced experimental parkinsonism in vivo and in vitro," *Pharmacology Biochemistry and Behavior*, vol. 92, no. 4, pp. 642–648, 2009.

[13] P. H. Wu, Y. C. Shen, Y. H. Wang, C. W. Chi, and J. C. Yen, "Baicalein attenuates methamphetamine-induced loss of dopamine transporter in mouse striatum," *Toxicology*, vol. 226, no. 2-3, pp. 238–245, 2006.

[14] X. L. He, Y. H. Wang, M. Gao, X. X. Li, T. T. Zhang, and G. H. Du, "Baicalein protects rat brain mitochondria against chronic cerebral hypoperfusion-induced oxidative damage," *Brain Research*, vol. 1249, pp. 212–221, 2009.

[15] L. Cui, X. Zhang, R. Yang et al., "Baicalein is neuroprotective in rat MCAO model: role of 12/15-lipoxygenase, mitogen-activated protein kinase and cytosolic phospholipase A2," *Pharmacology Biochemistry and Behavior*, vol. 96, no. 4, pp. 469–475, 2010.

[16] C. Liu, J. Wu, J. Gu et al., "Baicalein improves cognitive deficits induced by chronic cerebral hypoperfusion in rats," *Pharmacology Biochemistry and Behavior*, vol. 86, no. 3, pp. 423–430, 2007.

[17] Y. W. Xu, L. Sun, H. Liang, G. M. Sun, and Y. Cheng, "12/15-Lipoxygenase inhibitor baicalein suppresses PPARγ expression and nuclear translocation induced by cerebral ischemia/reperfusion," *Brain Research*, vol. 1307, pp. 149–157, 2010.

[18] H. Z. Piao, I. Y. Choi, J. S. Park et al., "Wogonin inhibits microglial cell migration via suppression of nuclear factor-kappa B activity," *International Immunopharmacology*, vol. 8, no. 12, pp. 1658–1662, 2008.

[19] H. G. Park, S. Y. Yoon, J. Y. Choi et al., "Anticonvulsant effect of wogonin isolated from Scutellaria baicalensis," *European Journal of Pharmacology*, vol. 574, no. 2-3, pp. 112–119, 2007.

[20] W. Tang, X. Sun, J. S. Fang, M. Zhang, and N. J. Sucher, "Flavonoids from *Radix Scutellariae* as potential stroke therapeutic agents by targeting the second postsynaptic density 95 (PSD-95)/disc large/zonula occludens-1 (PDZ) domain of PSD-95," *Phytomedicine*, vol. 11, no. 4, pp. 277–284, 2004.

[21] R. Liang, C. H. Chen, X. C. Ai, and J. P. Zhang, "Structural origins of the differential antioxidative activities between baicalein and baicalin," *Chinese Journal of Magnetic Resonance*, vol. 27, pp. 132–140, 2010.

[22] Z. Gao, K. Huang, and H. Xu, "Protective effects of flavonoids in the roots of Scutellaria Baicalensis Georgi against hydrogen peroxide-induced oxidative stress in HS-SY5Y cells," *Pharmacological Research*, vol. 43, no. 2, pp. 173–178, 2001.

[23] M. Letiembre, W. Hao, Y. Liu et al., "Innate immune receptor expression in normal brain aging," *Neuroscience*, vol. 146, no. 1, pp. 248–254, 2007.

[24] B. J. Marsh, R. L. Williams-Karnesky, and M. P. Stenzel-Poore, "Toll-like receptor signaling in endogenous neuroprotection and stroke," *Neuroscience*, vol. 158, no. 3, pp. 1007–1020, 2009.

[25] G. J. del Zoppo, "Inflammation and the neurovascular unit in the setting of focal cerebral ischemia," *Neuroscience*, vol. 158, no. 3, pp. 972–982, 2009.

[26] B. W. McColl, S. M. Allan, and N. J. Rothwell, "Systemic infection, inflammation and acute ischemic stroke," *Neuroscience*, vol. 158, no. 3, pp. 1049–1061, 2009.

[27] D. A. Ridder and M. Schwaninger, "NF-κB signaling in cerebral ischemia," *Neuroscience*, vol. 158, no. 3, pp. 995–1006, 2009.

[28] P. Rosenstiel, G. Jacobs, A. Till, and S. Schreiber, "NOD-like receptors: ancient sentinels of the innate immune system," *Cellular and Molecular Life Sciences*, vol. 65, no. 9, pp. 1361–1377, 2008.

[29] V. S. Chauhan, D. G. Sterka, S. R. Furr, A. B. Young, and I. Marriott, "NOD2 plays an important role in the inflammatory responses of microglia and astrocytes to bacterial CNS pathogens," *GLIA*, vol. 57, no. 4, pp. 414–423, 2009.

[30] K. Geddes, J. G. Magalhães, and S. E. Girardin, "Unleashing the therapeutic potential of NOD-like receptors," *Nature Reviews Drug Discovery*, vol. 8, no. 6, pp. 465–479, 2009.

[31] H. Li, J. Hu, L. Ma et al., "Comprehensive study of baicalin down-regulating NOD2 receptor expression of neurons with

oxygen-glucose deprivation in vitro and cerebral ischemia-reperfusion in vivo," *European Journal of Pharmacology*, vol. 649, no. 1–3, pp. 92–99, 2010.

[32] Y. Chen, N. Lu, Y. Ling et al., "Wogonoside inhibits lipopolysaccharide-induced angiogenesis *in vitro* and *in vivo* via toll-like receptor 4 signal transduction," *Toxicology*, vol. 259, no. 1-2, pp. 10–17, 2009.

[33] Y. G. Wang, H. Wu, Z. Meng et al., "Effect of total flavonoids of Radix Scutellariae on TLR2/Nod2 expression in lung after infection of staphylococcus aureus in vivo and in vitro," *Chinese Pharmacological Bulletin*, vol. 25, no. 7, pp. 866–870, 2009.

[34] E. F. Schippers, C. van't Veer, S. van Voorden, C. A. E. Martina, S. le Cessie, and J. T. van Dissel, "TNF-α promoter, Nod2 and toll-like receptor-4 polymorphisms and the in vivo and ex vivo response to endotoxin," *Cytokine*, vol. 26, no. 1, pp. 16–24, 2004.

[35] X. F. Xu, B. L. Cai, B. Liu et al., "Baicalin induces human mucoepidermoid carcinoma Mc3 cells apoptosis in vitro and in vivo," *Investigational New Drugs*, vol. 29, pp. 637–645, 2010.

[36] J. F. Zhang, R. Huang, Y. J. Yang, R. Z. Huang, and Y. M. Su, "Effect of baicalin preconditioning on neuron apoptosis in the rats with experimental autoimmune encephalomyelitis," *Chinese Pediatric Emergency Medicine*, vol. 16, pp. 564–567, 2009.

[37] J. Q. Yin, H. M. Chen, W. M. Luo, J. N. Shen, X. Y. Zheng, and Q. Jia, "In vitro studies of baicalein and baicalin mediated apoptosis in human osteosarcoma cell line U—2OS and U—2OS/MTX~(300)," *West China Journal of Pharmaceutical Sciences*, vol. 26, pp. 133–135, 2011.

[38] Z. Gong, Y. X. Cheng, M. Zhang, T. T. Song, J. F. Lv, and K. J. Ning, "Effects of baicalin on anti-oxidation function in liver of liver injury mice," *Journal of Anhui Science and Technology University*, vol. 25, pp. 5–8, 2011.

[39] J. Tao, Q. Hu, J. Yang et al., "In vitro anti-HIV and -HSV activity and safety of sodium rutin sulfate as a microbicide candidate," *Antiviral Research*, vol. 75, no. 3, pp. 227–233, 2007.

[40] H. H. Lee, L. L. Yang, C. C. Wang, S. Y. Hu, S. F. Chang, and Y. H. Lee, "Differential effects of natural polyphenols on neuronal survival in primary cultured central neurons against glutamate-and glucose deprivation-induced neuronal death," *Brain Research*, vol. 986, no. 1-2, pp. 103–113, 2003.

[41] R. V. Macri, J. Karlovská, G. F. Doncel et al., "Comparing anti-HIV, antibacterial, antifungal, micellar, and cytotoxic properties of tricarboxylato dendritic amphiphiles," *Bioorganic and Medicinal Chemistry*, vol. 17, no. 8, pp. 3162–3168, 2009.

[42] F. López-Neblina and L. H. Toledo-Pereyra, "Anti-ischemic effect of selectin blocker through modulation of tumor necrosis factor-α and interleukin-10," *Journal of Surgical Research*, vol. 138, no. 2, pp. 275–283, 2007.

[43] J. Hao, W. Shen, C. Tian et al., "Mitochondrial nutrients improve immune dysfunction in the type 2 diabetic Goto-Kakizaki rats," *Journal of Cellular and Molecular Medicine*, vol. 13, no. 4, pp. 701–711, 2009.

[44] C. Li, L. Zhou, G. Lin, and Z. Zuo, "Contents of major bioactive flavones in proprietary traditional Chinese medicine products and reference herb of *Radix Scutellariae*," *Journal of Pharmaceutical and Biomedical Analysis*, vol. 50, no. 3, pp. 298–306, 2009.

[45] K. L. Li and S. J. Sheu, "Determination of flavonoids and alkaloids in the scute-coptis herb couple by capillary electrophoresis," *Analytica Chimica Acta*, vol. 313, no. 1-2, pp. 113–120, 1995.

[46] N. Inohara and G. Nuñez, "NODS: intracellular proteins involved in inflammation and apoptosis," *Nature Reviews Immunology*, vol. 3, no. 5, pp. 371–382, 2003.

[47] C. Eskes, L. Juillerat-Jeanneret, G. Leuba, and P. Honegger, "Involvement of microglia-neuron interactions in the tumor necrosis factor-α release, microglial activation, and neurodegeneration induced by trimethyltin," *Journal of Neuroscience Research*, vol. 71, no. 4, pp. 583–590, 2003.

[48] E. Meylan, J. Tschopp, and M. Karin, "Intracellular pattern recognition receptors in the host response," *Nature*, vol. 442, no. 7098, pp. 39–44, 2006.

[49] K. B. Vartanian and M. P. Stenzel-Poore, "Toll-Like receptor tolerance as a mechanism for neuroprotection," *Translational Stroke Research*, vol. 1, no. 4, pp. 252–260, 2010.

[50] Y. Cao, X. Mao, C. Sun et al., "Baicalin attenuates global cerebral ischemia/reperfusion injury in gerbils via anti-oxidative and anti-apoptotic pathways," *Brain Research Bulletin*, vol. 85, no. 6, pp. 396–402, 2011.

[51] H. Takahashi, M. C. Chen, H. Pham et al., "Baicalein, a component of Scutellaria baicalensis, induces apoptosis by Mcl-1 down-regulation in human pancreatic cancer cells," *Biochimica et Biophysica Acta*, vol. 1813, no. 8, pp. 1465–1474, 2011.

[52] S. T. Huang, C. Y. Wang, R. C. Yang, C. J. Chu, H. T. Wu, and J. H. S. Pang, "Wogonin, an active compound in Scutellaria baicalensis, induces apoptosis and reduces telomerase activity in the HL-60 leukemia cells," *Phytomedicine*, vol. 17, no. 1, pp. 47–54, 2010.

18

Screening of α-Glucosidase Inhibitory Activity from Some Plants of Apocynaceae, Clusiaceae, Euphorbiaceae, and Rubiaceae

Berna Elya, Katrin Basah, Abdul Mun'im, Wulan Yuliastuti, Anastasia Bangun, and Eva Kurnia Septiana

Department of Pharmacy, Faculty of Mathematics and Sciences, University of Indonesia, Depok 16424, Indonesia

Correspondence should be addressed to Berna Elya, elya64@yahoo.com

Academic Editor: Munekazu Iinuma

Diabetes mellitus (DM) is recognized as a serious global health problem that is characterized by high blood sugar levels. Type 2 DM is more common in diabetic populations. In this type of DM, inhibition of α-glucosidase is a useful treatment to delay the absorption of glucose after meals. As a megabiodiversity country, Indonesia still has a lot of potential unexploited forests to be developed as a medicine source, including as the α-glucosidase inhibitor. In this study, we determine the α-glucosidase inhibitory activity of 80% ethanol extracts of leaves and twigs of some plants from the Apocynaceae, Clusiaceae, Euphorbiaceae, and Rubiaceae. Inhibitory activity test of the α-glucosidase was performed *in vitro* using spectrophotometric methods. Compared with the control acarbose (IC_{50} 117.20 μg/mL), thirty-seven samples of forty-five were shown to be more potent α-glucosidase inhibitors with IC_{50} values in the range 2.33–112.02 μg/mL.

1. Introduction

Diabetes mellitus (DM) is the most common endocrine disease worldwide. About 173 million people suffer from diabetes mellitus. The number of people with diabetes mellitus will more than double over the next 25 years to reach a total of 366 million by 2030 [1]. In 2000, Indonesia is ranked the fourth largest number of people with DM, after India, China, and the United States, which is about 8.4 million people. The amount is expected to rise to 21.3 million in 2030 [2].

DM consists of several types, one of which is noninsulin-dependent diabetes mellitus (type 2 DM). This type of DM is more common, reaching 90–95% of the population with DM [3]. This increasing trend in type 2 DM has become a serious medical concern worldwide that prompts every effort in exploring for new therapeutic agents to stem its progress.

In type 2 DM, inhibition of α-glucosidase therapy is beneficial to delay absorption of glucose after a meal [4]. α-glucosidase plays a role in the conversion of carbohydrates into glucose. By inhibiting α-glucosidase, glucose levels in the blood can be returned within normal limits [5].

Natural resources provide a huge and highly diversified chemical bank from which we can explore for potential therapeutic agents by bioactivity-targeted screenings [6]. As a megabiodiversity country, Indonesia still has a lot of potential unexploited forests to be developed as a source phytopharmaca or modern medicine [7]. Opportunity exploration of medicinal plants is still very wide open in line with the development of herbal industry, herbal medicine, and phytopharmaca. Therefore, researchers try to explore the potential antidiabetic agents with the mechanism of action of α-glucosidase inhibition in several plant species from four families: Apocynaceae, Clusiaceae, Euphorbiaceae, and Rubiaceae. The four families were chosen because members of some species have been scientifically proven to have antidiabetic activity. Based on the theory of kinship through a systematic approach to plant (chemotaxonomy), plants with the same family generally have similar chemical content,

Table 1: Phytochemical screening of 80% ethanol extracts from some plants of Apocynaceae, Clusiaceae, Euphorbiaceae, and Rubiaceae.

Simplicia	Chemical contents						
	Alkaloid	Flavonoid	Terpenoid	Tannin	Glycoside	Saponin	Anthraquinone
			Apocynaceae				
Beaumontia multiflora Teijsm. & Binn. Folium	+	+	−	+	+	+	+
Beaumontia multiflora Teijsm. & Binn. Cortex	−	−	−	−	+	+	−
Carissa carandas L. Folium	−	+	+	+	+	+	+
Carissa carandas L. Cortex	−	−	−	+	+	+	+
Ochrosia citrodora Lauterb. & K. Schum. Folium	+	−	+	+	+	+	+
Rauvolfia sumatrana Jack Folium	+	−	+	−	+	+	−
Strophanthus caudatus (Blume.f.) Kurz Folium	−	−	+	−	+	+	+
Strophanthus caudatus (Blume.f.) Kurz Cortex	+	−	+	+	+	+	−
Strophanthus gratus Baill. Folium	−	−	+	−	−	+	−
Strophanthus gratus Baill. Cortex	+	−	+	−	+	+	−
Tabernaemontana sphaerocarpa Blume Folium	+	−	+	−	+	+	−
Willughbeia tenuiflora Dyer ex Hook.f Folium	−	−	+	+	+	+	−
Willughbeia tenuiflora Dyer ex Hook.f Cortex	+	−	+	+	+	+	−
			Clusiaceae				
Calophyllum tomentosum Wight. Folium	+	+	+	+	+	+	−
Garcinia bancana Miq. Folium	+	−	+	+	+	+	−
Garcinia daedalanthera Pierre. Folium	−	+	+	+	+	+	+
Garcinia daedalanthera Pierre. Cortex	−	−	+	+	+	+	+
Garcinia hombroniana Pierre. Folium	+	−	+	+	+	+	+
Garcinia kydia Roxb. Folium	−	+	+	+	+	+	+
Garcinia rigida Miq. Folium	+	+	+	+	+	+	+
			Euphorbiaceae				
Antidesma bunius (L.) Spreng Folium	−	−	+	+	+	+	+
Antidesma bunius (L.) Spreng Cortex	+	−	+	+	+	+	−
Antidesma celebicum Cortex	−	−	−	+	+	+	−
Antidesma celebicum Folium	−	+	−	+	+	+	+
Antidesma montanum (Blume) Folium	+	−	+	+	+	+	−
Antidesma neurocarpum Miq. Folium	+	+	−	+	+	−	+
Blumeodendron toksbrai (Blume.) Kurz. Cortex	+	−	−	−	+	+	−
Blumeodendron toksbrai (Blume.) Kurz. Folium	+	−	+	−	+	−	−
Croton argyratus Blume. Folium	−	−	+	−	+	−	−

Table 1: Continued.

Simplicia	Chemical contents						
	Alkaloid	Flavonoid	Terpenoid	Tannin	Glycoside	Saponin	Anthraquinone
Cephalomappa malloticarpa J.J.Sm. Cortex	−	−	+	+	+	+	+
Cephalomappa malloticarpa J.J.Sm. Folium	−	−	+	+	+	−	+
Galearia filiformis Blume. Folium	+	−	+	+	+	−	+
Sumbaviopsis albicans (Blume) J.J.Sm. Cortex	−	−	+	−	+	+	−
Sumbaviopsis albicans (Blume) J.J.Sm. Folium	−	−	+	−	+	+	−
Suregada glomerulata (Blume) Baill. Folium	+	−	+	−	+	−	−
Rubiaceae							
Adina trichotoma Zoll. & Moritzi. Folium	+	−	+	−	+	−	+
Amaracarpus pubescens Blume. Folium	+	+	+	−	+	−	+
Canthium glabrum Blume. Folium	+	+	+	+	+	−	+
Chiococca javanica Blume. Folium	+	+	+	−	+	−	+
Hydnophytum formicarum Folium	+	−	+	+	+	+	−
Hydnophytum formicarum Cortex	+	+	+	−	+	−	−
Nauclea calycina (Batrl.ex DC.) Merr. Folium	+	−	−	+	+	−	−
Nauclea calycina (Batrl.ex DC.) Merr. Cortex	−	+	+	+	+	−	+
Posoqueria latifolia (Lam.) Roem. & Schult. Folium	−	−	+	+	+	−	−

Key: +: present; −: absent.

so it may just have the same potential for the treatment of a disease [8].

2. Method and Material

2.1. Plant Material. The stem bark and leaves of plants material were collected in November 2010 and identified by Center for Plant Conservation-Bogor Botanical Garden.

2.2. Extraction. Each dried powdered of wood bark, twig and leaves (20 g) were extracted by reflux with ethanol 80% then evaporated.

2.3. Inhibition Assay for α-Glucosidase Activity. The inhibition of α-glucosidase activity was determined using the modified published method [9]. One mg of α-glucosidase (*Saccharomyces cerevisiae*, Sigma-Aldrich, USA) was dissolved in 100 mL of phosphate buffer (pH 6.8) containing 200 mg of bovine serum albumin (Merck, German). The reaction mixture consisting 10 μL of sample at varying concentrations (0.52 to 33 μg/mL) was premixed with 490 μL phosphate buffer pH 6.8 and 250 μL of 5 mM *p*-nitrophenyl α-D-glucopyranoside (Sigma-Aldrich, Switzerland). After preincubating at 37°C for 5 min, 250 μL α-glucosidase (0.15 unit/mL) was added and incubated at 37°C for 15 min. The reaction was terminated by the addition of 2000 μL Na_2CO_3 200 mM. α-glucosidase activity was determined spectrophotometrically at 400 nm on spectrophotometer UV-Vis (Shimadzu 265, Jepang) by measuring the quantity of *p*-nitrophenol released from p-NPG. Acarbose was used as positive control of α-glucosidase inhibitor. The concentration of the extract required to inhibit 50% of α-glucosidase activity under the assay conditions was defined as the IC_{50} value.

2.4. Kinetics of Inhibition against α-Glucosidase. Inhibition modes of sample that had the best α-glucosidase inhibiting activity in Clusiaceae, Euphorbiaceae, and Rubiaceae were measured with increasing concentration of *p*-nitrophenyl α-D-glucopyranoside as a substrate in the absence or presence of ethanolic extract at different concentrations. Inhibition type was determined by the Lineweaver-Burk plots analysis of the data, which were calculated from the result according to the Michaelis-Menten kinetics.

2.5. Phytochemistry Test. In this research we performed phytochemistry test which consists of alkaloid test with Mayer, Dragendorff, and Bouchardat reagents; Flavonoid test with Shinoda and Wilson Töubock reaction; tannin test with

TABLE 2: IC_{50} values of rude extracts against α-glucosidase.

Number	Sample	IC_{50} (μg/mL)
(1)	Acarbose	117.20
	Apocynaceae	
(2)	*Beaumontia multiflora Teijsm. & Binn.* Folium	79.80
(3)	*Beaumontia multiflora Teijsm. & Binn.* Cortex	130.20
(4)	*Carissa carandas* L.Folium	21.14
(5)	*Carissa carandas L.*Cortex	20.44
(6)	*Ochrosia citrodora Lauterb. & K. Schum.* Folium	112.02
(7)	*Rauvolfia sumatrana* Jack Folium	174.27
(8)	*Strophanthus caudatus* (Blume.f.) Kurz Folium	706.81
(9)	*Strophanthus caudatus* (Blume.f.) Kurz Cortex	13.93
(10)	*Strophanthus gratus* Baill.Folium	50.61
(11)	*Strophanthus gratus* Baill. Cortex	202.17
(12)	*Tabernaemontana sphaerocarpa* Blume Folium	554.32
(13)	*Willughbeia tenuiflora* Dyer ex Hook.f Folium	8.16
(14)	*Willughbeia tenuiflora* Dyer ex Hook.f Cortex	42.11
	Clusiaceae	
(15)	*Calophyllum tomentosum* Wight. Folium	15.83
(16)	*Garcinia bancana* Miq. Folium	22.41
(17)	*Garcinia daedalanthera* Pierre. Folium	2.33
(18)	*Garcinia daedalanthera* Pierre. Cortex	3.71
(19)	*Garcinia hombroniana* Pierre. Folium	11.30
(20)	*Garcinia kydia* Roxb. Folium	3.88
(21)	*Garcinia rigida* Miq. Folium	24.48
	Euphorbiaceae	
(22)	*Antidesma bunius* (L.) Spreng Folium	7.94
(23)	*Antidesma bunius* (L.) Spreng Cortex	3.90
(24)	*Antidesma celebicum* Cortex	3.93
(25)	*Antidesma celebicum* Folium	2.34
(26)	*Antidesma montanum* (Blume) Folium	2.83
(27)	*Antidesma neurocarpum* Miq. Folium	4.22
(28)	*Blumeodendron toksbrai* (Blume.) Kurz. Cortex	22.82
(29)	*Blumeodendron toksbrai* (Blume.) Kurz. Folium	64.78
(30)	*Croton argyratus* Blume. Folium	366.07
(31)	*Cephalomappa malloticarpa* J.J.Sm. Cortex	12.22
(32)	*Cephalomappa malloticarpa* J.J.Sm. Folium	2.66
(33)	*Galearia filiformis* Blume. Folium	21.54
(34)	*Sumbaviopsis albicans* (Blume) J.J.Sm. Cortex	42.66
(35)	*Sumbaviopsis albicans* (Blume) J.J.Sm. Folium	43.40
(36)	*Suregada glomerulata* (Blume) Baill. Folium	57.46
	Rubiaceae	
(37)	*Adina trichotoma Zoll. & Moritzi. Folium*	28.22
(38)	*Amaracarpus pubescens* Blume. Folium	3.64
(39)	*Canthium glabrum Blume.* Folium	117.85
(40)	*Chiococca javanica Blume.* Folium	23.86
(41)	*Hydnophytum formicarum* Folium	181.90
(42)	*Hydnophytum formicarum* Cortex	11.04

TABLE 2: Continued.

Number	Sample	IC_{50} (μg/mL)
(43)	*Nauclea calycina (Batrl.ex DC.) Merr.* Folium	18.81
(44)	*Nauclea calycina (Batrl.ex DC.) Merr.* Cortex	25.99
(45)	*Posoqueria latifolia (Lam.) Roem. & Schult.* Folium	80.27

gelatin test, gelatin-salt test, and test with ferrous (III) chloride; glycoside test with Molisch reaction; saponin test with honeycomb froth test; anthraquinone test with Bornträger reaction; terpenoid test with Liebermann-Burchard reagent.

3. Results and Discussion

3.1. Phytochemistry Test. Compounds with α-glucosidase inhibitory activity were preliminary identificated by the existence of alkaloid, terpene, saponin, tannin, glycoside, flavonoid, and quinone (Table 1).

3.2. Assay for α-Glucosidase Inhibitory Activity. The α-glucosidase of *S. cerevisiae* is used to investigate the inhibitory activity of the rude extracts. α-glucosidase inhibitory activity of rude extracts compounds against α-glucosidases were determined using *p*-nitrophenyl-α-D-glucopyranoside (p-NPG) as a substrate and these were compared with acarbose (Table 2). The IC_{50} values of compounds range from 2.33 μg/mL to 706.81 μg/mL. There are thirty-seven of samples which have IC_{50} lower than acarbose. Extracts derived from leaves of *Garcinia daedalanthera* showed inhibitory activity against α-glucosidase enzyme significantly, with IC_{50} value of 2.33 μg/mL. Inhibitory activity of the enzyme α-glucosidase at forty-five extracts may be due to the glycoside content in each extract. Glycosides consist of sugars that may be structurally similar to carbohydrate which is a substrate of the enzyme α-glucosidase [10]. IC_{50} value of samples of plant extracts are lower than acarbose because their active chemical compounds have no further fractionation and may have a synergistic effect in inhibiting α-glucosidase [11].

Inhibition mode of leaves extract of *Antidesma celebicum* from Euphorbiaceae was investigated. Inhibition mode of 80% ethanol extract showed competitive inhibitory mode. This mode may have been due because the structure is similar with glucose. This result is similar with inhibition mode of Nojirimycin which has a competitive inhibition against α-glucosidase [9] (Figure 1).

Inhibition mode of leaves extract of *Garcinia kydia* from Clusiaceae was investigated. Inhibition mode of 80% ethanol extract showed noncompetitive inhibitory mode [12] (Figure 2).

Inhibition mode of 80% ethanol extract from *Amaracarpus pubescens* Blume. leaves had a combination of competitive and uncompetitive inhibition. Combination of competitive and noncompetitive may have been due to the extract having more than one compound that has α-glucosidase inhibitory activity [13] (Figure 3).

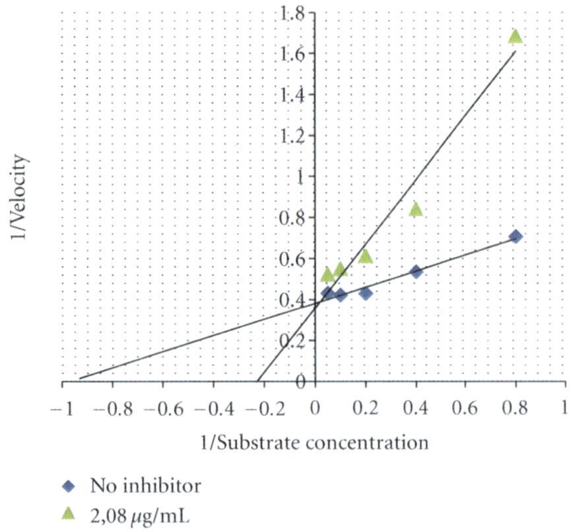

FIGURE 1: Lineweaver-Burk plot of 80% ethanol extract of leaves of *Antidesma celebicum* with concentration of 2.08 μg/mL with pNPG substrate concentration of 1.25, 2.5, 5, 10, and 20 mM.

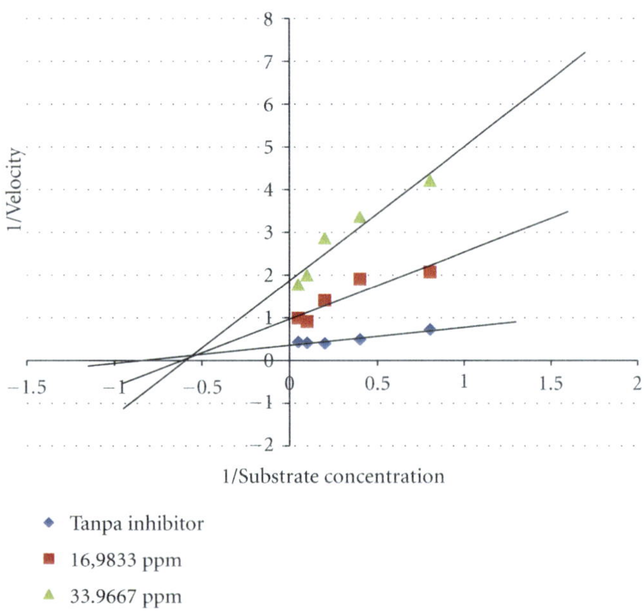

FIGURE 2: Lineweaver-Burke plot of the reaction α-glucosidase in the presence of 80% ethanol extract from *Garcinia kydia* Roxb. Leaves.

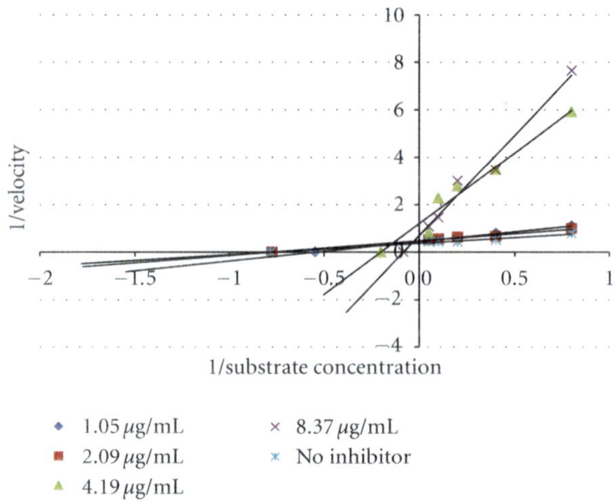

FIGURE 3: Lineweaver-Burke plot of the reaction α-glucosidase in the presence of 80% ethanol extract from *Amaracarpus pubescens* Blume.

4. Conclusion

In vitro assays of α-glucosidase activity showed thirty-seven of forty-five samples had IC_{50} values of between 2.33 μg/mL and 112.02 μg/mL, which were lower than that of acarbose (117.20 μg/mL). Based on family, 80% ethanol extract from *Garcinia daedalanthera* Pierre. leaves (Clusiaceae), *Antidesma celebicum* leaves (Euphorbiaceae), *Amaracarpus pubescens* Blume. leaves (Rubiaceae), and *Willughbeia tenuiflora* Dyer ex Hook.f leaves (Apocynaceae) had the highest α-glucosidase inhibiting activity with IC_{50} of 2.33 μg/mL, 2.34 μg/mL, 3.64 μg/mL, and 8,16 μg/mL. Meanwhile, types of enzyme inhibition mechanism from *Garcinia kydia* Roxb. leaves (Clusiaceae), *Antidesma celebicum* leaves (Euphorbiaceae), and *Amaracarpus pubescens* Blume. leaves (Rubiaceae) were noncompetitive inhibitor, competitive inhibitor, and mixed inhibitor. Currently attempts to purify the active compound from leaves extract of *Garcinia kydia* Roxb. (Clusiaceae), *Antidesma celebicum* (Euphorbiaceae), and *Amaracarpus pubescens* Blume. (Rubiaceae) are conducted to understand the inhibitory mechanisms more clearly. Moreover, further *in vivo* study is also required.

Acknowledgment

The authors would like thank to Department of Pharmacy, Faculty of Mathematics and Natural Sciences, University of Indonesia for supporting this project.

References

[1] I. Funke and M. F. Melzig, "Traditionally used plants in diabetes therapy—phytotherapeutics as inhibitors of α-amylase activity," *Revista Brasileira de Farmacognosia Brazilian Journal of Pharmacognosy*, vol. 16, no. 1, pp. 1–5, 2006.

[2] S. Wild, G. Roglic, A. Green, R. Sicree, and H. King, "Global prevalence of diabetes: estimates for the year 2000 and projections for 2030," *Diabetes Care*, vol. 27, no. 5, pp. 1047–1053, 2004.

[3] Department of Health Republic of Indonesia, *Pharmaceutical Care for Diabetes Mellitus*, Department of Health Republic of Indonesia, Kurihara, Indonesia, 2008.

[4] K. Y. Kim, K. A. Nam, H. Kurihara, and S. M. Kim, "Potent α-glucosidase inhibitors purified from the red alga Grateloupia elliptica," *Phytochemistry*, vol. 69, no. 16, pp. 2820–2825, 2008.

[5] L. H. Bösenberg and D. G. Van Zyl, "The mechanism of action of oral antidiabetic drugs: a review of recent literature," *Journal of Endocrinology, Metabolism and Diabetes of South Africa*, vol. 13, no. 3, pp. 80–88, 2008.

[6] S. H. Lam, J. M. Chen, C. J. Kang, C. H. Chen, and S. S. Lee, "α-Glucosidase inhibitors from the seeds of Syagrus romanzoffiana," *Phytochemistry*, vol. 69, no. 5, pp. 1173–1178, 2008.

[7] M. S. H. Wahyuningsih, S. Wahyuono, D. Santosa et al., "Plants exploration from central kalimantan forest as a source of bioactive compounds," *Biodiversitas*, vol. 9, pp. 169–172, 2008.

[8] L. S. De Padua, N. Bunyapiaphatsara, and R. H. M. J. Lemmens, *Plant Resources of South-East Asia: Medicinal and Poisonous Plants 1*, Prosea Foundation, Bogor, Indonesia, 1999.

[9] R. T. Dewi, Y. M. Iskandar, M. Hanafi et al., "Inhibitory effect of Koji Aspergillus terreus on α-glucosidase activity and postprandial hyperglycemia," *Pakistan Journal of Biological Sciences*, vol. 10, no. 18, pp. 3131–3135, 2007.

[10] S. Sugiwati, S. Setiasi, and E. Afifah, "Antihyperglycemic activity of the mahkota dewa [*Phaleria macrocarpa* (scheff.) boerl.] leaf extracts as an alpha-glucosidase inhibitor," *Makara Kesehatan*, vol. 13, no. 2, pp. 74–78, 2009.

[11] A. Andrade-Cetto, J. Becerra-Jiménez, and R. Cárdenas-Vázquez, "Alfa-glucosidase-inhibiting activity of some Mexican plants used in the treatment of type 2 diabetes," *Journal of Ethnopharmacology*, vol. 116, no. 1, pp. 27–32, 2008.

[12] D. S. Lee and S. H. Lee, "Genistein, a soy isoflavone, is a potent α-glucosidase inhibitor," *FEBS Letters*, vol. 501, no. 1–3, pp. 84–86, 2001.

[13] K. B. Storey, *Functional Metabolism: Regulation and Adaptation*, Wiley-Interscience, Hoboken, NJ, USA, 2004.

19

Pharmacokinetic Models for FcRn-Mediated IgG Disposition

Jim J. Xiao

Department of Clinical Pharmacology, Genentech Inc., 1 DNA Way, MS 463A, South San Francisco, CA 94080, USA

Correspondence should be addressed to Jim J. Xiao, xiao.jim@gene.com

Academic Editor: Dobromir Dobrev

The objectives were to review available PK models for saturable FcRn-mediated IgG disposition, and to explore an alternative semimechanistic model. Most available empirical and mechanistic PK models assumed equal IgG concentrations in plasma and endosome in addition to other model-specific assumptions. These might have led to inappropriate parameter estimates and model interpretations. Some physiologically based PK (PBPK) models included FcRn-mediated IgG recycling. The nature of PBPK models requires borrowing parameter values from literature, and subtle differences in the assumptions may render dramatic changes in parameter estimates related to the IgG recycling kinetics. These models might have been unnecessarily complicated to address FcRn saturation and nonlinear IgG PK especially in the IVIG setting. A simple semimechanistic PK model (cutoff model) was developed that assumed a constant endogenous IgG production rate and a saturable FcRn-binding capacity. The FcRn-binding capacity was defined as MAX, and IgG concentrations exceeding MAX in endosome resulted in lysosomal degradation. The model parameters were estimated using simulated data from previously published models. The cutoff model adequately described the rat and mouse IgG PK data simulated from published models and allowed reasonable estimation of endogenous IgG turnover rates.

1. Introduction

Under physiological conditions, IgG has prolonged half-life ($t_{1/2}$) relative to other plasma proteins, while IgG elimination is faster at much higher concentrations. These observations prompted Brambell et al. to propose a theoretical saturable protective Fc receptor in 1964 [1]. Subsequently, Brambell demonstrated that a neonatal intestinal receptor (FcRn) is responsible for maternal-to-infant IgG transport [2]. Waldmann and Strober later showed that FcRn preferentially binds to IgG Fc at lower pH [3]. The expression of FcRn in neonatal gut is transient [4], while in adults FcRn is expressed primarily in muscle, skin, vascular endothelium at relatively high levels [5–8]. The FcRn-mediated IgG recycling can be described as a 3-step process: (1) passive pinocytosis of IgG into endothelial cells; (2) acidification in endosome by H^+ ATPase to approximately pH 6 allowing IgG binding to FcRn; (3) unbound IgG is destined to lysosomal degradation while bound IgG is diverted back to circulation. Fc-FcRn binding in endosome may change FcRn distribution and intracellular trafficking of FcRn-coated endosome vesicles [9]. This directed endosome trafficking mechanism may further explain the high efficiency of IgG recycling.

FcRn is similar to the MHC class I molecule, consisting of a three-domain alpha subunit coupled with β-2 microglobulin. Mutation of the FcRn β-2 microglobulin in mice (β2m −/−) led to approximately 8–15-fold increase in IgG clearance [4, 6, 10]. This more-than-8-fold lower IgG clearance due to FcRn protection implies that an IgG molecule undergoes multiple cycles of FcRn-mediated endosomal recycling before its degradation in lysosome in mice.

Quantitative understanding of IgG recycling has been evolving. The first attempts in the 1960s by Brambell et al. [1] and Waldmann and Strober [3] were empirical by correlating fraction catabolic rate with plasma IgG concentrations. In 1966, Wochner et al. studied IgG disposition in patients with myotonic dystrophy, a hereditary error resulting in plasma deficiency of IgG but not albumin [11]. In 1990, Waldmann and Terru published IgG disposition in two patients with familial hypercatabolic hypoproteinemia [12]. These data provided insightful human kinetic data of the impact of FcRn on IgG disposition. In 2006, Kim et al. developed a mechanistic PK model for FcRn-mediated IgG PK in human [13]. The paper was an elegant review of available quantitative human IgG data in this field; it was also the first attempt to quantitatively assess IgG homeostasis and its disturbance by genetic FcRn diseases. Despite the several identified gaps due to limited available experimental data [14], the proposed model seems to be so far the best mechanistic model in human.

Saturation of FcRn by intravenous administration of high doses of pooled immunoglobulin (IVIG) has been a successful approach to clear pathogenic autoimmune antibodies from circulation, especially in patients with immune thrombocytopenia (ITP) [15]. Several semimechanistic models have been proposed to describe IgG disposition in IVIG setting in experimental animal models [16–19]. These models are discussed in detail in this paper. Quantitative models in clinical IVIG settings have not been published.

In addition, physiologically based PK (PBPK) models have been developed [20–23]. The models included multiple organs/tissues of interest, investigated the kinetics and determinants of IgG tissue distribution, and allowed studying the nonlinear FcRn and IgG recycling kinetics. However, these models are complicated in nature, and interpretations of FcRn-mediated IgG recycling seem very different among the models.

A new semimechanistic PK model is proposed. In this model, the saturable FcRn binding in endosome and subsequent IgG degradation are captured using a simple cutoff approach. The model avoided several questionable assumptions in previous work and adequately described data simulated from a previously published rat and mouse IVIG model.

2. Methods

2.1. Source IgG PK Data for Model Fitting. The rat and mouse semimechanistic IgG PK models [24] developed by Hansen and Balthasar were reconstructed in NONMEM (version 6.2.0; Icon Development Solutions, Ellicott City, MD). Since Hansen's model was derived from [17, 25] and adequately described [24] the experimental data, Hansen's models were used to simulate (reconstruct) the rat and mouse PK data according to the designs of the original experiments. Intersubject variability was fixed to 0. The simulated data were then used as source data to estimate the PK parameters in the new proposed rat and mouse cutoff models.

The rat experimental designs were as follows. In Study 1, an IV bolus dose of a monoclonal antibody 7E3, a platelet-binding antibody, was given to rats at 0.8, 4, or 8 mg/kg. Plasma PK was determined at 1, 3, 6, 12, 24, 48, 72, 96, and 168 hours after dose. In Study 2, rats received a single high dose IVIG at 0.4, 1, or 2 g/kg, followed by a single IV bolus dose of 7E3 at 8 mg/kg. Plasma PK was determined at 1, 3, 6, 12, 24, 48, 96, and 168 hours after dose. The simulated PK profiles using the reconstructed Hansen's model looked identical to the published results [24]. Both 7E3 and endogenous IgG concentration-time profiles were simulated, but only the plasma 7E3 PK data was used to estimate the parameter values of the new models.

The mouse study was as follows: an IV bolus dose of 7E3 was given to FcRn wild-type (WT) mice with or without concomitant dosing of 1 g/kg IVIG. PK plasma samples were collected at 1 and 12 hour, and 1, 2, 4, 7, 14, 23, 30, and 60 days after dose. Similarly, an IV bolus dose of 7E3 was given to FcRn knockout (KO) mice with or without concomitant dosing of 1 g/kg IVIG. PK plasma samples were collected at 1 and 12 hour, and 1, 2, 3, and 4 days after dose. Note that the mouse PK sampling time points were estimated based on the published figures [24] and may be slightly different from the original designs.

2.2. Full Mechanistic PK Model. The concept of the model is presented in Figure 1. In the full model scheme (upper panel), IgG disposition involves 3 compartments, that is, a central (plasma) compartment, a peripheral (tissue) compartment, and an endosome compartment nested in the peripheral compartment. As in Hansen's paper, IgG of different sources (i.e., 7E3, IVIG, and endogenous) were assumed to follow the same disposition kinetics [24]. In addition to first-order distribution (Q) between the central and peripheral compartments and first-order elimination (CL) from the central compartment, IgGs in the peripheral compartment also undergo endosome circulation/degradation. This starts with a nonspecific uptake by pinocytosis of first-order kinetics (CL_U), and followed by two transient steps governed by transit time τ_1 and τ_2. During τ_1, the endosomal pH decreases to approximately 6 by H^+ ATPase in parallel to IgG sorting when IgG molecules compete for FcRn. During τ_2, unbound IgGs get degraded. The FcRn-bound IgG is then recycled to circulation. A convenient assumption was made that the endosome vesicle volume does not change from the initial pinocytosis to the final fusion to plasma membrane. This allowed inferring FcRn saturation and fraction of unbound drug (f_U) using the total IgG concentration in the peripheral compartment. The total volume of endosome at a given time is determined by CL_U and the transit time τ_1 and τ_2.

2.3. Reduced Semimechanistic PK Model (Cutoff Model). It was reported that the endosome transit time is about 7 min [26, 27]. The whole recycling cycle can be instantaneously compared with the relatively slow elimination phase. For this reason, a simplified model was proposed where the endosome process collapsed into a nonlinear elimination directly from the peripheral compartment, that is, $\mathrm{CL}_U \times f_U$ (Figure 1, lower panel).

The cutoff model has 6 compartments (CMTs). All the three sources of IgGs (i.e., 7E3, IVIG, and endogenous IgGs) were incorporated in the model and share the same PK parameters including CL, Q, CL_U, the central compartment volume ($V_C = V_1 = V_3 = V_5$), and the peripheral compartment volume ($V_P = V_2 = V_4 = V_6$). In addition, it was assumed that k_{in} is the same regardless of the FcRn status in mice.

A key assumption was made for the f_U calculation. A hypothetical FcRn capacity parameter (Max) was proposed, $f_U = (C_{P,T} - \mathrm{Max})/C_{P,T}$, where $C_{P,T}$ is the total IgG concentration in the peripheral compartments (CMTs 2, 4, and 6). When $C_{P,T} \leq \mathrm{Max}$, $f_U = 0$. In FcRn KO

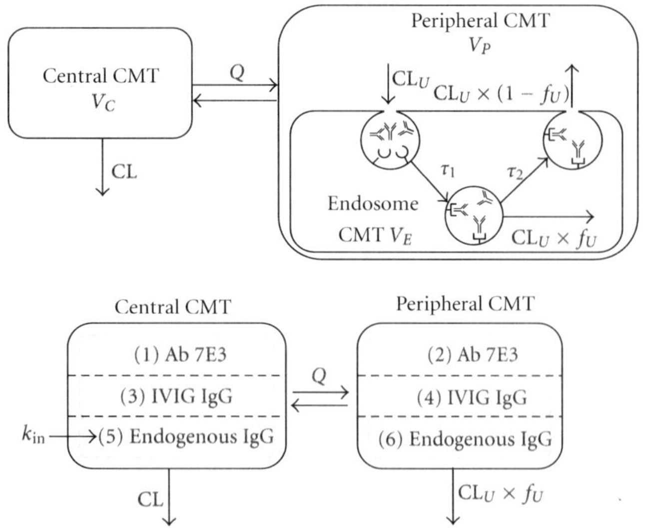

FIGURE 1: The proposed cutoff PK models. The full physiological model scheme (upper panel) describes physical processes, including IgG distribution in central, peripheral, and endosome compartments, nonspecific elimination from central compartment (CL), and FcRn-mediated endosomal IgG recycling and elimination in the endosome. The endosome space is nested in the peripheral compartment. In the reduced cutoff PK model scheme (lower panel), the endosome compartment is collapsed. The net endosomal IgG clearance is determined by endosomal uptake clearance (CL_U) from the peripheral compartment, the FcRn capacity (Max), the total IgG concentration in peripheral compartment ($C_{P,T}$), and the unbound fraction (f_U), where $f_U = (C_{P,T} - \text{Max})/C_{P,T}$ if $C_{P,T} > \text{Max}$; $f_U = 0$ if $C_{P,T} < \text{Max}$ or in FcRn KO mice.

mice (i.e., MAX = 0), $f_U = 1$. It was assumed that 7E3, IVIG, and endogenous IgGs have similar binding affinity for FcRn. In addition, instead of assuming that the microrate constants for endosome uptake (k_{up}) and return rate (k_{ret}) are equal as in other semimechanistic models [13, 16–19], a constant intercompartment clearance was assumed where the pinocytosis uptake clearance (CL_U) is the sum of endosome degradation clearance ($CL_U \times f_U$) and the returning clearance ($CL_U \times (1 - f_U)$).

The baseline endogenous plasma IgG concentrations in FcRn WT animals ($C_{5,\mathrm{WT},0}$) were fixed to 103 μM and 14.7 μM for rats and mice, respectively [24], where the subscript 5 is the compartment number (Figure 1, lower panel), WT stands for FcRn WT, and 0 represents time 0 (baseline). Since the endosome recycling and elimination are linked to the peripheral compartments (CMTs 2, 4, and 6), $C_{6,\mathrm{WT},0}$ may be lower than $C_{5,\mathrm{WT},0}$ if $f_U > 0$. As a result, conditional equations were derived to calculate secondary parameters, including $C_{6,\mathrm{WT},0}$, the endogenous IgG production rate (k_{in}), and baseline f_U ($f_{U,\mathrm{WT},0}$)

$$C_{6,\mathrm{WT},0} = \frac{C_{5,\mathrm{WT},0} \times Q + CL_U \times \mathrm{MAX}}{Q + CL_U}, \tag{1}$$

$$k_{in} = C_{5,\mathrm{WT},0} \times CL + CL_U \times C_{6,\mathrm{WT},0} - CL_U \times \mathrm{MAX}, \tag{2}$$

$$f_{U,\mathrm{WT},0} = \frac{C_{6,\mathrm{WT},0} - \mathrm{MAX}}{C_{6,\mathrm{WT},0}}. \tag{3}$$

However, when $C_{6,\mathrm{WT},0} \le \mathrm{MAX}$,

$$C_{6,\mathrm{WT},0} = C_{5,\mathrm{WT},0}, \tag{4}$$

$$k_{in} = C_{5,\mathrm{WT},0} \times CL, \tag{5}$$

$$f_{U,\mathrm{WT},0} = 0. \tag{6}$$

Note that (1)–(6) rely on the $C_{5,\mathrm{WT},0}$ values reported in the literature with normal FcRn expressions. In order to allow the model to predict endogenous IgG levels in FcRn KO mice, baseline endogenous IgG levels need to be defined independent of $C_{5,\mathrm{WT},0}$

$$A_{6,0} = V_P \times \frac{k_{in} \times Q + CL_U \times CL \times \mathrm{MAX} + CL_U \times Q \times \mathrm{MAX}}{Q \times CL + CL_U \times CL + CL_U \times Q}, \tag{7}$$

$$A_{5,0} = V_C \times \frac{k_{in} - CL_U \times (A_{6,0}/V_P) + CL_U \times \mathrm{MAX}}{CL}, \tag{8}$$

$$f_U = \frac{A_{6,0} - \mathrm{MAX} \times V_P}{A_{6,0}}, \tag{9}$$

where $A_{5,0}$ and $A_{6,0}$ are the endogenous IgG levels at baseline in the central and peripheral compartment, respectively.

In FcRn KO animals, MAX = 0 and the baseline can be simplified to the following:

$$A_{6,0} = V_P \times \frac{k_{in} \times Q}{Q \times CL + CL_U \times CL + CL_U \times Q}, \tag{10}$$

$$A_{5,0} = V_C \times \frac{k_{in} - CL_U \times (A_{6,0}/V_P)}{CL}, \tag{11}$$

$$f_U = 1. \tag{12}$$

When $A_{6,0}/V_P \le \mathrm{MAX}$, there is no IgG elimination from the peripheral compartment, and the baseline condition is defined as follows:

$$A_{6,0} = V_P \times \frac{k_{in}}{CL}, \quad A_{5,0} = V_C \times \frac{k_{in}}{CL}, \quad f_U = 0. \tag{13}$$

The derivations of the above equations are provided in the appendix.

The PK of 7E3, IVIG, and endogenous IgGs were further defined by differential equations:

$$\frac{dA_1}{dt} = -\frac{CL \times A_1}{V_C} - \frac{Q \times A_1}{V_C} + \frac{Q \times A_2}{V_P}, \tag{14}$$

$$\frac{dA_2}{dt} = \frac{Q \times A_1}{V_C} - \frac{Q \times A_2}{V_P} - \frac{CL_U \times f_U \times A_2}{V_P}, \tag{15}$$

$$\frac{dA_3}{dt} = -\frac{CL \times A_3}{V_C} - \frac{Q \times A_3}{V_C} + \frac{Q \times A_4}{V_P}, \quad (16)$$

$$\frac{dA_4}{dt} = \frac{Q \times A_3}{V_C} - \frac{Q \times A_4}{V_P} - \frac{CL_U \times f_U \times A_4}{V_P}, \quad (17)$$

$$\frac{dA_5}{dt} = -\frac{CL \times A_5}{V_C} - \frac{Q \times A_5}{V_C} + \frac{Q \times A_6}{V_P} + k_{in}, \quad (18)$$

$$\frac{dA_6}{dt} = \frac{Q \times A_5}{V_C} - \frac{Q \times A_6}{V_P} - \frac{CL_U \times f_U \times A_6}{V_P}, \quad (19)$$

where $C_{P,T} = (A_2 + A_4 + A_6)/V_P$, and $f_U = (C_{P,T} - \text{MAX})/C_{P,T}$.

2.4. Cutoff Model Parameter Estimation and Simulation. The models were coded in NONMEM (version 6.2.0) with FOCE method. A total of 6 model parameters (i.e., V_C, V_P, CL, Max, Q, and CL_U) were estimated by fitting the model with the simulated rat or mouse 7E3 plasma PK data. A constant coefficient of variation error model was used. Model performance was assessed visually by diagnostic plots. The model was then used to simulate 7E3, IVIG, and endogenous IgG concentrations under the experimental conditions. A sensitivity test was conducted to assess the effects of Max and CL_U on the 7E3 PK profile in the presence or absence of IVIG (2 g/kg) using the rat model.

3. Results

The parameter estimates of the reduced models are summarized in Table 1.

The rat cutoff model adequately described the simulated plasma 7E3 concentrations with or without IVIG using Hansen's model (Figures 2(a) and 2(b)). The estimated V_C and V_P values were 39.8 and 29.3 mL/kg, respectively, comparable to typical values for IgG reported in the literature [27]. The Cutoff Max was estimated to be 108 μM (16.2 mg/mL). With the endogenous IgG level of 103 μM, rat FcRn should not be saturated at baseline, that is, $f_U = 0$. CL_U, CL, and Q were estimated to be 2580, 24.5, and 81.0 mL/d/kg, respectively. The high CL_U value was somewhat unexpected, but physiologically it may make sense because a big component of the empirical peripheral compartment is comprised of endothelial cells expressing FcRn. As schematically shown in Figure 1, the nested structure and the fast CL_U suggest high intracompartment trafficking rate and endosomal recycling rate. Since FcRn was not saturated at baseline, the zero-order k_{in} was estimated to be 2.52 μmol/d/kg (or 378 μg/d/kg) using (5) instead of (2). All disposition PK parameters were estimated with good precisions (%RSE $\leq$ 6.7%). However, cautions should be used in interpreting the %RSE values because of the use of simulated data in the model fitting.

The plasma and peripheral concentration profiles of 7E3, IVIG, and endogenous IgGs were simulated using the rat cutoff model (Figure 3). Similar to plasma 7E3 PK profiles, the peripheral 7E3 exposures were lower with the increasing IVIG. The IVIG exposures increased at higher dose levels, with the highest plasma IVIG IgG concentration of 336 μM following 2 g/kg IVIG, approximately 3.3 times the endogenous level. This increased the total IgG concentration above MAX and was the driver for the nonlinear 7E3 PK. The endogenous IgG PK was minimally impacted by 7E3 alone (8 mg/kg), but decreased following IVIG treatment in an IVIG-dose-dependent manner, reaching maximum suppression of 13%, 28%, and 42% with 0.4, 1, and 2 g/kg IVIG, respectively. The extent of endogenous IgG suppression was similar to the values estimated using Hansen's model (differences within $\pm$2%) [24].

Similarly, the mouse cutoff model adequately described the simulated plasma 7E3 concentrations using Hansen's model (Figure 2(c)), with or without IVIG, and in FcRn WT or KO mice. The estimated V_C and V_P values were 66.8 and 65.5 mL/kg, respectively, larger than the estimates in the rat cutoff model. The CL_U, CL, and Q values were 564, 5.63, and 72.1 mL/d/kg, respectively, similar to the rat estimates. FcRn was not expected to be saturated at the baseline as MAX was estimated to be 20.1 μM, higher than the mouse baseline endogenous IgG concentration of 14.7 μM. Consistent with Hansen's model, the levels of 7E3 were eliminated monoexponentially in FcRn KO mice regardless of IVIG dose as IgGs were no longer protected by FcRn (Figure 2(c)). The endogenous IgG production rate was estimated to be 0.0827 μmol/d/kg. All PK parameters were estimated with reasonable precisions except Q that had a %RSE of 29.8% (Table 1).

The mouse cutoff model was then used to simulate the plasma and peripheral concentration profiles of 7E3, IVIG, and endogenous IgG under the experimental conditions (Figure 4). Similar to plasma 7E3 PK profiles, the peripheral 7E3 exposures were lower with IVIG in FcRn WT mice. The highest plasma IVIG IgG concentration following 1 g/kg IVIG was approximately 100 μM (7.8 times the endogenous level), thus transiently decreased the endogenous IgG level by up to 62%. In FcRn KO mice, IgG is not protected by FcRn (MAX = 0 and $f_U = 1$) while k_{in} remained the same as in FcRn WT mice. As a result, the plasma endogenous IgG levels at the baseline were 14.7 and 1.19 μM in WT and KO mice, respectively.

Sensitivity test was conducted with the rat model to evaluate the effects of Max and CL_U on plasma 7E3. In the absence of IVIG, the plasma 7E3 level increased with increasing Max when Max was less than total IgG level, but remained superimposable as Max was $\geq$108 μM and $f_U = 0$ (Figure 5). Concomitant 2 g/kg IVIG potentiated the effect of Max, and plasma 7E3 levels increased with the increasing Max throughout the tested Max range. On the other hand, changes in CL_U did not show appreciable impact on 7E3 PK profiles (data not shown), indicating that CL_U could not be well estimated. This is consistent with the higher %RSE values for CL_U in both species (Table 1) and is likely due to lack of informative data about endosomal IgG elimination kinetics.

Table 1: Summary of the cutoff PK model parameter estimates in rats and mice based on the PK data simulated by using Hansen's PK models.

Parameter	Rat		Mouse	
	Estimate	%RSE	Estimate	%RSE
V_C (mL/kg)	39.8	0.563%	66.8	1.46%
Max (μM)	108	0.0756%	20.1	0.557%
Q (mL/d/kg)	81.0	0.519%	72.1	3.47%
CL_U (mL/d/kg)	2580	6.7%	564	29.8%
V_P (mL/kg)	29.3	0.594%	65.5	7.43%
CL (mL/d/kg)	24.5	0.420%	5.63	12.5%
C_0 (μM)	103 (fixed)	—	14.7 (fixed)	—
EPS	0.000302	43.7%	0.00289	68.5%

In the mouse model, the MAX estimate is for FcRn WT mice; MAX is 0 in FcRn KO mice.

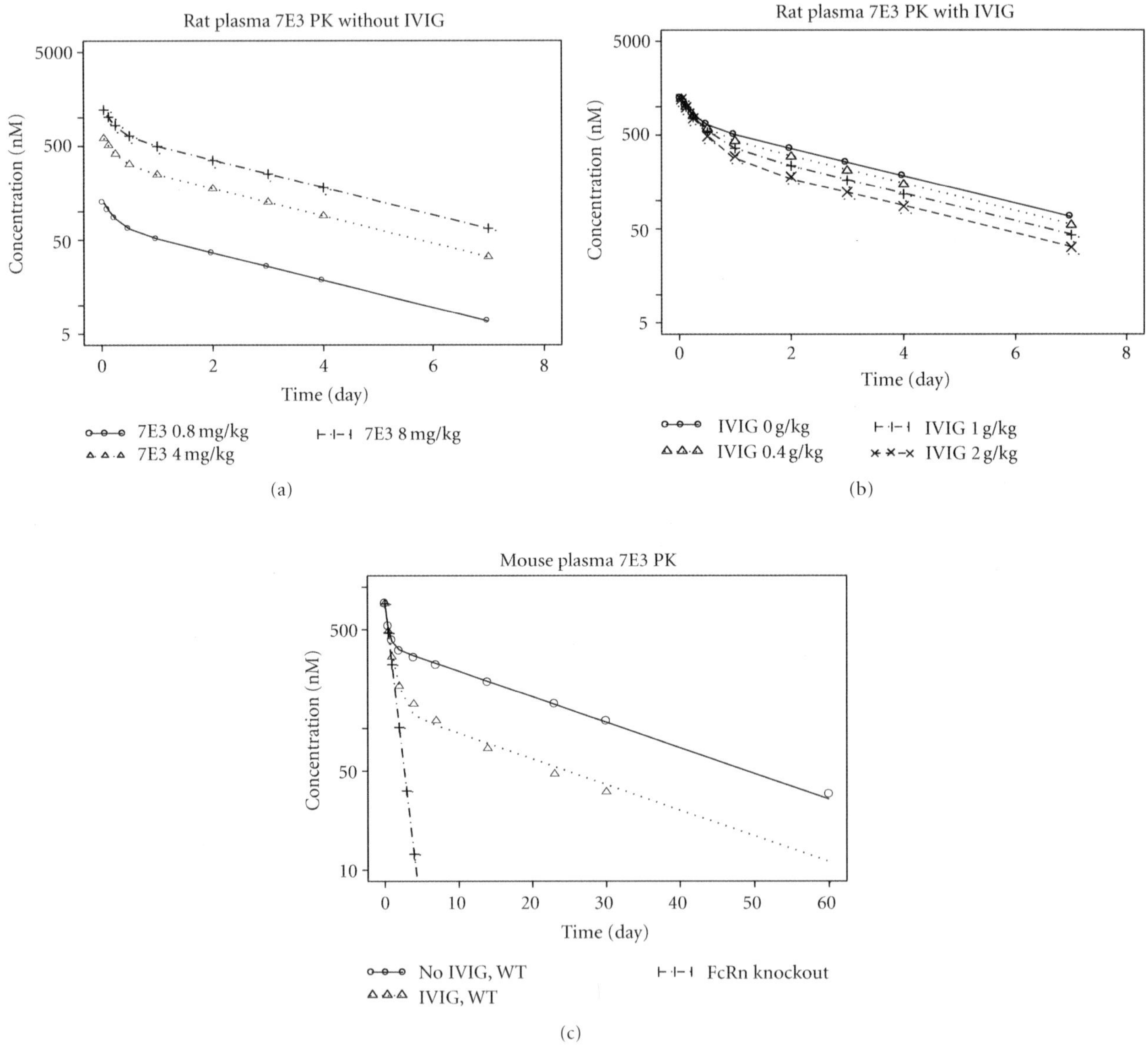

Figure 2: Cutoff model fitting of plasma 7E3 PK data that were simulated using Hansen's models. (a) Rat 7E3 PK data fitting at indicated dose levels without IVIG. (b) Rat 7E3 PK data fitting when 8 mg/kg 7E3 were dosed concomitant with IVIG of indicated dose levels. (c) Mouse 7E3 PK data fitting when 8 mg/kg 7E3 was given to FcRn WT or KO mice, with or without 1 g/kg IVIG.

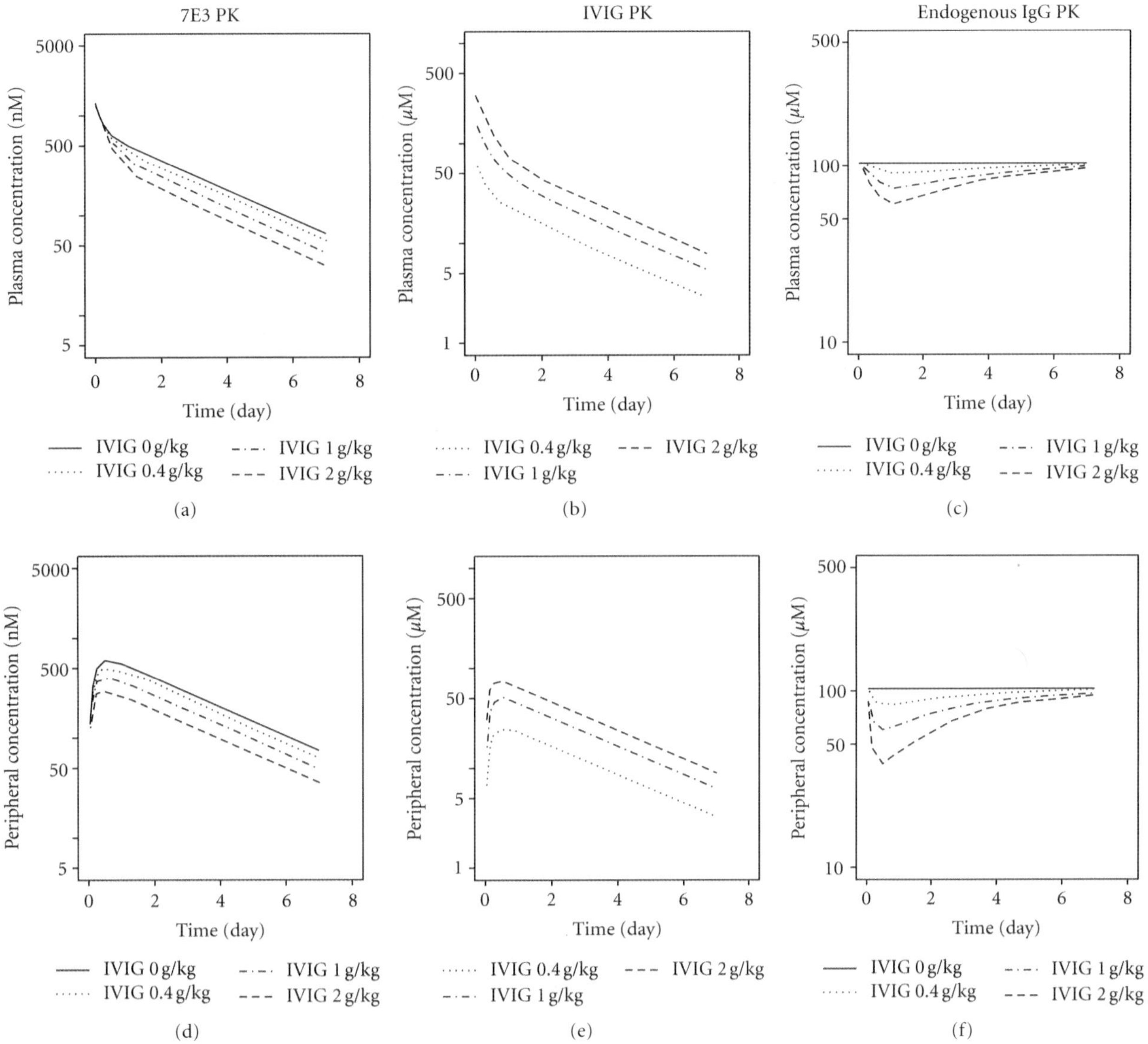

FIGURE 3: Simulated PK profiles using the rat cutoff model. All rats receive 8 mg/kg 7E3, as well as IVIG at indicated dose levels. Plasma and peripheral concentrations of 7E3, IVIG IgG, and endogenous IgG are plotted.

In most published models, the FcRn-IgG binding and FcRn saturation were based on either multiexponent functions [1, 3, 20], Langmuir-type binding isotherm, and quadratic equation solution of unbound concentration [16, 19, 24], or Michaelis-Menten kinetics [13]. In this proposed model, a simplified cutoff concept was introduced to describe the saturable FcRn-mediated kinetics. The relationship between the model estimated f_U and total peripheral IgG concentration is plotted in Figure 6. Under the simulated experimental conditions, the f_U ranged from 0 to 0.076 in rats, 0 to 0.25 in FcRn WT mice, and remained 1 in FcRn KO mice. For both species (FcRn WT), the cutoff model estimated f_U-total peripheral IgG concentration profiles are in parallel with the f_U-total plasma IgG concentration profiles estimated using Hansen's models. The difference is largely due to the different model structures and the additional nonspecific linear IgG elimination (CL) in the cutoff models which is absent in Hansen's models.

4. Discussion

4.1. Bleeker's Model [28]. The relationship between fraction clearance rate (FCR) and plasma IgG concentration was described by exponential equations in both human and mice using previously published data. This approach was empirical and did not allow physiological interpretation such as recycling rate and efficiency [13]. A mammillary PK model coupled with the predicted FCR was used for simulation and the results were consistent with IgG $t_{1/2}$ under physiological conditions and some clinical data. However, it underestimated IVIG effect on autoantibody suppression and overpredicted IgG exposures in FcRn KO model [18].

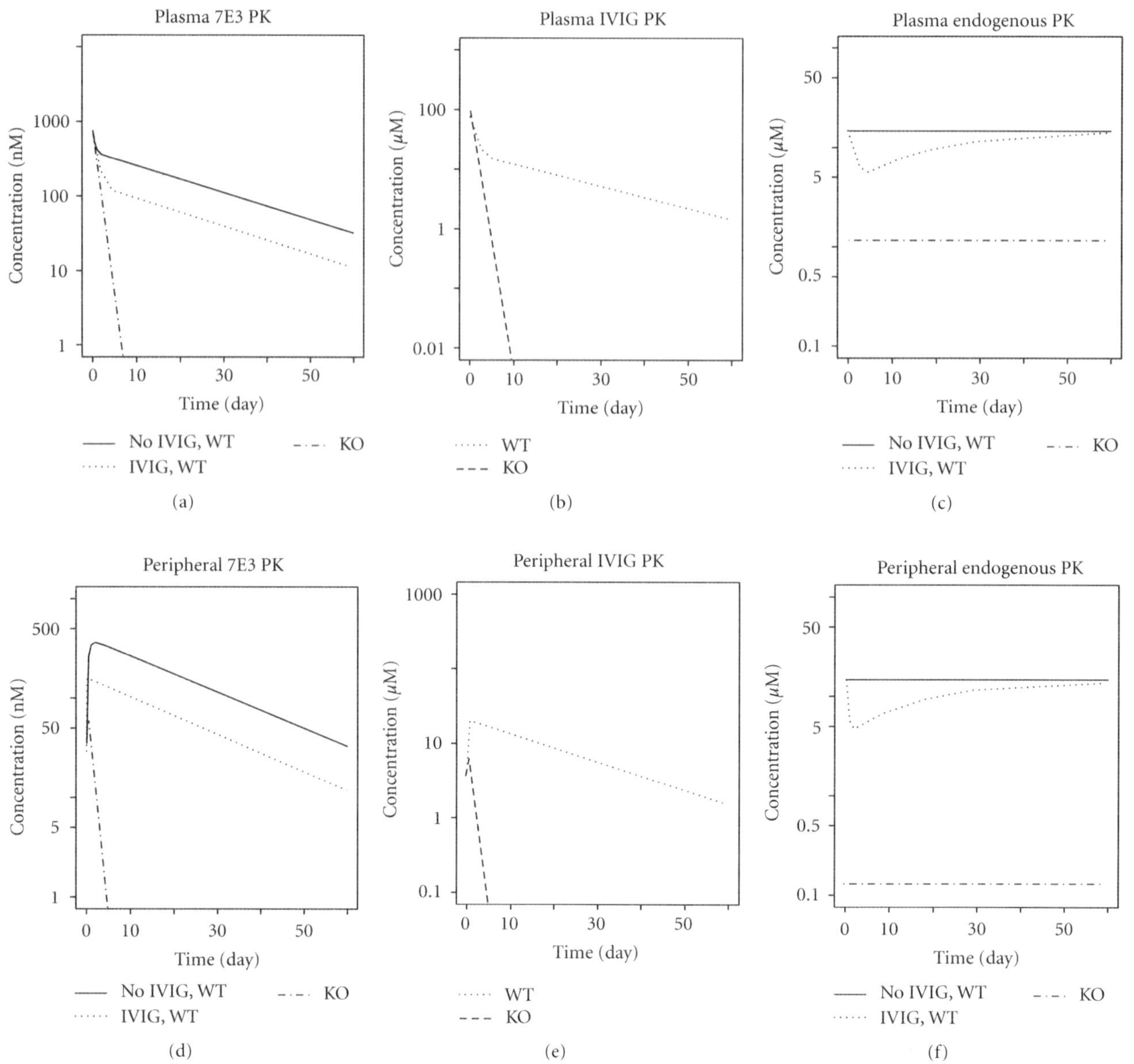

FIGURE 4: Simulated PK profiles using the mouse cutoff model. All mice receive 8 mg/kg 7E3 with or without concomitant 1 g/kg IVIG in either FcRn WT or KO mice. Plasma and peripheral concentrations of 7E3, IVIG IgG, and endogenous IgG are plotted.

4.2. Hansen's Model [24]. The model was comprised of the central and endosomal compartments (Figure 7(a)). It considered endogenous IgG, autoantibody (7E3), and IVIG simultaneously. The strengths of the model include simplicity, mechanistic basis, and ability to adapt to different situations. The model adequately described 7E3 PK data in normal and FcRn KO mice, and 7E3 PK data in rats with or without IVIG. The model was also used to infer the total FcRn-binding capacity and endogenous IgG turnover rate. However, the assumption of $k_{up} = k_{ret}$ is questionable. At steady-state in endosome, $C_1 \times k_{up} = C_E \times k_{ret}(1 - f_U) + C_E \times k_{deg} \times f_U$. It implied that $V_1 = V_E$ when the equation was to be scaled from concentration to amount. This may not be likely as it was estimated by the same group later that endosomal space volume is approximately 5 mL/kg in mice [21], much smaller than the plasma volume of 50 mL/kg [29].

According to Hansen's model, it appears that the endosome compartment has dual functions, that is, to explain the saturable elimination of IgG and to serve as a distribution compartment. The PK profiles of 7E3 in the absence of IVIG in the central and the endosome compartments look like typical 2-compartment PK model [24]. In the presence of IVIG, the PK profiles of 7E3 were lowered due to FcRn saturation [24]. While it is theoretically sound and practically convenient to assume that IgG concentration in the early endosome is the same as that in the circulation, dual functions of the endosome compartment had implication on

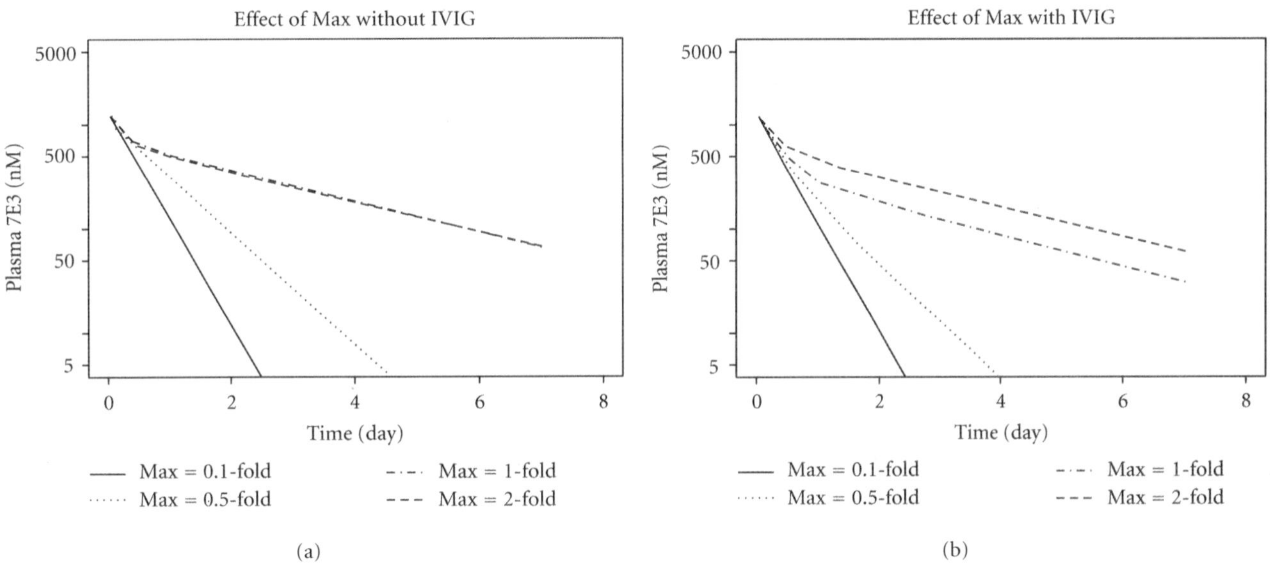

FIGURE 5: Sensitivity tests for Max. The effect of different MAX values on the plasma 7E3 pharmacokinetics was simulated in the presence or absence of IVIG (2 g/kg) using the rat PK model. The tested range was 0.1- to 2-fold the estimated Max (108 μM).

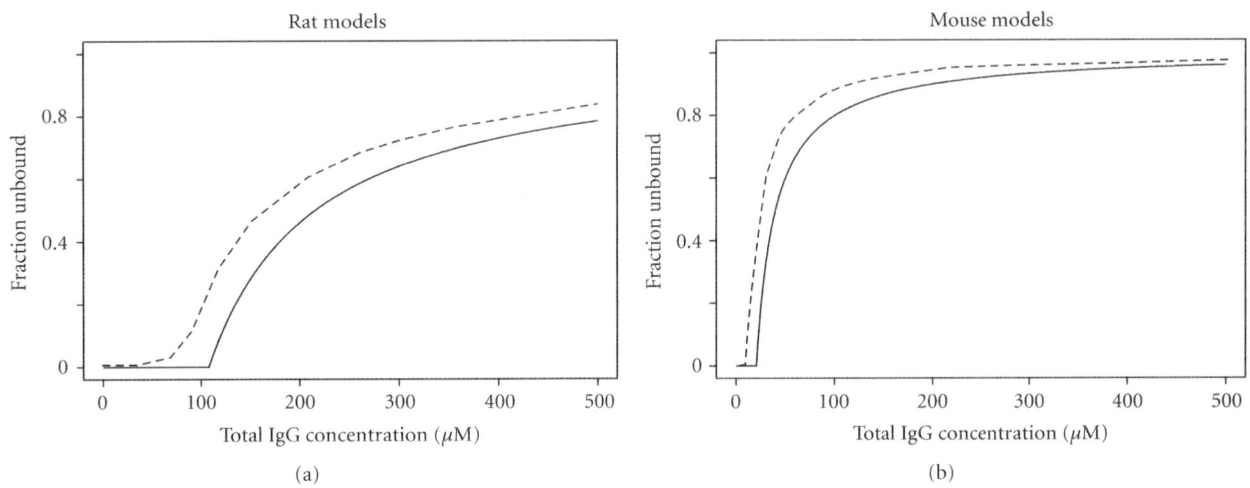

FIGURE 6: Relationship between f_U and total peripheral IgG concentration (cutoff models, solid lines) or total plasma IgG concentration (Hansen's models, dashed lines). The f_U values for Hansen's models were calculated according to the published models [4]. The f_U values for the cutoff models were based on the model parameters in Table 1.

the f_U estimation. To illustrate this, two sets of f_U values were calculated using the plasma or endosome total IgG concentrations simulated with Hansen's model, and plotted in Figure 8. The significant discrepancies and hysteresis indicate that it may not be appropriate to infer FcRn saturation using plasma total IgG concentrations under the particular model assumptions.

In addition, f_U was first calculated with the total plasma IgG concentration under the assumption that the total concentrations in plasma and endosome were the same. On the other hand, the steady-state endosome IgG concentration was redefined differently based on endosomal mass balance of IgG at steady state. These different definitions and empirical assumptions reflect the lack of informative experimental data of the endosome compartment and casts doubt in the interpretation of the model-derived parameter values. For example, the rat endogenous IgG production rate was estimated to be 62.9 μmol/d/kg in Hansen's model based on steady-state condition [24], while it was reported that the endogenous IgG CL in rats is only 1.9 μmol/d/kg (ranged from 1 to 2.9 μmol/d/kg) following a dose of ^{131}I-labeled rat IgGs [30].

Since the only mechanism of IgG elimination is through the endosome pathway (Figure 6(a)) in Hansen's model, the total FcRn-binding capacity (R_t) had to be smaller than the endogenous levels of IgG in order to describe the PK data (i.e., R_t = 83 μM and 12.2 μM for mice and rats, resp.) [24]. In other words, the model structure predetermined

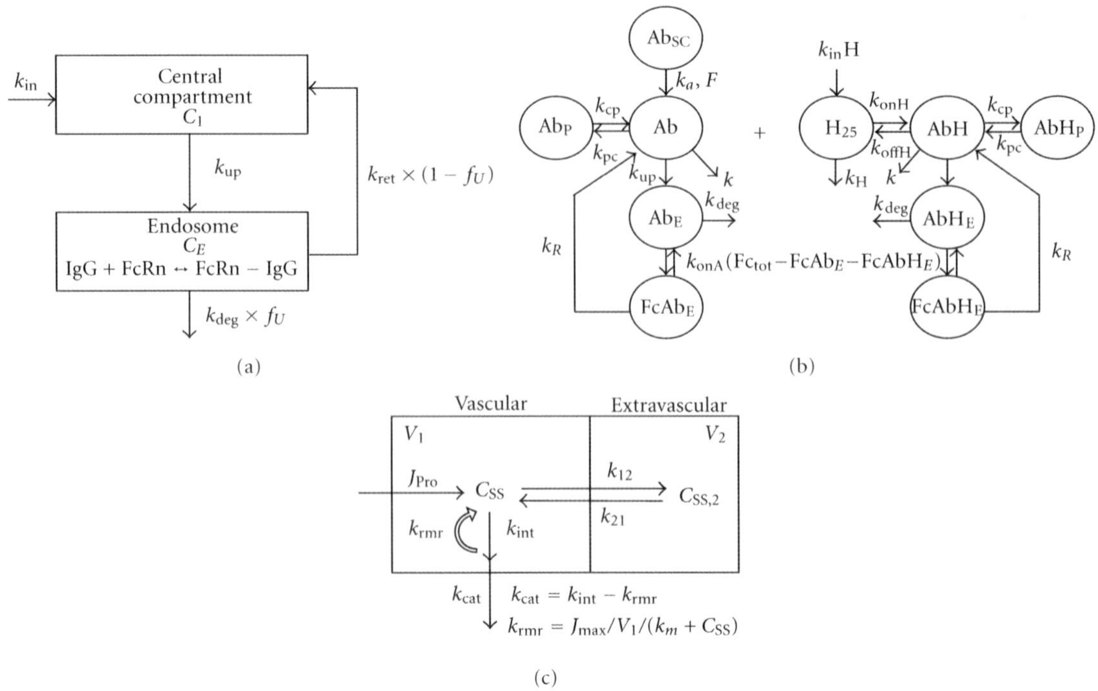

Figure 7: Published semimechanistic PK models. (a) Hansen's model; (b) Xiao's model; (c) Kim's model. Models schemes are redrawn based on published papers.

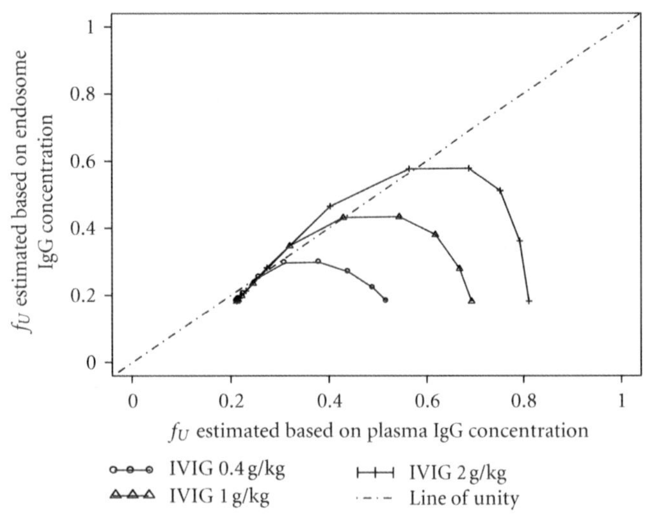

Figure 8: Comparison of f_U values derived from IgG concentrations in endosome and plasma using Hansen's rat model after a single IV dose of 8 mg/kg 7E3 in the presence or absence of IVIG. Significant counter clockwise hysteresis was observed due to IgG distribution delays. In the absence of IVIG, the line visually collapsed into a short line at the ending point of the counter-clockwise hysteresis loop as the lack of significant change in total IgG level kept f_U relatively constant.

that FcRn had to be saturated at physiological condition. Furthermore, simulations using the mouse model showed an accumulation of IgGs in the endosomal compartment in FcRn KO mice, and the same endogenous IgG concentrations at the baseline between FcRn WT and KO mice (data not shown). These indicate inappropriate model assumptions, and cautions should be used when interpreting the modeling results.

An improved PK/PD model was developed to describe the IVIG effect on the disposition of MWReg30, an anti-platelet antibody, and on MWReg30-induced thrombocytopenia in mice [16]. The PK model was similar to Hansen's model except that the PK data of both MWReg30 and IVIG were available, and the differential equations were written with respect to amounts of MWReg30 and IVIG as opposed to concentrations in Hansen's model. This avoided some of the confusion of distribution volume in Hansen's model. However, the differential equations for endogenous IgGs were still written with respect to concentration. This was probably for model simplification purpose and due to the lack of endogenous IgG PK data. Although this hybrid model offered some improvement, it was still subject to similar concerns.

4.3. Xiao's Model [19]. Another mechanistic FcRn-IgG model was developed by Xiao et al. recently [19] based on total hepcidin and an antihepcidin mAb (Ab 12B9m) concentrations (unbound + complex) in cynomolgus monkeys after single or multiple doses of Ab 12B9m (Figure 7(b)). Higher clearance of Ab 12B9m was observed after multiple weekly IV and SC doses of 300 mg/kg Ab 12B9m and was attributed to FcRn saturation. In addition, target-mediated IgG disposition (TMDD) was incorporated in order to infer the unbound hepcidin and unbound Ab 12B9m concentrations.

The model was a modified version of Hansen's model by inheriting the assumption of Langmuir-type FcRn-IgG interaction and $k_{up} = k_{ret}$. The model had a peripheral compartment, so that the endosomal compartment did not have to bear the dual functions as discussed in Hansen's model. Because it included unbound Ab 12B9m and its complex with hepcidin, endogenous IgG was not considered in the model to minimize the model complexity. As a result, interpretation of FcRn saturation should be viewed with caution. Another difference was that the endosome compartment volume (V_E) was included in the model to allow a better sense of mass transfer. However, the endosomal volume V_E and the dissociation constant k_D for FcRn-IgG binding were estimated as a product rather than separately since they operated in the model only as a product.

4.4. Kim's Model [13]. A mechanism-based PK model for human IgG was developed based on saturable kinetics and data from the literature using easily measurable plasma concentrations (Figure 7(c)). This appeared to be the first paper that addressed FcRn-mediated IgG recycling kinetics quantitatively in human. Note that this model was designed for endogenous IgG only although it may be adapted for therapeutic IgG and/or IVIG. All parameter values, with exception of k_m, were borrowed from the literature. It was recognized that the plasma concentration was not identical too but as an index for endosomal unbound IgG concentration. In addition, as an improvement from previous models, $k_{up} = k_{ret}$ was no longer assumed.

In this model, the rate constants for IgG internalization, catabolism, and recycling were defined as k_{int}, k_{cat}, and k_{rmr}, respectively. Because the plasma compartment (V_1) and the endosome compartment (V_E) were collapsed as the vascular space in the simplified model, the IgG concentrations became the same (C_{SS}). Although the k_{int} retained its physiological meaning to describe the IgG catabolism and trafficking within vascular space, that is, $k_{int} = k_{cat} + k_{rmr}$, according to equations $J_{rmr} = J_{max} \times C_{SS}/(k_m + C_{SS})$ and $J_{cat} = k_{cat} \times C_{ss} \times V_1$, the recycling rate J_{rmr} and the catabolic rate J_{cat} were directly linked to the vascular space, and no longer rely on k_{int} despite of the sequential events as shown in the model scheme (Figure 7(c)). As a result, k_{int} is not kinetically informed by other processes in the model, and obtaining k_{int} value solely relied on the literature. This might be a problem especially when the values of most parameters were borrowed from literature where different physiological and/or mechanistic assumptions might have been made. Probably because of this, the model did not seem to be able to explain the high fractional catabolic rate of IgG in patients with familial hypercatabolic hypoproteinemia.

In addition, as the author pointed out, the estimated rate of pinocytosis (k_{up}) was smaller in magnitude than the real unidirectional uptake rate, so the daily fractional uptake rate (18%), the fractional recycling rate (10.6%), and the fraction catabolic rate (7.4%) should be interpreted with cautions. Indeed, the inferred efficiency of FcRn-mediated IgG recycling (~60%) was lower than what can be inferred from the IgG PK data from two reported cases of familial hypercatabolic hypoproteinemia with non-functional FcRn due to a mutant β2m gene. In these patients with normal IgG synthesis rates, IgG survival was short. The IgG fractional catabolic rates increased fivefold to 31% and 36% of the intravenous pool per day (normal 6.7 ± 2%/d) [12]. This approximate 5-fold increase in FCR suggested that under normal physiological conditions, an average IgG molecule is degraded after approximately 5 times endothelial pinocytosis, or approximately 80% efficiency of FcRn-mediated IgG recycling.

Another difference between Kim's model and previously discussed models was the empirical E_{max} model for FcRn-IgG binding. It was equivalent to early regression models by Brambell and Waldmann [1, 3]. k_m was defined as the serum IgG concentration at which a half maximal IgG recycling was achieved and was estimated to be 21 mg/mL. Choosing the total serum IgG concentration for FcRn-binding estimation might have been a convenient approximation; however, cautions should be used when comparing results from models with different structures.

4.5. Physiological Models. Several physiologically based PK (PBPK) models were developed for anticarcinoembryonic antigen (CEA) antibodies [20, 22] or 7E3 [21] in mice. The models included organs/tissues of interest, lymphatic circulation, FcRn-IgG binding, and IgG-CEA binding (if applicable). Most physiological parameters regarding plasma flow rate, vascular, interstitial, and total tissue volume were available from the literature. Lymphatic circulation rate was either assumed [21] or estimated [20, 22]. Endosome update and return rates were either fixed to be the same value [22] or estimated [20, 21]. In general, the models described/predicted the anti-CEA antibody PK reasonably well. However, depending on the model assumptions, the FcRn or endosome-related parameter values might be very different. For example, Ferl's estimations of k_{int} and k_{rec} were 1.38 day^{-1} and 0.5 day^{-1}, respectively [20], while in Garg's model, the values were 1.96 day^{-1} and 20.4 day^{-1}, respectively [21, 24]. In a recent revision of the model, target-mediated disposition was included in addition to the FcRn-IgG binding, where k_{int} and k_{rec} were assumed to be the same and estimated to be 0.715 day^{-1} [22]. In addition, the percentage and mechanism of IgG elimination in each organ were interpreted differently. According to Ferl's model, approximately 40% of IgG eliminated was attributed to linear elimination kinetics in liver and other organs, while in Garg's model, skin, muscle, liver, and gut were the major organs responsible for 33, 24, 16, and 12% of total IgG elimination, respectively.

It is well recognized that the PBPK models have the potential to better describe the physiological processes, and thus may allow more meaningful interpretations. On the other hand, it should be noted that these models usually have complicated structures and heavily depend on available data from the literature. The complexity as an effort to best describe the physiological processes came with the need for more sophisticated modeling assumptions. Multiplicity of assumptions and potential error prorogation may lead to liabilities to model misspecification and result in misinterpretation. The routinely performed "model validation" using a small experimental data set might not be sufficient for model testing and assumption justification, as the inherent model flexibility may sometimes allow apparent good data fitting even when some inappropriate assumptions were made.

4.6. The Proposed Semimechanistic Cutoff Model. It has been reported that some IgGs with higher affinity for FcRn showed prolonged $t_{1/2}$ [31, 32]. However, affinity for FcRn may not be the only major contributor to IgG catabolic rate [33]. Physiological PK models have been proposed, including the one in Figure 1(a), to depict the saturable FcRn-mediated IgG kinetics based on known physiology. However, in a strict sense, quantitative physiological models have not been published. The reason might be twofold. First, there is insufficient understanding of the intracellular events and difficulty in scaling data from in vitro to in vivo (e.g., volume, rate, and transit time). In addition, there is insufficient or uninformative in vivo PK data to develop and differentiate such PK models. The simulated data using Hansen's model was easily described by the new cutoff model. The model parameters were estimated fairly precisely (Table 1). However, other models with different structural assumptions might be able to describe the data equally well. To better test a model, additional PK data are required, for example, PK of total IgG.

It is fair to say that none of the available models (including the cutoff model) adequately mimicked the physiology of FcRn-mediated IgG recycling, and more sophisticated physiological models cannot be developed simply because the lack of informative experimental data in the endosome compartment. For example, the rate of pinocytosis at a whole body level is difficult to measure experimentally. In addition, although the mean transit time of endosome was inferred to be about 7 min [26, 27], it remains largely unknown how endosome is destined to lysosome kinetically and how IgG degradation changes as a function of the mean transit. For example, it was reported that FcRn-IgG binding in endosome triggers more efficient intracellular trafficking and transcytosis [9], but the quantitative impact on the endosomal recycling is not clear. And the dynamics of pH lowering in early endosome is not easy to describe mathematically. Furthermore, it was realized that FcRn saturation estimated based on plasma IgG levels may not approximate the real situation in endosome as discussed for Hansen's model. The technical difficulties in estimating the parameters governing the FcRn-mediated IgG recycling process prevent developing models that truly resembles the physiology.

Taken together, it might be practically justified to utilize simple models of FcRn-mediated IgG disposition such as the cutoff model, especially in the IVIG setting, and leave more sophisticated models for later optimization when cumulative understanding of this physiological process allows so.

The proposed cutoff model has only 6 parameters (Table 1). The distribution volume parameters V_C and V_P were clearly defined. The collapsed IgG recycling was based on the relative short endosome mean transit time, and the assumption that FcRn-IgG dissociation did not happen, or more appropriately, only happened to a constant extent. It allows estimation of nonspecific linear CL and nonlinear endosomal elimination. At baseline level in both rats and FcRn WT mice, the linear CL accounted for 100% of endogenous IgG elimination. The apparent nonspecific linear CL at baseline should be further discussed. Mathematically, CL accounted for the linear portion of IgG elimination, but it did not necessarily imply endosome-unrelated processes. For example, a fraction of IgG in endosome could end up in the lysosome degradation pathway even when FcRn is not saturated. This is possible considering variability in the biological processes such as the endosome acidification dynamics, transit time of endosome intracellular trafficking, and conversion to lysosome, as well as proteolysis kinetics. At a whole-body level, the above could have led to an apparent nonspecific linear. It is also important to realize that although several organs and tissues have been identified to express FcRn, the expression levels may be different. It has been reported that the dispersed pinocytotic activities of virtually all cells capture and process all soluble plasma proteins at a rate of ≈2x per day with equivalent degradative rates unless they are protected by specific mechanisms [4]. This high pinocytosis rate not only explains the nonspecific linear CL, but also is consistent with the high CL_U values in both species estimated by the cutoff models (Table 1).

In rats, the estimated production rate of endogenous IgGs in rats was 2.52 μmol/d/kg using the cutoff model, slightly lower than the measured value of 1.9 μmol/d/kg (ranged 1 to 2.9 μmol/d/kg) [30]. In FcRn WT mice, the endogenous production rate was estimated to be 0.0827 μmol/d/kg, lower than previously reported value 0.132 μmol/d/day (assumed 50 mL/kg plasma) [4, 34]. Apparently, there is room for further model improvement and more precise parameter estimation (e.g., CL_U) with emerging experimental data and better understanding of the physiology. However, it is important to note there has been a big improvement from in the previous model [24], where the k_{in} estimates were 62.9 and 1.21 μmol/d/kg in rats and FcRn WT mice, respectively.

Different plasma endogenous IgG levels were reported between rats (103 μM) and mice (14.7 μM) at the baseline [24]. According to the cutoff model results, FcRn was almost saturated in rats (MAX = 108 μM) at the baseline but not in FcRn WT mice (MAX = 20.1 μM). In addition, rats seemed to have higher CL and CL_U than mice according to the cutoff models (Table 1). These differences translated to an estimated 30-fold faster k_{in} in rats than in mice versus approximately a 14-fold difference reported in the literature [4, 30, 34]. Further investigation would help understand the between-species difference in endogenous IgG turnover.

According to the cutoff model, FcRn should not be saturated at baseline, and the baseline total IgG clearance was determined solely by the nonspecific linear CL. The total body IgG clearance started to increase when the total peripheral IgG concentration exceeded MAX. In both rats and FcRn WT mice, the 7E3 plasma exposure decreased with the concomitant IVIG (Figures 2(b) and 2(c)). This is different from Hansen's model which predicted FcRn saturation at the baseline [24]. In addition, the mouse cutoff model is able to predict the endogenous IgG concentrations for FcRn WT and KO mice. The estimated baseline endogenous IgG concentrations in plasma were estimated to be 14.7 and 1.19 μM for FcRn WT and KO mice, respectively. This 12-fold decrease in the baseline IgG level reflects accelerated IgG catabolism in the absence of FcRn, consistent with reported values of 8–15-fold [4, 6, 10]. On the other hand, Hansen's model infers that the baseline endogenous IgG level remains the same in FcRn WT and KO mice [24].

In conclusion, A simple cutoff model was proposed for IgG PK modeling with saturable FcRn-mediated IgG disposition in rats and mice.

Appendix

Detailed Derivation of Equations

(1) Derivation of secondary PK parameters with the baseline plasma endogenous IgG concentration in rats and FcRn WT mice.

Based on mass balance of endogenous IgGs between CMT5 and CMT6, $C_{5,\mathrm{WT},0} \times Q = C_{6,\mathrm{WT},0} \times Q + C_{6,\mathrm{WT},0} \times \mathrm{CL}_U \times f_U$, where $f_U = (C_{6,\mathrm{WT},0} - \mathrm{MAX})/C_{6,\mathrm{WT},0}$.

So $C_{5,\mathrm{WT},0} \times Q = C_{6,\mathrm{WT},0} \times Q + \mathrm{CL}_U \times (C_{6,\mathrm{WT},0} - \mathrm{MAX})$,

If $C_{6,\mathrm{WT},0} > \mathrm{MAX}$,

then $C_{6,\mathrm{WT},0} = (C_{5,\mathrm{WT},0} \times Q + \mathrm{CL}_U \times \mathrm{MAX})/(Q + \mathrm{CL}_U)$ and $f_{U,\mathrm{WT},0} = (C_{6,\mathrm{WT},0} - \mathrm{MAX})/C_{6,\mathrm{WT},0}$

If $C_{6,\mathrm{WT},0} \le \mathrm{MAX}$, then $C_{6,\mathrm{WT},0} = C_{5,\mathrm{WT},0}$ and $f_{U,\mathrm{WT},0} = 0$.

For endogenous IgGs at baseline, production rate = elimination rate,

$$k_{\mathrm{in}} = C_{5,\mathrm{WT},0} \times \mathrm{CL} + C_{6,\mathrm{WT},0} \times \mathrm{CL}_U \times f_U. \tag{A.1}$$

If $C_{6,\mathrm{WT},0} > \mathrm{MAX}$, $k_{\mathrm{in}} = C_{5,\mathrm{WT},0} \times \mathrm{CL} + \mathrm{CL}_U \times (C_{6,\mathrm{WT},0} - \mathrm{MAX})$;

If $C_{6,\mathrm{WT},0} \le \mathrm{MAX}$, $k_{\mathrm{in}} = C_{5,\mathrm{WT},0} \times \mathrm{CL}$.

(2) Derivation of baseline endogenous IgG levels. The key is to allow model prediction of baseline plasma and peripheral IgG levels in both FcRn WT and KO animals.

With mass balance at baseline,

$$\begin{aligned} k_{\mathrm{in}} &= \frac{A_{5,0}}{V_C} \times \mathrm{CL} + \frac{A_{6,0}}{V_P} \times \mathrm{CL}_U \times f_U, \\ \frac{A_{5,0}}{V_C} \times Q &= \frac{A_{6,0}}{V_P} \times Q + \frac{A_{6,0}}{V_P} \times \mathrm{CL}_U \times f_U, \end{aligned} \tag{A.2}$$

Solve the above equations for $A_{5,0}/V_C$ and $A_{6,0}/V_P$,

$$\frac{A_{6,0}}{V_P} = \frac{k_{\mathrm{in}} \times Q}{Q \times \mathrm{CL} + \mathrm{CL}_U \times \mathrm{CL} \times ((A_{6,0}/V_P - \mathrm{MAX})/(A_{6,0}/V_P)) + \mathrm{CL}_U \times Q \times ((A_{6,0}/V_P - \mathrm{MAX})/(A_{6,0}/V_P))}. \tag{A.3}$$

If $A_{6,0}/V_P > \mathrm{MAX}$,

then $A_{6,0}/V_P = (k_{\mathrm{in}} \times Q + \mathrm{CL}_U \times \mathrm{CL} \times \mathrm{MAX} + \mathrm{CL}_U \times Q \times \mathrm{MAX})/(Q \times \mathrm{CL} + \mathrm{CL}_U \times \mathrm{CL} + \mathrm{CL}_U \times Q)$,

and $A_{5,0}/V_C = (k_{\mathrm{in}} - \mathrm{CL}_U \times (A_{6,0}/V_P - \mathrm{MAX}))/\mathrm{CL}$.

If $A_{6,0}/V_P \le \mathrm{MAX}$,

then $A_{6,0}/V_P = k_{\mathrm{in}} \times Q/(Q \times \mathrm{CL}) = k_{\mathrm{in}}/\mathrm{CL}$,

and $A_{5,0}/V_C = k_{\mathrm{in}}/\mathrm{CL}$.

In FcRn KO mice, $A_{6,0}/V_P$ and $A_{5,0}/V_C$ do not need to be separately coded. Instead, an NONMEM input data entry has FCRN = 0 for KO mice or FCRN = 1 for WT mice. MAX is defined as $\mathrm{MAX}_0 \times$ FCRN, where MAX_0 is the MAX in FcRn WT mice. So MAX = 0 for KO mice, and $A_{6,0}/V_P$ and $A_{5,0}/V_C$ equations can be simplified as

$$\frac{A_{6,0}}{V_P} = \frac{k_{\mathrm{in}} \times Q}{Q \times \mathrm{CL} + \mathrm{CL}_U \times \mathrm{CL} + \mathrm{CL}_U \times Q}, \tag{A.4}$$

$$\frac{A_{5,0}}{V_C} = \frac{k_{\mathrm{in}} - \mathrm{CL}_U \times (A_{6,0}/V_P)}{\mathrm{CL}}. \tag{A.5}$$

Acknowledgment

The author is an employee of Genentech Inc. and has no conflict of interests to declare.

References

[1] F. W. R. Brambell, W. A. Hemmings, and I. G. Morris, "A theoretical model of γ-globulin catabolism," *Nature*, vol. 203, no. 4952, pp. 1352–1355, 1964.

[2] F. W. Brambell, "The transmission of immunity from mother to young and the catabolism of immunoglobulins.," *The Lancet*, vol. 2, no. 7473, pp. 1087–1093, 1966.

[3] T. A. Waldmann and W. Strober, "Metabolism of immunoglobulins," *Progress in Allergy*, vol. 13, pp. 1–110, 1969.

[4] R. P. Junghans and C. L. Anderson, "The protection receptor for IgG catabolism is the β2-microglobulin-containing neonatal intestinal transport receptor," *Proceedings of the National Academy of Sciences of the United States of America*, vol. 93, no. 11, pp. 5512–5516, 1996.

[5] J. Borvak, J. Richardson, C. Medesan et al., "Functional expression of the MHC class I-related receptor, FcRn, in endothelial cells of mice," *International Immunology*, vol. 10, no. 9, pp. 1289–1298, 1998.

[6] V. Ghetie, J. G. Hubbard, J. K. Kim, M. F. Tsen, Y. Lee, and E. S. Ward, "Abnormally short serum half-lives of IgG

in β2-microglobulin-deficient mice," *European Journal of Immunology*, vol. 26, no. 3, pp. 690–696, 1996.

[7] R. M. Campbell, D. P. Cuthbertson, C. M. Matthews, and A. S. McFarlane, "Behaviour of 14C- and 131I-labelled plasma proteins in the rat," *The International Journal of Applied Radiation and Isotopes*, vol. 1, no. 1-2, pp. 66–84, 1956.

[8] A. S. McFarlane, "The behavior of I 131-labeled plasma proteins in vivo," *Annals of the New York Academy of Sciences*, vol. 70, no. 1, pp. 19–25, 1957.

[9] T. S. Ramalingam, S. A. Detmer, W. L. Martin, and P. J. Bjorkman, "IgG transcytosis and recycling by FcRn expressed in MDCK cells reveals ligand-induced redistribution," *The EMBO Journal*, vol. 21, no. 4, pp. 590–601, 2002.

[10] E. J. Israel, D. F. Wilsker, K. C. Hayes, D. Schoenfeld, and N. E. Simister, "Increased clearance of IgG in mice that lack β2-microglobulin: possible protective role of FcRn," *Immunology*, vol. 89, no. 4, pp. 573–578, 1996.

[11] R. D. Wochner, G. Drews, W. Strober, and T. A. Waldmann, "Accelerated breakdown of immunoglobulin G (IgG) in myotonic dystrophy: a hereditary error of immunoglobulin catabolism.," *The Journal of Clinical Investigation*, vol. 45, no. 3, pp. 321–329, 1966.

[12] T. A. Waldmann and W. D. Terru, "Familial hypercatabolic hypoproteinemia. A disorder of endogenous catabolism of albumin and immunoglobulin," *The Journal of Clinical Investigation*, vol. 86, no. 6, pp. 2093–2098, 1990.

[13] J. Kim, W. L. Hayton, J. M. Robinson, and C. L. Anderson, "Kinetics of FcRn-mediated recycling of IgG and albumin in human: pathophysiology and therapeutic implications using a simplified mechanism-based model," *Clinical Immunology*, vol. 122, no. 2, pp. 146–155, 2007.

[14] B. Gurbaxani, "Mathematical modeling as accounting: predicting the fate of serum proteins and therapeutic monoclonal antibodies," *Clinical Immunology*, vol. 122, no. 2, pp. 121–124, 2007.

[15] P. Imbach, S. Barandun, V. d'Apuzzo et al., "High-dose intravenous gammaglobulin for idiopathic thrombocytopenic purpura in childhood," *The Lancet*, vol. 1, no. 8232, pp. 1228–1231, 1981.

[16] R. Deng and J. P. Balthasar, "Pharmacokinetic/pharmacodynamic modeling of IVIG effects in a murine model of immune thrombocytopenia," *Journal of Pharmaceutical Sciences*, vol. 96, no. 6, pp. 1625–1637, 2007.

[17] R. J. Hansen and J. P. Balthasar, "Pharmacokinetics, pharmacodynamics, and platelet binding of an anti-glycoprotein IIb/IIIa monoclonal antibody (7E3) in the rat: a quantitative rat model of immune thrombocytopenic purpura," *Journal of Pharmacology and Experimental Therapeutics*, vol. 298, no. 1, pp. 165–171, 2001.

[18] F. Jin and J. P. Balthasar, "Mechanisms of intravenous immunoglobulin action in immune thrombocytopenic purpura," *Human Immunology*, vol. 66, no. 4, pp. 403–410, 2005.

[19] J. J. Xiao, W. Krzyzanski, Y. M. Wang et al., "Pharmacokinetics of anti-hepcidin monoclonal antibody Ab 12B9m and hepcidin in cynomolgus monkeys," *AAPS Journal*, vol. 12, no. 4, pp. 646–657, 2010.

[20] G. Z. Ferl, A. M. Wu, and J. J. DiStefano, "A predictive model of therapeutic monoclonal antibody dynamics and regulation by the neonatal Fc receptor (FcRn)," *Annals of Biomedical Engineering*, vol. 33, no. 11, pp. 1640–1652, 2005.

[21] A. Garg and J. P. Balthasar, "Physiologically-based pharmacokinetic (PBPK) model to predict IgG tissue kinetics in wild-type and FcRn-knockout mice," *Journal of Pharmacokinetics and Pharmacodynamics*, vol. 34, no. 5, pp. 687–709, 2007.

[22] S. R. Urva, V. C. Yang, and J. P. Balthasar, "Physiologically based pharmacokinetic model for T84.66: a monoclonal anti-CEA antibody," *Journal of Pharmaceutical Sciences*, vol. 99, no. 3, pp. 1582–1600, 2010.

[23] J. P. Davda, M. Jain, S. K. Batra, P. R. Gwilt, and D. H. Robinson, "A physiologically based pharmacokinetic (PBPK) model to characterize and predict the disposition of monoclonal antibody CC49 and its single chain Fv constructs," *International Immunopharmacology*, vol. 8, no. 3, pp. 401–413, 2008.

[24] R. J. Hansen and J. P. Balthasar, "Pharmacokinetic/pharmacodynamic modeling of the effects of intravenous immunoglobulin on the disposition of antiplatelet antibodies in a rat model of immune thrombocytopenia," *Journal of Pharmaceutical Sciences*, vol. 92, no. 6, pp. 1206–1215, 2003.

[25] R. J. Hansen and J. P. Balthasar, "Effects of intravenous immunoglobulin on platelet count and antiplatelet antibody disposition in a rat model of immune thrombocytopenia," *Blood*, vol. 100, no. 6, pp. 2087–2093, 2002.

[26] C. R. Hopkins and I. S. Trowbridge, "Internalization and processing of transferrin and the transferrin receptor in human carcinoma A431 cells," *Journal of Cell Biology*, vol. 97, no. 2, pp. 508–521, 1983.

[27] R. J. Ober, C. Martinez, C. Vaccaro, J. Zhou, and E. S. Ward, "Visualizing the site and dynamics of IgG salvage by the MHC class I-related receptor, FcRn," *Journal of Immunology*, vol. 172, no. 4, pp. 2021–2029, 2004.

[28] W. K. Bleeker, J. L. Teeling, and C. Erik Hack, "Accelerated autoantibody clearance by intravenous immunoglobulin therapy: studies in experimental models to determine the magnitude and time course of the effect," *Blood*, vol. 98, no. 10, pp. 3136–3142, 2001.

[29] B. Davies and T. Morris, "Physiological parameters in laboratory animals and humans," *Pharmaceutical Research*, vol. 10, no. 7, pp. 1093–1095, 1993.

[30] S. F. Cure and N. E. Cremer, "Decreased rate of synthesis of immunoglobulin (IgG) in rats infected with moloney leukemia virus.," *Journal of Immunology*, vol. 102, no. 6, pp. 1345–1353, 1969.

[31] V. Ghetie, S. Popov, J. Borvak et al., "Increasing the serum persistence of an IgG fragment by random mutagenesis," *Nature Biotechnology*, vol. 15, no. 7, pp. 637–640, 1997.

[32] P. R. Hinton, M. G. Johlfs, J. M. Xiong et al., "Engineered human IgG antibodies with longer serum half-lives in primates," *The Journal of Biological Chemistry*, vol. 279, no. 8, pp. 6213–6216, 2004.

[33] B. Gurbaxani, L. L. Dela Cruz, K. Chintalacharuvu, and S. L. Morrison, "Analysis of a family of antibodies with different half-lives in mice fails to find a correlation between affinity for FcRn and serum half-life," *Molecular Immunology*, vol. 43, no. 9, pp. 1462–1473, 2006.

[34] R. P. Junghans, "IgG biosynthesis: no 'immunoregulatory feedback'," *Blood*, vol. 90, no. 10, pp. 3815–3818, 1997.

20

In Vivo Clearance of Alpha-1 Acid Glycoprotein Is Influenced by the Extent of Its N-Linked Glycosylation and by Its Interaction with the Vessel Wall

Teresa R. McCurdy,[1,2,3] Varsha Bhakta,[2] Louise J. Eltringham-Smith,[1] Sharon Gataiance,[1] Alison E. Fox-Robichaud,[4] and William P. Sheffield[1,2]

[1] *Department of Pathology and Molecular Medicine, McMaster University, Hamilton, ON, Canada L8N 3Z5*
[2] *Canadian Blood Services, Research and Development, Hamilton, ON, Canada L8N 3Z5*
[3] *School of Nursing, McMaster University, Hamilton, ON, Canada L8N 3Z5*
[4] *Department of Medicine, McMaster University, Hamilton, ON, Canada L8N 3Z5*

Correspondence should be addressed to William P. Sheffield, sheffiel@mcmaster.ca

Academic Editor: Saulius Butenas

Alpha-1 acid glycoprotein (AGP) is a highly glycosylated plasma protein that exerts vasoprotective effects. We hypothesized that AGP's N-linked glycans govern its rate of clearance from the circulation, and followed the disappearance of different forms of radiolabeled human AGP from the plasma of rabbits and mice. Enzymatic deglycosylation of human plasma-derived AGP (pdAGP) by Peptide: N-Glycosidase F yielded a mixture of differentially deglycosylated forms (PNGase-AGP), while the introduction of five Asn to Gln mutations in recombinant *Pichia pastoris*-derived AGP (rAGP-N(5)Q) eliminated N-linked glycosylation. PNGase-AGP was cleared from the rabbit circulation 9-fold, and rAGP-N(5)Q, 46-fold more rapidly than pdAGP, primarily via a renal route. *Pichia pastoris*-derived wild-type rAGP differed from pdAGP in expressing mannose-terminated glycans, and, like neuraminidase-treated pdAGP, was more rapidly removed from the rabbit circulation than rAGP-N(5)Q. Systemic hyaluronidase treatment of mice transiently decreased pdAGP clearance. AGP administration to mice reduced vascular binding of hyaluronic acid binding protein in the liver microcirculation and increased its plasma levels. Our results support a critical role of N-linked glycosylation of AGP in regulating its *in vivo* clearance and an influence of a hyaluronidase-sensitive component of the vessel wall on its transendothelial passage.

1. Introduction

Alpha-1 acid glycoprotein (AGP; also known as orosomucoid) is a 44 kDa, heavily glycosylated protein synthesized primarily by hepatocytes and secreted into the plasma, where it circulates under normal conditions in humans at 8–30 μM [1, 2]. During the acute phase response, circulating levels of human AGP are elevated over baseline values by 2- to 7-fold [3]; in rats, rabbits, and mice, the elevation of either circulating AGP or hepatic AGP mRNA ranges from 10- to 200-fold [4–8]. The biological function of AGP is unclear. Suggested roles for this plasma protein include the modulation of the immune response [9]; the stabilization of plasminogen activator inhibitor-1 (PAI-1) functional activity [10]; and the maintenance of normal capillary permeability and selectivity [11].

Evidence from perfusion or cell culture systems supports a role for AGP in maintaining capillary permselectivity. Perfusion studies using isolated rat skeletal muscle [12] or kidneys [13] or frog mesenteric preparations [14] initially showed that the rate of negatively charged protein loss from the perfusate (e.g., albumin or lactalbumin) was reduced in the presence of AGP. These findings lead to the hypothesis that AGP binds to the capillary vessel wall and increases its negative charge [14]. AGP binding to endothelial cells in culture has also been demonstrated [15–17]. The protein has furthermore been suggested to form part of the glycocalyx, a dynamic endothelial surface layer of glycosaminoglycans, proteoglycans, and adsorbed plasma proteins deduced by indirect examination, for instance as a red cell exclusion zone in intravital microscopy [18]. Most recently, transfused human AGP was shown to exert renal effects by restoring normal glomerular filtration rates in rats rendered nephrotic by puromycin aminoglycoside administration [19].

It has long been known that enzymatic removal of terminal sialic acid residues, and exposure of terminal galactose moieties, converts AGP into a high-affinity ligand of the asialoglycoprotein receptor, leading to its rapid removal from the mammalian circulation [20–23]. Relatively few studies, however, have examined the *in vivo* clearance of the unmodified plasma glycoprotein [24–26], and none have examined the consequences of complete removal of glycans on the clearance and catabolism of AGP. Since AGP is a relatively small protein of approximately 43 kDa, with 45% of its mass being contributed by its carbohydrates, we hypothesized that removal of its sugars would render it filterable in the kidneys and accelerate its clearance from the circulation[27]. In the current study, we tested this hypothesis and in addition investigated the consequences to AGP clearance of systemic disruption of the glycocalyx.

2. Materials and Methods

2.1. Materials. Affi-Gel Blue chromatography resin and Bio-Gel HT hydroxyapatite resin were purchased from Bio-Rad Laboratories (Hercules, CA). Concanavalin A (Con A), Sepharose 4B, and T4 DNA ligase were from GE Healthcare (Piscataway, NJ). Reverse transcription reagents RNEasy and Sensiscript RT kits and heat-stable HotStarTaq DNA polymerase were from Qiagen (Chatsworth, CA). Neuraminidase, peptide N-glycosidase : F (PNGase F), and Phusion heat-stable DNA polymerase were purchased from New England BioLabs (Ipswich, MA). *Streptomyces* hyaluronidase, commercial AGP, goat antihuman AGP antibodies, and alkaline phosphatase conjugated anti-goat IgG were from Sigma (St. Louis, MO). A Glycan Differentiation kit was purchased from Roche Applied Science (Mannheim, Germany). Biotinylated hyaluronic acid binding protein was from Associates of Cape Cod (East Falmouth, MA). Alexa Fluor 488 labeling kits, streptavidin conjugated Alexa Fluor 647, Alexa Fluor 488-*Griffonia simplicifolia* lectin-1B_4(GS-1B_4), *Pichia pastoris* strain X-33 and Zeocin, ThermalAce high fidelity DNA polymerase, the pcDNA 3.1 vector, and *E. coli* DH5α cells were all purchased from Invitrogen Corporation (Carlsbad, CA). Restriction and DNA modification enzymes were supplied by either Fermentas Life Sciences (Burlington, ON), or Fisher Scientific (Unionville, ON). HepG2 (human hepatocellular carcinoma) cells were obtained from the American Type Culture Collection (Manassas, VA). $Na^{125}I$ for radioiodination was from Perkin Elmer Life Sciences (Boston, MA).

2.2. Experimental Animals. Experiments involving animals were carried out under the terms of Animal Utilization Protocols approved by the Animal Research Ethics Board of the Faculty of Health Sciences of McMaster University. Rabbits (New Zealand White, 2.1 to 2.8 kg, male and female, specific pathogen-free) were purchased from Charles River (St. Constant, Quebec), as were C57 Black 6 (C57Bl/6) male mice of 20–30 g body weight.

2.3. Purification of AGP from Human Plasma. AGP was purified exactly as described by Hervé et al. [28] from citrated plasma obtained from healthy volunteer donors, collected with informed consent using a protocol approved by the Hamilton Health Sciences Research Ethics Board. The plasma pool was combined, using equal volumes from each donor, aliquoted and frozen at −80°C until use; the same five donors (4 Caucasian, 1 Black) were used for all preparations employed in this study.

2.4. Enzymatic Modification of AGP. The terminal sialic acid chains of purified AGP were removed by treatment with *Clostridium perfringens* neuraminidase, using 5 units of enzyme per μg of AGP in 50 mM sodium citrate, pH 6.0, overnight at 37°C. Entire N-linked glycan chains were removed from AGP using Peptide: N-Glycosidase F (PNGase F). For electrophoretic use, AGP (0.02 mg) was denatured by boiling in 0.5% SDS, 80 mM dithiothreitol for ten minutes, then reacted with 2500 units PNGase F at 37° for one hour, after dilution into 1% NP-40, 50 mM sodium phosphate pH 7.5. For radiolabeling and *in vivo* use, 0.2 mg AGP in 5.0 M urea was incubated for one hour at room temperature, then diluted 1 : 1 with 10,000 units of PNGase F in 0.1 M sodium phosphate pH 7.5, and incubated overnight at 37°C, prior to dialysis against phosphate buffered saline.

2.5. DNA Manipulations. A human AGP cDNA was obtained by reverse transcription/PCR of HepG2 cell mRNA, employing RNEasy and Sensiscript RT kits (Qiagen) and oligonucleotide primers ML13047 (5′-GAATGGATCCAAGGT-GACTGCACCCTGC-3′) and ML13048 (5′-ATCGAATTCG GTACACATGT CGGGTTGG-3′). The product was subcloned into pUC19, yielding plasmid pUC19-AGP. The latter plasmid was amplified using Phusion polymerase under conditions recommended by the manufacturer (New England Biolabs), and sense oligonucleotide primer 07-1495 (5′ ACGTCTCGAGAAAAGACAGATCCCATTGTGTGC-CAACC-3′) and antisense oligonucleotide primer 07-1493 (5′ CAGTGAATTC CTAGTGATGG TGATGGGATTCCCC-CTCCTC CTGTTT-3′). The resulting PCR product was restricted with XhoI and EcoRI and inserted between these sites in yeast expression vector pPICZ9ssamp [29] to form pPICZ9ssAGPH6. This plasmid was modified by PCR in site-directed mutagenesis reactions that altered 5 Asn (N) codons 15, 38, 54, 75, and 85 to Gln (Q), forming pPIC-Z9ssAGP-N(5)Q-H6. All DNA constructs were verified by DNA sequencing (MOBIX, McMaster University) prior to expression and utilization of recombinant AGP.

2.6. Expression and Purification of Recombinant AGP. Plasmids pPICZ9ssAGPH6 and pPICZ9ssAGP-N(5)Q-H6 were separately used to transform *Pichia pastoris* X33 yeast to Zeocin resistance, and resulting cell lines were cultured and induced with methanol; conditioned media was neutralized and secreted recombinant proteins were purified by nickel affinity chromatography, as previously described [30].

2.7. In Vivo Clearance of AGP in Rabbits. Purified plasma-derived, enzymatically treated, or recombinant forms of AGP were iodinated using the Iodogen method [31] and injected into the marginal ear vein of rabbits, as previously described [32]. At timed intervals (0.083, 0.5, 1, 2, 4, 6, 8, 24, 48, 72, 96, and 168 hours or until the recovered radioactivity declined lower than 0.1% of the injected dose) blood samples were taken from the marginal vein of the other ear, centrifuged to obtain plasma, and the trichloroacetic acid-precipitable radioactivity was determined by γ counting. For each rabbit, semilogarithmic substrate disposition graphs of residual plasma radioactivity against time were generated, and analyzed using PK Solutions version 2.0 software (Summit Research Services, Montrose, CO, USA). Briefly, the software was employed to fit the data using noncompartmental (area) methods based on the trapezoid rule. For this purpose, radioactive doses were converted into pmoles using the measured specific activity of radiolabeling, and molecular weights of 43, 33, and 23 kDa for pdAGP, PNGase-AGP, and rAGP N(5)Q, respectively. The specific activity of radiolabeling was similar for all three proteins, ranging from 3.94 to 7.05 X 10^6cpm/μg. In some experiments, the tissue distribution of radioactivity 30 minutes after intravenous injection of radioiodinated AGP or derivatives was measured as described [33]; briefly, organs were excised, rinsed in ice cold saline, weighed, and either a portion or the entire organ, depending on its size, was γ counted. Results were expressed as a fraction of the total radioactive dose injected. In other experiments, either 4.0 g of α-methyl-D-mannopyranoside (α-methyl-mannoside) in 20 mL sterile saline, or 0.54 g of D-galactose in 10 mL sterile saline, was injected intraperitoneally immediately prior to intravenous injection of radioiodinated protein in an effort to block glycan-dependent uptake via hepatic receptors.

2.8. In Vivo AGP Clearance in Mice. Clearance of radiolabeled human AGP in C57Bl/6 mice was followed as previously described [30, 34] by measuring acid-precipitable plasma radioactivity in plasma samples. Plasma radioactivity was reported as percentage of the injected dose, using as a dilution factor the plasma volume divided by the sample volume. Plasma volume was calculated as the product of the weight of the mouse in grams X 0.078 mL blood volume per gram body weight X (1-the hematocrit), using a hematocrit of 0.44 (US NIH reference values from http://oacu.od.nih.gov/ARAC/). In some experiments the mice were treated with *Streptomyces* hyaluronidase (Sigma-Aldrich, St. Louis, MO, USA) by intravenous injection of 47 U (to deliver 30 U/mL estimated plasma volume) of the enzyme in 0.1 mL sterile saline coinjected with iodinated human AGP.

2.9. Intravital Microscopy. Anesthetized mice (20–30 g body weight) were cannulated via the right jugular vein, the abdomen opened, and a lobe of the liver placed on the heated Plexiglas stage of a Leica DMI 6000 B confocal microscope. The liver microvasculature was photographed using a Hamamatsu C9100-12 back-thinned EMCCD camera attached to a Leica DMI 6000 B confocal microscope using the 63X objective. Either 15 μg biotinylated bovine hyaluronic acid binding protein (bHABP) complexed to streptavidin-conjugated Alexa Fluor 647 (Associates of Cape Cod, Falmouth, MA, USA) or 40 μg *Griffonia simplicifolia* $1B_4$ (GS-$1B_4$,) lectin directly conjugated to Alexa Fluor 488 (Invitrogen, Carlsbad, CA, USA) was injected through the cannula into the vasculature. Baseline images were obtained over the next 15 minutes, then hyaluronidase was injected as described above, and images were acquired for an additional hour. In some experiments purified human AGP (165 mg/kg body weight) was injected after bHABP:streptavidin Alexa Fluor 647 administration and baseline image capture and 15 minutes prior to hyaluronidase treatment. Fluorescent intensity was quantified using ImageJ software (http://rsb.info.nih.gov/ij/).

2.10. Ligand Blotting. The ability of various forms of AGP to react with digoxigenin-labeled lectins was assessed following SDS-PAGE and electrical transfer of proteins to nitrocellulose; blots were analyzed using a DIG Glycan Differentiation Kit as suggested by the manufacturer (Roche Diagnostics, Mississauga, ON, Canada).

2.11. Statistical Analysis. Data are reported as the mean ± the standard deviation in all cases. Statistical analysis was performed using GraphPad Instat version 3.06 software (GraphPad Software Inc, San Diego, CA), using one-way Analysis of Variance (ANOVA) for multiple comparisons and Student's *t*-tests for paired comparisons. Nonparametric methods were employed if data did not pass tests of normality and equivalence of standard deviation; further details are provided in Figures 1–6 and Table 1.

3. Results

The *in vivo* clearance of AGP treated with neuraminidase to remove the terminal sialic acid residues has been widely investigated, to a greater extent than that of the unmodified protein [21, 24, 35, 36]. We first ensured that our purified AGP behaved as expected following this enzymatic modification. As shown in Figure 1(a), neuraminidase treatment increased the electrophoretic mobility of AGP and eliminated its recognition by *Sambucus nigra* agglutinin (SNA), which binds to sialic acid linked to galactose. Five minutes after injection, 45.5 ± 4.0% of the injected AGP was detected in plasma, compared to 0.77 ± 0.36% of neuraminidase-treated AGP, a difference of 82-fold. By fifteen minutes, the proportion of AGP remaining in the circulation was unchanged for native AGP (42.0 ± 5.5%) but had further declined to 0.25 ± 0.5% in the case of the neuraminidase-treated form (Figure 1(b)).

Enzymatic and recombinant DNA methods were used to reduce or eliminate the number of N-linked glycan chains

Table 1: Pharmacokinetic parameters relating to AGP clearance in rabbits.

	Form of AGP		
	pdAGP	PNGase-AGP (PNGase-treated)	rAGP N(5)Q
Area under the curve (AUC 0-∞) (in pmol-hr/mL)	11 ± 1	5.8 ± 0.9	0.74 ± 0.07***
Mean residence time (MRT; in hr)	73 ± 6	57 ± 3	23 ± 6***
Volume of distribution (V_{diss}; in mL/kg)	190 ± 20	700 ± 100***	6000 ± 1000***
Steady state volume of distribution (V_{ss}; in mL/kg)	160 ± 20	550 ± 90***	2000 ± 500***
Clearance (CL; mL/hr/kg)	2.23 ± 0.03	11 ± 2***	100 ± 10***
Half-life calculated from V_{diss} and CL (hours)	58 ± 4	50 ± 3	42 ± 9**

The mean ± the standard deviation is shown ($n = 6$). Derivatives of AGP were compared to the corresponding AGP value using one-way ANOVA with Tukey's post-test; **indicates $P < 0.01$, ***indicates $P < 0.001$.

attached to AGP. Denaturation of AGP was required to obtain any significant reduction in its extent of glycosylation using PNGase F, which removes glycan chains in their entirety at their point of attachment to asparagine residues on the polypeptide backbone of AGP. Enzymatic deglycosylation following denaturation of AGP with urea or SDS was compared. As shown in Figure 2, transient denaturation with urea allowed the partial removal of 0–5 glycans per AGP molecule; full denaturation with SDS removed all glycans. That the most rapidly migrating PNGase F reaction product of AGP was fully deglycosylated was indicated by its comigration both with SDS and PNGase F-treated AGP, and with a form of recombinant AGP mutated to abrogate N-linked glycosylation (rAGP N(5)Q) (Figure 1(a)), and by the loss of recognition of all of these putatively deglycosylated species with SNA lectin (data not shown). In keeping with its intermediate state of deglycosylation, PNGase F-treated AGP exhibited more rapid clearance in rabbits than unmodified AGP, but was retained in the circulation to a greater extent than rAGP N(5)Q; these differences were apparent as early as 30 minutes after injection (Figure 2(b)). Electrophoresis and autoradiography of postinjection plasma samples revealed that the most rapidly migrating deglycosylated forms of AGP (e.g., "1" versus "2" in Figure 3(b)) were lost from plasma more rapidly than less rapidly migrating forms (e.g., "3" or "4" in Figure 3(b)). In terms of organ distribution, both PNGase F-treated AGP and rAGP N(5)Q were found in the kidney to a greater extent than native AGP, the effect being more pronounced for the fully deglycosylated form (Figure 3(d)).

The differences in clearance of the three forms of AGP were apparent not only on substrate disposition versus time graphs, such as those shown in Figure 2, in which the proteins were compared on the basis of residual radioactivity, but also following pharmacokinetic analysis, in which the proteins were compared based upon their dose in pmoles and their residual plasma concentration in pmol/mL (Table 1). PNGase-AGP and rAGP N(5)Q exhibited decreased areas under the clearance curve, decreased mean retention times, and decreased half-lives, but the decreases were only statistically significant for rAGP N(5)Q. The volumes of distribution and clearance rates were significantly increased for both altered forms (e.g., mean CL was increased 4.9-fold for PNGase-AGP and 45-fold for rAGP N(5)Q, $P < 0.001$ versus pdAGP in both cases).

We produced recombinant nonglycosylated AGP N(5)Q in a *Pichia pastoris* yeast expression system [29]. The disappearance of injected radiolabeled rAGP-WT from the rabbit circulation, which like rAGP-N(5)Q, was C-terminally hexahistidinylated to facilitate purification, but which unlike the mutated AGP, retained all five sites of N-linked glycosylation, was also examined. As shown in Figure 4(a), rAGP-WT was much more rapidly removed from the circulation than its mutant rAGP-N(5)Q counterpart. Thirty minutes after injection of equal doses of either radiolabeled rAGP-WT or rAGP N(5)Q, the residual plasma concentration of the latter exceeded the former by more than 10-fold (Figure 4(a); 2.2 ± 0.5% versus 26 ± 3%, $P < 0.0001$ by unpaired t-test, Welch corrected). Coadministration of α-methylmannoside, but not galactose, significantly reduced the loss of rAGP-WT from the circulation (to 6 ± 1%, $P < 0.05$ by Kruskal-Wallis test); neither sugar significantly altered the concentration of rAGP N(5)Q in the circulation, suggesting that the yeast glycans contained terminal mannose residues (Figure 4(a)). Electrophoresis showed that rAGP-WT migrated more rapidly than pdAGP, consistent with its modification with shorter N-linked glycans than in plasma-derived AGP (Figure 4(b)), and ligand blotting showed that rAGP-WT, but not plasma-derived human AGP, bound *Galanthus nivalis* agglutinin (GNA), which is a lectin specific for glycans terminating in mannose residues (Figure 4(b)). In contrast, rAGP-N(5)Q was unreactive with all lectins, consistent with its intended lack of glycosylation (data not shown).

Intravenous administration of hyaluronidase prior to injection of radiolabeled AGP changed both its recovery and distribution in mice for several hours after treatment. Initially, the recovery of AGP rose from 80.2 ± 5.8 in the absence of hyaluronidase to 96.8 ± 6.0 ($P = 0.0007$ by two-tailed unpaired t-test); as seen in Figure 5, the elevation of AGP in the plasma in hyaluronidase-treated mice remained detectable until 3 hours after treatment. The area under the observed curve ($t = 0$ to $t = 6$ hours) was increased from 250 ± 30%-hr to 300 ± 30%-hr ($P = 0.037$ by two-tailed unpaired t-test) by hyaluronidase treatment. We next sought independent confirmation that hyaluronidase was having its intended effect on the murine vasculature, using intravital confocal microscopy of livers of mice treated with or without hyaluronidase. Treatment with the enzyme reduced sinusoidal vessel staining with fluorescently labeled HABP but left vascular binding by fluorescent GS-1B_4 unchanged (Figure 6,

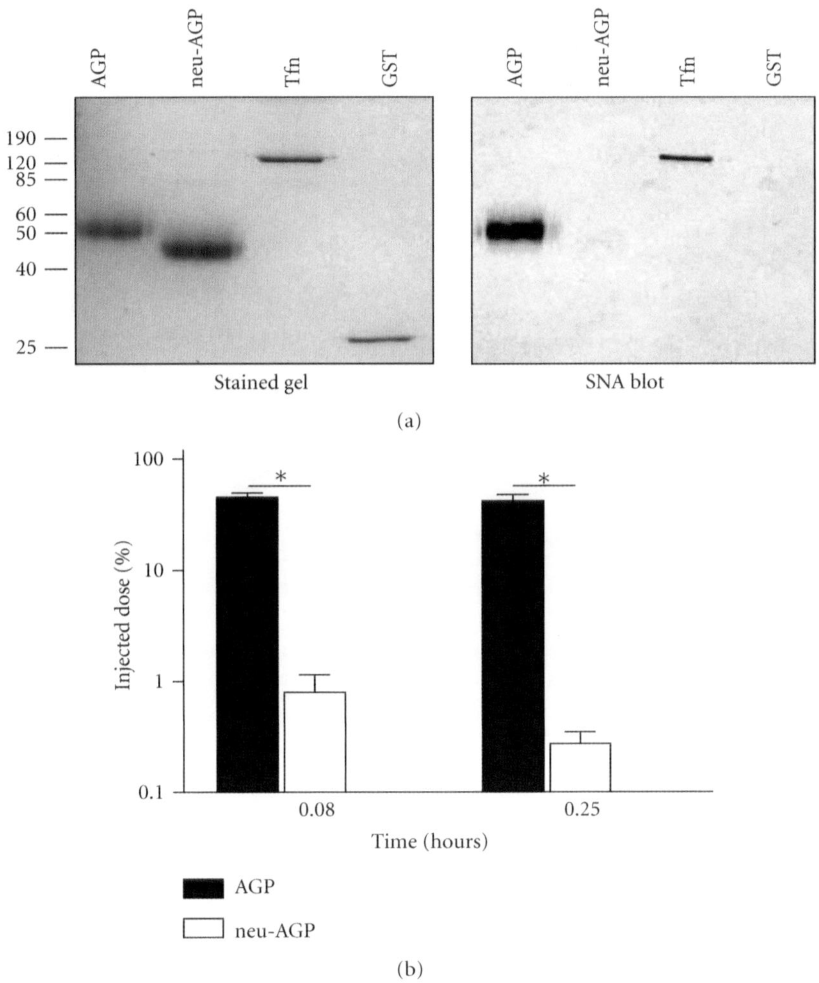

FIGURE 1: Neuraminidase treatment of human AGP increases its clearance from the rabbit circulation. Plasma-derived AGP with (neu-AGP) or without (AGP) neuraminidase treatment was examined on a 12% SDS reducing gel, either by Coomassie Blue staining ((a), left, stained gel) or by ligand blotting with SNA ((a), right, SNA blot). The position of molecular mass markers is shown in kDa, at left. Tfn: transferrin; GST: glutathione sulfotransferase. (b) Shows the recovery (% injected dose) of acid-precipitable radioactivity in plasma at different times following injection of radioiodinated AGP (solid bar) or neu-AGP (open bar) into rabbits. *Indicates $P < 0.05$ versus corresponding AGP value by unpaired t-test, Welch corrected. The mean of 7 determinations ± SD is shown.

compare (a) to (b) and (d) to (e)). The distribution of HABP was also altered by administration of 3.3 mg intravenous human AGP (10-20 times endogenous AGP levels) without hyaluronidase treatment. This intervention left 5- to 6-fold more HABP in the plasma column than in the absence of AGP treatment (Figures 6(c) and 6(f)). Although hyaluronidase treatment altered the clearance and distribution of AGP, and AGP injection increased HABP retention in plasma, AGP did not bind to immobilized hyaluronan *in vitro* in microtiter plates, unlike HABP, which demonstrated avid binding (data not shown).

4. Discussion

In this study we explored the effects of altered, diminished, or absent glycosylation of AGP on its *in vivo* clearance. Although neuraminidase-treated AGP (also called asialoAGP or asialoorosomucoid) has been widely employed for many years as an injectable ligand and competitor for the hepatic asialoglycoprotein receptor *in vivo* [21, 24, 35, 36], the clearance of glycosylated AGP has been less extensively examined. Regoeczi et al. [24] reported a terminal catabolic half-life of 68.5 hours for iodinated human AGP injected into a single 3.8 kg rabbit; this value is similar to our finding of 59 ± 4 hours (mean ± SD, $n = 6$, range 53–65 hours, weight range 2.52–2.79 kg). Some of the difference may derive from our use of noncompartmental modeling and pharmacokinetic software, as opposed to the compartmental model and manual calculation employed in the older report; alternatively, our use of lighter rabbits may also be a contributing factor. In this regard, others employing noncompartmental analysis of AGP clearance in rats reported steady state weight-adjusted volumes of distribution similar to that observed in rabbits in this study. For pdAGP in rabbits, we observed 160 ± 20 mL/kg, while others reported 150 mL/kg [37] and 90 ± 30 mL/kg [26]. Taken together, these comparisons suggest

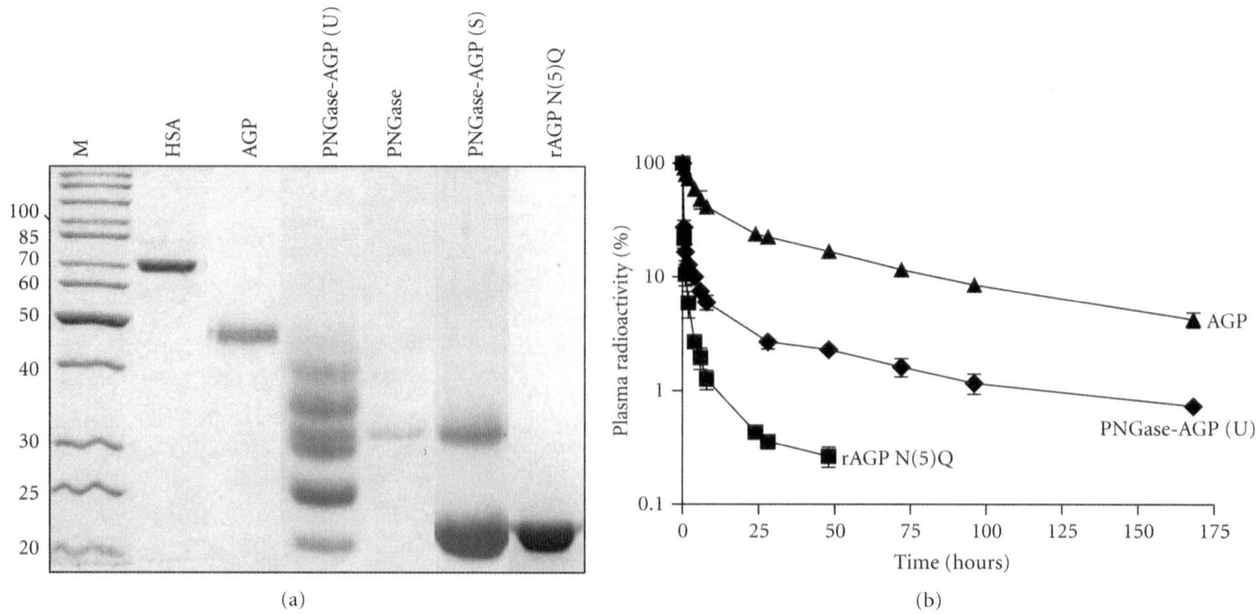

Figure 2: Forms of AGP with reduced or absent N-linked glycosylation are cleared from the rabbit circulation more rapidly than native AGP following intravenous injection. (a) Shows a Coomassie blue-stained 12% SDS reducing gel loaded with 5–10 μg per lane of human serum albumin, HSA; AGP; AGP treated with PNGase F (PNGase) in the presence of either urea (PNGase-AGP (U) or SDS (PNGase-AGP (S); or recombinant yeast-derived nonglycosylated AGP (rAGP N(5)Q). (b) Depicts the residual acid-precipitable radioactivity remaining in the plasma of rabbits after intravenous injection of the indicated radiolabeled proteins as a function of time; for each protein, plasma radioactivity is presented as the percentage of the injected radioactive dose recovered in plasma at the indicated time after injection. Each point is the mean ± SD of 6 determinations; in most instances error bars are smaller than the symbol that denotes the mean.

that our clearance findings with respect to pdAGP are reasonable in light of previous reports in the literature and form a sound basis for comparison to the novel deglycosylated forms of AGP that we generated.

We used two strategies to reduce or eliminate entire N-linked glycans from AGP: enzymatic treatment with PNGase F, or mutation of the five asparagine residues to which the glycans are ordinarily attached. The enzymatic strategy was complicated by the resistance of AGP to deglycosylation in the absence of treatment with SDS. We elected to employ urea, since it could be removed by dialysis, promoting refolding, as opposed to SDS, which binds tightly to proteins and cannot readily be removed. PNGase F treatment was only partially effective in altering AGP clearance, likely due to the presence of some unaltered, multiply glycosylated AGP in the mixture; however, the least glycosylated forms of AGP in that mixture were most rapidly removed from the circulation. A more convincing difference between native AGP and nonglycosylated AGP was achieved via the mutational strategy; nonglycosylated rAGP-N(5)Q exhibited a 15-fold decrease in area under the clearance curve (extrapolated to infinity) and a 45-fold increase in clearance rate compared to plasma-derived AGP. Although it was not possible to control the rAGP-N(5)Q experiments with wild-type recombinant AGP made in the same experimental system, due to the high mannose-type glycosylation typical of yeast, our results were consistent with previous data. These data were obtained by investigators who employed metabolic labeling of rat hepatocytes in the presence of an inhibitor of N-linked glycosylation (tunicamycin) and immunoaffinity purification to obtain nonglycosylated rat AGP [38]. Although the difficulty in obtaining radiolabeled AGP by this route prevented replication and kinetic analysis in this study, the 50% dose retention time was noted to decrease from 100 minutes to 5 minutes for nonglycosylated AGP, as compared with native AGP, consistent with our findings, as was increased renal clearance of nonglycosylated AGP [39].

Having shown that appropriately terminated N-linked glycans keep AGP from exhibiting accelerated clearance either via glomerular filtration or via hepatic receptors specific for abnormal glycosylation, we turned to the issue of AGP interaction with the vessel wall. Intravenous administration of hyaluronidase to hamsters led to a decrease in the FITC-Dextran 70 permeation zone defined using intravital microscopy [40], one consistent with degradation of the glycocalyx, a surface layer of glycosaminoglycans, proteoglycans, and adsorbed plasma proteins [18, 41] thought to contain AGP [42, 43]. While hyaluronidase treatment of rabbits would have been ideal in the context of this study, we found such treatment impractical in this larger laboratory animal. In mice, we found that hyaluronidase treatment decreased the initial clearance of AGP, an effect consistent with an AGP-glycocalyx action as a normal part of its distribution. Hyaluronidase treatment appeared to be specific in that HABP binding to liver sinusoidal vessels was reduced, but that of GS-1B_4, an α-galactose-specific lectin that mainly binds to animal endothelial cells [44], was unaffected. AGP administration also increased the amount of HABP found in the plasma column within liver sinusoids. This increase could have occurred due to AGP binding to hyaluronan in

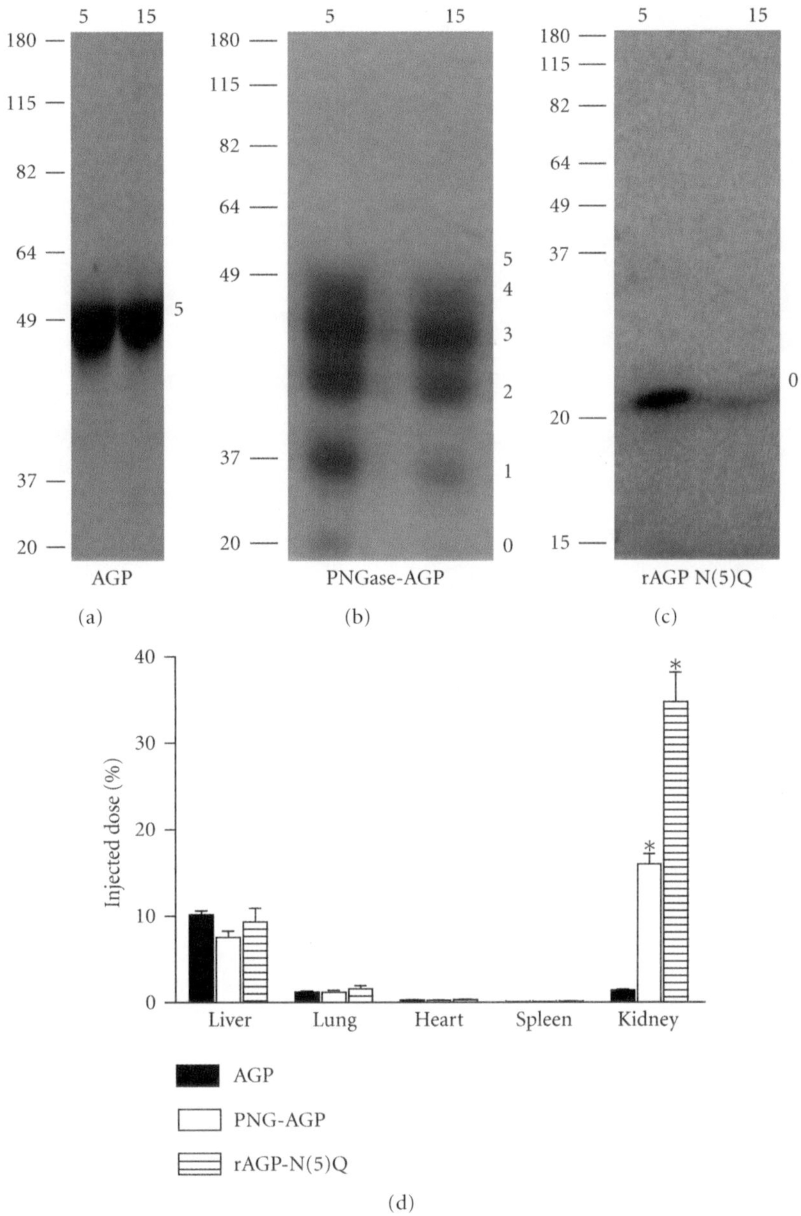

FIGURE 3: Forms of AGP with reduced glycosylation are cleared from the rabbit circulation and distribute to the kidneys more rapidly than native AGP. Plasma from rabbit injected with radioiodinated proteins (identified below (a)–(c)) was electrophoresed on reduced SDS-PAGE gels; autoradiograms of samples taken 5 and 15 minutes after injection are shown. Molecular mass markers in kDa are shown at left, and the deduced number of N-linked glycan chains at right. (d) Shows the percentage of the total radioactive dose of injected radioactivity found in the organs (identified below the panels) 30 minutes after injection of AGP (solid bars) or PNGase F-treated AGP (PNGase-AGP, open bars) or rAGP-N(5)Q (stippled bars). The mean of 6 determinations ± SD is shown. *Indicates $P < 0.001$ versus AGP value for the other two proteins within each organ sampled; all other comparisons to AGP values within organs are not significant.

the glycocalyx, or its binding to a component of the glycocalyx that affected the access of HABP to hyaluronan. We favour the second explanation because we were unable to detect AGP-hyaluronan binding *in vitro*; nevertheless, we cannot exclude the possibility that this interaction occurs *in vivo*. Although our primary reason for examining the liver microcirculation was technical in that this organ is amenable to intravital microscopy [45], it has also been shown that this microcirculatory bed is greatly enriched in hyaluronan as opposed, for instance, to those of lung or heart [46]. Our results support the suggestion that AGP is a component of the glycocalyx, as previously suggested [17, 42, 47, 48].

From a biotechnological point of view, our results also provide novel information with respect to targeting of recombinant AGP to either renal or hepatic destinations. AGP is a member of a protein family known as the lipocalins [49]. Lipocalins bind many drugs and metabolites within a central binding pocket of the polypeptide. Interestingly,

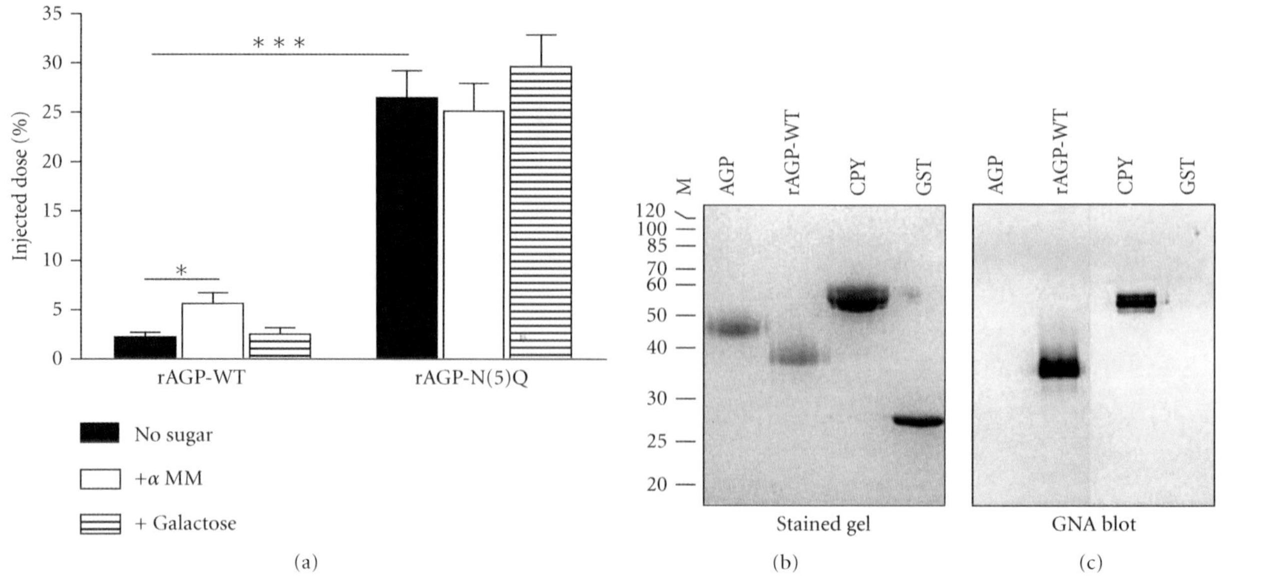

FIGURE 4: Recombinant AGP glycosylated in *Pichia pastoris* yeast is rapidly removed from the rabbit circulation via mannose receptors. (a) Shows the radioiodinated rAGP-WT or rAGP N(5)Q remaining in the plasma of rabbits 30 minutes after injection, without (no sugar) or with coadministered α-methylmannoside (+α MM) or D-galactose (+ Galactose). The mean and SD of 5–7 determinations are shown; *indicates $P < 0.05$ versus the corresponding "no sugar" condition by Kruskal-Wallis test. The proportion of the two proteins remaining in plasma in the absence of added sugar was also compared; ***indicates $P < 0.001$ by unpaired t-test, Welch corrected. (b) (Gel) shows a Coomassie blue-stained 12% SDS reducing gel loaded with 5–10 μg per lane of AGP (plasma-derived); rAGP-WT; carboxypeptidase Y (CPY); and glutathione sulfotransferase (GST). Molecular mass marker positions, shown at left, correspond to: 100; 90; 80; 70; 60; 50; 40; 30; 25; and 20 kDa. (c) (GNA blot) is a blotted replicate of the gel shown in (b), probed with GNA lectin.

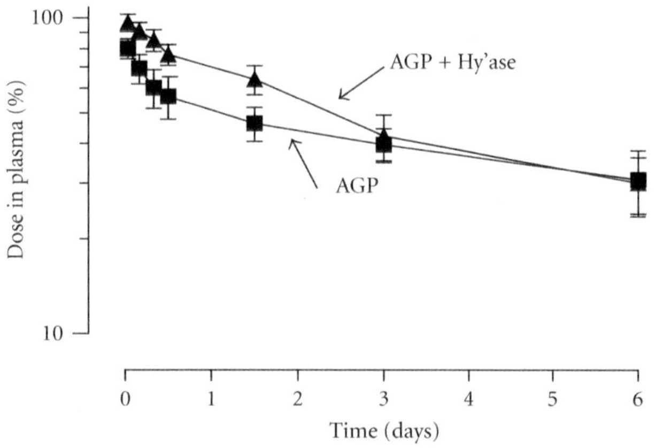

FIGURE 5: The disappearance of injected AGP from the plasma of mice following intravenous injection is altered by systemic hyaluronidase treatment. Radioiodinated AGP was injected into mice with (AGP + hy'ase) or without (AGP) concurrent hyaluronidase treatment, and acid-precipitable radioactivity, shown as the percentage of the dose remaining in plasma, was followed over time, $n = 6 \pm$SD.

in this regard lipocalin libraries have been described with engineered binding properties [50]. Our biological distribution results raise the possibility that engineered AGPs with defined ligand binding specificities could be directed to renal or hepatic destinations using either the N(5)Q mutant, or mannosylated rAGP-WT produced in yeast. In the latter instance, producing AGP (e.g., for conjugation to DNA, as has been previously reported for gene targeting [51, 52]) or an AGP fusion protein in *Pichia pastoris* could provide hepatic targeting in a single step, without the need for neuraminidase treatment.

This study had several limitations. It would have been preferable to use homologous rabbit AGP or murine AGP in rabbits and mice, respectively, but our efforts to isolate rabbit AGP by adapting a protocol designed for the purification of rat AGP [53] were not successful, and it was impractical to purify sufficient quantities of murine AGP from murine plasma for our purposes. Our study was also limited to human AGP purified from the plasma of healthy individuals, and clearance was similarly investigated in healthy animals. As such, our results do not address the possibility that AGP glycosylation or clearance properties are altered during inflammation, as has been suggested [54–56]. Our use of plasma purified from a small pool of healthy donors to purify AGP was aligned with the concept that this material might be a future therapeutic product of plasma fractionation [57, 58].

Our results show that N-linked glycosylation of AGP is a critical contributor to its plasma residency, in that reducing the number of glycans accelerated clearance; this was most clearly demonstrated for a mutant AGP completely lacking N-linked glycans. In this regard, AGP resembles antithrombin, in which mutation of any one of four sites of N-linked glycosylation has been shown to lead to accelerated clearance *in vivo* in rabbits [59], but not albumin, in which either naturally occurring [60] or engineered sites of N-linked glycosylation accelerate the clearance of the plasma protein [33].

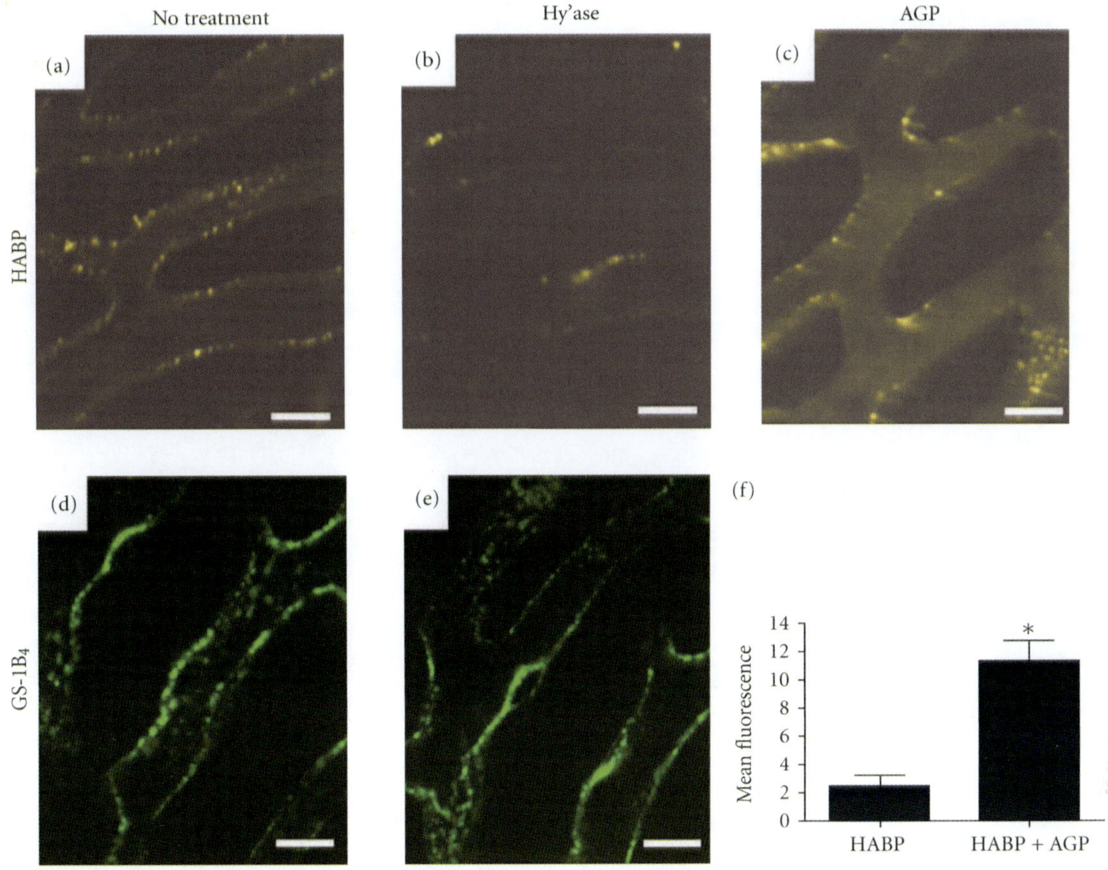

FIGURE 6: Either systemic hyaluronidase treatment or AGP administration reduces HABP binding to the vessel wall of mouse liver sinusoids *in vivo*. Mice were treated with hyaluronidase (Hy'ase; (b) and (e)) or without hyaluronidase (no treatment; (a) and (d)) after injection of either fluorescent HABP complex or fluorescent GS-1B_4 and visualization of liver sinusoids by confocal intravital microscopy. (c) Is an image of an experiment in which AGP intravenous injection was substituted for hyaluronidase. (f) (Mean of $n = 3 \pm$ SD) quantifies the intrasinusoidal HABP fluorescence in the experiment shown in (c) and in three additional replicates; each replicate is the mean of four intravascular samples within microscopic fields similar to that seen in (c); *signifies $P < 0.05$ by unpaired t-test, Welch corrected.

Glycosylation thus contributes to maintaining a circulating pool of AGP for exchange into the glycocalyx, where it may contribute to the maintenance of vascular permeability.

Acknowledgments

The authors thank Dr. Mark Hatton, Professor Emeritus, McMaster University, for helpful discussions during the course of this work. The authors declare that they have no competing financial interests in any aspect of the work described in this paper.

References

[1] P. G. Blain, J. C. Mucklow, and M. D. Rawlins, "Determinants of plasma α1-acid glycoprotein (AAG) concentrations in health," *British Journal of Clinical Pharmacology*, vol. 20, no. 5, pp. 500–502, 1985.

[2] T. Fournier, N. Medjoubi-N, and D. Porquet, "Alpha-1-acid glycoprotein," *Biochimica et Biophysica Acta*, vol. 1482, no. 1-2, pp. 157–171, 2000.

[3] J. M. H. Kremer, J. Wilting, and L. H. M. Janssen, "Drug binding to human alpha-1-acid glycoprotein in health and disease," *Pharmacological Reviews*, vol. 40, no. 1, pp. 1–47, 1988.

[4] G. A. Ricca, R. W. Hamilton, and J. W. McLean, "Rat α1-acid glycoprotein mRNA. Cloning of double-stranded cDNA and kinetics of induction of mRNA levels following acute inflammation," *Journal of Biological Chemistry*, vol. 256, no. 20, pp. 10362–10368, 1981.

[5] R. Cooper and J. Papaconstantinou, "Evidence for the existence of multiple α1-acid glycoprotein genes in the mouse," *Journal of Biological Chemistry*, vol. 261, no. 4, pp. 1849–1853, 1986.

[6] B. K. Ray, "Molecular cloning and nucleotide sequence of complementary DNA encoding rabbit α1-acid glycoprotein," *Biochemical and Biophysical Research Communications*, vol. 178, no. 2, pp. 507–513, 1991.

[7] H. Baumann and J. Gauldie, "The acute phase response," *Immunology Today*, vol. 15, no. 2, pp. 74–80, 1994.

[8] G. A. Clawson, J. Button, C. H. Woo, Y. C. Liao, and E. A. Smuckler, "In vitro release of α1-acid glycoprotein RNA sequences shows fidelity with the acute phase response in vivo," *Molecular Biology Reports*, vol. 11, no. 3, pp. 163–172, 1986.

[9] T. Hochepied, F. G. Berger, H. Baumann, and C. Libert, "α1-acid glycoprotein: an acute phase protein with inflammatory and immunomodulating properties," *Cytokine and Growth Factor Reviews*, vol. 14, no. 1, pp. 25–34, 2003.

[10] K. Smolarczyk, A. Gils, J. Boncela, P. J. Declerck, and C. S. Cierniewski, "Function-stabilizing mechanism of plasminogen activator inhibitor type 1 induced upon binding to α1-acid glycoprotein," *Biochemistry*, vol. 44, no. 37, pp. 12384–12390, 2005.

[11] T. Fournier, N. Medjoubi-N, and D. Porquet, "Alpha-1-acid glycoprotein," *Biochimica et Biophysica Acta*, vol. 1482, no. 1-2, pp. 157–171, 2000.

[12] B. Haraldsson and B. Rippe, "Orosomucoid as one of the serum components contributing to normal capillary permselectivity in rat skeletal muscle," *Acta Physiologica Scandinavica*, vol. 129, no. 1, pp. 127–135, 1987.

[13] B. S. Haraldsson, E. K. A. Johnsson, and B. Rippe, "Glomerular permselectivity is dependent on adequate serum concentrations of orosomucoid," *Kidney International*, vol. 41, no. 2, pp. 310–316, 1992.

[14] F. E. Curry, J. C. Rutledge, and J. F. Lenz, "Modulation of microvessel wall charge by plasma glycoprotein orosomucoid," *American Journal of Physiology*, vol. 257, no. 5, pp. H1354–H1349, 1989.

[15] J. E. Schnitzer and E. Pinney, "Quantitation of specific binding of orosomucoid to cultured microvascular endothelium: role in capillary permeability," *American Journal of Physiology*, vol. 263, no. 1, pp. H48–H55, 1992.

[16] D. Predescu, S. Predescu, T. Mcquistan, and G. E. Palade, "Transcytosis of α1-acidic glycoprotein in the continuous microvascular endothelium," *Proceedings of the National Academy of Sciences of the United States of America*, vol. 95, no. 11, pp. 6175–6180, 1998.

[17] J. Sörensson, M. Ohlson, A. Björnson, and B. Haraldsson, "Orosomucoid has a cAMP-dependent effect on human endothelial cells and inhibits the action of histamine," *American Journal of Physiology*, vol. 278, no. 5 47-5, pp. H1725–H1731, 2000.

[18] A. R. Pries, T. W. Secomb, and P. Gaehtgens, "The endothelial surface layer," *Pflugers Archiv European Journal of Physiology*, vol. 440, no. 5, pp. 653–666, 2000.

[19] C. Hjalmarsson, M. E. Lidell, and B. Haraldsson, "Beneficial effects of orosomucoid on the glomerular barrier in puromycin aminonucleoside-induced nephrosis," *Nephrology Dialysis Transplantation*, vol. 21, no. 5, pp. 1223–1230, 2006.

[20] W. E. Pricer Jr., R. L. Hudgin, G. Ashwell, R. J. Stockert, and A. G. Morell, "A membrane receptor protein for asialoglycoproteins," *Methods in Enzymology*, vol. 34, no. C, pp. 688–691, 1974.

[21] E. Regoeczi, M. T. Debanne, M. W. C. Hatton, and A. Koj, "Elimination of asialofetuin and asialoorosomucoid by the intact rat. Quantitative aspects of the hepatic clearance mechanism," *Biochimica et Biophysica Acta*, vol. 541, no. 3, pp. 372–384, 1978.

[22] W. M. Pardridge, A. J. Van Herle, and R. T. Naruse, "In vivo quantification of receptor-mediated uptake of asialoglycoproteins by rat liver," *Journal of Biological Chemistry*, vol. 258, no. 2, pp. 990–994, 1983.

[23] G. Ashwell and J. Harford, "Carbohydrate-specific receptors of the liver," *Annual Review of Biochemistry*, vol. 51, pp. 531–554, 1982.

[24] E. Regoeczi, M. W. C. Hatton, and P. A. Charlwood, "Carbohydrate mediated elimination of avian plasma glycoprotein in mammals," *Nature*, vol. 254, no. 5502, pp. 699–701, 1975.

[25] F. Hervé, P. D'Athis, D. Tremblay, J.-P. Tillement, and J. Barré, "Glycosylation study of the major genetic variants of human α 1-acid glycoprotein and of their pharmacokinetics in the rat," *Journal of Chromatography B*, vol. 798, no. 2, pp. 283–294, 2003.

[26] K. Parivar, L. Tolentino, G. Taylor, and S. Oie, "Elimination of non-reactive and weakly reactive human α1-acid glycoprotein after induction of the acute phase response in rats," *Journal of Pharmacy and Pharmacology*, vol. 44, no. 5, pp. 447–450, 1992.

[27] W. P. Sheffield, "Modification of clearance of therapeutic and potentially therapeutic proteins," *Curr Drug Targets Cardiovasc Haematol Disord*, vol. 1, no. 1, pp. 1–22, 2001.

[28] F. Hervé, M.-C. Millot, C. B. Eap, J.-C. Duché, and J.-P. Tillement, "Two-step chromatographic purification of human plasma α1-acid glycoprotein: its application to the purification of rare phenotype samples of the protein and their study by chromatography on immobilized metal chelate affinity adsorbent," *Journal of Chromatography B*, vol. 678, no. 1, pp. 1–14, 1996.

[29] W. P. Sheffield, T. R. McCurdy, and V. Bhakta, "Fusion to albumin as a means to slow the clearance of small therapeutic proteins using the *Pichia pastoris* expression system: a case study," *Methods in Molecular Biology*, vol. 308, pp. 145–154, 2005.

[30] W. P. Sheffield, L. J. Eltringham-Smith, S. Gataiance, and V. Bhakta, "A long-lasting, plasmin-activatable thrombin inhibitor aids clot lysis in vitro and does not promote bleeding in vivo," *Thrombosis and Haemostasis*, vol. 101, no. 5, pp. 867–877, 2009.

[31] P. J. Fraker and J. C. Speck Jr., "Protein and cell membrane iodinations with a sparingly soluble chloroamide, 1,3,4,6-tetrachloro-3a,6a-diphenylglycoluril," *Biochemical and Biophysical Research Communications*, vol. 80, no. 4, pp. 849–857, 1978.

[32] W. P. Sheffield, I. J. Smith, S. Syed, and V. Bhakta, "Prolonged in vivo anticoagulant activity of a hirudin—albumin fusion protein secreted from Pichia pastoris," *Blood Coagulation and Fibrinolysis*, vol. 12, no. 6, pp. 433–443, 2001.

[33] W. P. Sheffield, J. A. Marques, V. Bhakta, and I. J. Smith, "Modulation of clearance of recombinant serum albumin by either glycosylation or truncation," *Thrombosis Research*, vol. 99, no. 6, pp. 613–621, 2000.

[34] M. E. Begbie, A. Mamdani, S. Gataiance et al., "An important role for the activation peptide domain in controlling factor IX levels in the blood of haemophilia B mice," *Thrombosis and Haemostasis*, vol. 94, no. 6, pp. 1138–1147, 2005.

[35] D. A. Wall, G. Wilson, and A. L. Hubbard, "The galactose-specific recognition system of mammalian liver: the route of ligand internalization in rat hepatocytes," *Cell*, vol. 21, no. 1, pp. 79–93, 1980.

[36] C. J. Steer and G. Ashwell, "Studies on a mammalian hepatic binding protein specific for asialoglycoproteins. Evidence for receptor recycling in isolated rat hepatocytes," *Journal of Biological Chemistry*, vol. 255, no. 7, pp. 3008–3013, 1980.

[37] D. E. Keyler, P. R. Pentel, and D. B. Haughey, "Pharmacokinetics and toxicity of high-dose human α1-acid glycoprotein infusion in the rat," *Journal of Pharmaceutical Sciences*, vol. 76, no. 2, pp. 101–104, 1987.

[38] V. Gross, K. Steube, and T. A. Tran-Thi, "The role of N-glycosylation for the plasma clearance of rat liver secretory glycoproteins," *European Journal of Biochemistry*, vol. 162, no. 1, pp. 83–88, 1987.

[39] V. Gross, P. C. Heinrich, D. vom Berg et al., "Involvement of various organs in the initial plasma clearance of differently glycosylated rat liver secretory proteins," *European Journal of Biochemistry*, vol. 173, no. 3, pp. 653–659, 1988.

[40] C. B. S. Henry and B. R. Duling, "Permeation of the luminal capillary glycocalyx is determined by hyaluronan," *American Journal of Physiology*, vol. 277, no. 2, pp. H508–H514, 1999.

[41] S. H. Platts and B. R. Duling, "Adenosine A3 receptor activation modulates the capillary endothelial glycocalyx," *Circulation Research*, vol. 94, no. 1, pp. 77–82, 2004.

[42] J. Sörensson, G. L. Matejka, M. Ohlson, and B. Haraldsson, "Human endothelial cells produce orosomucoid, an important component of the capillary barrier," *American Journal of Physiology*, vol. 276, no. 2, pp. H530–H534, 1999.

[43] J. Boncela, I. Papiewska, I. Fijalkowska, B. Walkowiak, and C. S. Cierniewski, "Acute phase protein α1-acid glycoprotein interacts with plasminogen activator inhibitor type 1 and stabilizes its inhibitory activity," *Journal of Biological Chemistry*, vol. 276, no. 38, pp. 35305–35311, 2001.

[44] I. J. Goldstein and H. G. Winter, "The Griffonia simplicifolia I-B4 isolectin. A probe for alpha-D-galactosyl end groups," *Sub-Cellular Biochemistry*, vol. 32, pp. 127–141, 1999.

[45] H. K. Ondiveeran and A. E. Fox-Robichaud, "Pentastarch in a balanced solution reduces hepatic leukocyte recruitment in early sepsis," *Microcirculation*, vol. 11, no. 8, pp. 679–687, 2004.

[46] B. McDonald, E. F. McAvoy, F. Lam et al., "Interaction of CD44 and hyaluronan is the dominant mechanism for neutrophil sequestration in inflamed liver sinusoids," *Journal of Experimental Medicine*, vol. 205, no. 4, pp. 915–927, 2008.

[47] A. I. De Agostini, S. C. Watkins, H. S. Slayter, H. Youssoufian, and R. D. Rosenberg, "Localization of anticoagulantly active heparan sulfate proteoglycans in vascular endothelium: antithrombin binding on cultured endothelial cells and perfused rat aorta," *Journal of Cell Biology*, vol. 111, no. 3, pp. 1293–1304, 1990.

[48] V. Fridén, E. Oveland, O. Tenstad et al., "The glomerular endothelial cell coat is essential for glomerular filtration," *Kidney International*, vol. 79, no. 12, pp. 1322–1330, 2011.

[49] D. R. Flower, "The lipocalin protein family: structure and function," *Biochemical Journal*, vol. 318, no. 1, pp. 1–14, 1996.

[50] D. Schönfeld, G. Matschiner, L. Chatwell et al., "An engineered lipocalin specific for CTLA-4 reveals a combining site with structural and conformational features similar to antibodies," *Proceedings of the National Academy of Sciences of the United States of America*, vol. 106, no. 20, pp. 8198–8203, 2009.

[51] G. Y. Wu and C. H. Wu, "Receptor-mediated gene delivery and expression in vivo," *Journal of Biological Chemistry*, vol. 263, no. 29, pp. 14621–14624, 1988.

[52] D. Y. Yang, C. H. Ouyang, F. G. Lu, X. W. Liu, and L. Q. Huang, "Targeting specificity and pharmacokinetics of asialoorosomucoid, a specific ligand for asialglycoprotein receptor on hepatocyte," *Journal of Digestive Diseases*, vol. 8, no. 2, pp. 89–95, 2007.

[53] K. Shibata, H. Okubo, H. Ishibashi, and K. Tsuda, "Rat α1-acid glycoprotein. Purification and immunological estimation of its serum concentration," *Biochimica et Biophysica Acta*, vol. 495, no. 1, pp. 37–45, 1977.

[54] E. C. M. Brinkman-Van der Linden, R. Mollicone, R. Oriol, G. Larson, D. H. Van Den Eijnden, and W. Van Dijk, "A missense mutation in the FUT6 gene results in total absence of α3-fucosylation of human α1-acid glycoprotein," *Journal of Biological Chemistry*, vol. 271, no. 24, pp. 14492–14495, 1996.

[55] H. G. Jørgensen, M. A. Elliott, R. Priest, and K. D. Smith, "Modulation of sialyl Lewis X dependent binding to E-Selectin by glycoforms of alpha-1-acid glycoprotein expressed in rheumatoid arthritis," *Biomedical Chromatography*, vol. 12, no. 6, pp. 343–349, 1998.

[56] I. Rydén, P. Påhlsson, A. Lundblad, and T. Skogh, "Fucosylation of α1-acid glycoprotein (orosomucoid) compared with traditional biochemical markers of inflammation in recent onset rheumatoid arthritis," *Clinica Chimica Acta*, vol. 317, no. 1-2, pp. 221–229, 2002.

[57] E.-M. Muchitsch, W. Auer, and L. Pichler, "Effects of α1-acid glycoprotein in different rodent models of shock," *Fundamental and Clinical Pharmacology*, vol. 12, no. 2, pp. 173–181, 1998.

[58] E.-M. Muchitsch, H. P. Schwarz, M. D. Ginsberg, L. Belayev, and R. Busto, "Beneficial effect of albumin therapy attributable to α1-acid glycoprotein?" *Stroke*, vol. 34, no. 1, pp. 4–5, 2003.

[59] H. Ni, M. A. Blajchman, V. S. Ananthanarayanan, I. J. Smith, and W. P. Sheffield, "Mutation of any site of N-linked glycosylation accelerates the in vivo clearance of recombinant rabbit antithrombin," *Thrombosis Research*, vol. 99, no. 4, pp. 407–415, 2000.

[60] R. J. Peach and S. O. Brennan, "Structural characterization of a glycoprotein variant of human serum albumin: albumin Casebrook (494 Asp $\rightarrow$ Asn)," *Biochimica et Biophysica Acta*, vol. 1097, no. 1, pp. 49–54, 1991.

21

Fructation *In Vivo*: Detrimental and Protective Effects of Fructose

H. M. Semchyshyn

Department of Biochemistry and Biotechnology, Vassyl Stefanyk Precarpathian National University, 57 Shevchenko Street, Ivano-Frankivsk 76025, Ukraine

Correspondence should be addressed to H. M. Semchyshyn; semchyshyn@pu.if.ua

Academic Editor: Francieli Moro Stefanello

There is compelling evidence that long-term intake of excessive fructose can have deleterious side effects in different experimental models. However, the role of fructose *in vivo* remains controversial, since acute temporary application of fructose is found to protect yeast as well as animal tissues against exogenous oxidative stress. This review suggests the involvement of reactive carbonyl and oxygen species in both the cytotoxic and defensive effects of fructose. Potential mechanisms of the generation of reactive species by fructose in the nonenzymatic reactions, their implication in the detrimental and protective effects of fructose are discussed.

1. Introduction

Over the past decade, considerable scientific debate and controversy have arisen regarding the biological role of the reducing monosaccharides, and fructose in particular [1, 2]. Since many nutritionists believe that fructose is safer and healthier than glucose, fructose often is advocated as a glucose substitute by diabetes mellitus patients and a preferred sweetener for different population groups. At the same time, numerous epidemiological, clinical, and experimental studies demonstrate strong positive relationship between the intake of fructose and the development of metabolic disturbances [3–16]. Although consumption of fructose may have the adverse side effects and some authors state that there are no data showing a protective effect of fructose [3], it should also be mentioned that acute temporary application of fructose is found to be beneficial under some conditions [17–23].

Potential mechanisms underlying both detrimental and protective effects of fructose are under debate. Nonenzymatic reactions of fructose and higher production of reactive carbonyls (RCS) and oxygen species (ROS) compared with glucose are believed to be causative in negative effects of fructose [24–26]. However, ROS and RCS are found to play a dual role *in vivo*, which appears to be dose and time dependent [23, 27–32]. Therefore, we suggest the involvement of reactive species in both the cytotoxic and defensive effects of fructose. This review examines some of the potential mechanisms of ROS and RCS generation by the nonenzymatic reactions of fructose, their implication in the detrimental and defensive effects of fructose *in vivo*, and some of the differences between the long-term and short-term applications of fructose.

2. Involvement of Fructose in the Maillard Chemistry

The nonenzymatic reaction between amino acids and reducing monosaccharides was first described by Maillard a century ago [33, 34]. 40 years later, the Maillard reaction was recognized as one of the main reasons for the occurrence of the nonenzymatic food browning demonstrating an importance in food science [35, 36]. In late 1960s, the products of nonenzymatic glycosylation similar to the products of food browning were detected in human organism [37, 38]. It took several decades to realize the physiological significance of the reaction described by Maillard, which received renewed attention in biochemistry and medicine. The nonenzymatic glycosylation has been named "glycation" in order to differentiate it from the enzymatic glycosylation, an important posttranslation modification of proteins [39]. In 1980s, Monnier and Cerami postulated that glycation had a causative role in aging and age-related pathologies [40, 41]. Today, their theory called the "glycation hypothesis of aging" is at the origin of the growing interest in the field of *in vivo* glycation, aging, and age-related diseases.

Glycation is a process in which various compounds, including RCS and advanced glycation end-products (AGEs), are produced [36, 42–45]. An increase in the RCS and AGEs steady-state levels may result in so-called carbonyl stress. The concept of "carbonyl stress" was introduced by Miyata and colleagues in late 1990s [46]. The authors have defined carbonyl stress as a situation "resulting from either increased oxidation of carbohydrates and lipids (oxidative stress) or inadequate detoxification or inactivation of reactive carbonyl compounds derived from both carbohydrates and lipids by oxidative and non-oxidative chemistry." RCS are mainly known for their damaging effects. At the molecular level, RCS are found to modify the structure of proteins, nucleic acids, lipids, and carbohydrates. As a consequence, the loss of functions and even viability can occur at the cellular and organismal levels. These harmful effects of RCS are mainly linked to the initiation of glycation [36, 43, 47]. Therefore, a vicious cycle can be created *in vivo* when RCS serve as either the initiators or products of glycation.

It should be noted that reactive carbonyls are commonly generated *in vivo* as metabolic products [36, 44, 45, 48]. For example, oxidation of such amino acids as threonine and glycine can lead to RCS formation under physiological conditions [49]. Different RCS can be generated *in vivo* by activated human phagocytes. It has been found that stimulated neutrophils employed the myeloperoxidase-H_2O_2-chloride system to produce α-hydroxy and α,β-unsaturated aldehydes from hydroxy amino acids in high yield [49].

Besides highly reactive RCS, carbohydrates are important glycating agents. In general, RCS may demonstrate 20,000-fold higher reactivity than some reducing monosaccharides [48]; however the latter are more abundant intra- and extracellular glycation agents. The contribution of carbohydrates to nonenzymatic processes has been extensively investigated over few last decades. This may be attributed to either beneficial or detrimental effects of reducing carbohydrates *in vivo*, and most studies in the field of glycation are focused on glucose (glucation). Fructose is another reducing monosaccharide, a common component of honey, fruit juice concentrates, table sugar, and high-fructose corn syrup. It has been excessively consumed in human diets over the last decades, despite the evidence implicating fructose in the development of metabolic and other disorders [3–6]. However, glycation by fructose (fructation) has not been as thoroughly investigated as that of glucose.

The initial step of fructation is the covalent interaction between free carbonyl group of open-chain fructose and amino group of biomolecule, producing the Schiff base (Figure 1). The latter is an unstable compound that can be subjected to further isomerization (Heyns rearrangement) and form more stable Heyns adducts. The Heyns compounds as well as Amadori products derived from glucation are known as "early glycation products" or "fructosamines." The fructose moiety of the Heyns products can undergo enolization followed by dehydration, oxidation, and/or fragmentation reactions, consequently producing a variety of RCS [36, 50–52].

RCS can also be formed due to enzymatic reactions of reducing carbohydrates (e.g., glucose or fructose). For example, polyol pathway may be associated with the production of glyoxal, methylglyoxal, glucosone, and 3-deoxyglucosone [49]. Effective steady-state concentration of such RCS metabolites as acetaldehyde, glyceraldehyde-3-phosphate, and dihydroxyacetone phosphate is typically low in the cell because of their rapid utilization by the next step of the pathway [49]. However, the concentration of such by-products of glycolysis, polyol pathway, or enzymatic oxidation of ketone bodies as glyoxal, methylglyoxal, glucosone, and 3-deoxyglucosone is not so tightly controlled [48, 49]. In general, unlike enzymatic reactions, nonenzymatic processes are not tightly controlled, and therefore they can be harmful.

Oxidation reactions and ROS have been shown to be involved and frequently accelerate the fructation, glucation, and other nonenzymatic processes [24, 36]. In order to reflect the interplay between glycation and oxidative steps the "glycoxidation" term has been introduced [53]. Figure 1 shows the mechanism of fructation followed by the generation of reactive di- and tricarbonyls as well as such ROS as superoxide, hydrogen peroxide, and hydroxyl radical. Slow oxidative degradation of monosaccharides under physiological conditions also leads to the formation of α-dicarbonyls and some ROS. This process has been called monosaccharide autoxidation or the Wolff pathway [44, 54, 55]. Figure 2 demonstrates the mechanism of fructose autoxidation. Like other early glycation products, the Heyns compounds may undergo autoxidation (Figure 3). This process leading to the formation of RCS and ROS has been called the Hodge pathway [35, 56, 57]. In addition, there is an evidence for the fragmentation of the Schiff base that results in RCS and ROS generation (Figure 4). The series of reaction pathways in glycation established the Schiff base fragmentation to RCS and ROS now collectively called the Namiki pathway [44, 51, 58, 59]. Thus, some stages of glycoxidation demonstrate a strong relationship between carbonyl and oxidative stress (Figure 5). Interestingly, some compounds were simultaneously identified as the intermediates or end-products of glycoxidation and lipid peroxidation that confirms an interplay between both the nonenzymatic processes [49].

In the late stage of glycation, the reactive carbonyls and the Heyns compounds again interact with free amino, sulfhydryl, and guanidine functional groups of intracellular or extracellular biomolecules like proteins, nucleic acids, and aminophospholipids, resulting in their nonenzymatic, irreversible modification and formation of a variety of adducts and crosslinks collectively named advanced glycation end products (AGEs) [44, 45]. Therefore, the Heyns products and RCS formed during fructation are believed to be important precursors of nonenzymatic adduct formation in biological systems. In general, AGEs are poorly degraded complexes (Figure 6) accumulation of which increases with aging. They were detected in a variety of human tissues and serve as biomarkers of aging and age-related disorders [36]. Interestingly, the comparison of nutrition and plasma AGEs in vegetarian and omnivorous groups showed that the higher

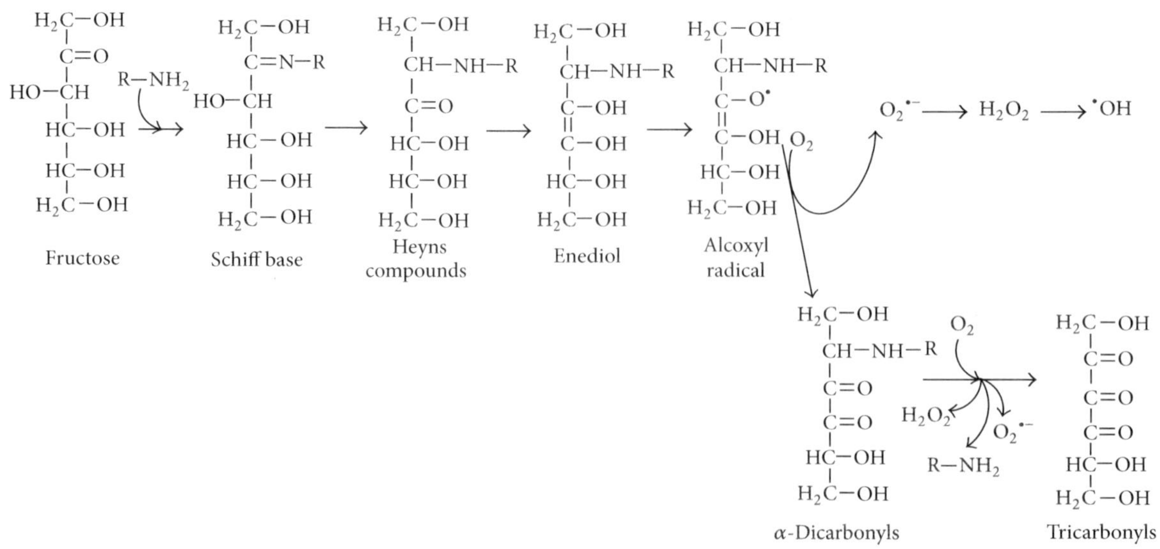

FIGURE 1: Suggested mechanism for the production of reactive carbonyl and oxygen species by the fructation.

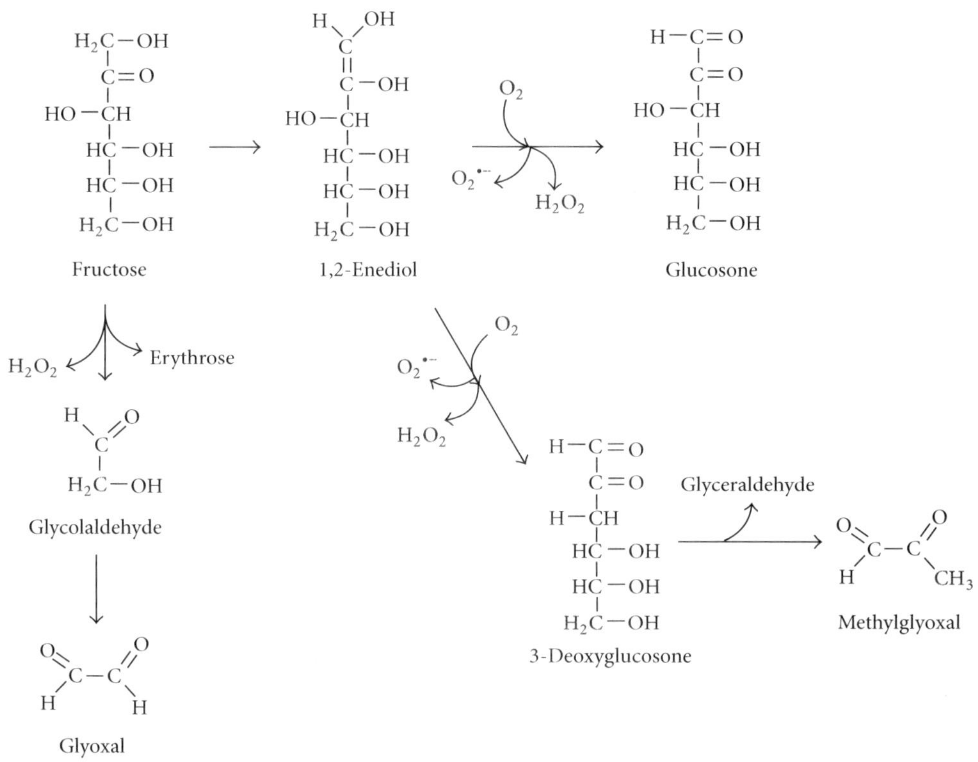

FIGURE 2: Fructose autoxidation (Wolff pathway).

intake of fructose in alternative nutrition of healthy subjects may cause an increase of AGE levels [60].

It should be noted that AGEs may undergo covalent interactions with biomolecules giving more complex cross-links. In addition, AGEs are efficient *in vivo* sources of RCS and ROS [44, 51, 61–63]. Like free-radical chain reaction, glycation is characterized by unpredictable direction and a wide variety of intermediates and end-products. That is why the term "Maillard chemistry" is widely used to describe the complicity of glycation [36, 43–45, 49].

3. Adverse Side Effects of Long-Term Consumption of Fructose

Fructose is commonly used as a sweetener and its intake has quadrupled since the early 1900s, in part because of

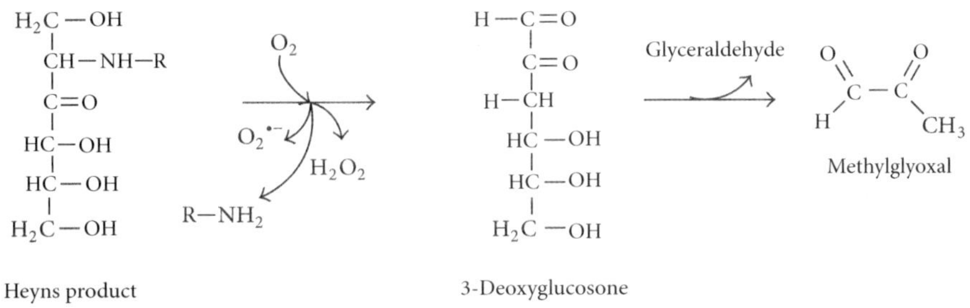

FIGURE 3: Autoxidation of Heyns compounds (Hodge pathway).

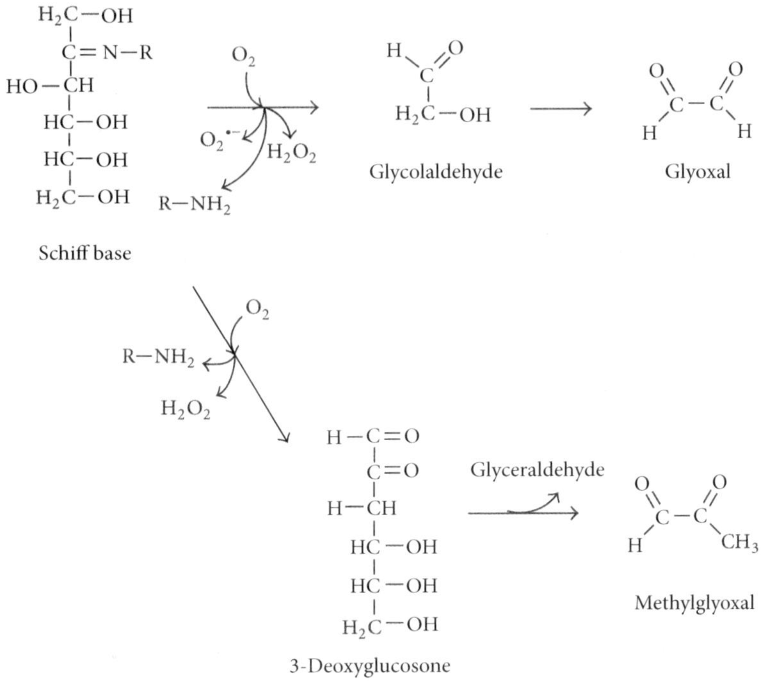

FIGURE 4: Oxidative fragmentation of Schiff base (Namiki pathway).

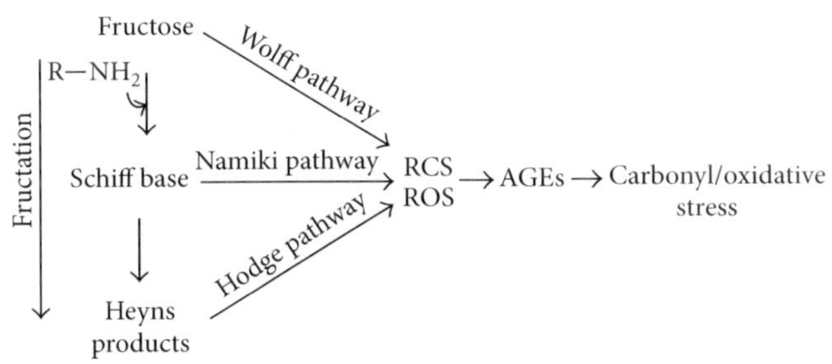

FIGURE 5: Formation of reactive species by the fructation leading to carbonyl/oxidative stress.

the introduction of high-fructose corn syrup [1]. This phenomenon parallels the development and progression of such disorders as obesity, type 2 diabetes mellitus and its complications, cardiovascular and neurodegenerative diseases, hypertension, and gout, liver, and kidney disease [1, 3, 7–16]. Experimental studies on animals have shown that chronic intake of excessive fructose can induce most features of the metabolic syndrome, including hypertriglyceridemia, fatty liver, nonalcoholic steatohepatitis, glucose intolerance, hyperglycemia, abdominal obesity, elevated blood pressure, microvascular disease, endothelial dysfunction, inflammation, hyperuricemia, glomerular hypertension, and renal injury [9, 16, 64–66].

Although the consumption of large amounts of dietary fructose can rapidly induce insulin resistance, most nutritionists believe that fructose is safer and healthier than glucose; therefore, fructose is advocated as a preferred sweetener, particularly for diabetes mellitus patients. Chronic hyperglycemia that in part can result from glucose intolerance induced by long-term consumption of fructose is a major inducer of vascular complications in diabetes (e.g., heart disease, stroke, blindness, and end-stage renal failure) which are responsible for disabilities and high mortality rates in patients with diabetes. The increased production of ROS, RCS, and AGEs as a result of glycoxidation is most preferable among the various mechanisms, which are supposed to be involved in vascular complications in diabetes. In general,

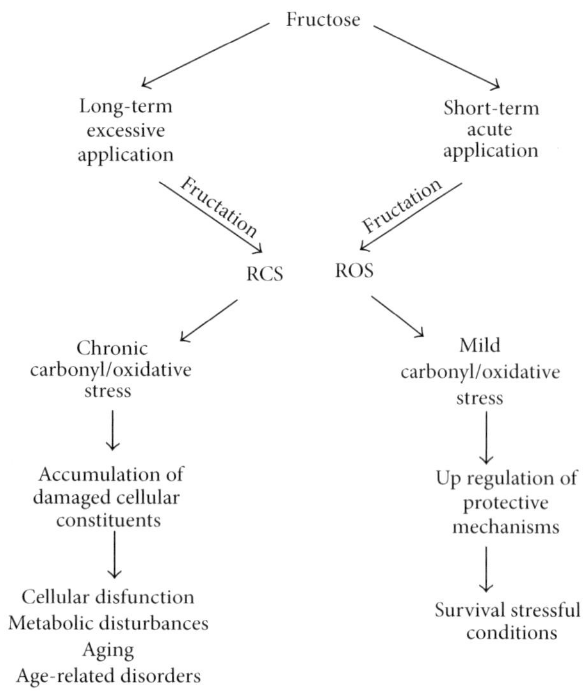

FIGURE 6: Involvement of reactive oxygen and carbonyl species in cytotoxic and defensive effects of fructose.

the enhanced levels of glycoxidation products can explain the detrimental effects of fructose due to its long-term application in different experimental models [67–71].

To compare glucose and fructose involvement in the generation of glycoxidation products, recently we used baker's yeast as a model and found higher level of carbonyl/oxidative stress markers, which were correlated with a higher aging rate of fructose-grown compared with glucose-grown yeast at stationary phase (long-term model) [25, 26]. We suggested that fructose rather than glucose is more extensively involved in glycoxidation *in vivo*, yeast aging, and development of carbonyl/oxidative stress. O'Brien with colleagues found that excessive fructose intake in animal models caused tissue damage associated with carbonyl/oxidative stress [72, 73]. *In vitro* experiments also demonstrated that fructose produced greater amounts of ROS and RCS than did glucose [24, 68, 69, 74].

At the first glance, from the point of view of basic organic chemistry it may seem surprising, since due to a greater electrophilicity and accessibility of the carbonyl group of aldoses (e.g., glucose), their reactivity is believed to be higher than that of respective ketoses (e.g., fructose). There is some information confirming higher reactivity of glucose versus fructose in nonenzymatic processes *in vitro* [75–77], while the opposite is reported in numerous *in vitro* and *in vivo* studies [24, 74, 78–80]. Possible explanation is that glucose is less reactive due to formation of very stable ring structures in aqueous solutions (glucopyranose and glucofuranose) which retards its reactivity. Generally, glucose is the least reactive monosaccharide and this characteristic can be considered to the emergence of glucose as the primary metabolic fuel [36, 81, 82]. Fructose also forms both pyranose and furanose structures [83] but exists to a greater extent in the open-chain active form than does glucose. The proportion of acyclic forms of glucose and fructose in aqueous solution accounts for 0.001–0.002% and 0.7%, respectively [48, 84]. Thus fructose is a more potent glycoxidation agent as compared with glucose that can explain its detrimental effects.

4. Short-Term Application of Fructose Protects against Oxidative Stress

Although a long-term consumption of excessive fructose may have adverse side effects, its acute temporary ingestion can be beneficial under some circumstances. For example, short-term application of fructose has been found to protect astroglial C6 cells against peroxide-induced stress [21]. In contrast to glucose, fructose inhibited apoptosis induced by reoxygenation in rat hepatocytes by decreasing the level of ROS [17]. Fructose has also been found to defend rat hepatocytes against exogenous oxidative stress [18, 20]. It has been demonstrated that fructose and its phosphorylated derivatives such as fructose-1,6-bisphosphate had significantly higher antioxidant capacities against ROS than other carbohydrates [22]. Based on these phenomena, it was suggested that acute infusion or ingestion of fructose could be of benefit in the cytoprotective therapy of disorders related to oxidative stress [21]. According to homeostasis theory, the steady-state concentration of oxidants as well as antioxidants is maintained at the limited range [85]. That is why antioxidant therapy is generally found to be ineffective [30, 31]. In contrast to strong antioxidants, fructose and its phosphorylated derivatives (e.g., fructose-1,6-bisphosphate) being important energy substrates are not "fought" by redox homeostatic mechanisms. The beneficial effects of fructose-1,6-bisphosphate have been documented in different tissues, including the heart, liver, kidney, brain, and small intestine [86–89]. The cytoprotective mechanisms underlying fructose-1,6-bisphosphate are believed to be involved in its intervention in the glycolytic pathway, as a metabolic regulator or substrate, as well as an agent modifying the ion permeability of cell membrane transporters.

Recently we have demonstrated that fructose-grown yeast at exponential phase (short-term model) exposed to hydrogen peroxide demonstrated higher survival compared to glucose-grown cells [23]. In this study, significantly higher total level of ROS was observed in fructose-grown than that in glucose-grown cells under control conditions (without H_2O_2). However, under peroxide-induced stress ROS amount significantly decreased in yeast grown on fructose, whereas it increased in glucose-grown cells, which was very consistent with the work of Spasojević et al. [21]. The authors demonstrated a significant increase in oxidative status of astroglial C6 cells under treatment with hydrogen peroxide in glucose medium, but it was not the case in a fructose-containing medium. At the same time, hydrogen peroxide led to a decrease of C6 cell viability in both media investigated; however, the survival was higher in fructose-containing medium. In accordance with another work by

Spasojević et al. [22], we demonstrated that hydrogen peroxide did not markedly change hydroxyl radical level in glucose-grown cells but it did decrease it significantly in fructose-grown cells [23].

An obvious question arises: what mechanism(s) is (are) responsible for the protective effect of fructose short-term application? Analysis of the literature data leads us to propose several mechanisms responsible for the defensive effect of fructose: (1) iron binding and prevention of the Fenton reaction [18, 21]; (2) stabilization of the glutathione pool in the cell [17]; (3) upregulation of the pentose phosphate pathway producing NADPH [22]; and (4) production of fructose-1,6-bisphosphate, the compound with cytoprotective and antioxidant mechanisms [86–89].

Our study extended the earlier findings with the involvement of SOD and catalase in the reduction of ROS level in fructose-grown yeast exposed to H_2O_2 [23]. It was shown that a reduced ROS level in fructose-grown cells was consistent with a broad peak of SOD and catalase activation by hydrogen peroxide, whereas cells grown on glucose demonstrated a sharp rise of the enzyme activities. We also found that fructose more markedly than glucose activated glyoxalases, the fundamental function of which is the metabolism of reactive α-dicarbonyl metabolites in most living organisms [43, 90–92].

These findings prompted us to propose additional explanation of fructose protective effect—a short-term application of fructose induces a mild carbonyl/oxidative stress-stimulating cellular defensive mechanisms responsible for cell survival under lethal stress [23]. The last mechanism can be posited from the *in vitro* and *in vivo* studies reporting that fructose is a much more potent glycoxidation agent, capable of producing greater amounts of RCS and ROS than glucose [21, 23–26, 68, 74]. Generally, ROS and RCS are found to play a dual role *in vivo*, which appears to be concentration dependent [23, 27–32]. At high concentrations, reactive species are potentially dangerous, as they can cause damage to cell constituents that, in turn, accompany aging and age-related disorders. In contrast, the beneficial effects of ROS and RCS occur at low concentrations and involve physiological roles in cellular signaling pathways, responses to environmental challenges, and so forth. It is also well documented that mild stress caused by low doses of reactive species can result in the acquisition of cellular resistance to lethal stress [28, 93–96].

5. Conclusion

Considering the literature data it can be supposed that at long-term consumption of excessive fructose chronic increase in the levels of reactive species leads to the accumulation of damaged cellular constituents resulting in cellular disfunction, whereas short-term application of fructose provokes a mild stress, resulting in the acquisition of cellular cross-resistance to lethal stress (Figure 6). Therefore, we suggest the involvement of reactive species like RCS and ROS in both the cytotoxic and defensive effects of fructose. Thus, depending on conditions, fructose can play a dual role in the living cell. Long-term application of excessive fructose leads to glycoxidation, generation of ROS and RCS, and accumulation of damaged cellular constituents which is suggested to accompany the aging process, cellular dysfunction. and age-related disorders. In opposite, short-term application of fructose provokes a mild carbonyl/oxidative stress, resulting in the acquisition of cellular cross-resistance to lethal stress. Generally, a long-term consumption of excessive fructose is found to have adverse side effects; however acute temporary application of fructose can be beneficial under some pathophysiological conditions.

References

[1] J. S. White, "Challenging the fructose hypothesis: new perspectives on fructose consumption and metabolism," *Advances in Nutrition*, vol. 4, no. 2, pp. 246–256, 2013.

[2] J. M. Rippe and T. J. Angelopoulos, "Sucrose, high-fructose corn syrup, and fructose, their metabolism and potential health effects: what do we really know?" *Advances in Nutrition*, vol. 4, no. 2, pp. 236–245, 2013.

[3] G. A. Bray, "Energy and fructose from beverages sweetened with sugar or high-fructose corn syrup pose a health risk for some people," *Advances in Nutrition*, vol. 4, no. 2, pp. 220–225, 2013.

[4] V. P. Karalius and D. A. Shoham, "Dietary sugar and artificial sweetener intake and chronic kidney disease: a review," *Advances in Chronic Kidney Disease*, vol. 20, no. 2, pp. 157–164, 2013.

[5] M. J. Dekker, Q. Su, C. Baker, A. C. Rutledge, and K. Adeli, "Fructose: a highly lipogenic nutrient implicated in insulin resistance, hepatic steatosis, and the metabolic syndrome," *The American Journal of Physiology—Endocrinology and Metabolism*, vol. 299, no. 5, pp. E685–E694, 2010.

[6] L. Tappy, "Q&A: "toxic" effects of sugar: should we be afraid of fructose?" *BMC Biology*, vol. 10, article 42, 2012.

[7] A. R. Gaby, "Adverse effects of dietary fructose," *Alternative Medicine Review*, vol. 10, no. 4, pp. 294–306, 2005.

[8] R. J. Johnson, M. S. Segal, Y. Sautin et al., "Potential role of sugar (fructose) in the epidemic of hypertension, obesity and the metabolic syndrome, diabetes, kidney disease, and cardiovascular disease," *The American Journal of Clinical Nutrition*, vol. 86, no. 4, pp. 899–906, 2007.

[9] L. G. Sánchez-Lozada, M. Le, M. Segal, and R. J. Johnson, "How safe is fructose for persons with or without diabetes?" *The American Journal of Clinical Nutrition*, vol. 88, no. 5, pp. 1189–1190, 2008.

[10] K. L. Stanhope, J. M. Schwarz, and P. J. Havel, "Adverse metabolic effects of dietary fructose: results from the recent epidemiological, clinical, and mechanistic studies," *Current Opinion in Lipidology*, vol. 24, no. 3, pp. 198–206, 2013.

[11] K. L. Stanhope, J. M. Schwarz, N. L. Keim et al., "Consuming fructose-sweetened, not glucose-sweetened, beverages increases visceral adiposity and lipids and decreases insulin sensitivity in overweight/obese humans," *Journal of Clinical Investigation*, vol. 119, no. 5, pp. 1322–1334, 2009.

[12] L. Tappy, K. A. Lê, C. Tran, and N. Paquot, "Fructose and metabolic diseases: new findings, new questions," *Nutrition*, vol. 26, no. 11-12, pp. 1044–1049, 2010.

[13] L. Tappy and K. Lê, "Metabolic effects of fructose and the worldwide increase in obesity," *Physiological Reviews*, vol. 90, no. 1, pp. 23–46, 2010.

[14] M. A. Lanaspa, E. Tapia, V. Soto, Y. Sautin, and L. G. Sánchez-Lozada, "Uric acid and fructose: potential biological mechanisms," *Seminars in Nephrology*, vol. 31, no. 5, pp. 426–432, 2011.

[15] M. Soleimani, "Dietary fructose, salt absorption and hypertension in metabolic syndrome: towards a new paradigm," *Acta Physiologica*, vol. 201, no. 1, pp. 55–62, 2011.

[16] A. Rebollo, N. Roglans, M. Alegret, and J. C. Laguna, "Way back for fructose and liver metabolism: bench side to molecular insights," *World Journal of Gastroenterology*, vol. 18, no. 45, pp. 6552–6559, 2012.

[17] J. Frenzel, J. Richter, and K. Eschrich, "Fructose inhibits apoptosis induced by reoxygenation in rat hepatocytes by decreasing reactive oxygen species via stabilization of the glutathione pool," *Biochimica et Biophysica Acta*, vol. 1542, no. 1–3, pp. 82–94, 2002.

[18] F. Valeri, F. Boess, A. Wolf, C. Göldlin, and U. A. Boelsterli, "Fructose and tagatose protect against oxidative cell injury by iron chelation," *Free Radical Biology and Medicine*, vol. 22, no. 1-2, pp. 257–268, 1996.

[19] J. Bogdanović, M. Mojović, N. Milosavić, A. Mitrović, Z. Vucinić, and I. Spasojević, "Role of fructose in the adaptation of plants to cold-induced oxidative stress," *European Biophysics Journal*, vol. 37, no. 7, pp. 1241–1246, 2008.

[20] S. L. MacAllister, J. Choi, L. Dedina, and P. J. O'Brien, "Metabolic mechanisms of methanol/formaldehyde in isolated rat hepatocytes: carbonyl-metabolizing enzymes versus oxidative stress," *Chemico-Biological Interactions*, vol. 191, no. 1–3, pp. 308–314, 2011.

[21] I. Spasojević, A. Bajić, K. Jovanović, M. Spasić, and P. Andjus, "Protective role of fructose in the metabolism of astroglial C6 cells exposed to hydrogen peroxide," *Carbohydrate Research*, vol. 344, no. 13, pp. 1676–1681, 2009.

[22] I. Spasojević, M. Mojović, D. Blagojević et al., "Relevance of the capacity of phosphorylated fructose to scavenge the hydroxyl radical," *Carbohydrate Research*, vol. 344, no. 1, pp. 80–84, 2009.

[23] H. M. Semchyshyn and L. M. Lozinska, "Fructose protects baker's yeast against peroxide stress: potential role of catalase and superoxide dismutase," *FEMS Yeast Research*, vol. 12, no. 7, pp. 761–773, 2012.

[24] M. Sakai, M. Oimomi, and M. Kasuga, "Experimental studies on the role of fructose in the development of diabetic complications," *Kobe Journal of Medical Sciences*, vol. 48, no. 5-6, pp. 125–136, 2002.

[25] L. M. Lozinska and G. M. Semchyshyn, "Fructose as a factor of carbonyl and oxidative stress development and accelerated aging in the yeast *Saccharomyces cerevisiae*," *Ukrainian Biochemical Journal*, vol. 83, no. 4, pp. 67–76, 2011.

[26] H. M. Semchyshyn, L. M. Lozinska, J. Miedzobrodzki, and V. I. Lushchak, "Fructose and glucose differentially affect aging and carbonyl/oxidative stress parameters in *Saccharomyces cerevisiae* cells," *Carbohydrate Research*, vol. 346, no. 7, pp. 933–938, 2011.

[27] A. Mesquita, M. Weinberger, A. Silva et al., "Caloric restriction or catalase inactivation extends yeast chronological lifespan by inducing H_2O_2 and superoxide dismutase activity," *Proceedings of the National Academy of Sciences of the United States of America*, vol. 107, no. 34, pp. 15123–15128, 2010.

[28] H. Semchyshyn, "Hydrogen peroxide-induced response in *E. coli* and *S. cerevisiae*: different stages of the flow of the genetic information," *Central European Journal of Biology*, vol. 4, no. 2, pp. 142–153, 2009.

[29] H. J. Forman, "Reactive oxygen species and α,β-unsaturated aldehydes as second messengers in signal transduction," *Annals of the New York Academy of Sciences*, vol. 1203, pp. 35–44, 2010.

[30] I. Spasojević, D. R. Jones, and M. E. Andrades, "Hydrogen peroxide in adaptation," *Oxidative Medicine and Cellular Longevity*, vol. 2012, Article ID 596019, 4 pages, 2012.

[31] K. Brieger, S. Schiavone, F. J. Miller Jr., and K. H. Krause, "Reactive oxygen species: from health to disease," *Swiss Medical Weekly*, vol. 142, Article ID w13659, 2012.

[32] M. Pohanka, "Role of oxidative stress in infectious diseases. A review," *Folia Microbiologica*, 2013.

[33] L. C. Maillard, "Action des acides aminés sur les sucres: formation des mélanoïdines par voie méthodique," *Comptes Rendus de l'Academie des Sciences*, vol. 154, pp. 66–68, 1912.

[34] L. C. Maillard, "Formation d'humus et de combustibles mineraux sans intervention de l'oxygene atmospherique des microorganismes, des hautes temperatures, ou des fortes pressions," *Comptes Rendus de l'Academie des Sciences*, vol. 155, pp. 1554–1556, 1912.

[35] J. E. Hodge, "Dehydrated foods: chemistry of browning reactions in model systems," *Journal of Agricultural and Food Chemistry*, vol. 1, no. 15, pp. 928–943, 1953.

[36] F. J. Tessier, "The Maillard reaction in the human body. The main discoveries and factors that affect glycation," *Pathologie Biologie*, vol. 58, no. 3, pp. 214–219, 2010.

[37] S. Rahbar, "Hemoglobin H disease in two Iranian families," *Clinica Chimica Acta*, vol. 20, no. 3, pp. 381–385, 1968.

[38] S. Rahbar, O. Blumenfeld, and H. M. Ranney, "Studies of an unusual hemoglobin in patients with diabetes mellitus," *Biochemical and Biophysical Research Communications*, vol. 36, no. 5, pp. 838–843, 1969.

[39] R. W. Yatscoff, G. J. Tevaarwerk, and J. C. MacDonald, "Quantification of nonenzymically glycated albumin and total serum protein by affinity chromatography," *Clinical Chemistry*, vol. 30, no. 3, pp. 446–449, 1984.

[40] V. M. Monnier and A. Cerami, "Nonenzymatic browning *in vivo*: possible process for aging of long-lived proteins," *Science*, vol. 211, no. 4481, pp. 491–493, 1981.

[41] A. Cerami, "Hypothesis: glucose as a mediator of aging," *Journal of the American Geriatrics Society*, vol. 33, no. 9, pp. 626–634, 1985.

[42] P. A. Finot, "Nonenzymatic browning products: physiologic effects and metabolic transit in relation to chemical structure. A review," *Diabetes*, vol. 31, pp. 22–28, 1982.

[43] E. M. Ellis, "Reactive carbonyls and oxidative stress: potential for therapeutic intervention," *Pharmacology and Therapeutics*, vol. 115, no. 1, pp. 13–24, 2007.

[44] X. Peng, J. Ma, F. Chen, and M. Wang, "Naturally occurring inhibitors against the formation of advanced glycation end-products," *Food and Function*, vol. 2, no. 6, pp. 289–301, 2011.

[45] L. Robert, A. M. Robert, and J. Labat-Robert, "The Maillard reaction—illicite (bio)chemistry in tissues and food," *Pathologie Biologie*, vol. 59, no. 6, pp. 321–328, 2011.

[46] T. Miyata, C. van Ypersele de Strihou, K. Kurokawa, and J. W. Baynes, "Alterations in nonenzymatic biochemistry in uremia: origin and significance of "carbonyl stress" in long-term uremic complications," *Kidney International*, vol. 55, no. 2, pp. 389–399, 1999.

[47] F. Moheimani, P. E. Morgan, D. M. van Reyk, and M. J. Davies, "Deleterious effects of reactive aldehydes and glycated proteins on macrophage proteasomal function: possible links between

diabetes and atherosclerosis," *Biochimica et Biophysica Acta*, vol. 1802, no. 6, pp. 561–571, 2010.

[48] Z. Turk, "Glycotoxines, carbonyl stress and relevance to diabetes and its complications," *Physiological Research*, vol. 59, no. 2, pp. 147–156, 2010.

[49] H. M. Semchyshyn and V. I. Lushchak, "Interplay between oxidative and carbonyl stresses: molecular mechanisms, biological effects and therapeutic strategies of protection," in *Oxidative Stress—Molecular Mechanisms and Biological Effects*, V. I. Lushchak and H. M. Semchyshyn, Eds., pp. 15–46, InTech, Rijeka, Croatia, 2012.

[50] O. Reihl, T. M. Rothenbacher, M. O. Lederer, and W. Schwack, "Carbohydrate carbonyl mobility—the key process in the formation of α-dicarbonyl intermediates," *Carbohydrate Research*, vol. 339, no. 9, pp. 1609–1618, 2004.

[51] P. J. Thornalley, "Dicarbonyl intermediates in the Maillard reaction," *Annals of the New York Academy of Sciences*, vol. 1043, pp. 111–117, 2005.

[52] M. Smuda and M. A. Glomb, "Novel insights into the Maillard catalyzed degradation of maltose," *Journal of Agricultural and Food Chemistry*, vol. 59, no. 24, pp. 13254–13264, 2011.

[53] D. G. Dyer, J. A. Blackledge, B. M. Katz et al., "The Maillard reaction *in vivo*," *Zeitschrift fur Ernahrungswissenschaft*, vol. 30, no. 1, pp. 29–45, 1991.

[54] P. J. Thornalley, S. P. Wolff, J. Crabbe, and A. Stern, "The autoxidation of glyceraldehyde and other simple monosaccharides under physiological conditions catalysed by buffer ions," *Biochimica et Biophysica Acta*, vol. 797, no. 2, pp. 276–287, 1984.

[55] S. P. Wolff, Z. Y. Jiang, and J. V. Hunt, "Protein glycation and oxidative stress in diabetes mellitus and ageing," *Free Radical Biology and Medicine*, vol. 10, no. 5, pp. 339–352, 1991.

[56] J. V. Hunt, R. T. Dean, and S. P. Wolff, "Hydroxyl radical production and autoxidative glycosylation. Glucose autoxidation as the cause of protein damage in the experimental glycation model of diabetes mellitus and ageing," *Biochemical Journal*, vol. 256, no. 1, pp. 205–212, 1988.

[57] C. J. Mullarkey, D. Edelstein, and M. Brownlee, "Free radical generation by early glycation products: a mechanism for accelerated atherogenesis in diabetes," *Biochemical and Biophysical Research Communications*, vol. 173, no. 3, pp. 932–939, 1990.

[58] T. Hayashi and M. Namiki, "Formation of two-carbon sugar fragments at an early stage of the browning reaction of sugar and amine," *Agricultural Biology and Chemistry*, vol. 44, no. 11, pp. 2575–2580, 1980.

[59] M. Namiki and T. Hayashi, "A new mechanism of the Maillard reaction involving sugar fragmentation and free radical formation," in *The Maillard Reaction in Foods and Nutrition*, G. R. Waller and M. S. Feather, Eds., ACS Symposium Series 215, American Chemical Society, Washington, DC, USA, 1983.

[60] M. Krajcovicová-Kudlácková, K. Sebeková, R. Schinzel, and J. Klvanová, "Advanced glycation end products and nutrition," *Physiological Reviwes*, vol. 51, no. 3, pp. 313–316, 2002.

[61] M. B. Yim, H. S. Yim, C. Lee, S. O. Kang, and P. B. Chock, "Protein glycation: creation of catalytic sites for free radical generation," *Annals of the New York Academy of Sciences*, vol. 928, pp. 48–53, 2001.

[62] R. Takamiya, M. Takahashi, T. Myint et al., "Glycation proceeds faster in mutated Cu, Zn-superoxide dismutases related to familial amyotrophic lateral sclerosis," *The FASEB Journal*, vol. 17, no. 8, pp. 938–940, 2003.

[63] K. B. Shumaev, S. A. Gubkina, E. M. Kumskova, G. S. Shepelkova, E. K. Ruuge, and V. Z. Lankin, "Superoxide formation as a result of interaction of L-lysine with dicarbonyl compounds and its possible mechanism," *Biochemistry*, vol. 74, no. 4, pp. 461–466, 2009.

[64] M. Alegret, N. Roglans, and J. C. Laguna, "Fructose consumption and leptin resistance: what have we learnt from animal studies?" in *Leptin: Hormonal Functions, Dysfunctions and Clinical Uses*, R. M. Hemling and A. T. Belkin, Eds., pp. 210–230, Nova Science Publishers, Hauppauge, NY, USA, 2011.

[65] L. Vilà, N. Roglans, V. Perna et al., "Liver AMP/ATP ratio and fructokinase expression are related to gender differences in AMPK activity and glucose intolerance in rats ingesting liquid fructose," *Journal of Nutritional Biochemistry*, vol. 22, no. 8, pp. 741–751, 2011.

[66] B. P. Cummings, K. L. Stanhope, J. L. Graham et al., "Dietary fructose accelerates the development of diabetes in UCD-T2DM rats: amelioration by the antioxidant, α-lipoic acid," *The American Journal of Physiology—Regulatory Integrative and Comparative Physiology*, vol. 298, no. 5, pp. R1343–R1350, 2010.

[67] B. Levi and M. J. Werman, "Long-term fructose consumption accelerates glycation and several age-related variables in male rats," *Journal of Nutrition*, vol. 128, no. 9, pp. 1442–1449, 1998.

[68] B. Levi and M. J. Werman, "Fructose triggers DNA modification and damage in an *Escherichia coli* plasmid," *Journal of Nutritional Biochemistry*, vol. 12, no. 4, pp. 235–241, 2001.

[69] B. Levi and M. J. Werman, "Fructose and related phosphate derivatives impose DNA damage and apoptosis in L5178Y mouse lymphoma cells," *Journal of Nutritional Biochemistry*, vol. 14, no. 1, pp. 49–60, 2003.

[70] O. Lee, W. R. Bruce, Q. Dong, J. Bruce, R. Mehta, and P. J. O'Brien, "Fructose and carbonyl metabolites as endogenous toxins," *Chemico-Biological Interactions*, vol. 178, no. 1–3, pp. 332–339, 2009.

[71] O. V. Lushchak, B. M. Rovenko, D. V. Gospodaryov, and V. I. Lushchak, "Drosophila melanogaster larvae fed by glucose and fructose demonstrate difference in oxidative stress markers and antioxidant enzymes of adult flies," *Comparative Biochemistry and Physiology*, vol. 160, no. 1, pp. 27–34, 2011.

[72] Q. Dong, K. Yang, S. M. Wong, and P. J. O'Brien, "Hepatocyte or serum albumin protein carbonylation by oxidized fructose metabolites: glyceraldehyde or glycolaldehyde as endogenous toxins?" *Chemico-Biological Interactions*, vol. 188, no. 1, pp. 31–37, 2010.

[73] K. Yang, C. Feng, H. Lip, W. R. Bruce, and P. J. O'Brien, "Cytotoxic molecular mechanisms and cytoprotection by enzymic metabolism or autoxidation for glyceraldehyde, hydroxypyruvate and glycolaldehyde," *Chemico-Biological Interactions*, vol. 191, no. 1–3, pp. 315–321, 2011.

[74] G. Suarez, R. Rajaram, A. L. Oronsky, and M. A. Gawinowicz, "Nonenzymatic glycation of bovine serum albumin by fructose (fructation). Comparison with the Maillard reaction initiated by glucose," *The Journal of Biological Chemistry*, vol. 264, no. 7, pp. 3674–3679, 1989.

[75] A. N. Wijewickreme, D. D. Kitts, and T. D. Durance, "Reaction conditions influence the elementary composition and metal chelating affinity of nondialyzable model Maillard reaction products," *Journal of Agricultural and Food Chemistry*, vol. 45, no. 12, pp. 4577–4583, 1997.

[76] F. K. Yeboah, I. Alli, and V. A. Yaylayan, "Reactivities of D-glucose and D-fructose during glycation of bovine serum albumin," *Journal of Agricultural and Food Chemistry*, vol. 47, no. 8, pp. 3164–3172, 1999.

[77] J. Rangsansarid, N. Cheetangdee, N. Kinoshita, and K. Fukuda, "Bovine serum albumin-sugar conjugates through the Maillard reaction: effects on interfacial behavior and emulsifying ability," *Journal of Oleo Science*, vol. 57, no. 10, pp. 539–547, 2008.

[78] G. Suarez, J. Maturana, A. L. Oronsky, and C. Raventos-Suarez, "Fructose-induced fluorescence generation of reductively methylated glycated bovine serum albumin: evidence for nonenzymatic glycation of Amadori adducts," *Biochimica et Biophysica Acta*, vol. 1075, no. 1, pp. 12–19, 1991.

[79] L. Robert, J. Labat-Robert, and A. M. Robert, "The Maillard reaction. From nutritional problems to preventive medicine," *Pathologie Biologie*, vol. 58, no. 3, pp. 200–206, 2010.

[80] G. D. Lawrence, A. Mavi, and K. Meral, "Promotion by phosphate of Fe(III)- and Cu(II)-catalyzed autoxidation of fructose," *Carbohydrate Research*, vol. 343, no. 4, pp. 626–635, 2008.

[81] H. F. Bunn and P. J. Higgins, "Reaction of monosaccharides with proteins: possible evolutionary significance," *Science*, vol. 213, no. 4504, pp. 222–224, 1981.

[82] W. L. Dills Jr., "Protein fructosylation: fructose and the Maillard reaction," *The American Journal of Clinical Nutrition*, vol. 58, no. 5, pp. 779S–787S, 1993.

[83] E. J. Cocinero, A. Lesarri, P. Ecija et al., "Free fructose is conformationally locked," *Journal of the American Chemical Society*, vol. 135, no. 7, pp. 2845–2852, 2013.

[84] L. D. Hayward and S. J. Angyal, "A symmetry rule for the circular dichroism of reducing sugars, and the proportion of carbonyl forms in aqueous solutions thereof," *Carbohydrate Research*, vol. 53, no. 1, pp. 13–20, 1977.

[85] V. I. Lushchak, "Adaptive response to oxidative stress: bacteria, fungi, plants and animals," *Comparative Biochemistry and Physiology C*, vol. 153, no. 2, pp. 175–190, 2011.

[86] J. Muntané, "Multiple beneficial actions of fructose 1,6-biphosphate in sepsis-associated liver injury," *Critical Care Medicine*, vol. 34, no. 3, pp. 927–929, 2006.

[87] P. J. Marangos, A. W. Fox, B. J. Riedel, D. Royston, and Z. E. Dziewanowska, "Potential therapeutic applications of fructose-1,6-diphosphate," *Expert Opinion on Investigational Drugs*, vol. 7, no. 4, pp. 615–623, 1998.

[88] R. P. Lopes, A. Lunardelli, T. Preissler et al., "The effects of fructose-1,6-bisphosphate and dexamethasone on acute inflammation and T-cell proliferation," *Inflammation Research*, vol. 55, no. 8, pp. 354–358, 2006.

[89] B. J. Riedel, J. Gal, G. Ellis, P. J. Marangos, A. W. Fox, and D. Royston, "Myocardial protection using fructose-1,6-diphosphate during coronary artery bypass graft surgery: a randomized, placebo-controlled clinical trial," *Anesthesia and Analgesia*, vol. 98, no. 1, pp. 20–29, 2004.

[90] P. J. Thornalley, "The glyoxalase system: new developments towards functional characterization of a metabolic pathway fundamental to biological life," *Biochemical Journal*, vol. 269, no. 1, pp. 1–11, 1990.

[91] Y. Inoue, K. Maeta, and W. Nomura, "Glyoxalase system in yeasts: structure, function, and physiology," *Seminars in Cell and Developmental Biology*, vol. 22, no. 3, pp. 278–284, 2011.

[92] M. Xue, N. Rabbani, and P. J. Thornalley, "Glyoxalase in ageing," *Seminars in Cell and Developmental Biology*, vol. 22, no. 3, pp. 293–301, 2011.

[93] L. P. Collinson and I. W. Dawes, "Inducibility of the response of yeast cells to peroxide stress," *Journal of General Microbiology*, vol. 138, no. 2, pp. 329–335, 1992.

[94] M. M. Bayliak, H. M. Semchyshyn, and V. I. Lushchak, "Possible accumulation of non-active molecules of catalase and superoxide dismutase in *S. cerevisiae* cells under hydrogen peroxide induced stress," *Central European Journal of Biology*, vol. 2, no. 3, pp. 326–336, 2007.

[95] H. M. Semchyshyn, O. B. Abrat, J. Miedzobrodzki, Y. Inoue, and V. I. Lushchak, "Acetate but not propionate induces oxidative stress in bakers' yeast *Saccharomyces cerevisiae*," *Redox Report*, vol. 16, no. 1, pp. 15–23, 2011.

[96] D. B. Berry and A. P. Gasch, "Stress-activated genomic expression changes serve a preparative role for impending stress in yeast," *Molecular Biology of the Cell*, vol. 19, no. 11, pp. 4580–4587, 2008.

Permissions

The contributors of this book come from diverse backgrounds, making this book a truly international effort. This book will bring forth new frontiers with its revolutionizing research information and detailed analysis of the nascent developments around the world.

We would like to thank all the contributing authors for lending their expertise to make the book truly unique. They have played a crucial role in the development of this book. Without their invaluable contributions this book wouldn't have been possible. They have made vital efforts to compile up to date information on the varied aspects of this subject to make this book a valuable addition to the collection of many professionals and students.

This book was conceptualized with the vision of imparting up-to-date information and advanced data in this field. To ensure the same, a matchless editorial board was set up. Every individual on the board went through rigorous rounds of assessment to prove their worth. After which they invested a large part of their time researching and compiling the most relevant data for our readers. Conferences and sessions were held from time to time between the editorial board and the contributing authors to present the data in the most comprehensible form. The editorial team has worked tirelessly to provide valuable and valid information to help people across the globe.

Every chapter published in this book has been scrutinized by our experts. Their significance has been extensively debated. The topics covered herein carry significant findings which will fuel the growth of the discipline. They may even be implemented as practical applications or may be referred to as a beginning point for another development. Chapters in this book were first published by Hindawi Publishing Corporation; hereby published with permission under the Creative Commons Attribution License or equivalent.

The editorial board has been involved in producing this book since its inception. They have spent rigorous hours researching and exploring the diverse topics which have resulted in the successful publishing of this book. They have passed on their knowledge of decades through this book. To expedite this challenging task, the publisher supported the team at every step. A small team of assistant editors was also appointed to further simplify the editing procedure and attain best results for the readers.

Our editorial team has been hand-picked from every corner of the world. Their multi-ethnicity adds dynamic inputs to the discussions which result in innovative outcomes. These outcomes are then further discussed with the researchers and contributors who give their valuable feedback and opinion regarding the same. The feedback is then collaborated with the researches and they are edited in a comprehensive manner to aid the understanding of the subject.

Apart from the editorial board, the designing team has also invested a significant amount of their time in understanding the subject and creating the most relevant covers. They scrutinized every image to scout for the most suitable representation of the subject and create an appropriate cover for the book.

The publishing team has been involved in this book since its early stages. They were actively engaged in every process, be it collecting the data, connecting with the contributors or procuring relevant information. The team has been an ardent support to the editorial, designing and production team. Their endless efforts to recruit the best for this project, has resulted in the accomplishment of this book. They are a veteran in the field of academics and their pool of knowledge is as vast as their experience in printing. Their expertise and guidance has proved useful at every step. Their uncompromising quality standards have made this book an exceptional effort. Their encouragement from time to time has been an inspiration for everyone.

The publisher and the editorial board hope that this book will prove to be a valuable piece of knowledge for researchers, students, practitioners and scholars across the globe.

List of Contributors

H. Rachmawati, A. Merika, R. A. Ningrum and D. S. Retnoningrum
Research group of Pharmaceutics, School of Pharmacy, Bandung Institute of Technology, Ganesha 10, Bandung 40132, Indonesia

K. Anggadiredja
Research group of Pharmacology and Clinical Pharmacy, School of Pharmacy, Bandung Institute of Technology, Bandung 40132, Indonesia

Muhammad Khan
Central Research Laboratory, Jilin University Bethune Second Hospital, Changchun 130041, China
Department of Zoology, University of the Punjab, Quaid-e-Azam Campus, Lahore 54590, Pakistan

Ting Li, Azhar Rasul, Meiyan Sun, Yongchen Zheng and Tonghui Ma
Central Research Laboratory, Jilin University Bethune Second Hospital, Changchun 130041, China

Muhammad Khalil Ahmad Khan
Department of Zoology, University of the Punjab, Quaid-e-Azam Campus, Lahore 54590, Pakistan

Faisal Nawaz
Key Laboratory of Inorganic Synthesis and Preparative Chemistry, Jilin University, Qianjin Street, Changchun 130012, China

Rong Guo, Baoxin Liu, Shunping Zhou, Buchun Zhang and Yawei Xu
Department of Cardiology, Shanghai Tenth People's Hospital, Tongji University School of Medicine, 301 Yan Chang Zhong Road, Shanghai 200072, China

Koji Yamamoto, Masatoshi Amako, Yasuo Yoshihara, Hiroshi Arino and Koichi Nemoto
Department of Orthopedic Surgery, National Defense Medical College, 3-2 Namiki, Tokorozawa, Saitama 359-8513, Japan

Masanori Fujita, Maki Uenoyama, Yoritsuna Yamamoto and Shoichi Tachibana
Division of Environmental Medicine, National Defense Medical College Research Institute, 3-2 Namiki, Tokorozawa, Saitama 359-8513, Japan

Toyokazu Tsuchihara
Orthopedic Surgery, Japan Self Defense Forces Central Hospital, 1-2-24 Ikejiri, Setagaya-ku, Tokyo 154-0001, Japan

Hitoshi Nukada
Department of Medicine, University of Otago Medical School, P.O. Box 913, Dunedin 9054, New Zealand
The Nukada Institute for Medical and Biological Research, 5-18 Inage-cho, Inage-ku, Chiba 263-0035, Japan

Somia A. Nassar, Hamdy Soufy and Soad M. Nasr
Department of Parasitology and Animal Diseases, National Research Center, El-Behouse Street, Dokki, P.O. Box 12622, Giza, Egypt

Amira H. Mohamed
Department of Clinical Pathology, Faculty of Veterinary Medicine, Cairo University, P.O. Box 12211, Giza, Egypt

Najihah Mohd Hashim, Mawardi Rahmani, Gwendoline Cheng Lian Ee, Mohd Aspollah Sukari, Maizatulakmal Yahayu and Winda Oktima
Department of Chemistry, Universiti Putra Malaysia, Selangor, 43400 Serdang, Malaysia

Abd Manaf Ali
Faculty of Agriculture and Biotechnology, Universiti Sultan Zainal Abidin, 20400 Kuala Terengganu, Malaysia

Rusea Go
Department of Biology, Universiti Putra Malaysia, Selangor, 43400 Serdang, Malaysia

Areum Cha, Youngshim Choi, Yoojeong Jin and Taesun Park
Department of Food and Nutrition, Yonsei University, 262 Seongsanno, Seodaemun-gu, Seoul 120-749, Republic of Korea

Mi-Kyung Sung
Department of Food and Nutrition, Sookmyung Women's University, 52 Hyochangwon-gil, Yongsan-gu, Seoul 140-742, Republic of Korea

Yun-Chang Koo and Kwang-Won Lee
Department of Food Science, College of Life Sciences and Biotechnology, Korea University, 1, 5-ga, Anam-dong, Sungbuk-ku, Seoul 136-701, Republic of Korea

Mervi Rokka and Kimmo Peltonen
Chemistry and Toxicology Unit, Research and Laboratory Department, Finnish Food Safety Authority Evira, Mustialankatu 3, 00790 Helsinki, Finland

Marika Jestoi
Product Safety Unit, Control Department, Finnish Food Safety Authority Evira, Mustialankatu 3, 00790 Helsinki, Finland

Anand Pandey, Rohit K. Mishra, Amit K. Tiwari and Anupam Dikshit
Biological Product Laboratory, Department of Botany, University of Allahabad, Allahabad 211002, India

Awadhesh Kumar
Department of Horticulture and Medicinal Plants, Mizoram University, Aizawl 796004, India

A. K. Bajaj
Department of Dermatology, Moti Lal Nehru Medical College, Allahabad 211002, India

Chun Yang, Xiang-Liu Liu, Zhi-Qiang Zhou and Jian-Jun Yang
Department of Anesthesiology, School of Medicine, Jinling Hospital, Nanjing University, No. 305 East Zhongshan Road, Jiangsu Nanjing 210002, China

Wen-Yuan Li
Department of Anesthesiology, Affiliated Drum-Tower Hospital of Medical College of Nanjing University, No. 321 Zhongshan Road, Jiangsu Nanjing 210008, China

Hai-Yin Yu and Zhi-Qin Gao
The PLA 102nd Hospital and Mental Health Center of Military, No. 55 North Heping Road, Jiangsu Changzhou 213000, China

Kamal M. Matar
Department of Pharmacology & □erapeutics, Faculty of Pharmacy, Kuwait University, P.O. Box 24923, Kuwait City 13110, Kuwait

Yousef Al-lanqawi
Department of Pharmacy, Al-Amiri Hospital, Ministry of Health, P.O. Box 491, Kuwait City 32005, Kuwait

Kefaya Abdul-Malek
Intensive Care Unit, Al-Amiri Hospital, Ministry of Health, P.O. Box 491, Kuwait City 32005, Kuwait

Roger Jelliffe
Laboratory of Applied Pharmacokinetics, School of Medicine, University of Southern California, Los Angeles, CA 90033, USA

Carlos E. Lanusse and Laura Moreno
Laboratorio de Farmacologıa, CIVETAN-CONICET, Facultad de Ciencias Veterinarias (UNCPBA), 7000 Tandil, Argentina

María J. Del Sole
Hospital de Pequenos Animales, CIVETAN-CONICET, Facultad de Ciencias Veterinarias (UNCPBA), Campus Universitario, Paraje Arroyo Seco s/n, 7000 Tandil, Buenos Aires, Argentina
Laboratorio de Farmacologıa, CIVETAN-CONICET, Facultad de Ciencias Veterinarias (UNCPBA), 7000 Tandil, Argentina

Paula Schaiquevich
Unidad de Farmacocinetica Clınica, CONICET, Hospital de Pediatrıa JP Garrahan, 1245 Buenos Aires, Argentina

Marcelo A. Aba
Laboratorio de Endocrinologıa, CIVETAN-CONICET, Facultad de Ciencias Veterinarias (UNCPBA), 7000 Tandil, Argentina

Young-Man Lee, Jun-Yeol Kim, Ha-Jin Jung and Eun-Cheol Kim
Department of Maxillofacial Tissue Regeneration and Research Center for Tooth & Periodontal Regeneration, School of Dentistry, Kyung Hee University, 1 Heogi-dong, Dongdaemun-gu, Seoul 130-701, Republic of Korea

Q-Schick Auh
Department of Oral Medicine, School of Dentistry, Kyung Hee University, Heogi-dong, Dongdaemun-gu, Seoul 130-701, Republic of Korea

Deok-Won Lee
Department of Oral and Maxillofacial Surgery, School of Dentistry, Kyung Hee University, Heogi-dong, Dongdaemun-gu, Seoul 130-701, Republic of Korea

Seung-Ho Lee
College of Pharmacy, College of Pharmacy, Yeungnam University, Gyeongsan 712-749, Republic of Korea

Maria P. Crespo-Ortiz
Department of Biomedical Science, Faculty of Basic and Health Science, Santiago de Cali University, Pampalinda Campus, Cali, Colombia

Ming Q. Wei
Division of Molecular and Gene Therapies, Griffith Health Institute and School of Medical Science, Griffith University, Gold Coast Campus, Southport, QLD 4222, Australia

Miroslav Radenković, Marko Stojanović and Milica Prostran
Department of Pharmacology, Clinical Pharmacology and Toxicology, Medical Faculty, University of Belgrade, P.O. Box 38, 11129 Belgrade, Serbia

Tatjana Potpara
Cardiology Clinic, Clinical Center of Serbia, Medical Faculty, University of Belgrade, 11000 Belgrade, Serbia

A. Lerner and M. Grafi-Cohen
Pediatric Gastroenterology and Nutrition Unit, Carmel Medical Center, Haifa 34362, Israel
B. Rappaport School of Medicine, Technion-Israel Institute of Technology, Haifa 31096, Israel

T. Napso
Department of Evolutionary and Environmental Biology, University of Haifa, Mount Carmel, Haifa 31905, Israel

N. Azzam
Department of Human Biology, University of Haifa, Mount Carmel, Haifa 31905, Israel

F. Fares
Department of Human Biology, University of Haifa, Mount Carmel, Haifa 31905, Israel
Department of Molecular Genetics, Carmel Medical Center, Haifa 34362, Israel

Hui-Ying Li, Jun Hu, Shuang Zhao, Zhi-Yi Yuan, Fan Lei, Dong-Ming Xing and Li-Jun Du
Protein Science Laboratory of the Ministry of Education, Laboratory of Pharmaceutical Sciences, School of Life Sciences and School of Medicine, Tsinghua University, Beijing 100084, China

Hong-Jiao Wan
Jiangxi University of Traditional Chinese Medicine, Nanchang 330004, China

Yi Ding
Drug Discovery Facility, School of Life Sciences, Tsinghua University, Beijing 100084, China

Berna Elya, Katrin Basah, AbdulMunim, Wulan Yuliastuti, Anastasia Bangun and Eva Kurnia Septiana
Department of Pharmacy, Faculty of Mathematics and Sciences, University of Indonesia, Depok 16424, Indonesia

Jim J. Xiao
Department of Clinical Pharmacology, Genentech Inc., 1 DNA Way, MS 463A, South San Francisco, CA 94080, USA

Louise J. Eltringham-Smith and Sharon Gataiance
Department of Pathology and Molecular Medicine, McMaster University, Hamilton, ON, Canada

Varsha Bhakta
Canadian Blood Services, Research and Development, Hamilton, ON, Canada

Teresa R. McCurdy
Department of Pathology and Molecular Medicine, McMaster University, Hamilton, ON, Canada
Canadian Blood Services, Research and Development, Hamilton, ON, Canada
School of Nursing, McMaster University, Hamilton, ON, Canada

William P. Sheffield
Department of Pathology and Molecular Medicine, McMaster University, Hamilton, ON, Canada
Canadian Blood Services, Research and Development, Hamilton, ON, Canada

Alison E. Fox-Robichaud
Department of Medicine, McMaster University, Hamilton, ON, Canada

H. M. Semchyshyn
Department of Biochemistry and Biotechnology, Vassyl Stefanyk Precarpathian National University, 57 Shevchenko Street, Ivano-Frankivsk 76025, Ukraine